Medical Family Therapy

Jennifer Hodgson • Angela Lamson •
Tai Mendenhall • D. Russell Crane
Editors

Medical Family Therapy

Advanced Applications

Springer

Editors
Jennifer Hodgson
Child Development & Family Relations
East Carolina University
Greenville, NC, USA

Angela Lamson
Child Development & Family Relations
East Carolina University
Greenville, NC, USA

Tai Mendenhall
Family Social Science Couple and Family Therapy Program
University of Minnesota
Saint Paul, MN, USA

D. Russell Crane
School of Family Life
Brigham Young University
Provo, UT, USA

ISBN 978-3-319-03481-2 ISBN 978-3-319-03482-9 (eBook)
DOI 10.1007/978-3-319-03482-9
Springer Cham Heidelberg New York Dordrecht London

Library of Congress Control Number: 2014931240

Printed on acid-free paper

Springer is part of Springer Science+Business Media (www.springer.com)

Jennifer Hodgson, Ph.D.
I dedicate this book to Steve (my husband), Lauren, Ava Lynn, and Brennon (our children). My family inspires me to dream big and allows me the privilege of enjoying the journey. They are the most precious people in my life. Without their love, understanding, and support I would not have realized the dream of this book. I also dedicate this book to the mentors, colleagues, and students whose passion for advancing Medical Family Therapy and improving health care has enriched my life and work. Medical Family Therapy is about valuing relationships, culture, community, and health simultaneously, for that I also share the success of this book with my patients and their loved ones who entrusted in me the privilege of their care.

Angela Lamson, Ph.D.
I dedicate this book to my wonderful husband, Brad, and our incredible son, Carter. You always believe in me, fill me with true love, and inspire me. I want to thank all of my parents, siblings, and friends for encouraging

me as I was writing or editing. Thanks also goes to my MFT and MedFT colleagues and students, ECU administrators, teachers who helped me find my way to MedFT, and all of the families that have allowed me the honor of coming into their lives as a therapist, researcher, and trainer. Thanks to each of you for giving meaning to my work.

Tai Mendenhall, Ph.D.
I dedicate this book to my family, my mentors, my students, and my patients. To my family, for loving and supporting me to follow my heart, chase my dreams, and never stop growing. To my mentors, for emboldening me to charge into the complex and uncharted territories of health care, build interdisciplinary bridges across education and treatment, and discover and advance new knowledge. I also dedicate it to my students, for challenging me with their curiosity and inspiring me with their passion. And to my patients, for keeping me humble and teaching me more than I have ever taught them.

D. Russell Crane, Ph.D.
I am personally indebted to my dear wife, Eileen Doyle Crane, J.D., for always supporting me and without whom, I would probably still be working for General Motors. Also to our children: Nathan, Keith, Benjamin, April, Michelle, Rachael, Sarah, and Scott, and their families for the joy they bring into my life. I would be egregiously ungrateful if I did not thank the faculty and administrators past and present of the College of Family, Home, and Social Sciences, the School of Family Life and the

Marriage and Family Therapy Program at Brigham Young University, who have made this research possible. Also, I have had a wonderful experience working with masters and doctoral students who help our research move forward in every way.

Foreword

Medical Family Therapy (MedFT) interweaves the biomedical and psychosocial by utilizing systems theory and interdisciplinary collaboration. Although its footprint is still small in the larger health care system, it is perfectly tailored to our twenty-first century web of interconnectedness where old orthodoxies (such as mind versus body, nature versus nurture, clinical care versus population care) are breaking down.

This book shows how far we have come since the introduction of the idea of MedFT in the early 1990s. Although the pioneers are still active in updating their work (McDaniel, Doherty, & Hepworth, 2014), there is a new generation taking MedFT to additional levels of depth and expansiveness. This generation came into the field already grounded in the biopsychosocial model and systems theory. They became "native speakers" more quickly than their predecessors and showed immediate confidence in their contributions. This impressive volume is one of the fruits of this second generation. It reflects experiential learning narrated by scholars and clinicians who recognize gaps in the care of people and their families and are determined to bridge them.

The areas of focus for this volume—training, research, policy, and finance—are exactly where the field needs further development. The first generation had to learn the ropes themselves without many teachers. The better-taught second generation is now crystallizing the pedagogy of MedFT. Given the historical context, the first generation did not have access to some of today's powerful research tools—such as well-accepted mixed methods designs and community-based participatory research—that fit MedFT so well. Likewise, public policy and economic issues were not at the forefront as the pioneers worked to establish a clinical foothold in health care.

In this single integrated volume, the editors and their colleagues have moved us forward and grounded us more fully in the world of health care and social change. Issues at the cutting-edge of this evolution such as scaling up and sustainability are boldly presented, as the country grapples with providing access for its population to health care services.

In some ways, the writing of this foreword is emblematic of the change that MedFT is bringing. We represent different generations and professions involved in primary care. After 25 years of practicing family medicine in Canada, and struggling with the lack of resources to address behavioral health needs of individuals and their families, A.J. discovered MedFT at the 2010 Collaborative Family Healthcare Association conference in Louisville, KY. She felt as if she had arrived at an oasis in a desert, but at first thought it was a mirage. At a subsequent conference in Philadelphia, PA, she met a therapist trained in MedFT who has since joined her practice. She now knows that the promise of MedFT and integrated care is not a mirage.

Bill is a first-generation medical family therapist. When he joined the faculty in a department of family medicine in 1979, he felt like an anthropologist in a foreign culture but without linguistic and observational skills to understand what was happening around him. He reflects that he earned a Ph.D. in family studies and family therapy without coming across the idea that families are made up of people with bodies. Family physician and family therapist Mac Baird introduced him to the depths and complexity of the culture of medicine. Bill was forever changed and later joined with colleagues Susan McDaniel and Jeri Hepworth to develop MedFT. He is thrilled to see the accomplishments of the next generation of medical family therapists represented in this book.

From a larger perspective, the future of health care will depend on therapists, medical providers, and other professionals learning to deliver the kind of care embodied in this therapeutic field. We know from chaos theory that subtle environmental shifts can lead eventually to major systemic changes. MedFT could turn out to be a "butterfly" in health care: may the flapping of its small wings turn into the tornado of change we badly need.

St. Paul, Minnesota, USA William J. Doherty
Halifax, Nova Scotia Ajantha Jayabarathan

Reference

McDaniel, S. H., Doherty, W. J., & Hepworth, J. (2014). *Medical family therapy and integrated care* (2nd ed.). Washington, DC: American Psychological Association.

Acknowledgements

> If you want to go fast, go alone. If you want to go far, go together.
> African Proverb

The editors would like to send a special thank-you to the following individuals for their time and endless energy on helping to review this text in preparation for publication:

Rola Aamar, M.S.
Brian Caples, B.S.
Meghan Lacks, M.S.
Aubry Koehler, M.A.
Irina Kolobova, M.S.
Ashley Maag, M.S.
Amelia Muse, M.S.
Kaitlyn Slight, B.S.

Contents

Chapter 1
Introduction to Medical Family Therapy: Advanced Applications

Jennifer Hodgson, Angela Lamson, Tai Mendenhall, and Lisa Tyndall

The first text on Medical Family Therapy (MedFT), entitled "*Medical Family Therapy: A Biopsychosocial Approach to Families with Health Problems*," was published in 1992. Its authors, Susan McDaniel, Jeri Hepworth, and Bill Doherty, shared a vision that it would be adopted by individuals from all different healthcare disciplines who practiced from a biopsychosocial (Engel, 1977, 1980) and family systems (von Bertalanffy, 1968) approach. Since then, a crescendo of literature has been introduced advocating for more systemic and family-centered approaches to healthcare practice. Their dream was achieved.

Then in 2014, McDaniel, Doherty, and Hepworth published their second edition, entitled "*Medical Family Therapy and Integrated Care*." In it they reinforced the importance of a family-centered clinical approach to a healthcare system in a state of flux and in need of reform. Throughout their second text, McDaniel, Doherty, and Hepworth highlight how MedFT has grown. They start at the inside jacket announcing MedFT as a "field" and carry this message throughout the text by proclaiming the numerous ways MedFT has grown beyond its original primary care incubator and into secondary and tertiary healthcare settings. The need for a more clinically robust and contemporary application of MedFT was reflected in their decision to publish a second edition.

While many of the original concepts, theories, and applications of MedFT have remained constant since McDaniel, Hepworth, and Doherty's (1992) primer, in 2012, Tyndall, Hodgson, Lamson, White, and Knight concurred with colleagues Linville, Hertlein, and Prouty Lyness (2007) to advance MedFT research literature, for an empirically rooted definition is needed. In 2010, Tyndall, Hodgson, Lamson, White, and Knight conducted a Delphi study to help resolve this issue. As a result of their research, the editors of this text have decided to adopt Tyndall et al.'s definition; it maintains that MedFT is

J. Hodgson (✉)
Department of Child Development & Family Relations, East Carolina University, Greenville, NC, USA
e-mail: hodgsonj@ecu.edu

J. Hodgson et al. (eds.), *Medical Family Therapy*, DOI 10.1007/978-3-319-03482-9_1,

> an approach to healthcare sourced from a BPSS [biopsychosocial-spiritual] perspective and marriage and family therapy, but also informed by systems theory. The practice of MedFT spans a variety of clinical settings with a strong focus on the relationships of the patient and the collaboration between and among the healthcare providers and the patient. MedFTs are endorsers of patient and family agency and facilitators of healthy workplace dynamics. (p. 68–69)

After years of publishing, presenting, researching, and teaching from the existing MedFT literature, the editors of this text respectfully determined that there was a need for a book that synthesizes contemporary advancements in training, research, policy, and financial models central to MedFT. Knowing that there are many cutting-edge thinkers who contribute to each of these areas, we opted to publish an edited text. Therefore, this book reflects more than the perspective of its editors, alone. It is a reflection of the work being done by MedFTs across the country. Each chapter can stand on its own; however, we believe that, as Aristotle said, "the whole is greater than the sum of its parts." Therefore, we encourage readers to consume it in its entirety.

The Medical Family Therapy Healthcare Continuum

There is no doubt that careers have been built upon the idea that health care needs people in it who think relationally, work systemically, and conduct research in manners that honor the complex biological, psychological, social, and spiritual dimensions of health. This text is the direct inspiration of big thinkers such as (a) von Bertalanffy (1968), who advocated for replacing the medical model with a more systemic one; (b) Engel (1977, 1980), who brought the biopsychosocial model to the attention of medicine; and (c) Wright, Watson, and Bell (1996), who advocated for the inclusion of spirituality in health care. We incorporated their transformative contributions as core theoretical components that are foundational to this text, henceforth referred to as the biopsychosocial-spiritual (BPSS) framework.

Building upon this foundation, the editors then thought about the potential for MedFT to be delivered by a variety of professional disciplines. McDaniel et al. (2014) suggested that there is room for a variety of clinical models and approaches to be used in the practice of MedFT as long as the healthcare provider identifies with the biopsychosocial-systemic approach. McDaniel et al. go on to specify, "Although primary care physicians and nurses may benefit, the strategies and techniques are intended primarily for therapists who are fully trained in family systems therapy" (p. xiv). As important as it is for relational and systemic thinking to span across all disciplines, the editors take the position that some MedFT clinical and research skill sets are more easily adapted with minimal training than others. For this reason, we have developed a continuum (i.e., Medical Family Therapy Healthcare Continuum) (Hodgson, Lamson, Mendenhall, & Tyndall, 2013), placing MedFT skills across five levels of application that range in proficiency and

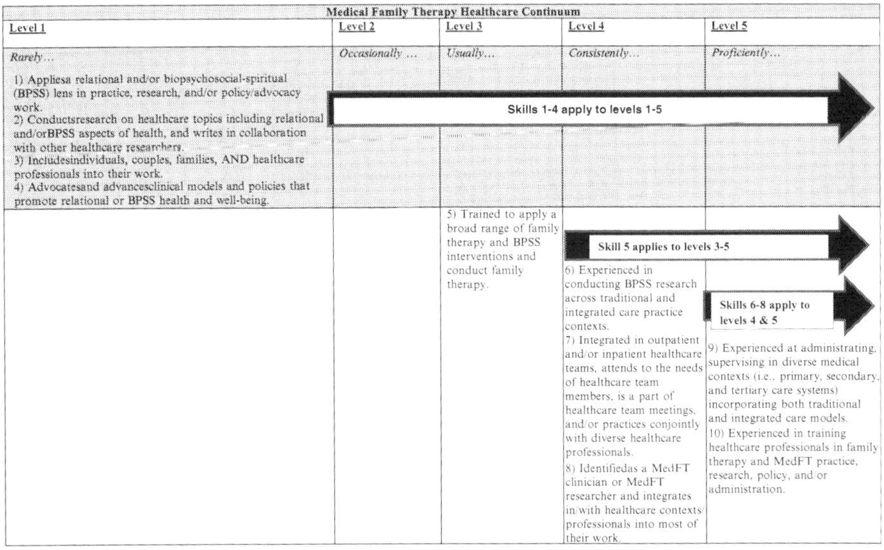

Fig. 1.1 Medical Family Therapy Healthcare Continuum

intensity. This allows readers to determine which level fits best with their respective experience(s) and level of training.

According to the Merriam-Webster dictionary, a continuum is a range or a series of things that are slightly different from each other and that exist between two different possibilities (Continuum, 2013). Hodgson et al. (2013) proposed that MedFT consists of a range of skills that different professionals, regardless of discipline, may execute depending on their preferences, training, and work contexts. Comprising five different levels across the continuum, MedFTs may find themselves aligning with a level that reflects their preparation and experience (Fig. 1.1).

The following descriptions of each level were developed by Hodgson et al. (2013) to help distinguish differences across skill sets depicted in the continuum.

Level 1. At this level MedFTs have an interest in BPSS healthcare models and have some experience or training with a relational and/or BPSS framework; however, he or she rarely applies either to his or her clinical, research, and/or policy and advocacy work. He or she may be a clinician who consults with other healthcare or spiritual professionals using a relational and/or BPSS framework on an "as-needed" basis and may be one who is consulted with if a patient is undergoing a relational crisis. He or she may be a researcher who has conducted one or more studies using one or more relational measures or questions but does not conduct interdisciplinary healthcare research routinely. He or she may be a policy maker who will integrate relational and/or BPSS issues into his or her work, but this is not a constant or a consistent focus.

Level 2. At this level MedFTs occasionally collaborate with healthcare providers from other disciplines (co-located or separate locations), patients, and patients' support system members. His or her clinical work reflects a relational or a BPSS focus less than 50 % of the time. When collaborating, this MedFT will occasionally incorporate the viewpoints of family/support system members, healthcare providers, and spiritual consultants into his or her treatment planning, particularly when the relational and/or BPSS issues are front and center (e.g., loss of loved one, caregiving). This MedFT may also be a researcher who has had multiple experiences investigating the relationships between patients' health status and couple/family support systems and/or the impact(s) of BPSS strengths and/or issues on health or well-being. He or she may be a policy maker who occasionally (less than 50 % of the time) advocates for healthcare policy that is inclusive of individuals, couples, families, and diverse populations and cultures across a wide range of BPSS issues.

Level 3. At this level MedFTs are trained to apply a broad range of family therapy and BPSS interventions and conduct family therapy. He or she usually collaborates with providers (co-located or separate locations), patients, and patients' support system members; uses MedFT techniques and family therapy interventions; incorporates family/support system members into treatment plans; and attends to relationships among healthcare team members and BPSS issues in health and well-being on up to 75 % of work scenarios. MedFT researchers with this skill set will usually assemble or be a part of multidisciplinary teams to study the reciprocal relationships between patients' health status and couple/family support systems and/or the impact(s) of aspects of BPSS in health and well-being. In his or her policy work he or she advocates for healthcare policy (75 % or less of his or her time) that is inclusive of individuals, couples, families, and diverse populations and cultures across a wide range of BPSS issues.

Level 4. At this level MedFTs identify as a MedFT clinician and/or researcher and integrate in/with healthcare contexts/professionals into most of his or her work. He or she is trained to apply a broad range of family therapy and BPSS interventions and conduct family therapy. He or she consistently collaborates at each encounter with providers (co-located or integrated), patients, and patients' support system members (if present). He or she uses MedFT techniques and family therapy theories, models, and interventions during each traditional and integrated care visit; prepares treatment plans that include a relational task/intervention; attends to relationships among healthcare team members; and strives to maintain wellness among the healthcare team. Researchers at this level consistently form multidisciplinary teams to study the reciprocal relationships between patients' BPSS health status and couple/family support systems and/or the impact(s) of a MedFT technique(s) or a family therapy intervention(s) in traditional and integrated care practice contexts. Practitioners, researchers, and policy makers consistently focus on the BPSS influence of health, illness, new diagnoses, trauma, and death of patients within healthcare or health policy systems.

Level 5. At this level MedFTs are experienced at administrating and supervising in diverse medical contexts (i.e., primary, secondary, and tertiary care systems) incorporating both traditional and integrated care models. He or she is also experienced in training healthcare professionals in family therapy and MedFT practice, research, policy, and/or administration. When in a clinical role, he or she collaborates routinely with providers, patients, and patients' support system members (when able to be present). He or she is proficient at family therapy theories, models, and interventions and uses MedFT techniques during traditional and integrated care visits; prepares treatment plans that include BPSS tasks/interventions; attends to relationships among healthcare team members; develops a curriculum for maintaining wellness among the healthcare team; advocates for family-centered and BPSS policy in health care; teaches, trains, and supervises family therapists and MedFTs; and administrates MedFT services in healthcare settings. Researchers at this level routinely form multidisciplinary teams to study the reciprocal relationships between patients' BPSS health status and couple/family support systems and/or the impact(s) of MedFT technique(s) or family therapy intervention(s), including outcome studies for patients and their families/support systems receiving brief and traditional family therapy in both integrated care and conventional mental health settings. Level 5 MedFT researchers study the influence of healthcare policy on patients, couples, families, and healthcare systems; conduct community-based participatory research or research that reflects an awareness of ethics and cultural humility around health concerns and systemic interventions; or study the roles, function, sustainability, or well-being of healthcare teams.

This continuum was designed by Hodgson et al. (2013) to assist MedFTs in understanding the depth and breadth of skills possible at different levels. It also aids the reader in determining what level of application he or she wants to engage in as a MedFT. Hodgson et al. take the perspective that while the title of MedFT should not rest within a specific discipline or healthcare specialization, the skills that fall under each level, particularly with regard to the provision, research, supervision, and teaching of family therapy, will depend on one's level of training. The authors noted that level 5 is not an ultimate goal for everyone, but instead to determine what is best based on needs and context and maximize one's skills within that level.

Layout of the Text

As stated above, this is an edited text and includes the professional contributions of cutting-edge theorists, practitioners, supervisors, leaders, administrators, researchers, policy makers, and up-and-coming professionals in MedFT. The text is divided into four distinct sections: (a) training, (b) research, (c) policy, and (d) finance. Each section has multiple chapters that are authored by some of the leading experts and emerging contributors in their areas. To assist the reader in applying the content in each chapter, each one concludes with discussion questions designed to help the reader apply and think critically about the written concepts and ideas. Chapter authors have also asterisked readings in their reference lists that they believe are critical works worthy of review. While not all contributors to this text would place themselves under "level 5" of the Medical Family Therapy Healthcare Continuum, the authors' diverse representation across the continuum reflects the importance of each level to the advancement of MedFT. The following is a brief description of each chapter included in the text.

Training

Chapter 1 sets the stage for the entire text; it takes the reader on a journey through the written history of MedFT and ends with questions about how advancements can be made in training, research, and policy to continue the field's growth and development. Chapter 2 addresses the importance of universally adopting a set of core competencies that reflect the skills needed to practice MedFT. The work in this chapter is built upon an empirical study and offers an example of competencies that can and should be expanded upon by proponents of MedFT. Chapter 3 offers invaluable contextual information relevant in assimilating successfully into healthcare settings. The authors offer concrete strategies for MedFTs to effectively enter and integrate themselves into traditional medical contexts. Chapter 4 introduces the reader to the practice of MedFT in an integrated primary care context and presents an innovative practice framework. The authors take the reader through interpersonal interactions and sequences that may occur between the MedFT and medical providers around patient care. Chapter 5 outlines the criticality for skills in developing relationships with and among members of the healthcare team and highlights how MedFTs are oftentimes the most skilled at seeing health care through a relational lens. The authors contend that until now practitioners and researchers have not adequately described the relational process(es) necessary to initiate and sustain integrated care models. Chapter 6 covers issues of burnout and compassion fatigue and offers recommendations that promote self-care in MedFTs and other healthcare staffs and providers who work in emotionally charged, psychologically draining, and oftentimes physically demanding settings. Chapter 7 takes the application of MedFT concepts and methods to the supervisory level. The authors provide specific recommendations on how supervisors can successfully guide and advise supervisees who are working in healthcare settings and with healthcare teams. It takes the reader through the process of choosing a supervisor, developing a supervision contract, recognizing potential supervision dynamics across the levels of integrated care, and assessing clinical and supervisorial productivity. Chapter 8 promises to inspire those who seek leadership roles in healthcare settings. Each author extends sage advice on their journey taken as well as opportunities for MedFTs in leadership roles. Chapter 9 helps MedFTs think about how they can adapt their skills to developing and leading a relationally enhanced behavioral medicine curriculum and teaching in family medicine residency settings. Chapter 10 provides information on how and why one should punctuate the spiritual dimension as a part of the biopsychosocial model. The authors address this topic from a clinical, teaching, and research perspective and offer specific recommendations on how to grow ones' skill set in this area.

Research

Chapter 11 describes MedFT's future as best advanced by professionals who simultaneously maintain skills and specialized efforts across both research and practice. Scientist-practitioner models are described, highlighting the respective journeys of several—ranging from new to seasoned—MedFT leaders. Chapter 12 makes a compelling case for how MedFTs can survive in today's healthcare climate. The authors suggest that MedFTs must produce empirical evidence that supports their work and earns their regard by policy makers, payers, providers, and educators. The authors propose a common lexicon from which to do this and outline concrete ways to advance the MedFT research agenda using qualitative, quantitative, and mixed-method approaches. Chapter 13 calls for increased involvement and active participation of patients, families, and communities in the construction, implementation, and evaluation of health interventions. The authors highlight several collaborative learning and investigatory methods—including Community-based Participatory Research and Citizen Health Care—that serve to flatten professional hierarchies as all participants in the research process work together to generate knowledge and solve local problems. Chapter 14 describes MedFTs as valuable contributors to program evaluation secondary to their purposeful attention to complex interactions and systemic/contextual sequences. The authors outline principal components, steps, and strategies for MedFTs to lead and/or take part in the clinical and program evaluation efforts advanced by the clinical sites in which they are positioned. Chapter 15 describes dissemination and implementation (D&I) science as an evolving field of models and methods aimed at closing the research–practice gap. The authors describe core characteristics of D&I science and illustrate its use with real-world examples relevant to MedFT. Chapter 16 calls for MedFT investigators to advance health equity through purposeful regard for issues of classism, racism, hetero-patriarchy, and colonialism. The authors highlight strategies, reflective work, and social insights helpful toward the conduct of ethical, humble, and collaborative research with patients, families, and communities.

Policy

Chapter 17 offers a primer on healthcare policy for MedFTs and describes current and proposed changes that will revolutionize the delivery of healthcare services to families in the United States. The authors identify ways that MedFTs can successfully integrate into the changing healthcare environment with particular attention given to work with children and youth, elderly and caregivers, and patients with disabilities. Chapter 18 provides MedFTs with an overview of the basic structure and barriers of integration, suggestions on how to deliver quality care despite barriers at the local level, and examples of key advocacy efforts representing possible entryways on a larger scale. Chapter 19 addresses some of the common ethical issues that arise within integrated care settings. The authors offer policy and practice implications for MedFTs who function in integrated care settings, including guidance via federal and state statutes as well as professional codes of ethics. Chapter 20 extends guidelines for constructing compelling policy briefs, including examples of briefs that address the benefits of MedFT as part of an integrated healthcare delivery system. This chapter describes what a policy brief is, how to strengthen the analysis using relevant and meaningful evidence, and how to convince target audiences that your desired policy is urgently needed and aligned with their priorities.

Finance

The chapters in this section take two very different approaches to thinking about financial sustainability in MedFT. Chapter 21 provides a summary of cost-effectiveness research in healthcare contexts. Outcomes from 21 unique studies are summarized, and the authors offer important recommendations for MedFTs who need to understand the value of medical offset, healthcare utilization, and cost-effective treatments and how they are relevant to their work. Chapter 22 opens with a discussion of the various payment modalities within the US healthcare system as well as specific reimbursement codes related to MedFT practices. Subsequently, two different clinical models are presented, one from the west coast and one from the east, along with a discussion regarding how services are provided at each site in order to maximize patient care while working toward financial sustainability.

The book concludes with an epilogue chapter that illuminates the editors' shared vision for the future of MedFT, alongside their sources of professional and personal inspiration. Ultimately, it has been our intent to edit a book that reflects how far MedFT has come and how much there is still to do to keep the psychological, social, and spiritual dimensions a part of the healthcare home. In the fast-paced world of health care, working systemically can be challenging. In addition, many remain uncertain about how big of a role families/support persons and spirituality should play in the day-to-day delivery of health care. There may be more questions than answers, but that is expected insofar as MedFT is still in its adolescence. This text was written to recognize and advance the work of MedFT teachers, leaders, supervisors, researchers, policy makers, and financial experts. It was also written to inspire the students and professionals who will be contributing to it. We believe that, ultimately, it is our shared responsibility in communion with one another to develop and study the products of these efforts so as to advance the art and science behind MedFT.

References

Continuum. (2013). In *Merriam-Webster.com*. Retrieved September 23, 2013, from http://www.merriam-webster.com/dictionary/continuum

Engel, G. L. (1977). The need for a new medical model: A challenge for biomedicine. *Science, 196*, 129–136. doi:10.1126/science.847460.

Engel, G. L. (1980). The clinical application of the biopsychosocial model. *American Journal of Psychiatry, 137*, 535–544. Retrieved from http://ajp.psychiatryonline.org/

Hodgson, J., Lamson, A., Mendenhall, T., & Tyndall, L. (2013, October). *The medical family therapy in healthcare continuum*. American Association for Marriage and Family Therapy Annual Conference, Portland, OR.

Linville, D., Hertlein, K. M., & Prouty Lyness, A. M. (2007). Medical family therapy: Reflecting on the necessity of collaborative healthcare research. *Families, Systems, and Health, 25*, 85–97. doi:10.1037/1091-7527.25.1.85.

McDaniel, S. H., Doherty, W. J., & Hepworth, J. (Eds.). (2014). *Medical family therapy and integrated care*. Washington, DC: American Psychological Association. doi:10.1037/14256-000; doi:10.1080/01926189208250882.

McDaniel, S. H., Hepworth, J., & Doherty, W. J. (Eds.). (1992). *Medical family therapy: A biopsychosocial approach to families with health problems*. New York, NY: Basic Books. doi:10.1080/01926189208250882.

Tyndall, L., Hodgson, J., Lamson, A., White, M., & Knight, S. (2012). Medical family therapy: A theoretical and empirical review. *Contemporary Family Therapy, 34*, 156–170. doi:10.1007/s10591-012-9183-9.

Tyndall, L., Hodgson, J., White, M., Lamson, A., & Knight, S. (2010). *Medical family therapy: Conceptual clarification and consensus for an emerging profession* (Unpublished doctoral dissertation). East Carolina University, Greenville, NC.

von Bertalanffy, L. (1968). *System theory: Foundations, development, applications*. New York, NY: George Braziller.

Wright, L. M., Watson, W. L., & Bell, J. M. (1996). *Beliefs: The heart of healing in families and illness*. New York, NY: Basic Books.

Part I
Training

Chapter 2
A Review of Medical Family Therapy: 30 Years of History, Growth, and Research

Lisa Tyndall, Jennifer Hodgson, Angela Lamson, Mark White, and Sharon Knight

Medical Family Therapy (MedFT) began developing in the 1980s in response to several opposing forces including the fragmented system of health care, disconnection between behavioral health and medical providers, separation of the treatment of the mind from the body, and extraction of the patient from the family/community. Clinicians, educators, healthcare administrators, and researchers began to address the importance of collaboration between the medical and behavioral health fields, and the relationship between family medicine and family therapy was born (McDaniel & Amos, 1983; McDaniel & Campbell, 1986; McDaniel, Campbell, & Seaburn, 1989). McDaniel, Hepworth, and Doherty (1992a) used the term Medical Family Therapy (MedFT) to refer to the "Biopsychosocial treatment of individuals and families who are dealing with medical problems. As we conceptualize it, MedFT works from a biopsychosocial systems model and actively encourages collaboration between therapists and other health professionals" (p. 2).

Fifteen years after McDaniel and colleagues' (1992a) groundbreaking text, in an effort to identify how MedFT has evolved since its inception, Linville, Hertlein, and Prouty Lyness (2007) reviewed the empirical research on its efficacy and effectiveness, as well as the research focusing on "family interventions and health." They expressed in their paper that they included other research on "family interventions and health" due to the challenges of identifying available research branded as MedFT. It appeared that researchers were using different variables to define MedFT at times, and without a universally agreed-upon definition in place, this made determining what could be classified as MedFT difficult.

A possible explanation for the lack of a concurrent definition is the developmental changes in MedFT across time. According to some proponents of MedFT, it has grown from being a clinical orientation, or framework, to a field that is making unique contributions to the research literature and serving as the foundation for

L. Tyndall (✉)
Department of Child Development & Family Relations, East Carolina University, Greenville, NC, USA
e-mail: tyndalll@ecu.edu

J. Hodgson et al. (eds.), *Medical Family Therapy*, DOI 10.1007/978-3-319-03482-9_2,

training programs, particularly in family therapy (Edwards & Patterson, 2003; Marlowe, 2011; Tyndall, Hodgson, Lamson, White, & Knight, 2014). The intention of this chapter is to review the literature where MedFT is mentioned by name and unveil its developmental trajectories for research, training, and practice.

Literature Review Method

This literature review process followed three phases. First, a search was conducted using several databases: Academic Search Premier, ProQuest, Psychological and Behavioral Sciences, PubMed, PsycINFO, PsycARTICLES, CINAHL, and EBSCOhost. The search included the following parameters: (a) English language, (b) all years since its inception (i.e., 1992), and (c) the full phrase "Medical Family Therapy" in the abstract or title. Second, a manual search of the journal of *Family Systems Medicine* (later renamed *Families, Systems, and Health*) was conducted to identify earlier works referencing MedFT in a section of the journal entitled, *Medical Family Therapy Casebook*. Third, several articles were found that were professional interviews of MedFT pioneers. A total of 96 articles from 1992 through 2012, empirical and nonempirical, fit the search criteria. The resulting literature was categorized into the following four themes: (a) historical emergence of MedFT, (b) contemporary MedFT skills and applications, (c) punctuating the "family therapy" in MedFT, and (d) MedFT effectiveness and efficacy research. Most of the literature is chronologically presented within each thematic category.

Emergence of MedFT in the Literature

While clinicians were already practicing MedFT in the 1980s (Ruddy & McDaniel, 2003), it was not until the early 1990s that the practice was formally introduced into Western literature (Doherty, McDaniel, & Hepworth, 1994; McDaniel, Hepworth, & Doherty, 1992a). The primer text by McDaniel and colleagues, *Medical Family Therapy*, was published in 1992 providing the first working definition, description, and text about MedFT. Six favorable reviews in peer-reviewed journals reinforced its unique and needed contribution to the healthcare industry (Anonymous, 1993; Fulton, 1996; Griffith, 1994; Kazak, 1993; Kelley, 1993; Shapiro, 1993). It was a time when a patient's autonomy and support system were treated as ancillary to health care and a group of systemic thinkers sought out to challenge this status quo thinking. McDaniel, Doherty, and Hepworth (2014) captured healthcare's movement in the integration of the patient and family with the publication of their second edition MedFT text entitled *Medical Family Therapy and Integrated Care*. In their second edition, they updated the definition of MedFT to read, "Medical family therapy is a form of professional practice that uses the biopsychosocial model and systemic family therapy principles in the collaborative treatment of individuals and families dealing with medical problems" (p. 9). However, the initial emergence of MedFT was not without controversy. Three articles were published within the next few years debating the need for and naming of MedFT. Family nurses, Wright, Watson, and Bell (1992) asserted that the word "medical" limited the focus on the biological and excluded work done in this area by nonphysician professionals. Lask (1994), a psychiatrist, argued that MedFT, as he understood it, was a biopsychosocial (BPS) approach to working with patients and their families that had been practiced for over 40 years in various forms in the United Kingdom (UK). While Czauderna and Tomson (1994) also mentioned the presence of MedFT in the UK, especially in secondary and hospital settings, they acknowledged that McDaniel and colleagues (1992a) introduced the idea of integrating family therapy into primary care, which is something that had not been done in the UK.

With continued reflection on the emergence and development of MedFT, interviews with several MedFT leaders surfaced (Burgess-Manning, 2007; Dankoski, 2003; Jencius, 2004; Pratt, 2003), populating the literature with information about this newly named way of doing family therapy in healthcare settings. In a 2012 special issue on MedFT published in the *Journal of Contemporary Family Therapy*, Dr. Barry Jacobs interviewed the pioneers of MedFT, McDaniel, Hepworth, and Doherty on the state of MedFT. They punctuated how advocates for MedFT have encouraged them to publish a second edition of their pioneering text due to continued growth and development in this area (McDaniel et al., 1992a). One of the debated topics in that interview included whether or not MedFT should be considered a subspecialty of a discipline (like Health Psychology or Medical Social Work) or a framework adoptable by any health professional operating from a systemic and BPS approach. As mentioned above, in 2012, a special edition of *Contemporary Family Therapy* was published focusing on MedFT. In it, Hodgson, Lamson, Mendenhall, and Crane (2012) described the current healthcare climate as rich with opportunity for Medical Family Therapists (MedFTs) trained in collaborative care and systemic thinking and urged those in the field to be purposeful in the training provided, research conducted, and integrating themselves into healthcare settings. This was the first special issue ever exclusively published on MedFT in any scholarly journal and marks its continued advancement since McDaniel and colleagues' (1992a) pioneering text.

Contemporary MedFT Skills and Applications

Dissemination and training. Since 1992, when McDaniel and colleagues published their landmark text, authors and researchers from a variety of disciplines have written about how they have applied MedFT concepts and ideas. A discussion of the clinical applications of MedFT with infertility issues was one of the earliest publications (McDaniel et al., 1992). In this article, McDaniel and colleagues (1992b) noted, "The roots of medical family therapy are intertwined with the origins of the field. Pioneers such as Whitaker, Auerswald, Bowen, Wynne, and Minuchin foresaw the use of family therapy for problems of both mental and physical health" (p.103). They reinforced the importance of using a collaborative, biopsychosocial, and family systems framework when treating medical and behavioral health conditions. They wrote, "Medical family therapy interweaves the biomedical and the psychosocial by utilizing a biopsychosocial/systems theory, with collaboration between medical providers and family therapists as a centerpiece of the approach" (p. 101). Infertility and reproductive issues continued to be fertile ground for the application of MedFT as a foundational theory (McDaniel, 1994). However, a need emerged for proponents of MedFT to have a place where they could disseminate their ideas and vision for the potential of MedFT in healthcare settings.

The initiation of the *Medical Family Therapy Casebook* section of the journal *Family Systems Medicine* (now renamed the journal of *Families, Systems, and Health*) began in 1993. The MedFT Casebook was intended to be a forum for clinicians to present a clinical case and commentary with the first article published in 1993 by Weiss and Hepworth. The MedFT Casebook was published through 2009 with a total of 18 articles, not inclusive of commentaries separately published from the main article (Altum, 2007; Bayona, 2007; Candib & Stovall, 2002; Harp, 1998; Siegel, 2009) illustrating how MedFT concepts could be applied clinically. Many of these articles were written to highlight collaborative and training opportunities (Weiner & Lorenz, 1994). For example, casebook authors advocated for clinical observation and immersion to serve as the two main mechanisms for building MedFT skills. They targeted application of skills across certain diagnostic areas, including, but not limited to, somatization disorders (Cohen, 1995), congestive heart failure (Clabby & Howarth, 2007), diabetes (Munshower, 2004), Munchausen (Kannai, 2009), fibromyalgia (Navon, 2005), neurologic impairment (Gellerstedt & Mauksch, 1993), parenting children with health challenges (Rosenberg, Brown, & Gawinski, 2008; Thomasgard, Boreman, & Metz, 2004), and HIV/AIDS (Lowe, 2007). MedFT Casebook authors also addressed navigating cultural differences in establishing care (Schirmer & Le, 2002), supporting the doctor–patient relationship (Knishkowy & Herman, 1998; Radomsky, 1996), and facilitating the act of collaboration (Leahy, Galbreath, Powell, & Shinn, 1994; Prest, Fitzgibbons, & Krier, 1996; Ruddy et al., 1994). A recent review of these casebook articles was conducted by Bischoff, Springer, Felix, and Hollist (2011). The review revealed that not all casebook articles were using the same language (i.e., lexicon) to describe MedFT, and over time, articles appeared to be written more about the act of collaboration rather than the practice of MedFT. Bischoff and colleagues (2011) noted, "It would be more appropriate to label what is reflected in the Casebooks as 'collaborative care'" (p. 195). This could explain why this section of the journal appears to change names from "Medical Family Therapy Casebook" to "Casebook" (Berkley, 2000; Fogarty, 2001; Riccelli, 2003; Souza, 2002) and then to "Family Therapy Casebook" (Edwards & Turnage, 2003) throughout the years. While the lack of consistency with titling may seem insignificant to some, it reflected a symptom of either uncertainty surrounding the definition and practice of MedFT (Bischoff et al., 2011; Linville et al., 2007) or its adoption as part of the collaborative care movement.

MedFT with diverse patient populations and diagnoses. The work of MedFT with diverse patient populations has been written about with particular respect for marginalized groups. In the early 2000s, family therapy and public policy journals published pieces that expanded the theoretical perspectives and practice of MedFT, while referencing stories of clinical success with highly complex patients and families (McDaniel, Harkness, & Epstein, 2001; Wissow, Hutton, & Kass, 2002). Around this time, *Feminist Perspectives in Medical Family Therapy* was published with articles that paid special attention to the role of gender and power dynamics in the medical environment (Bischof, Lieser, Taratua, & Fox, 2003; Dankoski, 2003; Edwards & Patterson, 2003; Hertlein, 2003; Pratt, 2003; Prouty Lyness, 2003; Smith-Lamson & Hodgson, 2003). Several largely favorable reviews of the compilation were published shortly thereafter (Burge, 2005; Degges-White, 2005; Oberman, 2006; Rosenberg, 2005; Trepal, 2005). Developmentally, MedFT was at the point where it was building general clinical skills, and thinking about how to do so with cultural sensitivity, while building a theoretical infrastructure central to its practice.

Over time, more literature emerged highlighting the skills and applications of MedFT with patients diagnosed with a variety of illnesses such as diabetes (Phelps et al., 2009; Robinson, Barnacle, Pretorius, & Paulman, 2004), pediatric HIV/AIDS (Wissow et al., 2002), fibromyalgia (Preece & Sandberg, 2005), somatoform and chronic fatigue syndrome (Szyndler, Towns, Hoffman, & Bennett, 2003), and cancer (Burwell, Templeton, Kennedy, & Zak-Hunter, 2008; Dankoski & Pais, 2007; Hodgson, McCammon, & Anderson, 2011; Hodgson, McCammon, Marlowe, & Anderson, 2012). Research was beginning to take a more central place in the evolution of MedFT as clinicians, educators, and scholars wanted to understand what was making the difference. For example, Robinson and colleagues (2004) wrote about how they incorporated a MedFT student in their work with patients on an interdisciplinary team. The medical family therapist was tasked with assessing for psychosocial strengths and or challenges related to the patient's health condition, as well as other life stressors that may also involve the family. The medical family therapist gained invaluable experience through cross-training and collaborating with medical and pharmacy students, and the medical students learned the value of the psychosocial aspects of the illness.

While researchers were beginning to think about how to study the effectiveness of MedFT with a variety of cultural groups and diagnoses, Willerton, Dankoski, and Sevilla Martir (2008) made the case for how MedFTs are well trained in a systems orientation and, therefore, afforded a skill set to better respect the cultural importance of the family in Latino communities. Willerton and colleagues (2008) also listed a variety of potential skills brought to the table by MedFTs, including conducting therapy with patients in a medical setting, consulting with healthcare teams in the care of patients, and providing education for medical students and residents. MedFT and collaborative care were becoming inseparable. Phelps and colleagues (2009) took it a step further and presented a culturally and spiritually sensitive integrated care model for working with underserved African–American and Hispanic patients with type 2 diabetes. In it they utilized a medical family therapist as a member of a community health center team who enacted his skill set as systems interventionist and collaborator and worked with each identified patient, their support system, nutritionist, and primary care provider collaboratively so that the patient could benefit from a more cohesive healthcare team. Included in the cultural competency skills noted by Phelps and colleagues (2009), the authors addressed the influence of spirituality and the impact it had on some patients' healthcare decisions.

One of the most recent articles applied the seven MedFT techniques developed by McDaniel and colleagues (1992a) to sexual dysfunction (Hughes, Hertlein, & Hagey, 2011). They presented MedFT as a framework that was previously shown to be helpful with chronic illness but had not yet been utilized to help couples cope with sexual dysfunction as a result of an illness. These techniques are as follows: (a) recognize the biological dimension, (b) solicit the illness story, (c) respect defenses and remove blame and unacceptable feelings, (d) maintain communication, (e) attend to developmental issues, (f) increase a sense of agency in the patient and the family, and (g) leave the door open for future contact. Hughes and colleagues (2011) provided a case example and outlined possible examples of how to employ these techniques; however, they did not specify any training necessary for a clinician to implement these techniques.

Lastly, Marlowe, Hodgson, Lamson, White, and Irons (2012) conducted a study using ethnography of communication to outline an integrated care framework for behavioral health providers functioning in a primary care setting where the behavioral health providers were trained marriage and family therapists and MedFTs. As primary care presents a wide range of possible patient interactions, this article was especially helpful in providing the interactional sequences between MedFTs, primary care providers, and patients that take place during the patient encounter. Also highlighted in this contribution was the importance of the relational training of a MedFT to the success of the integrated care framework. In a military healthcare setting, Lewis, Lamson, and Leseuer (2012) made the case for the inclusion of a BPS assessment to be done earlier and more regularly for veterans and their partners. Lewis and colleagues (2012) argued that MedFTs are the most prepared behavioral health clinicians to address the connection between relationships, stress, and health for military members.

While family therapy concepts and ideas have helped to form the basis of MedFT research and application, MedFT still remained something that only a subset of family therapists, and members of other behavioral health disciplines, did. Unfortunately, across the articles reviewed under this theme, there is not a consensus regarding what skills or training is required to become a medical family therapist (e.g., family therapists or systemic providers) or even on the definition of MedFT. For example, using MedFT as a framework (Hughes et al., 2011; McDaniel, Doherty, & Hepworth, 2013; Wissow et al.; 2002) alludes to the idea that MedFT can be used by a variety of healthcare clinicians and practitioners, but this then furthers the question: What are the required training components of MedFT? The constant through each article and research study reviewed was the endorsement of biopsychosocial and systemic intervention and adherence in varying degrees to family therapy principles and practices.

Punctuating the "Family Therapy" in Medical Family Therapy

The systemic nature of MedFT. Authors have demonstrated that the practice of MedFT can have an impact on the clinician as well as the family, illustrating the breadth of the treatment system and the bidirectional influences impacting it. For example, citing the application of family systems theory and MedFT, Streicher (1995) provided a case study of a patient with seizure disorder that highlighted a transformative process for her as a therapist and a transformative process for her client. She highlighted the importance of recognizing the limits of the therapist's power and control in the therapeutic process and how that might mirror a patient's experience with power and control in coping with an illness. McDaniel, Hepworth, and Doherty (1995) endorsed the importance of systemic thinking as a foundation for MedFT through their work with somaticizing patients. These same leading authors, McDaniel, Hepworth, and Doherty (1999), outlined emotional themes that patients and families may experience regardless of the illnesses and discussed ways that MedFTs can be useful in working through those challenges systemically.

After an introduction highlighting the benefits of family-centered care (Alvarez, 1996), Ragaisis (1996) referenced MedFT while using a combination of elements from systems theory, systemic belief theory, crisis theory, communication theory, developmental theory, structural–strategic theory, and Milton Erickson's work. Ragaisis (1996) articulated the application of MedFT by psychiatric consultation–liaison nurses (PCLN) due to their knowledge about diseases and the ability to move easily among the family, medical professionals, and staff. While Ragaisis (1996) noted that the PCLN would benefit from outside supervision by a colleague skilled particularly in family therapy, she saw MedFT as an orientation to be adopted by other professions and not necessarily belonging exclusively to the field of family therapy.

The case for MedFT as a subspecialty of family therapy. In 1995, Campbell and Patterson published an expansive literature review on family-based interventions that served as the foundation for MedFT. They defined MedFT based on the McDaniel and colleagues' (1992a) primer text and called for all family therapists in training to receive training in MedFT or, at the very least, training in how to operate from a BPS framework. They also recommended MedFTs complete academic courses via a traditional medical curriculum (e.g., psychopharmacology). Twelve years later Dankoski and Pais (2007) made a similar plea to all marriage and family therapists (MFT) to employ key MedFT techniques such as genograms, establishing a collaborative relationship with the patient's provider and addressing the biological needs of the patient. This workforce development need was recently reinforced in an editorial written by Hodgson and colleagues (2012) for the MedFT special issue published in the *Journal of Contemporary Family Therapy*. They called for more MFTs to specialize in MedFT as described by McDaniel and colleagues (1992a), particularly due to the opportunities created for behavioral health professionals as a result of healthcare reform. In what seems to be an effort to emphasize the importance of MFTs being trained in MedFT, throughout the years authors have also turned their attention toward field-based cross-training experiences with medical professionals (Edwards & Patterson, 2003; Harkness & Nofziger, 1998; Yeager et al., 1999). These publications appeared as integrated health care was beginning to take root (Blount, 1998). Articles reflecting the training process of MedFTs, with respect to training techniques (Smith-Lamson & Hodgson, 2003), also appeared in 2003. Soon after, Brucker and colleagues (2005) discussed existing MedFT internship experiences offered to marriage and family therapy doctoral students that outlined the importance of the development of a particular skill set needed to work in healthcare settings.

MedFT gained international recognition as authors paid special attention to the evolution of family therapy and application of the BPS approach in MedFT (Kojima, 2006; Pereira & Smith, 2006; Wirtberg, 2005). However, some differences or confusion regarding the definition and practice of MedFT became apparent. For example, Kojima (2006) mentioned that MedFT was conducted via co-therapy by a physician and a therapist in one room with the family. While Kojima (2006) did not illustrate specific MedFT skills, in the brief history and evolution of family therapy and MedFT, the importance of involving the family in the treatment of psychosomatic medicine and any healthcare practice was highlighted. Pereira and Smith (2006) argued that several of the seven techniques cited by McDaniel and colleagues (1992a) were not unique to MedFT and rather were very similar to traditional family therapy; however, they believed illness- and health-related techniques (recognize the biological dimension, solicit the illness story, and maintain communication), along with the focus of the presenting problem being illness or health related, were considered to set MedFT apart from other therapies. Pereira and Smith (2006) further stated that MedFT was a metaframework, in which family therapy is applied to medical problems.

In a clinical case study of a pediatric patient with HIV/AIDS, interventionists were designated as family therapists, rather than MedFTs, indicating a link between family therapy and MedFT but rendering the difference between family therapists and MedFTs unclear (Davey, Duncan, Foster, & Milton, 2008). In a clinical case illustration involving the application of MedFT with polytrauma rehabilitation, MedFT and ambiguous loss were cited as being helpful perspectives from which to work (Collins & Kennedy, 2008). These authors again referenced the influence of family systems by defining MedFT as a BPS and family systems perspective whose proponents utilize MedFT techniques authored by McDaniel and colleagues (1992a) (soliciting the illness story, respecting defenses, remove blame, and accepting unacceptable feelings). Furthermore, the concepts of agency and communion were referenced as important therapeutic goals, but the element of collaboration was largely absent. In an article written by Collins and Kennedy (2008), the words family therapy and MedFT were used interchangeably. The authors' heavy emphasis on family systems further supported the strong and developing epistemological connection between family therapy and MedFT.

Key elements of McDaniel and colleagues' (1992a) original definition of MedFT (i.e., BPS perspective, collaboration, and family systems) continued to be referenced in the literature. While another group noted that the practitioner's field did not matter as much as their skills in systemic orientation and thinking (Willerton et al., 2008), others like Marlowe (2011) contended that MedFT was an extension of family therapy using the same systemic and relational lens but in a different context. Marlowe (2011) also stated that family therapy was the professional home of MedFT drawing a very clear connection. These inconsistencies punctuate the need for a clear definition and set of core competencies for MedFT, as well as an agreed-upon list of metrics to help evaluate its outcomes.

MedFT Effectiveness and Efficacy Research

Campbell and Patterson (1995) discussed that family therapy research and family-based intervention research in the form of controlled trials were sparse. Only a few researchers have attempted to study the effectiveness of MedFT in healthcare settings (all of which were authored by family therapists); no known researchers have measured its efficacy. There are no known randomized control trials comparing the outcomes of family therapists practicing MedFT with other behavioral health disciplines. The first study to examine the MedFT skill set and its benefit was conducted on an outpatient medical oncology unit (Sellers, 2000). Quantitative surveys and qualitative interviews revealed that healthcare providers, patients, and their partners benefitted from the addition of MedFT services. The three most noted areas of benefit from the physicians and staff included the convenience of having the medical family therapist on-site, the support and hope provided to the patients, and the relief that was brought to the physicians and staff by having this support in place. Additionally, patients and their families were also surveyed and reported benefits included a 90 % reduction in emotional suffering due to the work with the MedFT, a 91 % increase in being able to access personal resources, and a 73 % increase in the ability to remain hopeful and maintain clarity about their cancer experience.

Hodgson and colleagues (2011) identified a need for delving further into the systemic interactions of the MedFT through a phenomenological study conducted in an oncology setting. Investigators interviewed patients and their partners. They identified some of the following characteristics of MedFTs to be most helpful: (a) ability to anticipate and address anxiety in a systemic manner, (b) ability to mobilize and go where the patient needed him/her to go in terms of physical setting or location, and (c) ability to provide and address the couple relationship. Participants particularly noted that the medical family therapist offered more than a patient-centered outcome—they offered a family-centered one.

Bischof and colleagues (2003) conducted a qualitative study of MedFTs' experiences working in a primary and secondary healthcare setting. While the researchers did not define MedFT, they did reference the foundational McDaniel and colleagues (1992a) text. Qualitative interview data revealed themes of power and gender dynamics in the healthcare setting, the ways in which MedFTs began and maintained collaborative relationships, practical and professional considerations, the need for MedFTs to accommodate to the healthcare system, and how they could be seen both as a potential threat to other healthcare providers and as an ally in helping providers care for themselves. Again, while this study is important to understanding the skills and value added by MedFTs, it does not demonstrate that their work resulted in outcomes similar to or different from other behavioral health disciplines.

In an attempt to further understand MedFTs' contributions in secondary care settings, Anderson, Huff, and Hodgson (2008) published a grounded theory study that specifically addressed the skills of MedFTs working in an inpatient psychiatric unit. Using a definition of MedFT consistent with McDaniel and colleagues (1992a), Anderson and colleagues (2008) referenced the systems framework, biopsychosocial–spiritual perspective, the importance of collaboration, and the concepts of agency and communion. However, one slight difference in their definition was the expansion of the BPS perspective to include spirituality. While Anderson and colleagues (2008) highlighted the collaborative model and approach used to integrate into an inpatient psychiatric setting, they did not report on the specific strategies MedFTs used to address the spiritual needs of their patients and patients' families. They deconstructed the timeline of the MedFTs' involvement in a patient care encounter into three phases: presession preparation, during session, and post-session follow-up. For each phase they included data evidencing the skills and applications of the MedFTs. This was the first field study of MedFTs in an inpatient behavioral health setting. A follow-up commentary on this article by psychiatrists Heru and Berman (2008) suggested that the addition of a medical family therapist to an inpatient unit would be beneficial, because historically families have sometimes been either avoided or demonized on these units by staff members.

In 2009, Harrington, Kimball, and Bean explored the inclusion of a medical family therapist on a pediatric oncology multidisciplinary team. While the authors did not define MedFT, they did reference McDaniel and colleagues' (1992a) guiding therapeutic principles when working with children diagnosed with a chronic illness. The researchers revealed that participants perceived relief in having the availability of a medical family therapist to assist patients and families with the systemic and emotional effects of cancer. MedFTs provided a sense of holistic treatment to patients and their families and enabled other team members to provide better patient and family care because they knew that families' emotional needs were being addressed. The authors reported the skills and possible interventions MedFTs could employ in oncology, but it was not clear if the MedFTs involved in the study actually do employ these interventions or how the interventions were perceived by other providers.

The above studies are foundational for MedFT and critical for identifying the variables needed for further study of the subdiscipline. The descriptions are helpful in clarifying MedFT practice. While such studies are invaluable to clinicians for their practice and academicians for their instruction of students, the research base must be strengthened with a wider variety of research methodologies that demonstrate the efficacy of MedFT. Mendenhall, Pratt, Phelps, and Baird (2012) outlined the variety of research methodologies that could be employed to deepen the MedFT research base. They included both quantitative, qualitative, and mixed-method designs, all while focusing on the importance of examining MedFT from a clinical, operational, and financial lens in health care.

Recommendations for Research, Practice, and Training

The following recommendations are suggested after a thorough review and analysis of the available literature. The three recommendations are (a) to establish a current definition of MedFT, (b) to implement effectiveness and efficacy studies of MedFTs and MedFT interventions, and (c) to develop a curriculum and core competencies for MedFT that are grounded in systemic skills and family therapy practice and research.

A Current Definition

Analysis of the literature reveals that the practice of MedFT has grown since its inception in the late 1980s (Ruddy & McDaniel, 2003). This was evidenced by the number of publications ($n = 96$) that have been produced since 1992 with the words "Medical Family Therapy" in the abstract or title. Given the absence of a consistent definition or agreement on its relationship to a specific discipline (i.e., family therapy), Linville and colleagues (2007) challenged MedFTs to operationalize their work to advance their science. To date, no one has accepted this challenge, despite evidence in the literature that McDaniel and colleagues' (1992a) original definition of MedFT continues to mature and develop. Though the differences in definitions of MedFT may be subtle, such variances can alter how MedFT is taught, practiced, and studied. It does not have a consistent lexicon, or language, used to describe it. For example, throughout the literature, the BPS perspective is pervasive (e.g., Burwell et al., 2008; McDaniel et al., 2001; Smith-Lamson & Hodgson, 2003), but the spiritual dimension endorsed by some proponents of the BPS model is mentioned less frequently (e.g., Linville et al., 2007; Phelps et al., 2009). Hodgson, Lamson, and Reese (2007) published a chapter attempting to help all behavioral health clinicians envision a method for including spirituality into their BPS interview, but this area still remains largely understudied.

A lack of a cohesive definition or core training standards compromises the ability to capture outcomes attributable to MedFTs. For example, a recent case study on the application of MedFT with polytrauma rehabilitation defined MedFT as an approach combining BPS and family systems perspectives with cognitive–behavioral and narrative methodologies (Collins & Kennedy, 2008). In this study, the intervention was conducted by a psychologist and social worker where training in MedFT or family therapy was unknown. In another recent article on the application of MedFT to address behavioral health disparities among Latinos (Willerton et al., 2008), the authors defined MedFT as "an attempt to better integrate the components of the BPS model in the delivery of mental health services through active collaboration of family therapists as members of health care teams" (p. 200). The former definition did not mention collaboration or the need for a family therapist, while the latter did not mention cognitive–behavioral and narrative methodologies. Consensus regarding the definition of MedFT and consistency in training would help to create a solid body of MedFT research with more established boundaries for those conducting the research and those practicing its interventions.

MedFT Intervention Studies

The MedFT literature references family interventions and their effectiveness (e.g., Campbell & Patterson, 1995) but does not demonstrate the effectiveness of a medical family therapist performing these interventions in a healthcare setting. Since 2000, there have been increased efforts to understand and study MedFT interventions. Researchers have reported perceived MedFT benefits in an inpatient psychiatric setting (Anderson et al., 2008), as part of a diabetic treatment team (Robinson et al., 2004), in primary care (Marlowe, 2011), and in oncology settings (Harrington, Kimball, & Bean, 2009; Sellers, 2000), but more detail is needed to understand exactly what MedFT interventions were conducted that were effective. Through a clinical case study, Rosenberg and colleagues (2008) illustrated the focus of MedFT sessions that included aiming to increase the patient's sense of agency, as well as facilitating and nurturing the relationship between the patient and the healthcare team. It is unclear, however, how or if it was these specific interventions that impacted the patient outcome, or if it was another element of treatment such as the collaboration that existed among the treatment team. Similarly, Robinson and colleagues (2004) included MedFTs as part of a treatment team for patients with diabetes, and while it was articulated that the medical family therapist was of value to the team, the overall goal of the article was the demonstration of the value of collaboration for treatment and training purposes. Therefore, the specific MedFT interventions were not outlined. MedFT researchers must focus on demonstrating that interventions conducted by trained MedFTs are effective either by comparing them to other treatment/control groups, exploring various patient and systemic outcomes, improving patient–provider communication, or benefitting the providers themselves. Additionally, these interventions must be employed with a larger population rather than single case studies to add weight to their generalizability. Researchers must continue to build on the descriptive, qualitative studies that have already been conducted to illuminate the practice and role of MedFT (e.g., Anderson et al., 2008; Harrington et al., 2009; Robinson et al., 2004; Rosenberg et al., 2008), thereby taking these descriptions and creating a body of interventions conducted by MedFT trained clinicians that can be studied further and integrated into a curriculum for the training of future MedFTs.

Most of the research studies have been done by family therapists in conjunction with academic programs and by MedFTs in training at the master's or doctoral levels. With the relative youth of MedFT, it is understandable that controlling for years in formal training may be a challenge as there are few clinicians who have received a doctorate, postdoctorate, master's, or certificate in MedFT as compared to those who have learned through experience in context. While several researchers have identified MedFT interventionists as being graduate-level students (e.g., Anderson et al., 2008; Davey et al., 2008; Marlowe et al., 2012; Robinson et al., 2004; Rosenberg et al., 2008), other researchers who have studied MedFT in action did not specify the background or type of training received (e.g., Harrington et al., 2009; Sellers, 2000). Efficacy research is needed to determine whether or not individuals who identify as MedFTs and hold degrees in family therapy apply MedFT concepts and applications differently than those who do not, whether or not those who identify as MedFTs and who have been trained to offer it yield different outcomes than those who do not, and whether or not MedFT produces results beyond treatment as usual.

MedFT Curriculum and Core Competencies

While most of the articles referenced in this review did not include material specific to MedFT training standards or competencies, a few authors noted some important concepts, skills, or practices such as immersion and observation (Weiner & Lorenz, 1994), family systems theory and the BPS approach (e.g., McDaniel et al., 1992b), spirituality associated with the BPS approach (e.g., Phelps et al., 2009), collaborative skills (e.g., Anderson et al., 2008), and psychopharmacology (Campbell & Patterson, 1995). MedFT training has grown from one summer institute in its early years (University of Rochester Medical Center, 2013) to eight training programs, including two doctoral programs (East Carolina University, 2013; University of Nebraska-Lincoln, 2013; please see Chap. 3 for a complete listing of academic institutions). With the expansion of training (Ungureanu & Sandberg, 2008), a need exists to establish a foundational curriculum. Published articles have focused on the availability (Brucker et al., 2005) and development of internship sites (Grauf-Grounds & Sellers, 2006), as well as specific skills needed to supervise students in healthcare settings (e.g., Edwards & Patterson, 2006; Hodgson, Boyd, Koehler, Lamson, & Rambo, 2013). However, there has not yet been an effort to elucidate core courses or core competencies pertaining to MedFT. No research has been done on level of training and clinical effectiveness among MedFT providers. Students who have graduated from a MedFT training institute or program may vary in their core training, theories, and practicum experiences. It is not known if a medical family therapist who received training in an intense workshop is any more or less effective, in practice, research, and training, than one trained through a master's or doctoral program. Agreement on core courses and the context for instruction would give credibility, improve fidelity, and increase opportunities to the study, practice, and research of MedFT.

Conclusion

The themes found through this review regarding the historical emergence of MedFT, the skill set and application of MedFT, the connection to family therapy, and the effectiveness of research all indicate signs of growth in MedFT. While growth seems apparent by both the total number of articles, the heightened interest from other disciplines, and the beginnings of effectiveness research, it is also clear that MedFT is still young in its development. It is the responsibility of current MedFTs to (a) clarify their role, scope, and unique skill set; (b) produce research demonstrating the efficacy and effectiveness of MedFT; and (c) identify and adopt core competencies that set standards for training of MedFTs. As a newer member to the healthcare team, it makes sense to not have these already established. Other disciplines such as Health Psychology and Medical Social Work are also pursuing this work. The development of MedFT as a specialization begins with a need and creative solutions and then moves into testing those solutions and implementing training programs to disseminate them. Reviews like this are important for highlighting the work that has been done and what has yet to be accomplished. While we recognize that a recommendation for a more contemporary definition is needed, at this time we refrain from providing one based on anecdotal evidence but prefer to report one grounded in empirical support. In 2010, a Delphi study was done surveying those with expertise in MedFT to take steps toward accomplishing this goal (Tyndall, Hodgson, Lamson, Knight, & White, 2010). Some of the outcomes of this study, particularly as related to the development of core competencies, are reported in Chap. 3 of this text. Researchers are encouraged to build on these results and conduct field research to confirm that what experts think MedFT should look like in its application is actually what is happening in the field. Lastly, future researchers should empirically examine the effectiveness of MedFT in primary, secondary, and tertiary care settings and identify a core curriculum that experts in MedFT share as fundamental to effective professional practice and the growth and advancement of the profession.

Reflective Questions

1.) How would you define MedFT to a client/patient? Healthcare provider? Healthcare administrator? Researcher? Legislator?
2.) What are some of the ways MedFTs can contribute innovation to clinical, political, training, and empirical work?
3.) What competencies do you believe all behavioral health professions integrating into healthcare settings should have and which ones do you identify as unique to MedFT?

References[1]

Altum, S. (2007). Commentary: Managing CHF and depression in an elderly patient: Being open to collaborative care. *Families, Systems, and Health, 25*, 465–467. doi:10.1037/1091 7527.25.4.465.

Alvarez, C. A. (1996). Medical family therapy: Therapeutic and financial benefits of family centered care in the hospital. *Clinical Nurse Specialist, 10*, 50–56. doi:10.1097/00002800-199601000-00017.

Anderson, R., Huff, N., & Hodgson, J. (2008). Medical family therapy in an inpatient psychiatric setting. *Families, Systems, and Health, 26*, 164–180. doi:10.1037/10917527.26.2.164.

Anonymous. (1993). Book reviews—medical family therapy: A biopsychosocial approach to families with health problems. *Adolescence, 28*, 753. Retrieved from http://www.vjf.cnrs.fr/clt/php/va/Page_revue.php?ValCodeRev=ADO.

Bayona, J. (2007). Finding hope in tragedy and chaos: A commentary on "I finally got real parents, and now they're gonna die. *Families, Systems, and Health, 25*, 234–235. doi:10.1037/1091-7527.25.2.234.

Berkley, M. (2000). Keith and Ashley: Treating a reluctant HIV+ client. *Families, Systems, and Health, 18*, 499–506. doi:10.1037/h0091897.

Bischof, G. H., Lieser, M. L., Taratua, C. G., & Fox, A. D. (2003). Power and gender issues from the voices of medical family therapists. *Journal of Feminist Family Therapy, 15*, 23–54. doi:10.1300/J086v15n02_02.

*Bischoff, R. J., Springer, P. R., Felix, D. S., & Hollist, C. S. (2011). Finding the heart of medical family therapy: A content analysis of medical family therapy casebook articles. *Families, Systems, and Health, 29*, 184–196. doi:10.1037/a0024637.

Blount, A. (Ed.). (1998). *Integrated primary care*. New York, NY: W. W. Norton. doi:10.1300/J086v15n02_03.

Brucker, P. S., Faulkner, R. A., Baptist, J., Grames, H., Beckham, L. G., Walsh, S., & Willert, A. (2005). The internship training experiences in medical family therapy of doctoral-level marriage and family therapy students. *The American Journal of Family Therapy, 33*, 131–146. doi:10.1080/01926180590915518.

Burge, B. (2005). Feminist perspectives in medical family therapy (book review). *Australian and New Zealand Journal of Family Therapy, 26*, 175–176. Retrieved from http://www.anzjft.com/pages/index.php.

[1] An asterisk has been use to note references that the chapter authors recommend for further reading.

Burgess-Manning, J. (2007). Bringing two worlds together: A collaborative interview with JoEllen Patterson. *Australian and New Zealand Journal of Family Therapy, 28*, 38–43. Retrieved from http://www.anzjft.com/pages/index.php.

Burwell, S. R., Templeton, B., Kennedy, K. S., & Zak-Hunter, L. (2008). Feminist-informed medical family therapy techniques across biopsychosocial. *Journal of Feminist Family Therapy, 20*, 99–125. doi:10.1080/08952830802023276.

*Campbell, T. L., & Patterson, J. M. (1995). The effectiveness of family interventions in the treatment of physical illness. *Journal of Marital and Family Therapy, 21*, 545–583. doi:10.1111/j.1752-0606.1995.tb00178.x.

Candib, L. M., & Stovall, J. G. (2002). Response to Schirmer and Le. *Families, Systems, and Health, 20*, 311–320. doi:10.1037/h0089586.

Clabby, J., & Howarth, D. (2007). Managing CHF and depression in an elderly patient: Being open to collaborative care. *Families, Systems, and Health, 25*, 457–464. doi:10.1037/1091-7527.25.4.457.

Cohen, J. L. (1995). Somatization revisited: A case of migraine headaches. *Family Systems Medicine, 13*, 395–404. doi:10.1037/h0089233.

Collins, R. C., & Kennedy, M. C. (2008). Serving families who have served: Providing family therapy and support in interdisciplinary polytrauma rehabilitation. *Journal of Clinical Psychology, 64*, 993–1008. doi:10.1002/jclp.20515.

Czauderna, J., & Tomson, D. (1994). Family therapy and primary care: Connections and challenges. *Journal of Family Therapy, 16*, 342–345. doi:10.1111/j.1467-6427.1994.00799.x.

Dankoski, M. E. (2003). An interview with Shobha Pais, PhD. *Journal of Feminist Family Therapy, 15*, 149–164. doi:10.1300/J086v15n02_11.

Dankoski, M. E., & Pais, S. (2007). What's love got to do with it? Couples, illness, and MFT. *Journal of Couple and Relationship Therapy, 6*, 31–43. Retrieved from http://www.tandfonline.com/loi/wcrt20.

Davey, M. P., Duncan, T. M., Foster, J., & Milton, K. (2008). Keeping the family in focus at an HIV/AIDS pediatric clinic. *Families, Systems, and Health, 26*, 350–355. doi:10.1037/a0013056.

Degges-White, S. (2005). Book review: Feminist perspectives in medical family therapy. *The Family Journal, 13*, 236–237. doi:10.1177/1066480704271117.

Doherty, W. J., McDaniel, S. H., & Hepworth, J. (1994). Medical family therapy: An emerging arena for family therapy. *Journal of Family Therapy, 16*, 31–46. doi:10.1111/j.1467-6427.1994.00775.x.

East Carolina University (ECU). (2013). *Doctor of philosophy in medical family therapy*. Retrieved from http://www.ecu.edu/che/cdfr/phdmft.html

Edwards, T. M., & Patterson, J. E. (2003). A "Golden Girl" tarnished: Amplifying one patient's (and family's) voice through collaborative care in a family medicine setting. *Journal of Feminist Family Therapy, 15*, 75–88. doi:10.1300/J086vI5n02_04.

Edwards, T. M., & Patterson, J. E. (2006). Supervising family therapy trainees in primary care medical settings: Context matters. *Journal of Marital and Family Therapy, 32*, 33–43. doi:10.1111/j.1752-0606.2006.tb01586.x.

Edwards, T., & Turnage, J. (2003). "Cheating almost killed me:" Collaborative care for a man who believed he had AIDS. *Families, Systems, and Health, 21*, 233–239. doi:10.1037/1091-7527.21.2.233.

Fogarty, C. T. (2001). Examining the influence of physicians in the lives of patients over time: Taking a history of the doctor-patient relationship. *Families, Systems, and Health, 19*, 221–226. doi:10.1037/h0089546.

Fulton, R. (1996). Medical family therapy: A biopsychosocial approach to families with health problems (book review). *Journal of Psychosomatic Research, 40*, 108–109. Retrieved from http://www.us.elsevierhealth.com/product.jsp?isbn=00223999.

Gellerstedt, M. E., & Mauksch, L. (1993). Chronic neurologic impairment: A family problem. *Family Systems Medicine, 11*, 425–431. doi:10.1037/h0089034.

Grauf-Grounds, C., & Sellers, T. S. (2006). Creating internships and potential jobs for medical family therapists: Lessons learned. *Families, Systems, and Health, 24*, 230–237. doi:10.1037/1091-7527.24.2.230.

Griffith, J. L. (1994). Review of "Medical family therapy". *Family Systems Medicine, 12*, 87–89. doi:10.1037/h0089245.

Harkness, J. L., & Nofziger, A. (1998). Medical family therapy casebook: Training in a collaborative context: What we did not know then. . .we know now. *Families, Systems, and Health, 16*, 443–450. doi:10.1037/1091-7527.24.2.230.

Harp, J. (1998). Ruth's dizziness: A commentary. *Families, Systems, and Health, 16*, 329–331. doi:10.1037/h0089944.

*Harrington, A. D., Kimball, T. G., & Bean, R. A. (2009). Families and childhood cancer: An exploration of the observations of a pediatric oncology treatment team. *Families, Systems, and Health, 27*, 16–27. doi:10.1037/a0014909.

Hertlein, K. M. (2003). Reflecting on feminist suggestions and the practice of medical family therapy: One therapist's personal framework. *Journal of Feminist Family Therapy, 15*, 127–136. doi:10.1300/J086v1502_08.

Heru, A., & Berman, E. (2008). Family meetings and integrated patient care. Commentary: Medical family therapy in an inpatient setting. *Families, Systems, and Health, 26*, 181–184. doi:10.1037/1091-7527.26.2.181 DOI:10.1037%2F1091-7527.26.2.181.

Hodgson, J., Lamson, A., Mendenhall, T., & Crane, R. (2012). Medical family therapy: Opportunity for workforce development in healthcare. *Contemporary Family Therapy, 34*, 143–146. doi:10.1007/s10591-012-9199-1.

*Hodgson, J., Lamson, A., & Reese, L. (2007). The biopsychosocial-spiritual interview method. In D. Linville, D. Lusterman, & K. Hertlein (Eds.), *Therapist notebook for family healthcare* (pp. 3–12). New York, NY: Hayworth Press.

*Hodgson, J. L., McCammon, S. L., & Anderson, R. J. (2011). A conceptual and empirical basis for including medical family therapy services in cancer care settings. *The American Journal of Family Therapy, 39*, 348–359. doi:10.1080/01926187.2010.537944.

*Hodgson, J. L., McCammon, S. L., Marlowe, D. P., & Anderson, R. J. (2012). Medical family therapy in cancer care: Patient and family experiences. *Contemporary Family Therapy, 40*, 258–266. doi:10.1080/01926187.2011.611783.

Hodgson, J., Boyd, T., Koehler, A., Lamson, A., & Rambo, A. (2013). Supervision in evolving contexts. In T. Todd & C. Storm (Eds.), *The complete systemic supervisor: Context, philosophy, and pragmatics* (2nd ed.). Bloomington, IN: iUniverse.

Hughes, A., Hertlein, K. M., & Hagey, D. W. (2011). A medft informed sex therapy for treating sexual problems associated with chronic illness. *Journal of Family Psychotherapy, 22*, 114–127. doi:10.1080/08975353.2011.577689.

Jacobs, B. J. (2012). "Here's how we're seeing it": An interview with Susan H. McDaniel, PhD, Jeri Hepworth, PhD, and William J. Doherty, PhD. *Contemporary Family Therapy, 34*, 147–155. doi:10.1007/s10591-012-9190-x.

Jencius, M. (2004). Citizen therapist: An interview with William Doherty. *The Family Journal, 12*, 82–88. doi:10.1177/1066480703258947.

Kannai, R. (2009). Munchausen by mommy. *Families, Systems, and Health, 27*, 105–112. doi:0.1037/a0015031.

Kazak, A. E. (1993). Medical family therapy: A biopsychosocial approach to families with health problems (book review). *Journal of Pediatric Psychology, 18*, 529–531. doi:10.1093/jpepsy/18.4.529.

Kelley, P. (1993). Medical family therapy: A biopsychosocial approach to families with health problems (book review). *Contemporary Psychology: APA Review of Books, 38*, 1071–1072. Retrieved from http://www.apa.org/pubs/journals/cnt/index.aspx.

Knishkowy, B., & Herman, J. (1998). Medical family therapy casebook: Ruth's dizziness. *Families, Systems, and Health, 16*, 325–327. doi:10.1037/h0089858.

Kojima, T. (2006). The development of family therapy in Japanese psychosomatic medicine. *International Congress Series, 1287*, 154–157. doi:10.1016/j.ics.2005.12.050.
Lask, B. (1994). The illness network. *Journal of Family Therapy, 16*, 47–51. Retrieved from http://www.wiley.com/bw/journal.asp?ref=0163-4445.
Leahy, D., Galbreath, L., Powell, R., & Shinn, M. A. (1994). A case of collaboration HMO style. *Family Systems Medicine, 12*, 437–449. doi:10.1037/h0089376.
Lewis, M., Lamson, A., & Leseuer, B. (2012). Healthy dynamics of military and veteran couples: A biopsychorelational overview. *Contemporary Family Therapy, 34*, 259–276. doi:10.1007/s10591-012-9193-7.
*Linville, D., Hertlein, K. M., & Prouty Lyness, A. M. (2007). Medical family therapy: Reflecting on the necessity of collaborative healthcare research. *Families, Systems, and Health, 25*, 85–97. doi:10.1037/1091-7527.25.1.85.
Lowe, W. (2007). "I finally got real parents, and now they're gonna die" – a case study of an adolescent with two HIV-positive parents. *Families, Systems, and Health, 25*, 227–233. doi:10.1037/1091-7527.25.2.227.
*Marlowe, D. (2011). Bridging conversations: Discussing the intra-professional relationship between medical family therapy and family therapy. *Journal of Family Therapy, 16*, 1–20.
*Marlowe, D., Hodgson, J., Lamson, A., White, M., & Irons, T. (2012). Medical family therapy in a primary care setting: A framework for integration. *Contemporary Family Therapy, 34*, 244–258. doi:10.1007/s10591-012-9195-5.
McDaniel, S. H. (1994). Within-family reproductive technologies as a solution to childlessness due to infertility: Psychological issues and interventions. *Journal of Clinical Psychology in Medical Settings, 1*, 301–308. doi:10.1007/BF01991074.
McDaniel, S. H., & Amos, S. (1983). The risk of change: Teaching family as the unit of care. *Family Systems Medicine, 1*, 25–30. doi:10.1037/h0090088.
McDaniel, S. H., & Campbell, T. (1986). Physicians and family therapists: The risks of collaboration. *Family Systems Medicine, 4*, 4–8. doi:10.1037/h0090176.
McDaniel, S. H., Campbell, T., & Seaburn, D. (1989). Somatic fixation in patients and physicians: A biopsychosocial approach. *Family Systems Medicine, 7*, 5–16. doi:10.1037/h0089761.
McDaniel, S. H., Doherty, W. J., & Hepworth, J. (2013). *Medical family therapy and integrated care* (2nd ed.). Washington, DC: American Psychological Association.
McDaniel, S. H., Doherty, W. J., & Hepworth, J. (2014). *Medical family therapy and integrated care* (2nd ed.). Washington, DC: American Psychological Association.
McDaniel, S. H., Harkness, J. L., & Epstein, R. M. (2001). Medical family therapy for a woman with end stage Crohn's disease and her son. *The American Journal of Family Therapy, 29*, 375–395. doi:10.1037/10395-027.
McDaniel, S. H., Hepworth, J., & Doherty, W. J. (1992a). Medical family therapy with couples facing infertility. *The American Journal of Family Therapy, 20*, 101–122. doi:10.1080/01926189208250882.
*McDaniel, S. H., Hepworth, J., & Doherty, W. J. (Eds.). (1992b). *Medical family therapy: A biopsychosocial approach to families with health problems*. New York, NY: Basic Books.
McDaniel, S. H., Hepworth, J., & Doherty, W. J. (1995). Medical family therapy with somaticizing patients: The co-creation of therapeutic stories. *Family Process, 34*, 349–361. doi:10.1111/j.1545-5300.1995.00349.x.
McDaniel, S. H., Hepworth, J., & Doherty, W. J. (1999). The shared emotional themes of illness. *Journal of Family Psychotherapy, 10*, 1–8. doi:10.1300/J085v10n04_01.
*Mendenhall, T. J., Pratt, K. J., Phelps, K. W., & Baird, M. A. (2012). Advancing medical family therapy through research: A consideration of qualitative, quantitative, and mixed-methods designs. *Contemporary Family Therapy, 34*, 187–203. doi:10.1007/s10591-012-9186-6.
Munshower, J. C. (2004). Group visits for diabetic patients: One physician's experience. *Families, Systems, and Health, 22*, 497–500. doi:10.1037/1091-7527.22.4.497.
Navon, S. (2005). Listening to illness/nonillness motifs: A case of fibromyalgia. *Families, Systems, and Health, 23*, 358–361. doi:10.1037/1091-7527.23.3.358.

Oberman, A. (2006). Review of feminist perspectives in medical family therapy. *The Family Journal, 14*, 453. doi:10.1177/1066480706289564.
Pereira, M. G., & Smith, T. E. (2006). Evolution of the biopsychosocial model in the practice of family therapy. *International Journal of Clinical and Health Psychology, 6*, 455–467. Retrieved from http://www.aepc.es/ijchp/index.php?coid=English.
Phelps, K. W., Howell, C. D., Hill, S. G., Seeman, T. G., Lamson, A. L., Hodgson, J. L., & Smith, D. A. (2009). A collaborative care model for patients with Type-2 diabetes. *Families, Systems, and Health, 27*, 131–141. doi:10.1037/a0015027.
Pratt, D. M. (2003). Interview with Dr Susan McDaniel: Medical family therapy and feminism. *Journal of Feminist Family Therapy, 15*, 137–147. doi:10.1300/J086v15n02_09.
Preece, J. C., & Sandberg, J. G. (2005). Family resilience and the management of fibromyalgia: Implications for family therapists. *Contemporary Family Therapy, 27*, 559–576. doi:10.1007/s10591-005-8242-x.
Prest, L. A., Fitzgibbons, P. M. R., & Krier, J. (1996). Head injury and decisions about care: A collaborative approach. *Families, Systems, and Health, 14*, 387–393. doi:10.1037/h0089923.
Prouty Lyness, A. M. (2003). Preface: Perspectives in medical family therapy. *Journal of Feminist Family Therapy, 15*, xvii. Retrieved from http://www.tandfonline.com/loi/wfft20.
Radomsky, N. A. (1996). The essence of family medicine: Story of a doctor-patient partnership. *Families, Systems, and Health, 14*, 497–502. doi:10.1037/h0089984.
Ragaisis, K. M. (1996). The psychiatric consultation-liaison nurse and medical family therapy. *Clinical Nurse Specialist, 10*, 50–56. doi:10.1097/00002800-199601000-00018.
Riccelli, A. (2003). Memoirs of a "poop lady". *Families, Systems, and Health, 21*, 109–117. doi:10.1037/h0089507.
Robinson, W. D., Barnacle, R. E. S., Pretorius, R., & Paulman, A. (2004). An interdisciplinary student-run diabetes clinic: Reflections on the collaborative training process. *Families, Systems, and Health, 22*, 490–496. doi:10.1037/1091-7527.22.4.490.
Rosenberg, M. (2005). Feminist perspectives in medical family therapy (book review). *Families, Systems, and Health, 23*, 113–114. doi:10.1037/1091-7527.23.1.113.
Rosenberg, T., Brown, E., & Gawinski, B. (2008). Multidisciplinary intervention for failure to thrive: Casebook. *Families, Systems, and Health, 26*, 365–371. doi:10.1037/a0013333.
Ruddy, N. B., & McDaniel, S. H. (2003). Medical family therapy. In T. Sexton, G. Weeks, & M. S. Robbins (Eds.), *Handbook of family therapy: The science and practice of working with families and couples* (pp. 418–436). New York, NY: Bruner-Rutledge.
Ruddy, N. (with Farley, T., Nymberg, J., & Hayden, K.) (1994). Multiple personality disorder in primary care: A collaboration. *Family Systems Medicine, 12*, 327–338. doi:10.1037/h0089056.
Schirmer, J. M., & Le, N. H. (2002). The Vietnam Family Medicine Development Project: A cross cultural collaboration. *Families, Systems, and Health, 20*, 303–311. doi:10.1037/h0089585.
*Sellers, T. S. (2000). A model of collaborative healthcare in outpatient medical oncology. *Families, Systems, and Health, 18*, 19–33. doi:10.1037/h0091851.
Shapiro, J. (1993). A book review. *Family Systems Medicine, 11*, 219–221. doi:10.1037/h0089192.
Siegel, D. M. (2009). Munchausen syndrome by proxy: A pediatrician's observations. *Families, Systems, and Health, 27*, 113–115. doi:10.1037/a0015030.
Smith-Lamson, A., & Hodgson, J. (2003). Medical family therapy: From the big screen to a collaborative learning environment. *Journal of Feminist Family Therapy, 15*, 165–169. doi:10.1300/J086v15n02_11.
Souza, J. M. (2002). End of life decision-making: An interdisciplinary perspective. *Families, Systems, and Health, 20*, 449–453. doi:10.1037/h0089596.
Streicher, P. J. (1995). A suicidal client: The limits of power and control. *Family Systems Medicine, 13*, 91–95. doi:10.1037/h0089343.
Szyndler, J. E., Towns, S., Hoffman, R. C., & Bennett, D. L. (2003). Clinical assessment, management and outcomes of a group of adolescents presenting with complex medico-

psychosocial conditions. *Annals of the Academy of Medicine Singapore, 32*, 51–57. Retrieved from http://www.annals.edu.sg/.

Thomasgard, M., Boreman, C., & Metz, W. P. (2004). A family under siege: Empathic mirroring and collaborative care. *Families, Systems, and Health, 22*, 245–254. doi:10.1037/1091-7527.22.2.245.

Trepal, H. C. (2005). Book review: Feminist perspectives in medical family therapy. *The Family Journal, 13*, 368. doi:10.1177/1066480704273644.

Tyndall, L., Hodgson, J., Lamson, A., Knight, S., & White, M. (2010). *Medical family therapy: Conceptual clarification and consensus for an emerging profession* (Doctoral dissertation). Retrieved from http://thescholarship.ecu.edu/handle/10342/2794

Tyndall, L., Hodgson, J., Lamson, A., White, M., & Knight, S. (2014). Medical family therapy: Charting a course in competencies. In J. Hodgson, A. Lamson, T. Mendenhall, & R. Crane (Eds.), *Medical family therapy: Advanced applications* (pp. 33–53). New York, NY: Springer.

Ungureanu, I., & Sandberg, J. G. (2008). Caring for dying children and their families: MFTs working at the gates of elysian fields. *Contemporary Family Therapy, 30*, 75–91. 10.1007/s10591-008-9059-1.

University of Nebraska-Lincoln (UNL). (2013). *Medical family therapy – PhD program*. Retrieved from http://cehs.unl.edu/cyaf/grad/mftPhD.shtml

University of Rochester Medical Center (URMC). (2013). *20th Annual medical family therapy intensive*. Retrieved from http://www.urmc.rochester.edu/psychiatry/institute-for-the-family/family-therapy/mfti.cfm

Weiner, E. L., & Lorenz, A. (1994). Initiation of a behavioral scientist: Lessons from a boy who wouldn't poop. *Family Systems Medicine, 12*, 73–79. doi:10.1037/h0089340.

Weiss, M., & Hepworth, J. (1993). A case for solutions. *Family Systems Medicine, 11*, 297–302. doi:10.1037/h0089301.

Willerton, E., Dankoski, M. E., & Sevilla Martir, J. F. (2008). Medical family therapy: A model for addressing mental health disparities among latinos. *Families, Systems, and Health, 26*, 196–206. doi:10.1037/1091-7527.26.2.196.

Wirtberg, I. (2005). Introduction to medical family therapy. *Acta Paediatrica, 94*, 45–46. doi:10.1080/08035320510035483.

Wissow, L. S., Hutton, N., & Kass, N. (2002). Preliminary study of a values-history advance directive interview in a pediatric HIV clinic. *AIDS and Public Policy Journal, 17*, 17–28. Retrieved from http://www.upgbooks.com/appj/.

Wright, L. M., Watson, W. L., & Bell, J. M. (1992). The medical map is not the territory: "Medical Family Therapy" watch your language. *Families, Systems, and Health, 10*, 35–39. doi:10.1037/h0089250.

Yeager, B., Auyang, M., Brown, D. L., Dickinson, P., Goldstein, J. A., Jaffe, N.,. . ., & Workman, G. (1999). MFT student training in medical family therapy: A collaborative hospital project with radiation oncology. *Families, Systems, and Health, 17*, 427–436. doi:10.1037/h0089894.

Chapter 3
Medical Family Therapy: Charting a Course in Competencies

Lisa Tyndall, Jennifer Hodgson, Angela Lamson, Mark White, and Sharon Knight

The first text on medical family therapy (MedFT) appeared in 1992 (McDaniel, Doherty, & Hepworth, 1992). Since that time there has been an increasing interest in MedFT as evidenced in the growing body of literature and in the increasing numbers of training and academic programs (Tyndall, Hodgson, Lamson, White, & Knight, 2012). Initially, MedFTs were trained through post-degree programs such as the pioneering MedFT intensive course offered at the University of Rochester Medical Center (URMC, 2013). Since then, this has expanded to include MedFT internships, workshops, and concentrations offered within already existing degree programs. Given the growth of MedFT and consequent increase in training opportunities, the researchers recognized a need for consensus among MedFT experts regarding academic courses and competencies that reflected requisite MedFT knowledge and skills.

Professional Competencies

While behavioral health disciplines are working individually to identify competencies for their professional members to practice in healthcare settings, researchers from medical disciplines have been leading the way to increase competency for their professional members in behavioral health. For example, Marvel and Major (1999) examined behavioral health competencies in family medicine physicians by surveying over 600 practicing family physicians and asking them to rate the importance of knowledge about various behavioral health domains. Baglia et al. (2011) built on these ideas and focused on the need to transform abstract medical competencies into more concrete observable behaviors among physicians

L. Tyndall (✉)
Department of Child Development & Family Relations, East Carolina University, Greenville, NC, USA
e-mail: tyndalll@ecu.edu

J. Hodgson et al. (eds.), *Medical Family Therapy*, DOI 10.1007/978-3-319-03482-9_3,

in the process of completing their residencies. As a result of their work, they concluded "the principles of outcomes-based assessment require that explicit efforts be directed toward identifying actual changes in learners' knowledge, behaviors, and attitudes rather than relying on completion of a time-based requirement as evidence of competence" (p. 90).

Both of the aforementioned studies incorporated content-expert opinions and reflected elements of a Delphi method (Dalkey, 1972). The researchers either asked field experts to rate various competencies on a Likert scale (Marvel & Major, 1999) or worked with a group of content-expert faculty to attain consensus regarding professional competencies (Baglia et al., 2011). While the methods used in these studies deviated from a Delphi method, as exemplified by the use of a face-to-face survey rather than an anonymous questionnaire (e.g., Baglia et al., 2011), some similarities to the Delphi method existed because the aims of the studies were to reach consensus and help direct future movement in the professions studied.

Members of behavioral health professions, such as Social Work and Psychology, have worked to identify competencies or standards of practice for those in their respective disciplines who practice in healthcare settings (APA, 2013; NASW, 2005). Social work began this discussion as early as 1977 and refined and expanded these standards in 2005 by means of expert consensus (NASW). Social work standards related to professional practice in healthcare settings include areas such as ethics, cultural competence, assessment, and treatment planning and intervention. The competencies for Psychology practice in primary care were developed as a result of representatives from nine national organizations meeting together to develop the competencies with a central focus on education or practice in primary care Psychology. The core competencies identified by the group included six broad domains with specific aptitudes under each domain that cover essential knowledge, skills, and attitudes, as well as example of what this looks like if observed (i.e., behavioral anchors).

While both medical and behavioral health providers have been working to better prepare their workforces for behavioral health integration in medical settings, competencies in interprofessional collaboration among healthcare professionals have seemingly increased both in the United States and abroad. In fact, the College of Health Disciplines at the University of British Columbia (2008), for example, developed a "Competency Framework for Interprofessional Collaboration" with the goal of informing the continuing education process for transdisciplinary healthcare professionals. Competencies included in the framework were organized into three domains: interpersonal and communication skills, patient-centered and family-focused care, and collaborative practice. Recognizing that identifying competencies for a relatively new professional emphasis such as interprofessional collaboration (IPC) can be difficult, members of The Canadian Interprofessional Health Collaborative (2010) developed a standard of interprofessional competencies for healthcare providers. Health practitioners in the United States have also examined IPC competencies, arguing that core competencies are needed to guide the professional and institutional development of learning approaches, coordinate the effort to identify essential knowledge and skills for all healthcare professions, and facilitate licensing and professional credentialing (IPEC, 2011).

It is clear that the identification and assessment of competencies present an ongoing discussion topic in a variety of health-related fields. The timing is also right for MedFT to begin a more formal process of identifying competencies and curricula to assure excellence in training and to improve the evaluation and measurement of MedFT training outcomes. At the same time that our expert consensus study on MedFT competencies was published in 2012 (Tyndall et al., 2012), Bischoff, Springer, Reisbig, Lyons, and Likcani (2012) recognized a similar need and conducted and published a survey-based qualitative study identifying skills needed for behavioral health professionals to practice integrated care successfully. They referred to MedFT specifically in the body of the document. However, despite these two emerging sets of competencies, without consensus via active discussion among the experts about what these competencies should be and what should be included in a standard training curriculum, MedFTs may be presenting a disparate image and set of skills.

Competencies not only help to strengthen a specialization but promote quality among those trained to do it. While training programs in MedFT have been in existence, or are being developed currently, there is no agreement among those groups on what training is required or competencies are needed to be effective in behavioral health positions.

Training Opportunities in MedFT

At the time this chapter was written, in the summer of 2013, 17 MedFT Professional Programs or other focused training opportunities were available in the United States (Table 3.1). Additionally, one doctoral program in MedFT was set to launch in the fall of 2014 (Saint Louis University, personal communication, July 8, 2013). Similarities among the programs occurred in both training opportunities in medical settings and across course topics. For example, coursework that addressed the intersection of families and illness and that focused on transdisciplinary collaborative processes was clearly evident across each program listed. Another similarity was clinical supervision typically offered through practicums/supervised clinical experiences. In contrast, lengths of clinical exposure and depth of submersion and supervision differed among varying graduate degree levels and certificates. Programs also included a variety of special topics, including psychopharmacology and children with special needs, provided varying levels of research training, and addressed the business side of MedFT clinical services. While several of the training programs use MedFT in their title, others have adopted a title reflecting specialized areas for the MedFT practitioner or researcher that included any combination of the following terms: families, systems, illness, collaboration, and health.

Table 3.1 Training in MedFT

Institution	Level of Training(s)	Program/ Certificate Name	Curriculum: Course Content and Field Work
Chicago Center for Family Health (2013)	Advanced certificate specialization/summer institute	Families, illness, and collaborative health care	Classes include impact of illness on family with developmental perspective, death and loss, family resiliency
	Doctoral fellowship		Participate in multidisciplinary teaching conferences, teaching residents and medical students about the integration of family systems approaches health care, collaboration with healthcare providers, and clinical research projects related to families and health care
Dartmouth Family Practice Residency, Concord Hospital	Doctoral internship	Community and family medicine	Clinical, teaching, and research experiences relevant to working in a family medicine residency setting
Drexel University (2012)	Online post-master's certificate	Medical family therapy	Classes include illness through a life-cycle perspective, analysis of healthcare policy, applying family systems work to families with healthcare challenges
Duke University Health System, Cancer Patient Support Program	Doctoral- and master's-level internships	Cancer patient support program	Doctoral internship involves clinical services and research Master's internship involves clinical services only
Duke/Southern Regional AHEC	Doctoral internship	Family medicine residency program	Clinical, teaching, and research experiences relevant to working in a family medicine residency setting
East Carolina University (2012)	Doctoral degree	Medical family therapy	Classes include research methods, theory (clinical, policy, and financial), illness and disability, healthcare economics, gender and ethnicity, supervision, master's and doctoral fieldwork in primary, secondary, and tertiary care settings
	Doctoral internships	Internships in adult and pediatric community healthcare centers	

(continued)

Table 3.1 (continued)

Institution	Level of Training(s)	Program/ Certificate Name	Curriculum: Course Content and Field Work
Loma Linda University	Doctoral degree in marriage and family therapy program with concentration	Concentration: Families, systems, and health	Classes include introduction to medical family therapy, families and illness, medicine and family therapy, and special projects. Clinical internships in primary, secondary, and tertiary care settings
	Post-master's certificate	Post-master's certificate: MedFT	Clinical internships in the following: community health center, kidney and liver transplantation institute, pediatrics, adult oncology center, and chaplaincy program
Northcentral University	Doctoral degree in marriage and family therapy with specialization	Medical family therapy	Classes include biopsychosocial connections and interventions; families with severe and chronic illness; death, dying, and bereavement; and medical family therapy; dissertation and internship focus on medical family therapy
	Master's degree in marriage and family therapy with specialization	Medical family therapy	Master's specialization program in development, enrollment scheduled for fall 2014
Nova Southeastern University (2011)	Post-master's certificate and specialized doctoral-level track	Family systems health care	Classes include systems theory, marital and family therapy theories, healthcare policy, optional practicum placements
Saint Louis University (2013)	Doctoral degree	Medical family therapy	Classes include models of medical family therapy; families, illness, and health; neurobiology of interpersonal behavior; behavioral medicine intervention; doctoral integrative care practicum for four semesters
	Master's degree in marriage and family therapy with MedFT concentration		

(continued)

Table 3.1 (continued)

Institution	Level of Training(s)	Program/ Certificate Name	Curriculum: Course Content and Field Work
Seattle Pacific University (2012)	Post-master's certificate	Medical family therapy	Classes include collaboration between therapist and physician, interviewing for biopsychosocial and spiritual care, motivational interviewing for patient and family health, marketing your practice to physicians, spirituality and health, family therapy tools for treating medical illness, psychopharmacology, brain-savvy therapist, supervision, and a 1-year-long internship in an integrated behavioral health position in a community-based outpatient primary and specialty care clinic
St. Mary's Family Medicine Residency/ University of Colorado School of Medicine	Doctoral internship/ postdoctoral fellowship	Medical family therapy advanced specialization training certificate	Advanced training in medical family therapy and integrated care; includes a balance of clinical work, teaching, research, and interdisciplinary supervision. This multisite program includes rotations in inpatient medicine, HIV specialty care, group medical appointments, and homeless outreach
University of Minnesota in Minneapolis-St. Paul	Doctoral internship	Family medicine and community health	Clinical, teaching, and research experiences relevant to working in a family medicine residency setting
University of Nebraska-Lincoln (UNL 2012; UNMC, 2011)	Post-master's/graduate certificate	Medical family therapy	Classes include psychopathology, ethics, sexual dysfunction, pharmacology, family therapy, collaborative health care; partnership with Department of Internal Medicine
University of Rochester (2014)	Post-masters certificate/week-long intensive	Medical family therapy	Curriculum emphasis on major family therapy models, family development theories, and research
	Doctoral-level internship	Family medicine	Clinical, teaching, and research experiences relevant to working in a family medicine residency setting

(continued)

Table 3.1 (continued)

Institution	Level of Training(s)	Program/ Certificate Name	Curriculum: Course Content and Field Work
University of San Diego (n.d.)	Master's degree in marriage and family therapy with MedFT emphasis	Medical family therapy	Classes include social neu roscience for family therapists, families of children with special needs, collaborative care, and psychopharmacology and the brain, and master's fieldwork in primary care settings
Northern Illinois University (2014)	Post-master's certificate	MedFT and Counseling	Course Content and Field Work: Courses include cultural and spiritual dimensions of medical family therapy and counseling, introduction to medical family therapy and counseling; with 6 credit hours of internship in a medical setting

Program information listed may not be a complete list of courses offered or required

Doctoral programs differ from master's degree and certificate programs largely around the areas of research and teaching preparedness. East Carolina University (ECU) launched the first MedFT doctoral program in the United States in August of 2005 (ECU, 2012). ECU requires doctoral students to conduct research and has strong research and clinical ties to local academic and community-based healthcare centers and hospitals. Its program heavily emphasizes the foundational underpinnings of the biopsychosocial-spiritual (BPSS) model and systems thinking (ECU, 2012). Loma Linda University (LLU) offers doctoral-level classes and internship experiences in MedFT, as well as a post-master's certificate program in it. Clinical healthcare placements include primary care, organ transplantation, trauma, spiritual care, oncology, and pediatric services (LLU, 2013). Some of the suggested courses of study for the Saint Louis University doctoral program include an integrative care practicum; families, health, and illness; and advanced couple and family therapy (C. Smith, personal communication, August 1, 2013). All three programs offer doctoral students the opportunity to gain research experience in a variety of integrated care medical contexts.

A majority of the MedFT post-master's certificate programs share similar foci as well, but differences also exist. For example, the University of San Diego (n.d.) offers a master's degree in marital family therapy with an optional practicum emphasis on MedFT (T. Edwards, personal communication, July 1, 2013). While all of their master's students take the same core courses, those core courses include Collaborative Care and Social Neuroscience for Family Therapists as well as Family Therapy Theories and Family Development. Nova Southeastern University (2011) offers a post-master's certificate that, while titled "Family Systems Health

Care Graduate Certificate," its courses reflect a focus similar to that of MedFT programs, such as biopsychosocial (BPS) and systemic theories and healthcare systems. Seattle Pacific University (2012) offers a MedFT certificate for both current master's students and post-master's students, with course offerings ranging from collaboration between therapists and physicians and extenders to spirituality and health. While differences exist among these master's and certificate programs, they share a similar goal of educating clinicians on the importance of using a BPS framework in working with patients (Engel, 1977, 1980) while also recognizing the systemic context within which patients are embedded.

Internships are essential in preparing MedFTs at the graduate level or employment in healthcare settings (Grauf-Grounds & Sellers, 2006). It is through immersion in the healthcare culture that students learn how biomedical contexts differ from traditional behavioral health contexts, how to interact and best collaborate with other healthcare professionals, how to speak the language of collaboration, and how to teach and conduct research using a BPS lens. MedFT internships and postdoctoral training take place in a variety of institutions and range from primary to tertiary care, with the availability of specific sites tending to change annually and the focus for the internships ranging from clinical to teaching and research experiences in health care. While master's-level internships mainly focus on clinical work, doctoral-level internships emphasize research and teaching in addition to clinical practice. Information gathered on MedFT internships is included in Table 3.1, sourced largely from institutional websites and personal communication with program faculty.

MedFT Core Competencies

As noted above, a lack of standardization in curricula and core competencies exists across various MedFT degrees and training opportunities. Training program descriptions, however, reveal some commonalities. For example, practicum sites included in various programs generally involve MedFT placement within a family medicine, primary care, or specialty setting to facilitate learning and immersion within a medical culture. Coursework tends to focus on intervention with individuals, couples, and families working toward a behavioral health goal and/or experiencing an acute or chronic illness, trauma, disability, or loss. All coursework appears to be informed by a BPS perspective (Engel, 1977, 1980). A theme of collaboration with healthcare professionals, patients, and families defines a majority of the programs. Programs differ, though, on the inclusion of specific training foci to develop student competency in areas such as spirituality, psychopharmacology, integrated care, and family resiliency but share a common view of MedFT as inclusive of those who are trained to apply a BPS, collaborative, and systemic lens in a variety of healthcare settings.

As a range of marriage and family therapy (MFT) skills may be evident in those practicing MedFT, in 2004, the American Association of Marriage and Family Therapy (AAMFT) published a core competencies update for the practice of MFT.

The competencies emerged from a partnership between AAMFT and interested stakeholders and were informed by a prior version of the competencies and several critical reports: *Mental Health: A Report of the Surgeon General* (SAMSHA/IOM, n.d.), *Achieving the Promise: Transforming Mental Health Care in America* (SAMSHA, 2003), and the Institute of Medicine's *Crossing the Quality Chasm* (2001). The authors of the update considered the impact of historical, political, social, and economic contexts on patients and treatment processes and aimed to use the competencies to focus on strengthening the services provided by marriage and family therapists (AAMFT, 2004). Therefore, when a professional identifies as an MFT, it is implied that he or she possesses basic competency in those areas. These competencies put forth by AAMFT have helped to identify the necessary skills sets for the practice of MFT.

Unlike the core competencies identified for MFT and the other behavioral health professions noted above (i.e., Social Work and Psychology), no core competencies had been identified for the practice of MedFT, leaving each training program to develop its own. Without a set of core competencies that is interinstitutional, those enrolled in varying MedFT degree or training programs would not have a shared skill set that could be communicated to other healthcare providers, used in formal evaluations of practitioners and programs, or marketed in the workplace.

Method

The Delphi Method

The authors conducted a research study approved by the East Carolina University Institutional Review Board using a Delphi method to identify the contemporary definition, scope, and practice of MedFT. Findings reported in this chapter are not inclusive of all findings that emerged from the study; data that are reported specifically pertain to expert panelists' perspectives on MedFT training and fundamental core competencies.

The Delphi method originated as a way for individuals with a particular shared knowledge and background to come together and discuss a topic related to their field of expertise without the undue influence of one another (Dalkey, 1972; Linstone & Turoff, 1975). It is designed so that panelists act independently, typically by means of surveys, without direct confrontation by an interviewer (Dalkey & Helmer, 1963). In this study, the Delphi technique was modified to include two, rather than three, phases of questionnaires, a decision made in an effort to reduce panelist attrition (Stone Fish & Busby, 2005). This modified format has also been utilized in other MFT-related Delphi studies (e.g., Godfrey, Haddock, Fisher, & Lund, 2006; Jenkins, 1996; Sori & Sprenkle, 2004; Stone Fish & Osborn, 1992; White, Edwards, & Russell, 1997; White & Russell, 1995).

Panelists

To meet the inclusion criteria for a Delphi study, participants must have content expertise in the topic being surveyed (Dalkey, 1972; Jenkins & Smith, 1994; Linstone & Turoff, 1975). As a result, panelists invited to participate were chosen purposively. Panelist criteria included one or more of the following: (a) self-identification as a MedFT, (b) current employment in a clinical or academic setting as a MedFT, or (c) self-identified healthcare provider who collaborated with a MedFT in his or her professional work.

Three primary sources were used to identify potential study participants. Panelists were identified through a review of the academic literature and by reviewing the faculty and doctoral student listings for institutions of higher education offering MedFT academic courses or educational programs. Individuals were then contacted via email for confirmation that they met the inclusion criteria and asked for their willingness to participate. Potential panelists were also contacted via an email message posted from the Collaborative Family Healthcare Association's (CFHA) membership listserv. CFHA was chosen as an appropriate listserv because it has historically been an outlet for scholarly work in MedFT.

Thirty-seven panelists (21 females and 16 males) ranging in age from 26 to 63 years (mean = 41 years) completed the first phase of the study. In the second phase, three panelists were lost to attrition; thus the final sample included 34 of the original 37 panelists. Panelists' terminal degrees included Marriage and Family Therapy (43 %, $n = 16$), MedFT (30 %, $n = 11$), nursing or medicine (11 %, $n = 4$), and other areas (10 %, theology, $n = 1$; Clinical Psychology, $n = 1$; Developmental Psychology, $n = 1$; Education, $n = 1$; and Family Studies, $n = 2$). Self-reported, formal training in MedFT (e.g., degrees, certificate, institute, and internship/fellowship training) was indicated for the majority of panelists (81 %, $n = 30$). Approximately 60 % of panelists identified themselves as faculty at an academic institution, while 16 % of master's-level providers were enrolled in doctoral programs. Panelists reported being employed in both medical and non-healthcare settings. For those employed in healthcare settings, workload distribution was reported as follows: clinical (68 %), teaching (57 %), and research (43 %). For panelists in non-healthcare settings, workloads were similar: teaching (57 %), clinical (46 %), and research (41 %).

Data Collection and Analysis

Data collection in this study occurred in two phases: Delphi Questionnaire I (DQ I) and Delphi Questionnaire II (DQ II). The DQ I included 8 open-ended questions and 12 demographic items. Findings from the analysis of seven of the eight questions are presented in a separate publication (Tyndall, Hodgson, Lamson, White, & Knight, 2010). The open-ended survey question forming the basis for this chapter is:

> What core courses, training and field experiences, and core competences (i.e., essential skills) do you believe MedFTs should have successfully completed as part of their MedFT curriculum? Indicate if courses should be taken at the MS or Ph.D. levels by inserting (MS) or (Ph.D.) after each course.

The statements rated in the DQ II were generated from panelists' responses to the DQ I. Wording of the statements was kept as closely to the original as possible. Consistent with the purpose of the Delphi method, the researchers' role in this study was to facilitate an asynchronous online conversation among experts (Dalkey, 1972; Linstone & Turoff, 1975) and then analyze the product of their participation.

Responses to the DQ I resulted in 600 statements. To help increase interrater reliability, three researchers assisted in the analysis process. Participant responses were individually read and each researcher noted his or her interpretation of its meaning. When clarification of a statement was needed, researchers followed up with panelists. This occurred three times. Researchers deleted redundant statements and then collapsed the remaining 552 statements into 17 distinct categories by thematic analysis. Researchers randomly distributed the 552 statements from each of the 17 categories into two separate DQ II surveys in an effort to reduce the total number of statements to be answered and avoid panelist attrition. At times, due to the length of statements, panelists' responses were divided into shorter statements for ease of ratings in the DQ II. The purpose of the DQ II was to take the initial series of statements (i.e., items) resulting from the DQ I and ask that participants rate their level of agreement with each item. The panelists were divided into two groups (DQ IIA, $n = 19$; DQ IIB, $n = 18$), based first on institutional affiliation and then randomly, in an effort to provide a variety of opinions for each question. The final DQ IIA contained 278 items and the DQ IIB contained 274 items. Panelists rated their responses for each item on a seven-point Likert scale, with seven indicating a strong level of agreement and one indicating a strong level of disagreement. There was a 92 % response rate on the DQ IIA and B combined with total of 34 of the 37 panelists responding.

Results

Consensus among panelists was determined by an analysis of the median and interquartile range of each survey item. The higher end of the Likert scale indicated the highest level of agreement, while the lower values of the scale indicated level of disagreement (Stone Fish & Busby, 2005). The interquartile range (a measure of variability) indicates how much the panelists differed in their responses. An item that had both a high median and a small IQR indicated that a majority of panelists agreed with the statement. Items from the DQ IIA and DQ IIB with a median of six or higher (agree/strongly agree) and an IQR of 1.5 or less were included in the final profile. The final academics and training profile included 175 items (i.e., variables) that were grouped under the two larger thematic categories of courses and competencies (Table 3.2). Also shown in the table is the level at which each course and

Table 3.2 Academics/training statements included in MedFT profile

$N = 175$							
Courses ($N = 100$)				Competencies ($N = 75$)			
	PhD	PM	MS		PhD	PM	MS
Field training	12	4	6	Clinical skills	–	17	–
Physiology/pharmacology	2	5	3	Medical culture and collaboration	1	14	3
Systems/relational theories	–	3	3	Treatment planning	1	1	1
Family and illness	5	2	8	Theoretical base	–	7	–
MedFT theory	3	1	1	Knowledge of health/ relationships	–	4	–
Research/stats	7	–	4	Knowledge of diseases	–	4	–
Medical culture and collaboration	4	2	3	Teaching	–	4	–
MFT training	–	–	3	Evidence base	–	3	–
Ethics	–	–	4	Administration	–	3	–
Behavioral health theory	–	1	–	Self-care	–	2	–
Special topics	5	1	7	DSM knowledge	–	2	–
Health policy	1	–	–	Family systems knowledge	1	1	2
				BPSS/applied MedFT	3	1	–

Note. Data reflect number of statements recognized in the final profile. PM statements reflect skills at the PM level minimally for those who did not study MedFT in their master's program curricula. It is assumed that doctoral-level programs build upon competencies and courses at the master's and post-master's levels

PhD, doctoral level; PM, post-master's level; MS, master's level

competency should be mastered. It was assumed that doctoral-level programs built upon the competencies and courses at the master's and post-master's levels.

Courses

Panelists revealed that MedFTs should complete 12 course content and fieldwork areas (Table 3.2) during their training. The area that generated the largest number of statements was the need for field training within healthcare settings. Panelists endorsed 22 statements in this area. Three statements, two referencing training at the doctoral level and one referencing an unspecified level of training, reflected the highest possible score (median = 7; IQR = 0.0). These statements generally emphasized the need for supervised practical experience in a medical setting, for example, "MedFTs should do internships in medical settings."

Research and statistics were viewed as important courses by panelists at both the master's and doctoral levels; however, more emphasis was given at the doctoral level with a higher number of statements endorsed ($n = 7$). It should be noted that "n" refers to the number of statements that met the "agreement" cutoff for inclusion. Four such courses were endorsed at the master's level. Doctoral courses reflected a greater diversity and sophistication in terms of including entire courses on qualitative research, integrated care research, and advanced statistics, while master's courses reflected a more basic and general research knowledge base.

Overall, the panelists approved 13 special topics courses. At both the master's and doctoral levels, panelists included courses on sexuality, gender and diversity, and death and dying. Substance abuse was included at both the master's and the post-master's levels. At the doctoral level, they recommended a course that addressed medical disparities. At the master's level, they identified courses related to community resources and crisis assessment.

Twelve of the course content areas approved by the panel focused on the theoretical underpinnings of MedFT. Panelists endorsed MedFT theory at all three levels ($n = 5$). Specifically, at the doctoral level, panelists gave the highest rating to a course entitled *Advanced Medical Family Therapy*. Systems, relational theories, behavioral health, and the biopsychosocial-spiritual perspective were only mentioned at the master's ($n = 3$) and post-master's levels ($n = 4$). This led us to assume that at the doctoral level, panelists believed that MedFTs would have already received training in these theories. At the master's level, also receiving the highest rating was the statement "MedFTs at the master's level should have a course in family therapy theory." Health policy theory ($n = 1$) was endorsed as a course at the doctoral level only.

Panelists ($n = 4$) identified ethics courses as important at the master's level of study: two general ethics, one working within a medical setting, and one research ethics. The researchers interpreted panelists' recommendations as the need for students to have completed ethics courses prior to enrolling in doctoral-level courses. No statements in this category received the highest score (median = 7; IQR of 0.0).

As a content area, panelists reached consensus that MedFTs at all three levels should take general courses on families and illness ($n = 15$). Examples of those course titles included *Advanced Families, Illness, and Disabilities*; *Chronic Illness and Families*; and *Illness Across the Life Cycle {Span}*. A statement at the post-master's level reflected the general necessity of a course on health and families received the highest level of endorsement "MedFTs should take courses in health and families" (median = 7; IQR = 0.0).

The presence of courses on marriage and family therapy (MFT) was indicated at the master's level only. In this content area, panelists strongly agreed with three statements reflecting the notion that a MedFT must have training in MFT. With a strong knowledge base in MFT, the panelists' statements also reflected the importance of the inclusion of courses more medical in nature. The statement that reflected that inclusion received the highest possible score (median = 7, IQR 0.0) was "MedFTs should have all the training one would get to be a family therapist, and then additional courses/training in appropriate medical issues and the related BPS issues that individuals/families face."

The panelists endorsed courses on human physiology and psychopharmacology at all three levels ($n = 10$). Panelists suggested a basic level for these courses that provides MedFTs with a foundation from which they can collaborate with medical providers. An example of the endorsed courses included "Psychopharmacology (basic knowledge of how drugs that treat physical illness can affect behavioral health and vice versa)." Panelists indicated that these courses were important for collaboration with physicians, "Ideally, MedFTs should take some kind of course in the brain and mental illness so that one can converse well with physicians."

The final content area, medical culture and collaboration, included courses that would be essential to the successful function of MedFTs in a medical system ($n = 9$). The courses endorsed by panelists addressed the importance of learning how to collaborate with medical professionals and work effectively within the medical system. Two statements at the doctoral level received the strongest endorsement (median = 7; IQR = 0.0). These statements focused heavily on collaboration: "Collaborating in medical settings" and "Advanced collaborative care with physicians including understanding and skills of relating with them."

Competencies

Panelists were asked to address the competencies that MedFTs should have at the master's, post-master's, and doctoral levels. Beginning with clinical competencies, the largest content area was medical culture and collaboration. While there were 18 statements where consensus was reached, 6 reflected the strongest possible ratings (median = 7; IQR = 0.0). These six statements included the following: the ability to communicate with providers ($n = 2$), act as a facilitator between providers and patients and their families ($n = 1$), and maintain an awareness of the cultural differences within a medical environment as compared to a traditional therapy setting ($n = 3$).

Regarding clinical care or therapy skills, panelists endorsed 17 statements related to MedFTs' clinical competencies with patients and their families. The statements that received the highest possible agreement (median = 7; IQR = 0.0) reflected being skilled at systemic therapy, integrated care, empowering patients, general family therapy skills, and being culturally competent. Closely related to clinical skills was treatment planning ($n = 3$), which was also identified by the panelists as a necessary competency for preparing MedFTs at all three levels of training.

Panelists agreed that the knowledge about family therapy and family systems was critical as a base at the master's, post-master's, and doctoral levels ($n = 4$). With family therapy established as its base, panelists agreed on four statements related to competency in advanced and applied MedFT built on family systems knowledge ($n = 4$). Of these four statements, the ones that received the strongest agreement included those related to levels of collaboration, coordinated/integrated delivery systems/services, and the overlap of medical and behavioral health problems (e.g., "MedFTs should have competency in advanced application of family systems concepts developmentally to acute, chronic, and terminal illness"; median = 7; IQR = 0.0).

Additional fundamental competencies at the post-master's level included training in health and relationships ($n = 4$), including knowledge of common diseases ($n = 4$), as well as proficiency in using the *DSM-IV-TR* ($n = 2$) *(at the time of this study, the DSM-IV-TR was the current version)*. Theoretical competencies ($n = 7$) at the post-master's level that were also included in the final profile included systems theory, the BPSS model, the three-world view ("clinical, operational, financial"), and the concepts of agency and communion. Panelists also reached consensus on the idea that being competent as a MedFT included being informed and knowledgeable about medical, psychological, social, and spiritual research ($n = 3$). For example, "MedFTs should know the research on interventions with health problems and with psychiatric problems." They approved four statements at the post-master's level reflecting the importance of MedFTs' ability to educate others about what they do to teach systems theory and the BPSS model (e.g., "MedFTs should have strong abilities to teach BPSS").

Lastly, panelists indicated that MedFTs should be competent in self-care ($n = 2$). These two statements were strongly endorsed and reflected that MedFTs should make an effort to avoid compassion fatigue and be aware of their own self-of-provider issues. MedFTs were held accountable to the administrative and business side of health care as well, with the inclusion of three statements reflecting the implementation of an integrated care practice, creating a niche for one's MedFT services within a healthcare system, and being skilled in conducting a marketing analysis for MedFT opportunities.

Discussion

The results of this study provide a comprehensive view of courses and competencies required of MedFTs. Previously published articles have focused on the availability (Brucker et al., 2005) and development of internship sites (Grauf-Grounds & Sellers, 2006), as well as specific skills needed to supervise students in medical settings (Edwards & Patterson, 2006; Hodgson, Rambo, Boyd, Koehler, & Lamson, 2013; Lamson, Pratt, Hodgson, & Koehler, 2014; Pratt & Lamson, 2011, 2012). Others have provided insight into the quality of training that can occur in a collaborative context (Gawinski, Edwards, & Speice, 1999; Harkness & Nofziger, 1998). With the expansion of training programs, this study addressed a need to initiate the establishment of a foundational curriculum base and identify core competencies. The effort is to enable students who receive training in MedFT to receive a curriculum informed by expert consensus. While it is not known if MedFTs who receive training via intense workshops or graduate degree programs are any more or less effective in their professional practice, agreement on competencies and curricula would give credibility and fidelity to the practice of MedFT.

Competencies

Participants in this study revealed that to be an effective collaborator, MedFTs must be comfortable educating themselves and becoming well versed in other disciplines' research and literature. When collaborating with other health professionals,

MedFTs should be current on relevant research from both a social sciences perspective and the perspectives of other healthcare professions. In fact, panelists agreed that MedFT programs should include basic human physiology and psychopharmacology in the curriculum, two areas not generally addressed in master's level behavioral health curricula. Additionally, MedFT core competencies identified by study participants not only included medical knowledge and collaboration but also held MedFTs accountable for competencies ranging from general therapy skills to self-care and implementing an integrated care business plan.

Panelists agreed that advanced training in MedFT (e.g., degree granting programs, extensive coursework, and field application) was critical to the development of MedFTs at the master's, post-master's, and doctoral levels. While those holding licensure in other behavioral health and medical fields may become trained in MedFT, panelists also agreed about the need for a solid foundation of knowledge and skills in marriage and family therapy theories, interventions, and research.

Panelists overwhelmingly agreed on the inclusion of a biopsychosocial and spiritual (BPSS) perspective and systems theory as the theoretical underpinnings of MedFT. McDaniel et al. (1992) first described MedFT as practiced by therapists who specialized in integrating BPS and systems theory perspectives. This initial definition and the focus of MedFT have evolved to include the spiritual dimension (Hodgson, Lamson, & Reese, 2007; Katerndahl, 2008; Onarecker & Sterling, 1995). While it seemed that BPS and BPSS were used interchangeably in panelists' statements, the spiritual component was included more often than it was absent. The frequent inclusion of spirituality within the BPS perspective suggests that trainers, clinicians, researchers, and supervisors should address spirituality in their MedFT curricula.

Based on the outcomes of this study, MedFT faculty members at East Carolina University (ECU) adopted a set of 26 MedFT competencies and offer it as an example of applying the findings from this study (see Appendix). The purpose of including them in this chapter is to serve as "an" example and not "the" example for how the findings of this study may be translated into training programs. The ECU MedFT competencies were modified slightly to fit the culture, context, and purpose of its doctoral program (e.g., advancement in areas of research, leadership, and policy as well as clinical expertise in healthcare settings). However, in the current study, a majority of the competencies recognized by the panelists were at a post-master's level. In fact, if a competency was indicated at either a doctoral or master's level, it was also indicated at a post-master's level. The difference in the level at which a particular competency was included was one of beginner versus advanced level of practice. These evidence-based competencies are offered with author permission for adoption consideration by other programs in an effort to develop and unify training curriculum, as well as help better advocate for more parsimonious student learning outcomes, research, and evidence for advancement of advocacy efforts and policy changes at the legislative level. Additionally, Bischoff et al. (2012) offered evidence-based competencies for behavioral health professionals operating in an integrated healthcare setting. These competencies ranged from skills specific to the setting itself as well as working with patients and understanding the interpersonal intricacies of working with medical providers.

As is true with all research studies, this study had limitations. The authors presented only a portion of the larger study in this chapter. The initial survey instrument included eight questions which led to the inclusion of over 500 items on the second survey instrument. As a result, the second instrument was lengthy and potentially associated with panelist fatigue and loss of interest. Delphi studies are generally used to provide broad suggestions rather than specifics (Godfrey et al., 2006); this study represents an initial effort that may influence the general direction of MedFT preparation and practice. The panelists who participated in this study were unique. Only 19 % of the 37 panelists had terminal degrees from fields other than MFT and MedFT and 14 % were senior-level doctoral students. While these doctoral students were considered to have expertise in MedFT as a consequence of their immersion in the current research and clinical experiences, it should also be noted that the majority of these individuals were drawn from the same institution. As a result, the panelists were similar in their educational backgrounds, and this attribute reflected a lack of professional diversity among them. Additional studies addressing these limitations will help to expand and enhance the competencies that were presented in this chapter. The next step would be to take the competencies identified in this study as well as in Bischoff et al. (2012) and conduct focus groups with content area experts to identify a unified set of competencies that may be used to drive workforce development. It is the next developmental step in the maturation of MedFT.

Summary

Until now, MedFT training programs have been operating and developing curricula based largely on educated assumptions regarding the important elements associated with MedFT training and practice. While those programs have had fundamental aspects in common, this work provides a cornerstone for programmatic growth. Incorporating findings from this study will assist MedFT clinicians, academicians, supervisors, and researchers in developing field-based training, curriculum, and MedFT effectiveness and efficacy research studies.

Reflection Questions

1. Given what we know about the courses outlined for MedFTs, is there a course or a body of knowledge that you feel has been left out of the training?
2. What are the next steps needed for further solidifying and operationalizing the MedFT competencies?
3. What other professional groups, as potential collaborators, would you have included in a similar study?
4. What are your thoughts on how research should inform MedFT domains and core competencies?

5. As MedFT moves forward with these competencies and courses now outlined, what future steps do you see in the development of MedFT? For example, do you see a future licensure, professional organization, or division within other larger organizations?
6. What are your thoughts on the type of assessments that might measure MedFT competencies?

Appendix: East Carolina University—Medical Family Therapy Competencies

1. Develop sufficient understanding of the relevant biomedical issues, language, culture, and providers in primary, secondary, and tertiary healthcare systems.
2. Apply MFT evidence-based models to medical family therapy cases.
3. Demonstrate skills in helping families manage the demands of acute and chronic illness.
4. Demonstrate skills in providing integrated case.
5. MedFTs should have a personal theoretical approach to working with individuals, couples, families, and larger systems.
6. Demonstrate the ability to empower patients to advocate for themselves in the healthcare system.
7. Demonstrate ability to motivate health-related behavior change.
8. Demonstrate awareness of and sensitivity to cultural and contextual variables pertaining to health, illness, loss, and trauma.
9. Recognize the various disciplines involved with medical care and their role in the healthcare environment.
10. Facilitate communication between patients, families, and healthcare providers and invite coordination of services.
11. Demonstrate the ability to refer, document, and communicate with healthcare professionals.
12. Understand the ethical issues of delivering mental health care within a healthcare system
13. Understand and apply the concepts of agency and communion.
14. Understand the clinical, operational, and financial elements of healthcare systems.
15. Understand the key historical figures, theoretical underpinnings, and empirical literature central to MedFT.
16. Understand the bidirectional relationship between health and wellness on mental health functioning.
17. Understand psychopharmacology and its systemic effects.
18. Understand disease processes and developmentally appropriate treatments.
19. Articulate clearly the difference between MedFT and other mental health professionals.

20. Apply systems theory and the biopsychosocial–spiritual approach to research, education, clinical, supervision, and/or consultation services.
21. Evaluate and design intervention and program research associated with biopsychosocial–spiritual health issues and collaborative care models.[1]
22. Demonstrate the ability to conduct a BPSS assessment.
23. Understand the impact of one's family illness stories, self-of-provider issues, and biases in relation to care delivery.
24. Recognize the importance of self-care and understand how to avoid burnout and compassion fatigue.
25. Integrate BPSS elements into treatment plans and other clinical documents.
26. Evidence skills in designing and building transdisciplinary collaborative care teams.

References[2]

American Association for Marriage and Family Therapy. (2004). *Marriage and family therapy core competencies.* Retrieved February 1, 2012, from http://www.aamft.org/imis15/Documents/MFT_Core_Competencie.pdf.

American Psychological Association Interorganizational Work Group on Competencies for Primary Care Psychology. (2013). *Competencies for psychology practice in primary care.* Retrieved from American Psychological Association website: http://www.apa.org/ed/resources/competencies-practice.pdf

*Baglia, J., Foster, E., Dostal, J., Keister, D., Biery, N., & Larson, D. (2011). Generating developmentally appropriate competency assessment at a family medicine residency. *Family Medicine, 43*, 90–98.

Bischoff, R. J., Springer, P. R., Reisbig, A. M. J., Lyons, S., & Likcani, A. (2012). Training for collaboration: Collaborative practice skills for mental health professionals. *Journal of Marital and Family Therapy, 38*, 199–210. doi:10.1111/j.1752-0606.2012.00299.x.

Brucker, P. S., Faulkner, R. A., Baptist, J., Grames, H., Beckham, L. G., Walsh, S., & Willert, A. (2005). The internship training experiences in medical family therapy of doctoral-level marriage and family therapy students. *The American Journal of Family Therapy, 33*, 131–146. doi:10.1080/01926180590915518.

Canadian Interprofessional Health Collaborative, Curriculum Committee. (2010). *A national interprofessional competency framework.* Retrieved from http://www.cihc.ca/files/CIHC_IPCompetencies_Feb1210r.pdf

Chicago Center for Family Health (CCFH). (2013). *Families, illness, and collaborative healthcare program offerings.* Retrieved July 2, 2013, from http://ccfhchicago.org/training/fichprogram/offerings/

College of Health Disciplines, & Interprofessional Network of British Columbia (CHD & INBC). (2008). *The British Columbia competency framework for interprofessional collaboration.* Retrieved from http://www.chd.ubc.ca/files/file/BC%20Competency%20Framework%20for%20IPC.pdf

Dalkey, N. (1972). *Studies in the quality of life.* Lexington, MA: Lexington Books.

[1] Suggested as a doctoral level competency only.

[2] An asterisk has been use to note references that the chapter authors recommend for further reading.

Dalkey, N., & Helmer, O. (1963). An experimental application of the Delphi method to the use of experts. *Management Science, 9*, 458–467. doi:10.1287/mnsc.9.3.458.

East Carolina University (ECU). (2012). *Doctor of philosophy in medical family therapy*. Retrieved January 15, 2012, from http://www.ecu.edu/che/cdfr/phdmft.html

*Edwards, T. M., & Patterson, J. E. (2006). Supervising family therapy trainees in primary care medical settings: Context matters. *Journal of Marital and Family Therapy, 32*, 33–43. doi:10.1111/j.1752-0606.2006.tb01586.x.

Engel, G. L. (1977). The need for a new medical model: A challenge for biomedicine. *Science, 196*, 129–136. doi:10.1126/science.847460.

Engel, G. L. (1980). The clinical application of the biopsychosocial model. *American Journal of Psychiatry, 137*, 535–544. Retrieved from http://ajp.psychiatryonline.org/.

Gawinski, B. A., Edwards, T. M., & Speice, J. (1999). A family therapy internship in a multidisciplinary healthcare setting: Trainees' and supervisor's reflections. *Journal of Marital and Family Therapy, 25*, 469–485. doi:10.1111/j.1752-0606.1999.tb00263.x.

Godfrey, K., Haddock, S. A., Fisher, A., & Lund, L. (2006). Essential components of curricula for preparing therapists to work effectively with lesbian, gay, and bisexual clients: A Delphi study. *Journal of Marital and Family Therapy, 32*, 491–504. doi:10.1111/j.1752-0606.2006.tb01623.x.

*Grauf-Grounds, C., & Sellers, T. S. (2006). Creating internships and potential jobs for medical family therapists: Lessons learned. *Families, Systems & Health, 24*, 230–237. doi:10.1037/1091-7527.24.2.230.

Harkness, J. L., & Nofziger, A. (1998). Medical family therapy casebook: Training in a collaborative context: What we did not know then. . .we know now. *Families, Systems & Health, 16*, 443–450. doi:10.1037/h0089868.

Hodgson, J. L., Lamson, A., & Reese, L. (2007). The biopsychosocial-spiritual interview method. In D. Linville & K. M. Hertlein (Eds.), *The therapist's notebook for family health care: Homework, handouts, and activities for individuals, couples, and families coping with illness, loss, and disability* (pp. 3–12). New York, NY: Haworth Press.

*Hodgson, J., Rambo, A., Boyd, T., Koehler, A., & Lamson, A. (2013). Supervision in evolving contexts. In T. Todd & C. Storm (Eds.), *The complete systemic supervisor: Context, philosophy, and pragmatics* (2nd ed.). Bloomington, IN: iUniverse.

Institute of Medicine (IOM). (2001). *Crossing the quality chasm: A new health system for the 21st century*. Washington, DC: National Academy Press.

Interprofessional Education Collaborative Expert Panel (IPEC). (2011). *Core competencies for interprofessional collaborative practice: Report of an expert panel*. Washington, DC: Interprofessional Education Collaborative. Retrieved from http://www.aacn.nche.edu/education-resources/IPECReport.pdf.

Jenkins, D. (1996). A reflecting team approach to family therapy: A Delphi study. *Journal of Marital and Family Therapy, 22*, 219–238. doi:10.1111/j.1752-0606.1996.tb00200.x.

Jenkins, D. A., & Smith, T. E. (1994). Applying Delphi methodology in family therapy research. *Contemporary Family Therapy, 16*, 411–430. doi:10.1007/BF02197902.

Katerndahl, D. A. (2008). Impact of spiritual symptoms and their interactions on health services and life satisfaction. *Annals of Family Medicine, 6*, 412–420. doi:10.1370/afm.886.

Lamson, A., Pratt, K., Hodgson, J., & Koehler, A. (2014). MedFT supervision in context. In J. Hodgson, A. Lamson, T. Mendenhall, & R. Crane (Eds.), *Medical family therapy: Advanced applications* (pp. 125–146). New York, NY: Springer.

Linstone, H. A., & Turoff, M. (1975). Introduction. In H. A. Linstone & M. Turoff (Eds.), *The Delphi method: Techniques and applications* (pp. 1–14). Reading, MA: Addison-Wesley.

Loma Linda University. (2013). *Medical family therapy*. Retrieved June 29, 2013, from http://www.llu.edu/behavioral-health/cfs/medft.page

Marvel, K., & Major, G. (1999). What should we be teaching residents about behavioral science? Opinions of practicing family physicians. *Family Medicine, 31*, 248–251.

McDaniel, S. H., Hepworth, J., & Doherty, W. J. (Eds.). (1992). *Medical family therapy: A biopsychosocial approach to families with health problems*. New York, NY: Basic Books. doi:10.1080/01926189208250882.

National Association of Social Workers. (2005). *NASW standards for social work practice in health care settings*. Retrieved from http://www.socialworkers.org/practice/standards/NASWHealthCareStandards.pdf

Northern Illinois University (NIU). (2014). *Medical family therapy and counseling: Certificate of graduate study*. Retrieved February 24, 2014, from http://catalog.niu.edu/preview_program.php?catoid=21&poid=3778&hl=%22Medical+Fmily+herapy+and+Counseling%22&returnto=search
Nova Southeastern University (NSU). (2011). *Family systems health care graduate certificate*. Retrieved February 21, 2012, from http://shss.nova.edu/programs/certificate/family_systems.htm
Onarecker, C. D., & Sterling, B. C. (1995). Addressing your patient's spiritual needs. *Family Practice Management, 2*, 44–49.
Pratt, K., & Lamson, A. (2011). Supervision for the integrated behavioral health provider. In R. Curtis & E. Christian (Eds.), *Integrated Care: Creating a thriving practice*. New York, NY: Haworth Press.
Pratt, K., & Lamson, A. L. (2012). Supervision in behavioral health: Implications for students, interns, and new professionals. *Journal of Behavioral Health Services and Research, 39*(3), 285–294. doi:10.1007/s11414-011-9267-6.
Seattle Pacific University (SPU). (2012). *What is medical family therapy*. Retrieved January 15, 2012, from http://www.spu.edu/depts/spfc/mdft/program-overview/index.asp
Sori, C. F., & Sprenkle, D. H. (2004). Training family therapists to work with children and families: A modified Delphi study. *Journal of Marital and Family Therapy, 30*, 479–496. doi:10.1111/j.1752-0606.2004.tb01257.x.
Stone Fish, L. S., & Busby, D. (2005). The Delphi method. In D. H. Sprenkle & F. P. Piercy (Eds.), *Research methods in family therapy* (pp. 238–253). New York, NY: Guilford.
Stone Fish, L., & Osborn, J. L. (1992). Therapists' view of family life: A Delphi study. *Family Relations, 41*, 409–416. doi:10.2307/585583.
Substance Abuse and Mental Health Services (SAMHSA). (2003). *Achieving the promise: Transforming mental health care in America, executive summary* (Pub id SMA03-0831).
Substance Abuse and Mental Health Services, & National Institutes of Health. (n.d.). *Mental health: A report of the surgeon general*. Retrieved February 22, 2012, from http://www.surgeongeneral.gov/library/mentalhealth/home.html#forward
Tyndall, L., Hodgson, J., Lamson, A., White, M. & Knight, S. (2010). *Medical family therapy: Conceptual clarification and consensus of an emerging profession* (Doctoral dissertation). Retrieved from http://hdl.handle.net/10342/2794
Tyndall, L., Hodgson, J., Lamson, A., White, M., & Knight, S. (2012). Medical family therapy: Charting a course in competencies. *Contemporary Family Therapy, 34*, 171–186. doi:10.1007/s10591-012-9191-9.
University of Nebraska Medical Center (UNMC). (2011). Family Therapy Program. Retrieved January 30, 2012 from http://www.unmc.edu/familymed/familytherapy.htm
University of Nebraska-Lincoln (UNL). (2012). Graduate Certificate in Medical Family Therapy. Retrieved January 15, 2012 from http://www.unl.edu/gradstudies/prospective/programs/Cert_MedicalFamilyTherapy.shtml
University of Rochester Medical Center (URMC). (2013). *20th annual medical family therapy intensive*. Retrieved July 2, 2013, from http://www.urmc.rochester.edu/psychiatry/institute-for-the-family/familytherapy/mfti.cfm
University of Rochester Medical Center (URMC). (2014). *Family therapy training program*. Retrieved February 17, 2014, from https://www.urmc.rochester.edu/psychiatry/institute-for-the-family/family-therapy/
University of San Diego (USD). (n.d.). *Emphasis in medical family therapy*. Retrieved February 21, 2012, from http://www.sandiego.edu/soles/programs/marital_and_family_therapy/about_the_program/medical_family_therapy_emphasis.php
White, M. B., Edwards, S. A., & Russell, C. S. (1997). The essential elements of successful MFT: A modified Delphi study. *The American Journal of Family Therapy, 25*, 213–231. doi:10.1080/01926189708251068.
White, M. B., & Russell, C. S. (1995). The essential elements of supervisory systems: A modified Delphi study. *Journal of Marital and Family Therapy, 21*, 33–53. doi:10.1111/j.1752-0606.1995.tb00137.x.

Chapter 4
Preparing to Be a Medical Family Therapist: Bridging the Multiple Worlds of Health Care

Stephanie Trudeau-Hern, Tai Mendenhall, and Alison Wong

Medical family therapists (MedFTs) functioning as behavioral health providers (BHPs) within healthcare settings encounter unique cultural and contextual factors, as well as biopsychosocial-spiritual (BPSS) stressors, that are often more acute and intense than those experienced by providers in conventional freestanding behavioral health clinics/agency settings. In this chapter, the authors describe concrete strategies for MedFTs to effectively enter and integrate themselves into these complex healthcare contexts. Common experiences highlighted include both difficult (e.g., coping with a sense of not initially "fitting in" with traditional behavioral health providers or biomedical colleagues) and enriching (e.g., becoming valuable members of integrated healthcare teams) sequences.

Bridging the Distinct "Worlds" of Medicine and Behavioral Health

The respective "worlds" of behavioral health and medicine were separated long ago as Western paradigms of care began to (artificially) separate the "mind" from the "body" and set into motion the establishment of the myriad of specialties that we see today (Barondess, 2000; Ivbijaro, 2012; Magner, 2005). Medical students are asked from the moment they begin training what they want to "be," choosing from areas like Family Medicine, Cardiology, Neurology, or Dermatology. Those seeking a future in behavioral health are similarly asked to choose from a variety of professional homes, like Counseling, Marriage and Family Therapy, Psychology, and Social Work. Further, these professionals may develop clinical foci targeting children with developmental disabilities, families with adolescents who are acting out, or couples living with a chronic illness. "Generalists" like family practice

S. Trudeau-Hern (✉)
University of Minnesota, St Paul, MN, USA
e-mail: hernx002@umn.edu

J. Hodgson et al. (eds.), *Medical Family Therapy*, DOI 10.1007/978-3-319-03482-9_4,

doctors or BHPs, who will see anybody who walks through their door, are oftentimes seen by their colleagues as less focused or even less skilled, and they (the generalists) are usually paid less by insurance companies, employers, and patients/families themselves (Bodenheimer, Berenson, & Rudolf, 2007; Kane, 2012; Martin, Currie, & Finn, 2009; McGrath & Zimet, 1977; Pingitore, Scheffler, Sentell, & West, 2002).

As our healthcare contexts increasingly call for better integration of services, specialty providers and generalists are beginning to work together more than they have historically (Hodgson, Lamson, Mendenhall, & Crane, 2012; Ivbijaro, 2012; McDaniel, Doherty, & Hepworth, 2014). The more MedFTs integrate and partner with biomedically trained providers, the narrower the divide is that separates their professional worlds. This is not because BHPs or medical providers have insisted that the rules change to accommodate them. Rather, it is because both parties have decided to understand one another's culture and methods of providing patient care, working to rewrite the rules to create a new model of care: integrated care.

A Critical Evaluation of the Myths Dividing Our Worlds

A great deal has been written about commonplace myths and stereotypes regarding medical providers (e.g., Caspi et al., 2003; Greenhalgh, 2010; Jecker & Self, 1991; Young, 2011). Whether these relate to gendered stereotypes (e.g., caring and empathic female nurses; detached and hurried male physicians), positive and/or negative castings of sundry specialties (e.g., family physicians are cough-and-cold doctors who are easy to talk to, but not paid very well; radiologists are diagnosticians who do not treat, but are paid handsomely), or any variety of other characteristics, stereotypes, and myths can often serve to sabotage interdisciplinary collaboration.

As MedFTs get ready to enter the world(s) of health care, it is important to take a close and honest look at our own presumptions and biases about the very providers we would like to make our colleagues. In the authors' work with students, trainees, and other professionals who are integrating their efforts into healthcare contexts and/or increasing their collaborative work with healthcare providers, we facilitate the following exercise in brainstorming and critical reflection:

Take out a piece of paper and write down everything that comes to mind when thinking about "doctors," "medicine," "hospitals," or "clinics." As participants in the exercise do this, we encourage them to not hold back. What the authors find are relatively consistent lists that contain many of the following things: medical providers, as a whole, are often unfairly cast to (a) care only about the body; (b) not understand the mind/body connection; (c) be stoic and impersonal; (d) always be in a hurry; (e) not have time to collaborate; (f) not want to collaborate, i.e., we have to sell the idea to them; (g) be rich and have "cushy" lives; (h) be arrogant; and (i) think that their ideas are the best ideas. Medical specialists are often unfairly cast in ways that frame those lowest—in physicians' terms—in salary and compensation to be the most personable (e.g., family physicians, pediatricians). Medical specialists making the most money are unfairly cast as less personable (e.g., radiologists, surgeons).

Before discussing or outwardly challenging these global characterizations of our healthcare colleagues, the authors then ask students, trainees, and/or associates to brainstorm about the misconceptions often held about them. This is important to do because it represents the flip-side of the stereotypes-about-medical-providers-can-sabotage-collaboration argument. Indeed, many have written about the manners in which behavioral health providers are unfairly or sometimes accurately viewed by others (e.g., Orchowski, Spickard, & McNamara, 2006; Sydow, Henning, & Reimer, 1998; Tartakovsky, 2009; Waters, 2012). Whether they relate to global characterizations of therapists making patients do strange rituals or "homework assignments," images that cast us as perpetually happy, stories about diffuse interpersonal boundaries, or notions that we are always psychoanalyzing what friends and family members say, these images can get in the way of effective interdisciplinary work. Specifically, the authors facilitate the following exercise:

Write down everything that people think about when they hear things like "behavioral health," "therapists," "psychologists," "behavioral health providers," and the like. In a similar way to the first part of this brainstorming and reflection sequence, the authors encourage participants to not hold back. What they find are relatively consistent lists that contain many of the following things: therapists, as a group, are often unfairly cast to: (a) care only about the "warm and fuzzy" of human experience (e.g., emotions, feelings, personal growth, sense of balance); (b) have lots of time and are generally unhurried; (c) not understand the urgent pace of healthcare practice and many of the common situations/challenges therein; (d) not be economically productive; and (e) be eccentric and a bit "odd," themselves. Behavioral health providers are almost always seen as "less than" medical providers in terms of social status, professional regard, and income. Those with doctoral-level training (e.g., PhD, PsyD) are still not viewed as "real" doctors.

As participants in this exercise look at and discuss the two respective lists now constructed, they begin to understand how neither is a very fair portrayal, and how walking into any type of new collaboration could be derailed by espousing attitudes that demonize or trivialize the other in such a priori manners. And contrary to common stereotypes, most physicians do understand that the mind and body are in constant dialogue with each other and would welcome (if/when the "How do we do it?" questions can be answered) collaboration with another professional who maintains expertise in an area that they do not (Dowell, Morris, Dodd, & McLoughlin, 2012; McDaniel et al., 2014). Also, if most physicians lead "cushy" lives, why are their burnout rates equal to or higher than behavioral health providers' burnout rates (Dyrbye & Shanafelt, 2011a, 2011b; McCray, Cronholm, Bogner, Gallo, & Neill, 2008; Paris & Hoge, 2010)? Similarly, few therapists will tell you that they have lots of time on their hands or that all they care about are their patients' feelings (Clay, 2012; McDaniel et al., 2014; Timm & Blow, 1999).

A Critical Evaluation of the Realities Dividing Our Worlds

Moving past the myths that can work against us, we then must consider the realities that do (James & O'Donohue, 2009; McDaniel et al., 2014; Mendenhall, 2007). It is important for MedFTs to understand these contextual and cultural differences, insofar as this knowledge will equip them to effectively hit-the-ground-running and avoid making professional mistakes that might otherwise be easy to make.

Professional hierarchies. Health care as a "culture" is one wherein rigid and clear hierarchies are evident in almost every place you look (Bate, 2000; Lerner, 2007; Miedema et al., 2012; Starr, 1982). With dress, everyone in any hospital, anywhere, knows their professional standing by nature of whether they are wearing a short white coat (students) vs. a long white coat (physicians), light blue or green scrubs (physicians or physician extenders) vs. dark blue or white scrubs (nurses or medical assistants), or a suit-and-tie (administrator) vs. comparatively casual business attire (BHPs or other office personnel). The atmosphere of most spaces in which patients talk with healthcare providers reflects the providers' training (e.g., with different types of chairs for physicians to sit on vs. those for patients' use, with sterile-looking medical equipment on every wall and in every corner). In addition, language and terminology used by medical providers (e.g., HEENT, b.i.d., qhs) is often not comprehensible to lay persons. Power and status differences between specialists (e.g., a family practice physician vs. a neurosurgeon) are clear, alongside marked disparities in income and pay-grade (Bodenheimer et al., 2007; Kane, 2012).

Compare this to the world of behavioral health. In our dress, it is difficult to distinguish a BHP from anybody else attending to patients' and families' psychosocial lives (e.g., recreation therapists, pastoral counselors, peer specialists). Traditionally, a BHP's work space for meeting with patients and families is more home-like than medical-like, complete with comfortable furniture, soft lights, plants, and pleasant artwork. Our psychotherapy language (like "undifferentiated boundaries," "labile mood," or "anhedonia") is generally communicated between like-minded and similarly trained colleagues, and is comparatively easy to translate to those initially unfamiliar with our argot (Huang, 2007; Montalt & Davies, 2007; Paul, 1998). And while income and pay inequities exist between different BHP disciplines, they are not as marked as those dividing medical specialties (Bureau of Labor Statistics, 2012), and they are narrowing with research that demonstrates effectiveness and cost savings to be unrelated to professional license type (Crane & Christenson, 2012).

Patient–Provider interactions. The manners in which providers work and interact with those seeking their help are also considerably different when we compare conventional medical practice to the ways that therapists have tended to work (Britt, 2013; Ivbijaro, 2012; McDaniel et al., 2014). In health care, visits tend to last for 15–20 min. Continuity in care is not commonplace sans some family medicine and pediatric practices, insofar as patients will often see different providers each time they seek help. Physicians' and physician extenders' affect and personability are often formal, and they do not tend to disclose much about themselves in the contexts of care-provision (i.e., personal information goes only from patient to provider, while professional information goes from the provider to the patient). The equipment used is highly technical, and malpractice threats are always looming in the back of providers' and their employers' minds (i.e., screw anything up, and you will be sued for everything you've got) (MacDonald & Attaran, 2009; Wong et al., 2011).

Compare this to the ways in which BHPs conventionally interact with patients and their families (American Association for Marriage and Family Therapy [AAMFT], 2013; American Psychological Association [APA], 2011; Northey, 2002). Their standard visits are 50 min long, and a great deal of effort is put forth to maintain continuity in care (and indeed, patients and families would not dream of seeing a different therapist each time they came in). BHPs' affect and personability are generally warm and friendly, and we purposefully share personal information from time-to-time as a way to effectively negotiate "joining" or communicate empathy in-session. Our "equipment" is generally child-friendly (e.g., art supplies, flip-charts) and ambiance-/comfort-conscious (e.g., nice chairs and couches). We do not usually worry about malpractice threats, insofar as the most obvious ways to hurt people are easy to avoid (via commonsense), and suits brought against us are generally rare (and this is why we pay much lower premiums for malpractice insurance than medical providers) (Coombs, 2005; Gutheil & Drogin, 2013; Shapiro & Smith, 2011).

Professional training. Trainees' experiences in medical education (i.e., as medical students and/or residents) are remarkably different than those borne within behavioral health training programs (Accreditation Council for Graduate Medical Education [ACGME], 2011; Peets & Ayas, 2012; Schultz, 2012). Requisite hours spent studying or providing patient-care average more than 80 h per week, alongside on-call sequences that last up to 24 h in duration. Patient panels are often in the hundreds, with sometimes remarkably high stakes (e.g., lethal medical errors). Even when trainees do everything right, it is not uncommon for patients under their care to die. Maintaining professional composure from one care episode to another can be psychologically demanding (e.g., losing a baby in one delivery room secondary to birth-complications, and then moving to another delivery room to attend a birth only a few minutes later). Delivering bad news (e.g., a positive HIV diagnosis, no heartbeat on a prenatal visit ultrasound, telling family members their loved-one did not survive a motorcycle crash) can be a regular occurrence.

Researchers confirm that trainees in medicine maintain high rates of depression (e.g., Dahlin, Joneborg, & Runeson, 2005; Dyrbye, Thomas, & Shanafelt, 2006), suicidality (e.g., Schwenk, Davis, & Wimsatt, 2010), anxiety (e.g., Bunevicius, Katkute, & Bunevicius, 2008; Dyrbye et al., 2006), insomnia (e.g., Abdulghani et al., 2012), substance abuse (e.g., Frank, Elon, Naimi, & Brewer, 2008; Gutgesell, Reeve, Parsons, & Morse, 1999), and somatic troubles (e.g., Brimstone, Thistlethwaite, & Quirk, 2007; Roberts et al., 2000) that are directly attributable to the stressful nature of their work (Drolet & Rodgers, 2010; Dyrbye & Shanafelt, 2011a, 2011b; Dyrbye et al., 2010). Relationally, medical students and residents evidence higher divorce and break-up rates than the general population (Dyrbye, Shanafelt, Balch, Satele, & Freischlag, 2010; Woodford, 2006). Intergenerational patterns of abuse in education (e.g., being treated poorly—if not aggressively—by faculty and senior trainees) are longstanding and highly predictable (McKegney, 1989; Rees & Monrouxe, 2011), alongside financial aid debt upon graduation averaging in the hundreds-of-thousands of dollars (Greysen, Chen, & Mullan, 2011; Steinbrook, 2008).

Compare this to the experience of behavioral health trainees. Hours worked per week rarely come close to health care's 80 h cap. Clinical loads are usually between 10 and 20 patients or families at any given time (unless BHPs are practicing in an integrated care environment) (APA, 2008; Northey, 2002). The intensity of clinical presentations is variable, but rarely with life-or-death stakes connected to what we advise or how we intervene during the course of care-provision. As MedFTs, we are often drawn in to help deliver bad news with (or even instead of) medical providers, but outside of specialty contexts like Oncology or Emergency Medicine, doing this is not a very common sequence in baseline therapy training programs. Reported rates of poor behavioral health (e.g., depression, anxiety) and interpersonal problems (e.g., marital distress or dissolution) are higher for behavioral health trainees than the general population, but with more variability and less prevalence than medical trainees (Negash & Sahin, 2011; Pakenham & Stafford-Brown, 2012). Intergenerational transmission of abuse in graduate education has not been recognized as a pervasive problem in the behavioral health professions, and financial aid debt paired with one's degree is inconsistent from one graduate to the next (Caldwell, 2012).

Self-care. The culture of health care does not readily structure self-care into its training of students and residents (Cooke, Irby, & O'Brien, 2010), and systemically it is not structured into the healthcare contexts in which they function thereafter (Wallace, Lemaire, & Ghali, 2009). The theme felt by medical providers is often to function as "experts," to maintain mastery, and exhibit emotional control. In contrast, self-care and self-awareness in many behavioral health training programs is one of the first lessons learned, and it is something that is discussed in ongoing supervision (and persists long after graduation from a master's or doctoral program) (Baker, 2003; Shallcross, 2011; Skovholt & Trotter-Mathison, 2010; Tartakovsky, 2012). A theme felt by providers in behavioral health is one of awareness of self during and outside of clinical processes, and about recognizing one's reactions in context to the therapeutic response.

Strategies for MedFTs to Effectively Enter Healthcare Contexts

After MedFT trainees gain the knowledge outlined above about how their baseline orientation(s) in behavioral health differ from the uncharted territory before them, they are ready to begin their journey(s) into health care. Equipped with this understanding, they can effectively engage with new colleagues as active and collaborative learners, team members, and behavioral health providers.

Functioning with Humility, as an Anthropologist, and as a Learner

One of the easiest mistakes that a new MedFT can make is to enter a healthcare context over-zealously, touting his or her systems-paradigm as the panacea that everyone there has been missing until now. Understanding and respecting the rigid hierarchy of health care, the well-prepared trainee instead goes in with the understanding that he does not know very much yet, and that his first job is to learn the lay of the land upon which he has just arrived. Behavioral health providers function (especially at first) relatively low on the professional hierarchy vis-à-vis their biomedical counterparts, and it is important to interact with these colleagues in a manner(s) that communicates this understanding and respect.

Consistent with the adage that God gave us two ears and one mouth for a reason (Diogenes, 1901), it is important to engage in this new environment as a person eager to learn more than she wants to (or at least showing a desire to) teach. Observing precepting rotations in residency training sites (i.e., interactions between resident learners and faculty preceptors/supervisors), learning about patient presentations common to unique sites (e.g., diabetes or depression in primary care, end-of-life decisions and grief reactions in respite care, vaccination discussions or ADHD medication regimens in pediatrics), and asking questions when doing so is not disruptive to care-provision (e.g., in-between case consultations vs. as a provider is trying to catch up after getting behind with cases) are good ways to begin. Learning (if one has not already learned) biomedical language like MDD, qd, qhs, PRN, b.i.d., iii, ii, I, x, HEENT, A1c, BP, CQI, BPD, c, Cx, etc., facilitates these processes, alongside equipping the MedFT to read and understand patients' charts and/or communicate/describe her own care in patients' charts so that healthcare providers will read and understand them in return (Cohen & DePetris, 2013; Grauf-Grounds & Sellers, 2006).

Another way to effectively integrate one's self into a healthcare environment as a MedFT is to consciously seek, learn about, honor, and even embrace multiple evidence-based treatment approaches for patients' biopsychosocial presentations and behavioral health goals. While some nonmedical colleagues, for example, maintain that psychotropic medication is not necessary in treating mental disorders (Abraham, Ducharme, & Roman, 2009; Springer & Harris, 2010), MedFTs should become conversant with the use of this approach (and the many types of medications herein) in conjunction with other individual, couple, family, and group talk-therapies. This will help facilitate collaborative—vs. parallel or even contradictory—efforts in care as providers coordinate their work with patients and families. For example, researchers strongly support treatment approaches for major depression that combine both pharmaceutical and talk therapies (e.g., Blier et al., 2010; Cuijpers, Van Straten, Hollon, & Andersson, 2010; National Institute of Mental Health [NIMH], 2013); advancing best-practices requires mutual understanding and buy-in by providers representing different facets of this broader care framework.

MedFTs should attend conferences and read books across a wide variety of disciplines (e.g., Psychology, Family Medicine) and become articulate in explaining and discussing how multiple views regarding problem geneses and solutions fit (or do not fit) together. They must also be careful to not frame their way(s) as superior to those conventionally espoused by the colleagues with whom they wish to work. Key here, too, is to actively learn from clinic receptionists, care coordinators, medical assistants, and nurses. They often hold local and clinically indigenous information, are valuable resources regarding healthcare's culture, and can help decipher and translate the dialects that other providers speak (Allison, 2011; Myrick, Yonge, & Billay, 2010).

Aligning Practice-Patterns to Fit with the Culture of Health Care

While maintaining a clinical practice at the same address as a healthcare practice is better than trying to collaborate with medical providers from across town (Ivbijaro, 2012; McDaniel et al., 2014), the notion of "co-located" care is best seen as a step toward a more integrated model. Co-located practices are exactly that: co-located. BHPs and medical providers are working within the same facility but may or may not share the same practice space or actively collaborate with each other. If a MedFT only sees his patients and families for 50-min time-periods, charts his work electronically or in paper notes stored in his office, and does not regularly interact with colleagues, then integrated care is not going to happen very well. If a MedFT frequently communicates with other care providers, divides time across conventional therapy sessions and joint meetings involving multiple stakeholders (e.g., physicians, patients, family members), and shares in team-based problem-solving and electronic records and note-taking, then the co-located care provided is moving toward an integrated type (Peek, 2013; Peek & National Integration Academy Council, 2013).

If a MedFT is going to function as a collaborative colleague in a healthcare context, she must adjust her practice patterns away from conventional behavioral health service models and toward the mainstream culture(s) of healthcare practice. Purposefully scheduling "open" time to shadow, collaborate with, precept, and/or otherwise be available to healthcare colleagues is essential. If some clinical time is set-apart for standard 50-min patient visits, then it is imperative that healthcare colleagues understand—inconsistent with hallowed tenets or stereotypes regarding behavioral health visits—that you are very interrupt-able. Some of the authors'

MedFT colleagues even have signs on their office doors that say "Please Disturb" (i.e., it is okay to interrupt me when the door is closed). This sets a precedent for collaboration so MedFTs are always available. Just as the patients who are being seen by a physician or physician extender appreciate a BHP's ability to step-in and collaborate, so too will the patients that BHPs are seeing understand the need for healthcare providers to do so for others when and if indicated.

Sensitive Interpersonal Conduct with Medical Colleagues

Throughout the journey and as one advances through any and all of the strategies outlined so far, it is essential for the MedFT to be aware of how he is personally conducting himself with his healthcare colleagues. Equipped with a better understanding of how physicians, physician assistants, nurse practitioners, nurses, and other healthcare colleagues got there (and how they tend to function in their daily work), for example, the MedFT should be careful to not complain about how exhausted he is after a 10–12 h day. This type of day is normative for healthcare providers. Similarly, a MedFT who laments about the intensity of one of his sessions, time he is missing with his spouse or children, and/or financial stress that he is shouldering secondary to financial aid debt, etc., can easily elicit a negative reaction from medical colleagues. He, by nature of being a BHP at the healthcare site, has made a conscious decision to not work in a comfortable private practice where he can set his own hours and attend to a wealthy clientele. Communicating what could be interpreted by others as discontent or personal weakness can sabotage a MedFT's attractiveness as a member on a healthcare team.

Another important thing to understand as a MedFT interacts with healthcare colleagues is that they—the colleagues trained in the medical model—are often not aware of, or care about, the differences between a BHP trained in Medical Family Therapy vs. Psychology, Social Work, Pastoral Counseling, or any other behavioral health field. And if they are, it is likely that their familiarity with MedFT is comparatively less, insofar as MedFT is comparatively new. Being comfortable with being called a "counselor" or "social worker" for the 100th time is thereby important. In the larger scheme of integrated care, your healthcare colleague introducing you to a patient or family as a MedFT per se is less important than the fact that she is introducing you at all (i.e., it is a good sign that she is collaborating with you in the care she is providing). As your interprofessional relationships evolve, having others accurately refer to your disciplinary training and background is something that can catch up later.

Ultimately, the exact steps that a MedFT takes to gain entry into a healthcare practice will vary according to the practice that she is entering. Some sites will be familiar with and maintain strong buy-in for BHPs by nature of their unique history and development (e.g., a family practice site that has organized its services to align with contemporary developments in the medical home movement). Other sites may not have included a BHP in their ranks before but are open to the idea in light of the type of cases they see (e.g., an oncology department wherein patient declines and deaths are frequent and families' efforts in coping are clearly commonplace and relevant). Conversely, some sites may not be very interested in hiring a BHP, for reasons like not seeing any financial benefits for doing so, leadership that is unfriendly to "mental health" secondary to aforementioned negative stereotypes, or administrative discomfort with taking on new complexities in referral or billing systems. For some MedFTs, then, the experience of getting one's "foot in the door" will be relatively easy. For others, it may be remarkably difficult. Whether or not it occurs at either end of this continuum, or somewhere in the middle, the understandings (e.g., myths, realities) and strategies (e.g., being humble, adjusting practice style) outlined above will help.

You've Made It In. Now What?

After gaining entry into a healthcare setting, trainees are ready to begin putting into practice much of what they have learned during earlier phases of their professional preparation. As they become and function as members of integrated care teams, the following points and strategies are important to consider and advance.

Know Who Your On-site Champions Are

If you have integrated into the culture of medicine, you are in there for a reason. Part of that reason is because you have made an impact or an impression on a system that is looking to integrate a systemic perspective to working with patients and families. That person or groups of people are your champions. Find out ways that you can help those persons. By using your natural systemic perspective(s), be curious about ways in which you can be an asset to the healthcare team and not a hindrance to their professional flow (Patterson, Williams, Edwards, Chamow, & Grauf-Grounds, 2009). Along the way, it is important to maintain aforementioned connections with others who are on the frontlines. These are not typically the physicians or extenders; they are the receptionists, care coordinators, case managers, and medical assistants. By making yourself an asset to all parts of the clinical system, you create an expedited and more robust visibility to everyone on the team.

Communication Matters

Conventional therapists speak a language replete with words and descriptors about intergenerational structures, interpersonal boundaries, attunement, and affect. Healthcare providers speak a very different language, one defined by acronyms, short-hand measurements, and Latin-based terminologies. It is important for MedFTs to be conversant in medical language, while at the same time being able to translate conventional behavioral health dialects into language(s) that other team members can hear and understand. To be sure, the best way to function as a BHP in a healthcare context is to do so bilingually. This means being proficient in both psychotherapeutic and medical languages across both verbal (e.g., case consultation, team meetings) and written (e.g., electronic medical records, emails, text-pagers) mediums. Without this skill, the delivery and reception of our contributions may be misinterpreted, overlooked, or invalidated. Keeping statements succinct and of the native tongue(s) of the local culture (e.g., saying "p.r.n." instead of "if and when the patient feels like following-up in therapy would be helpful") will facilitate the healthcare provider to see that you are team member, an asset, and respectful of their limited time. And if in doubt, keep a medical terminology dictionary readily available (Mosby, 2012; Turley, 2013).

Educate and Advocate

As MedFTs continue to educate themselves, there are simultaneously ways in which they can educate others with whom they work. The authors encourage, for example, getting involved in national, regional, state, and local advocacy groups designed to promote the integration of behavioral health, nutrition, or pharmacy into healthcare settings. In turn, share what you are learning with your colleagues through volunteering to speak for a noon-conference forum about family-based approaches to managing chronic pain, for example, or about how to help parents support adolescents with diabetes without being overly intrusive or nagging. Write a post for the local hospital's newsletter focusing on relational and family health. Host a lunch-in for physicians and physician extenders to discuss and process ways to work together toward shared and overlapping clinical goals. Across any of these forums, too, it is important for a MedFT to understand (and be accommodating of) the natural "coming and going" of participants in healthcare meetings. Start on time, but be aware that people will continuously come in late and leave early. Do not take attendees looking at cell phones or answering pages personally; this is all normal within healthcare contexts.

Define Your Role

It is important for any BHP to establish clarity about the role(s) he is presuming within the setting he is entering early on. This will look different across different healthcare sites. For instance, a MedFT functioning as a liaison or consultant in primary care will not look like a MedFT who is functioning as the sole clinician in a pediatric clinic. Once clear about the roles he possesses, a MedFT can then define the boundaries that are going to keep him functioning optimally. For example, establishing that one cannot see every patient that another healthcare provider deems to be in crisis, or every family member who is loosely diagnosed as anxious and depressed, will better equip a MedFT to conduct high-quality work. A systematic referral system may need to be implemented as a way to guide healthcare providers regarding which patients and families should be seen in priority to others. Collaborating with local specialty behavioral health services can help to connect patients and families who are in need of focused or long-term therapy. This will help the MedFT to not overwhelm his schedule (thereby making him unavailable to collaborate) or himself (thereby making him less effective in care-provision).

Attend to Self-care

Emotions can run high in healthcare contexts (Kroenke, Spitzer, Williams, Monahan, & Löwe, 2007). The pace is typically fast, the patients are often uneasy, and providers' stress levels are regularly high. How can a MedFT function within this culture and not "catch" the institutionalized anxiety? There are a variety of ways that we can attend to ourselves so as to ideally function sans burnout or compassion fatigue; see Chap. 7 (Lamson, Meadors, & Mendenhall, 2014) in this book for a thorough review.

Know your triggers. As a MedFT strengthens and grows in her competencies, she must also recognize her limitations and triggers. Sometimes these triggers are unknown until they become roadblocks. For example, a MedFT who has a family history of diabetes may have one way of looking at family dynamics with that illness and its interactions within a healthcare system. While there may be strengths to having these personal experiences (e.g., internalized empathy for the challenges of living with a chronic illness), these same experiences may also hold blind spots that can hinder therapeutic relationships (e.g., personal reactivity to a patient not complying with indicated dietary recommendations). Constructing a health and illness genogram can reveal potential blind spots or triggers with particular clinical populations or presentations (Mendenhall & Trudeau-Hern, in press; Neumann & Gamble, 1995). By exploring her personal and intergenerational draws toward—and experiences within—health care and its intersection(s) with therapy, the MedFT can hone in on her strengths and step back when triggers cloud her therapeutic judgment.

When patients die. The culture of health care oftentimes does not allow providers to process severe incidents, such as a patient's death (Spencer, 1994; Ward, 2012). However, it is important for a provider (of any type) to think about. How you would like to be notified if (when) this occurs? Are you the type of person who wants to know when the news becomes available, or would rather find out the next time you are on-site? Whether unexpected or foreseen, death can be heartbreaking and sad. When hearing this news, it is important for providers to recognize and honor their own humanness, and to give themselves permission to grieve. If part of one's role is to assist in notifying and/or supporting the patient's family, understand that it is alright to grieve with them (Rubel, 2004). Do not hesitate to reschedule appointments for the rest of the day, talk with supportive colleagues, or take time to engage in self-care sequences that are personally unique and effective (e.g., exercise, meditation, church, family/friends).

Life After Graduate School: The New Professional

Opportunities for training in MedFT are rapidly growing, from internship experiences to MedFT certificates and program specialties (Brucker et al., 2005; Grauf-Grounds & Sellers, 2006; Tyndall, Hodgson, Lamson, White, & Knight, 2012). As students complete their training, the question "Now what?" can evoke both excitement and anxiety.

Laying the Groundwork

It is important for a new MedFT to establish his professional identity before exploring potential job opportunities. Take time to think about and articulate what it is that you do, what role(s) you play, and what you want to accomplish. MedFTs are valuable members of healthcare teams in general settings, such as primary care, and in specific settings like oncology (Hodgson, McCammon, Marlowe, & Anderson, 2012; Tyndall et al., 2012). Keep in mind, though, that MedFTs, like all the other BHPs, are working on expanding their presence in many healthcare settings. When searching for postgraduate clinical position and/or a postdoctoral fellowship, a MedFT should research the community, staff, and affiliated networks and consider the "fit" between his own and sites' respective values, philosophies, and approaches. He should remember, too, that different positions require different combinations of clinical, administrative, research, and/or teaching responsibilities, and thereby consider the commitments he is willing to make to each one.

When speaking to potential employers, applicants must be prepared to explain what a MedFT is and how MedFTs differs from other BHPs in action and approach. It is important to emphasize that the systemic framework from which MedFT orients itself contributes a valuable perspective in healthcare teams. At the same time, it is important to acknowledge and articulate similarities between MedFT and its sibling disciplines (e.g., Psychology, Social Work) with whom healthcare providers may be more familiar. Along the way, the MedFT should stress the clinical training and supervision he has received, his familiarity with and competence within healthcare settings, and his potential to obtain licensure and approved-supervisor credentials (if not already achieved).

Table 4.1 Professional organizations with high MedFT membership

American Association for Marriage and Family Therapy (AAMFT)
www.aamft.org
Collaborative Family Healthcare Association (CFHA)
www.cfha.net
Society of Behavioral Medicine (SBM)
www.sbm.org
Society of Teachers of Family Medicine (STFM)
www.stfm.org
Suggested job-search engines
The Career Network
www.Beyond.com
Career Builder
www.CareerBuilder.com
HigherEd Jobs
www.HigherEdJobs.com
Indeed
www.Indeed.com
LinkedIn
www.LinkedIn.com

Exploring the Options

One of the most useful tools when searching for a clinical position is one's professional network. The professionals within your network will serve as sources for information, consultation, and collaboration. Network development can happen in numerous ways, including formal and informal conversations with mentors and colleagues, utilizing social networking Web sites, and involvement in professional organizations.

To create a professional network, MedFTs must reach beyond their initial comfort zones and seek out colleagues from similar and different disciplines across clinical, research, and/or teaching interests. One way to do this is to become involved in various professional organizations, particularly those that will advance one's professional development in integrated care. Annual meetings serve as outlets for presenting one's work, learning from others' work, forums for consultation (i.e., receiving and providing feedback), and opportunities for service and learning. Organizations that have a large MedFT membership include the Collaborative Family Healthcare Association (CFHA), Society of Behavioral Medicine (SBM), Society for Teachers of Family Medicine (STFM), and numerous other state and local groups. Additional resources are available on each organization's Web site, including job opportunities, access to peer-reviewed journals, and social networking groups and blogs. Involvement in a professional organization takes commitment, but the opportunities and community it provides are invaluable (see Table 4.1).

Continued Professional Consultation

In this chapter, the authors have highlighted both rewards and challenges to working within healthcare settings. What we have not yet discussed is how to sustain our professional identities and continue our professional growth within systems that hold high potential for burnout (Balch, Shanafelt, Sload, Satele, & Kuerer, 2011). MedFTs—whether they are located within primary care, trauma/emergency centers, palliative care settings, etc.—are confronted with the potential to see cases that extend beyond what they were taught and prepared for in graduate training. Supervision, as we know, is an ongoing standard in graduate programs at the master's and doctoral levels (Brucker et al., 2005). However, once training is completed and licensure is secured, supervision is no longer a requirement (Edwards & Patterson, 2006; Gawinski, Edwards, & Speice, 1999).

Best practices in health care offer and provide a structure for healthcare professionals to meet and discuss cases as an ongoing process. Schwartz rounds and Balint groups are two modalities oftentimes used for training physicians, and are offered in many healthcare settings. The authors advocate for BHPs to follow a similar suit.

Schwartz rounds aim to foster compassionate caring between patients and providers (Schwartz Center, 2013). These sequences take place in settings wherein healthcare professionals come together to safely confer and express the feelings they have about patient care and interactions. All healthcare staff (e.g., physicians, nurses) are welcome. Researchers have shown that healthcare contexts that utilize Schwartz rounds to advance care are more sensitive and patient-centered (Lown & Manning, 2010; Pepper, Jaggar, Mason, Finney, & Dusmet, 2012).

Balint groups are traditionally held to focus on the details of the doctor–patient relationship as a therapeutic, healing tool (Balint, 1957). These forums are composed of physicians who regularly meet to discuss patients and cases that are directly or indirectly impacting them (the providers) personally. This peer support structure enables participants to discuss innate expectations in relation to patients in order to achieve a more balanced, realistic, and sustainable sense of purpose within work. Roberts (2012) reflected on his experiences as a physician who benefits greatly from participation in Balint groups. He stated...

> Over the years, we have discussed a spectrum of themes: the 'difficult' patient, making errors, work and home life balance, personal crisis and illnesses, office challenges, medical learners, the 'system,' the joys of practice, and the uniqueness of our relationship with our patients. (p. 246)

In a parallel vein to these forums, the authors encouraged and advocated for MedFTs to participate in ongoing consultation and support. Doing this purposively (e.g., creating and sustaining a group designed for behavioral health providers) is important, insofar as Schwartz rounds are often positioned as part of Grand Rounds sequences and Balint groups are generally open only to physicians. MedFTs may find it difficult to gain entry into these groups, and they may not find their structure to be beneficial to their unique professional and personal needs. At the second author's large University-based healthcare site, for example, behavioral medicine providers working across five Family Medicine residencies (representing MedFT, Psychology, Social Work, and Psychiatry) meet once per month for case consultation, self-of-provider discussions, and collegial support. All participants are licensed (i.e., formal supervision is not requisite), and range in professional experience from a few years to decades postgraduate training.

Conclusion

There are several ways to effectively prepare to learn about, integrate into, and function within healthcare contexts as a MedFT. From their baseline systemic sensitivities in care provision, MedFTs bring a skillset that readily connects the dots between patients' BPSS experiences, and between the members of interdisciplinary teams that collaborate with them in coping, healing, and/or maintaining health. Functioning within these contexts is more stressful, fast-paced, and higher-stakes than compared to the comfortable private practices of days gone-by. It is argued, however, that behavioral health care can also more rewarding, from the never-ending and reciprocal learning that MedFTs engage in with their colleagues, to the honor and privilege felt through being part of patients' and families' most intimate, difficult, and inspiring journeys.

Discussion Questions

1. What are your biases or perceptions about medically trained healthcare providers? About Medicine as a field?
2. How would you succinctly explain MedFT (e.g., at a job interview) to a healthcare provider or administrator who is not familiar with the field? What does a MedFT do? How is this similar and/or different from the work that hospital chaplains or medical social workers do?
3. What are you currently doing for self-care? What will you need to do (instead of, more of, or less of) in order to survive within a healthcare environment?
4. In what ways will you seek ongoing support and supervision/consultation from colleagues as you assimilate or help others to assimilate into a healthcare context?

References[1]

Abdulghani, H., Alrowais, N., Bin-Saad, N., Al-Subaie, N., Haji, A., & Alhaqwi, A. (2012). Sleep disorder among medical students: Relationship to their academic performance. *Medical Teacher, 34*(s1), S37–S41. doi:10.3109/0142159X.2012.656749.

Abraham, A., Ducharme, L., & Roman, P. (2009). Counselor attitudes toward pharmacotherapies for alcohol dependence. *Journal of Studies on Alcohol and Drugs, 70*, 628–635. Retrieved from http://www.ncbi.nlm.nih.gov/pmc/articles/PMC2696303/

Accreditation Council for Graduate Medical Education. (2011). *Common program requirements*. Retrieved from http://www.acgme.org/acgmeweb/Portals/0/PFAssets/ProgramResources/Common_Program_Requirements_07012011[1].pdf

Allison, E. (2011). Wisdom dressed in scrubs: A non-nurse offers insights to the caring profession. *Reflections of Nursing Leadership, 37*. Retrieved from http://www.reflectionsonnursingleadership.org/Pages/Vol37_3_Allison.aspx

American Association for Marriage and Family Therapy. (2013). *Marriage and family therapists: The friendly mental health professionals*. Retrieved from http://www.aamft.org/imis15/content/consumer_updates/Marriage_and_Family_Therapists.aspx

American Psychological Association. (2008). *2008 APA survey of psychology health service providers*. Retrieved from http://www.apa.org/workforce/publications/08-hsp/index.aspx

American Psychological Association. (2011). *What do practicing psychologists do*? Retrieved from http://www.apa.org/helpcenter/about-psychologists.aspx

Baker, E. K. (2003). *Tending to our self*. Arlington, VA: American Psychological Association.

Balch, C. M., Shanafelt, T. D., Sload, J., Satele, D. V., & Kuerer, H. M. (2011). Burnout and career satisfaction among surgical oncologists compared with other surgical specialties. *Annals of Surgical Oncology, 18*, 16–25. doi:10.1245/s10434-010-1369-5.

Balint, M. (1957). *The doctor, his patient and the illness*. London, UK: Churchill Livingstone.

Barondess, J. (2000). Specialization and the physician workforce: Drivers and determinants. *Journal of the American Medical Association, 284*, 1299–1301. doi:10.1001/jama.284.10.1299.

Bate, P. (2000). Changing the culture of a hospital: From hierarchy to networked community. *Public Administration, 78*, 485–512. doi:10.1111/1467-9299.00215.

Blier, P., Ward, H. E., Tremblay, P., Laberge, L., Hébert, C., & Bergeron, R. (2010). Combination of antidepressant medications from treatment initiation for major depressive disorder: A double-blind randomized study. *American Journal of Psychiatry, 167*, 281–288. doi:10.1176/appi.ajp.2009.09020186.

Bodenheimer, T., Berenson, R., & Rudolf, P. (2007). The primary care-specialty income gap: Why it matters. *Annals of Internal Medicine, 146*, 301–306. doi:10.7326/0003-4819-146-4-200702200-00011.

Brimstone, R., Thistlethwaite, J. E., & Quirk, F. (2007). Behavior of medical students in seeking mental and physical health care: Exploration and comparison with psychology students. *Medical Education, 41*, 74–83. doi:10.1111/j.1365-2929.2006.02649.x.

Britt, D. (2013). Healthcare professionalism: How important is bedside manner? *SouthSource*. Retrieved from http://source.southuniversity.edu/healthcare-professionalism-how-important-is-proper-bedside-manner-132067.aspx

Brucker, P., Faulkner, R., Baptist, J., Grames, H., Beckham, L., Walsh, S., & Willert, A. (2005). The internship training experiences in medical family therapy of doctoral-level marriage and therapy students. *American Journal of Family Therapy, 33*, 131–146. doi:10.1080/01926180590915518

Bunevicius, A., Katkute, A., & Bunevicius, R. (2008). Symptoms of anxiety and depression in medical students and in humanities students: Relationship with big-five personality dimensions

[1] An asterisk has been use to note references that the chapter authors recommend for further reading.

and vulnerability to stress. *International Journal of Social Psychiatry, 54*, 494–501. doi:10.1177/0020764008090843.
Bureau of Labor Statistics. (2012). *Occupational outlook handbook: Psychologists*. Retrieved from http://www.bls.gov/ooh/Life-Physical-and-Social-Science/Psychologists.htm#tab-1
Caldwell, B. (2012). *Choosing the MFT program that is right for you*. National Council on Family Relations. Retrieved from http://www.ncfr.org/professional-resources/career-resources/choosing-mft-program-s-right-you
Caspi, O., Sechrest, L., Pitluk, H. C., Marshall, C. L., Bell, I. R., & Nichter, M. (2003). On the definition of complementary, alternative, and integrative medicine: Societal mega-stereotypes vs. the patients' perspectives. *Alternative Therapies in Health and Medicine, 9*, 58–62.
Clay, R. (2012). *Is stress getting to you? Like their clients, psychologists struggle with work/life conflict. How can they help their clients and themselves*? American Psychological Association. Retrieved from http://www.apa.org/monitor/2011/01/stress.aspx
*Cohen, B. J., & DePetris, A. (2013). *Medical terminology: An illustrated guide* (7th ed.). Baltimore, MD: Wolters Kluwer Health.
Cooke, M., Irby, D., & O'Brien, B. (2010). *Educating physicians: A call for reform of medical school and residency*. Stanford, CA: Carnegie Foundation.
Coombs, R. H. (Ed.). (2005). *Family therapy review: Preparing for comprehensive and licensing examinations*. Mahwah, NJ: Psychology Press.
Crane, D., & Christenson, J. (2012). A summary report of the cost-effectiveness of the profession and practice of marriage and family therapy. *Contemporary Family Therapy, 34*, 204–216. doi:10.1007/s10591-012-9187-5.
Cuijpers, P., Van Straten, A., Hollon, S. D., & Andersson, G. (2010). The contribution of active medication to combined treatments of psychotherapy and pharmacotherapy for adult depression: A meta-analysis. *Acta Psychiatrica Scandinavica, 121*, 415–423. doi:10.1111/j.1600-0447.2009.01513.x.
Dahlin, M., Joneborg, N., & Runeson, B. (2005). Stress and depression among medical students: A cross-sectional study. *Medical Education, 39*, 594–604. doi:10.1111/j.1365-2929.2005.02176.x.
Diogenes, L. (1901). *The lives and opinions of eminent philosophers*. London, UK: George Bell & Sons.
*Dowell, T., Morris, C., Dodd, T., & McLoughlin, B. (2012). Psychological interventions in primary care mental health. In G. Ivbijaro (Ed.), *Companion to primary care mental health* (pp. 241–264). London, UK: Wonca and Radcliff Publishing.
Drolet, B., & Rodgers, S. (2010). A comprehensive medical student wellness program: Design and implementation at Vanderbilt School of Medicine. *Academic Medicine, 85*, 103–110. doi:10.1097/ACM.0b013e3181c46963.
Dyrbye, L., & Shanafelt, T. (2011a). Medical student distress: A call to action. *Academic Medicine, 86*, 801–803. doi:10.1097/ACM.0b013e31821da481.
Dyrbye, L., & Shanafelt, T. (2011b). Physician burnout. *Journal of the American Medical Association, 305*, 2009–2010. doi:10.1001/jama.2011.652.
Dyrbye, L., Shanafelt, T., Balch, C., Satele, D., & Freischlag, J. (2010). Physicians married or partnered to physicians: A comparative study in the American College of Surgeons. *Journal of the American College of Surgeons, 211*, 663–671. doi:10.1016/j.jamcollsurg.2010.03.032.
Dyrbye, L., Thomas, M., Huschka, M., Lawson, K., Novotny, P., Sloan, J., & Shanafelt, T. (2006). A multicenter study of burnout, depression, and quality of life in minority and nonminority US medical students. *Mayo Clinic Proceedings, 81*, 1435–1442. doi:10.4065/81.11.1435
Dyrbye, L., Thomas, M., Power, D., Durning, S., Moutier, C., Massie, St., . . . Shanafelt, T. (2010). Burnout and serious thoughts of dropping out of medical school: A multi-institutional study. *Academic Medicine, 85*, 94–102. doi:10.1097/ACM.0b013e3181c46aad
Dyrbye, L. N., Thomas, M. R., & Shanafelt, T. D. (2006). Systematic review of depression, anxiety, and other indicators of psychological distress among us and Canadian medical students. *Academic Medicine, 81*(4), 354–373.
Edwards, T., & Patterson, J. (2006). Supervising family therapy trainees in primary care medical settings: Context matters. *Journal of Marital and Family Therapy, 32*, 33–43. doi:10.1111/j.1752-0606.2006.tb01586.x.

Frank, E., Elon, L., Naimi, T., & Brewer, R. (2008). Alcohol consumption and alcohol counselling behaviour among US medical students: cohort study. *BMJ: British Medical Journal*. Retrieved from http://www.ncbi.nlm.nih.gov/pmc/articles/PMC2659955/

Gawinski, B., Edwards, T., & Speice, J. (1999). A family therapy internship in a multidisciplinary healthcare setting: Trainees' and supervisor's reflections. *Journal of Marital and Family Therapy, 25*, 469–484. doi:10.1111/j.1752-0606.1999.tb00263.x.

*Grauf-Grounds, C., & Sellers, T. S. (2006). Creating internships and potential jobs for medical family therapists: Lessons learned. *Families, Systems & Health, 24*, 230–237. doi:10.1037/1091-7527.24.2.230.

Greenhalgh, T. (2010). New images needed. *British Medical Journal, 340*, 660. http://dx.doi.org/10.1136/bmj.c1524.

Greysen, S., Chen, C., & Mullan, F. (2011). A history of medical student debt: Observations and implications for the future of medical education. *Academic Medicine, 86*, 840–845. doi:10.1097/ACM.0b013e31821daf03.

Gutgesell, M., Reeve, R., Parsons, B., & Morse, R. M. (1999). Exercise and alcohol consumption among medical students. *Academic Medicine, 74*, 750–751. doi:10.1097/00001888-199907000-00005.

Gutheil, T., & Drogin, E. (2013). *The mental health professional in court: A survival guide*. Arlington, VA: American Psychological Association.

*Hodgson, J., Lamson, A., Mendenhall, T., & Crane, R. (2012). Medical family therapy: Opportunity for workforce development in healthcare. *Contemporary Family Therapy, 34*, 143–146. doi:10.1007/s10591-012-9199-1.

Hodgson, J. L., McCammon, S. L., Marlowe, D. P., & Anderson, R. J. (2012). Medical family therapy in cancer care: Patient and family experiences. *American Journal of Family Therapy, 40*, 258–266. doi:10.1080/01926187.2011.611783.

Huang, J. (2007). Terminology issues unique to medical translation. *TeamCoord*. Retrieved from http://termcoord.wordpress.com/2013/06/11/terminology-issues-unique-to-medical-translation/

Ivbijaro, G. (Ed.). (2012). *Companion to primary care mental health*. London, UK: Radcliffe Publishing.

James, L., & O'Donohue, W. (Eds.). (2009). *The primary care toolkit: Practical resources for the integrated behavioral care provider*. New York, NY: Springer.

Jecker, N. S., & Self, D. J. (1991). Separating care and cure: An analysis of historical and contemporary images of nursing and medicine. *Journal of Medicine and Philosophy, 16*, 285–306. doi:10.1093/jmp/16.3.285.

Kane, L. (Ed.). (2012). Physician compensation report: 2012 results. *Medscape*. Retrieved from www.medscape.com/sites/physician-comp/2012

Kroenke, K., Spitzer, R., Williams, J., Monahan, P., & Löwe, B. (2007). Anxiety disorders in primary care: Prevalence, impairment, comorbidity, and detection. *Annals of Internal Medicine, 146*(5), 317–325. doi:10.7326/003-4819-146-5-200703060-00004.

Lamson, A., Meadors, P., & Mendenhall, T. (2014). Working with providers and healthcare systems experiencing compassion fatigue and burnout. In J. Hodgson, A. Lamson, T. Mendenhall, & R. Crane (Eds.), *Medical family therapy: Advanced applications* (pp. 107–124). New York, NY: Springer.

Lerner, B. (2007). In a hospital hierarchy, speaking up is hard to do. *New York Times*. Retrieved from http://www.nytimes.com/2007/04/17/health/17essa.html

Lown, B. A., & Manning, C. F. (2010). The Schwartz Center rounds: Evaluation of an interdisciplinary approach to enhancing patient-centered communication, teamwork, and provider support. *Academic Medicine, 85*, 1073–1081. doi:10.1097/ACM.0b013e3181dbf741.

MacDonald, N., & Attaran, A. (2009). Medical errors, apologies and apology laws. *Canadian Medical Association Journal, 180*, 11. doi:10.1503/cmaj.081997.

Magner, L. (Ed.). (2005). *A history of medicine* (2nd ed.). Boca Raton, FL: Taylor & Francis Group.

Martin, G. P., Currie, G., & Finn, R. (2009). Reconfiguring or reproducing intra-professional boundaries? Specialist expertise, generalist knowledge and the 'modernization' of the medical workforce. *Social Science & Medicine, 68*, 1191–1198. doi:10.1016/j.socscimed.2009.01.006.

McCray, L., Cronholm, P., Bogner, H., Gallo, J., & Neill, R. (2008). Resident physician burnout: Is there hope? *Family Medicine, 40*, 626–632. Retrieved from http://www.ncbi.nlm.nih.gov/pmc/articles/PMC2903755/

*McDaniel, S., Doherty, W., & Hepworth, J. (2014). *Medical family therapy and integrated care* (2nd ed.). Washington, DC: American Psychological Association.

McGrath, E., & Zimet, C. N. (1977). Female and male medical students: Differences in specialty choice selection and personality. *Academic Medicine, 52*, 293–300. doi:10.1097/00001888-197704000-00001.

*McKegney, C. (1989). Medical education: A neglectful and abusive family system. *Family Medicine, 21*, 452–457. Retrieved from http://europepmc.org/abstract/MED/2612802

*Mendenhall, T. (2007, May/June). Crisis land: A view from inside a behavioral health team. *Psychotherapy Networker*, 32–39.

*Mendenhall, T., & Trudeau-Hern, S. (in press). Developing self-awareness in clinicians who work in medical settings: A guide for using medical genograms in supervision. In R. Bean, S. Davis, & M. Davey (Eds.), *Increased self-awareness: Experiential exercises for dedicated clinicians and supervisors*. Thousand Oaks, CA: Sage Publications.

Miedema, B., MacIntyre, L., Tatemichi, S., Lambert-Lanning, A., Lemire, F., Manca, D., & Ramsden, V. (2012). How the medical culture contributes to coworker-perpetrated harassment and abuse of family physicians. *Annals of Family Medicine, 10*, 111–117. doi:10.1370/afm.1341

Montalt, V., & Davies, M. G. (2007). *Medical translation step by step: Learning by drafting*. Manchester, UK: St. Jerome Publishing.

Mosby. (2012). *Mosby's dictionary of medicine, nursing & health professionals* (8th ed.). Philadelphia, PA: Elsevier.

Myrick, F., Yonge, O., & Billay, D. (2010). Preceptorship and practical wisdom: A process of engaging in authentic nursing practice. *Nurse Education in Practice, 10*, 82–87. doi:10.1016/j.nepr.2009.03.018.

National Institute of Mental Health. (2013). *Depression*. Retrieved from http://www.nimh.nih.gov/health/publications/depression/index.shtml

Negash, S., & Sahin, S. (2011). Compassion fatigue in marriage and family therapy: Implications for therapists and clients. *Journal of Marital and Family Therapy, 37*, 1–13. doi:10.1111/j.1752-0606.2009.00147.x.

Neumann, D., & Gamble, S. (1995). Issues in the professional development of psychotherapists: Counter transference and vicarious traumatization in the new trauma therapist. *Psychotherapy, 32*, 341–347. doi:10.1037/0033-3204.32.2.341.

Northey, W. F. (2002). Characteristics and clinical practices of marriage and family therapists: A national survey. *Journal of Marital and Family Therapy, 28*, 487–494. doi:10.1111/j.1752-0606.2002.tb00373.x.

Orchowski, L. M., Spickard, B. A., & McNamara, J. R. (2006). Cinema and the valuing of psychotherapy: Implications for clinical practice. *Professional Psychology: Research and Practice, 37*, 506–514. doi:10.1037/0735-7028.37.5.506.

Pakenham, K., & Stafford-Brown, J. (2012). Stress in clinical psychology trainees: A review of current research and future directions. *Australian Psychologist, 47*, 147–155. doi:10.1111/j.1742-9544.2012.00070.x.

Paris, M., & Hoge, M. A. (2010). Burnout in the mental health workforce: A review. *The Journal of Behavioral Health Services & Research, 37*, 519–528. doi:10.1007/s11414-009-9202-2.

Patterson, J. E., Williams, L., Edwards, T., Chamow, L., & Grauf-Grounds, C. (2009). *Essential skills in family therapy: From the first interview to termination* (2nd ed.). New York, NY: Guilford Press.

Paul, A. (1998). Beyond psychobabble. *Psychology Today*. Retrieved from http://www.psychologytoday.com/articles/199807/beyond-psychobabble

Peek, C. J. (2013). Integrated behavioral health in primary care: A common language. In M. R. Talen & A. B. Valeras (Eds.), *Integrated behavioral health in primary care: Evaluating the evidence, identifying the essentials* (pp. 9–32). New York, NY: Springer.

*Peek, C. J., & National Integration Academy Council. (2013). *Lexicon for behavioral health and primary care integration: Concepts and definitions developed by expert consensus* (AHRQ Publication No. 13-IP001-EF). Retrieved from http://integrationacademy.ahrq.gov/sites/default/files/Lexicon.pdf

Peets, A., & Ayas, N. T. (2012). Restricting resident work hours: The good, the bad, and the ugly. *Critical Care Medicine, 40*, 960–966. doi:10.1097/CCM.0b013e3182413bc5.

Pepper, J. R., Jaggar, S. I., Mason, M. J., Finney, S. J., & Dusmet, M. (2012). Schwartz rounds: Reviving compassion in modern healthcare. *Journal of the Royal Society of Medicine, 105*, 94–95. doi:10.1258/jrsm.2011.110231.

Pingitore, D., Scheffler, R., Sentell, T., & West, J. (2002). Comparison of psychiatrists and psychologists in clinical practice. *Psychiatric Services, 53*, 977–983. doi:10.1176/appi.ps.53.8.977.

Rees, C. E., & Monrouxe, L. V. (2011). "A morning since eight of just pure grill": A multischool qualitative study of student abuse. *Academic Medicine, 86*, 1374–1382. doi:10.1097/ACM.0b013e3182303c4c.

Roberts, M. (2012). Balint groups: A tool for personal and professional resilience. *Canadian Family Physician, 58*, 245. Retrieved from http://www.cfp.ca/content/58/3/245.full.pdf+html

Roberts, L., Warner, T., Carter, D., Frank, E., Ganzini, L., & Lyketsos, C. (2000). Caring for medical students as patients: access to services and care-seeking practices of 1,027 students at nine medical schools. *Academic Medicine, 75*, 272–277. doi:10.1097/00001888-200003000-00019.

Rubel, R. (2004). When a client dies. *Psychoanalytic Social Work, 11*(1), 1–14. doi:10.1300/J032v11n01_01.

Schultz, D. (2012). Medical residents work long hours despite rules. *Health News from National Public Radio*. Retrieved from http://www.npr.org/blogs/health/2012/12/04/166477987/medical-residents-work-long-hours-despite-rules

Schwartz Center. (2013). *Schwartz Center Rounds*. Retrieved from http://www.theschwartzcenter.org/ourprograms/rounds.aspx

Schwenk, T., Davis, L., & Wimsatt, L. (2010). Depression, stigma, and suicidal ideation in medical students. *Journal of the American Medical Association, 304*, 1181–1190. doi:10.1001/jama.2010.1300.

Shallcross, L. (2011). Taking care of yourself as a counselor. *Counseling Today*. Retrieved from http://ct.counseling.org/2011/01/taking-care-of-yourself-as-a-counselor/

Shapiro, D. L., & Smith, S. R. (2011). *Malpractice in psychology: A practical resource for clinicians*. Arlington, VA: American Psychological Association.

*Skovholt, T., & Trotter-Mathison, M. J. (2010). *The resilient practitioner: Burnout prevention and self-care strategies for counselors, therapists, teachers, and health professionals*. New York, NY: Taylor & Francis.

Spencer, L. (1994). How do nurses deal with their own grief when a patient dies on an intensive care unit, and what help can be given to enable them to overcome their grief effectively? *Journal of Advanced Nursing, 19*, 1141–1150. doi:10.1111/j.1365-2648.1994.tb01198.x.

Springer, P. R., & Harris, S. M. (2010). Attitudes and beliefs of marriage and family therapists regarding psychotropic drugs and therapy. *Journal of Marital and Family Therapy, 36*, 361–375. doi:10.1111/j.1752-0606.2010.00200.x.

Starr, P. (1982). *The social transformation of American medicine*. New York, NY: Basic Books.

Steinbrook, R. (2008). Medical student debt—Is there a limit? *New England Journal of Medicine, 359*, 2629–2632. doi:10.1056/NEJMp0808520.

Sydow, K. V., Henning, T., & Reimer, C. (1998). Stereotypes of psychotherapists: A content-analytical study of medical and psychology students. *International Journal of Psychotherapy, 3*, 135–152.

Tartakovsky, M. (2009). Media's damaging depictions of mental illness. *Psych Central*. Retrieved from http://psychcentral.com/lib/2009/medias-damaging-depictions-of-mental-illness/

Tartakovsky, M. (2012). How clinicians practice self-care & 9 tips for readers. *Psych Central*. Retrieved from http://psychcentral.com/lib/how-clinicians-practice-self-care-9-tips-for-readers/00011200

Timm, T., & Blow, A. (1999). Self-of-the-therapist work: A balance between removing restraints and identifying resources. *Contemporary Family Therapy, 21*, 331–351. doi:10.1023/A:1021960315503.

Turley, S. (2013). *Medical language* (3rd ed.). Upper Saddle River, NJ: Prentice Hall.

Tyndall, L., Hodgson, J., Lamson, A., White, M., & Knight, S. (2012). Medical family therapy: Charting a course in competencies. *Contemporary Family Therapy, 34*, 171–186. doi:10.1007/s10591-012-9191-9.

Wallace, J., Lemaire, J., & Ghali, W. (2009). Physician wellness: A missing quality indicator. *The Lancet, 374*, 1714–1721. doi:10.1016/S0140-6736(09)61424-0.

Ward, J. (2012). Patient death: Supporting our colleagues. *NurseTogether*. Retrieved from http://www.nursetogether.com/patient-death-supporting-our-colleagues

Waters, B. (2012, August). 10 stereotypes of mental health professionals. *Psychology Today*. Retrieved from http://www.psychologytoday.com/blog/design-your-path/201208/10-stereotypes-mental-health-professionals

Wong, A., Kowalenko, T., Roahen-Harrison, S., Smith, B., Maio, R., & Stanley, R. (2011). A survey of emergency physicians' fear of malpractice and its association with the decision to order computed tomography scans for children with minor head trauma. *Pediatric Emergency Care, 27*, 182–185. doi:10.1097/PEC.0b013e31820d64f7.

Woodford, G. (2006). Doctors and D-I-V-O-R-C-E. *Physician Life*. Retrieved from http://www.nationalreviewofmedicine.com/issue/2006/03_15/3_physicians_life02_05.html

Young, M. (2011, December). Common stereotypes often cloud patients' perceptions of physicians. *Physicians Practice*. Retrieved from http://www.physicianspractice.com/blog/common-stereotypes-often-cloud-patients%E2%80%99-perception-physicians

Chapter 5
Medical Family Therapy in Integrated Primary Care: An Interactional Framework

Daniel Marlowe, Jennifer Hodgson, Angela Lamson, Mark White, and Tom Irons

The Institute of Medicine (IOM) has described primary health care as "the provision of *integrated, accessible healthcare services* by clinicians who are *accountable* for addressing a large *majority of personal healthcare needs*, developing a *sustained partnership* with *patients*, and practicing in the *context of family and community*" [*sic*] (1996, p. 31). Frontline primary care providers (e.g., physicians, nurse practitioners, physician assistants) typically work with patients who present with comorbidities that involve often complex and interrelated psychosocial and physiological health issues (Blount & Bayona, 1994; Ostbye, Yarnall, Pollak, Gradison, & Michener, 2005; Robinson & Reiter, 2007). Due to the complexity of patient health problems and the emergence of primary care as the de facto behavioral health system in the USA, providers often find themselves addressing a myriad of patient illnesses and psychosocial issues (Adler, Shaw, Sitt, Maya, & Morrill, 2009; O'Connor, Solberg, & Baird, 1998; Strosahl, 1996). As a consequence, primary care providers may experience role exhaustion (Bodenheimer, 2006).

The reality of role exhaustion has contributed to a scenario in which "primary care physicians are expressing frustration that the knowledge and skills they are expected to master exceed the limits of human capability" (Bodenheimer, 2006, p. 3). Brodenhemier's observation is echoed by Ostbye and colleagues (2005) whose research revealed that primary care physicians perceived a personal inability to manage chronic illness effectively due to training and time constraints. In response to practice overload, some primary care physicians (e.g., Baird, 1998) and behavioral healthcare providers (e.g., McDaniel, 1995; McDaniel, Hepworth, & Doherty, 1992; Miller, Mendenhall, & Malik, 2009; Strosahl, 2001) have merged behavioral and physical health care into a collaborative, holistic approach to patient care termed integrated care (Blount, 2003; Peek, 2003).

D. Marlowe (✉)
Campbell University School of Osteopathic Medicine, Buies Creek, NC, USA
e-mail: marlowed@campbell.edu

J. Hodgson et al. (eds.), *Medical Family Therapy*, DOI 10.1007/978-3-319-03482-9_5,

In the context of integrated care, physicians address their patients' presenting physical issues while working collaboratively with behavioral healthcare providers who screen for and treat patients' psychosocial issues. Widely published models of integrated primary care (IPC) have typically highlighted the use of psychologists (e.g., Hegel et al., 2002; Price, Beck, Nimmer, & Bensen, 2000; Robinson & Reiter, 2007; Robinson & Strosahl, 2009; Strosahl, 1996), primary care physicians (e.g., Baird, 1998; Oakley, Moore, Burford, Fahrenwald, & Woodard, 2005), social workers (e.g., Manoleas, 2008; Williams, Shore, & Foy, 2006), psychiatrists (e.g., Judd et al., 2004), and nurses (e.g., Gerada, Barrett, Betterton, & Tighe, 2000) as the primary providers of behavioral health care. However, a review of the literature revealed no other model or framework describing the role of Medical Family Therapists (MedFT) in an IPC setting other than the one presented in this chapter and initially published in 2012 by (Marlowe, Hodgson, Lamson, White, & Irons, 2012).

This chapter introduces a basic framework for understanding MedFTs' interpersonal communication as behavioral health providers (BHPs) in IPC settings; the Medical Family Therapy-Integrated Primary Care Framework (MedFT-IPCF). The MedFT-IPCF specifically addresses the culturally mediated interpersonal communication intersection of MedFTs with IPC providers and patients, thus affording an understanding of the interactions among this triad of individuals. In addition to gaining an awareness of the attributes of communication within the IPC culture, the authors intend for the MedFT-IPCF to serve as a catalyst for further conversation and exploration regarding how collaborative, systemically oriented professionals such as MedFTs function in IPC settings.

Integrated Care

Referred to by Doherty and colleagues (1996) as "the degree of involvement and sophistication in collaborative health care involving behavioral health professionals and other health professionals," integrated care reflects, in part, the ways in which behavioral health providers function in healthcare settings, given "the strengths and limitations of a variety of options" (p. 25). They along with Peek, and in collaboration with the National Integration Academy Council (2013) and Heath, Wise Romero, and Reynolds (2013), suggested that any involvement of BHPs enables a system of health care to be classified as integrated. However, these integrated healthcare systems, differ according to the degree to which BPHs are involved in care provision, proximal location to medical providers, type of case management process (i.e., shared or combined medical record charting), and degree of direct communication between BHPs and physician or physician extender providers.

Within the domain of integrated health systems, Doherty and colleagues (1996) originally delineated five levels of integrated care delivery, with higher levels equating to more integrated practice structures. Level one systems, for example, locate providers at different sites, maintain little or no structure in terms of on-going communication regarding patients, and rarely involve the cross-referral of patients among providers. In contrast, level five systems physically locate behavioral health and physician providers together, provide communication and case management structures that facilitate constant and continuous communication among providers, and involve cross-provider patient referrals (Doherty et al., 1996; Peek, 2003). Heath and colleagues (2013) added to this foundation a sixth level where sites not only have all of the above but have successfully resolved systemic/organizational issues, as well as blended roles and barriers in organizational culture. The level of integration may not only vary clinic to clinic, but provider to provider within the same clinic. This adds to the level of complexity in practice and program evaluation and leads some clinics to treat "targeted populations" (Blount, 2003) (i.e., vertical integration) versus the whole patient population (i.e., horizontal integration).

Primary Care Integration

In these early population-specific models of care, primary care physicians referred patients to a BHP for treatment of "mental illnesses" such as depression, anxiety, bipolar disorder, or post-traumatic stress disorder (e.g., Price et al., 2000; Reiss-Brennan, Briot, Daumit, & Ford, 2006; Rollman, Weinreb, Korsen, & Schulberg, 2006; Samson, Bensen, Beck, Price, & Nimmer, 1999) as found in previous versions to the 2013 edition of the DSM (APA). However, with increasing concerns about health and growing levels of diseases related to lifestyle, BHPs found their role expanding from one of an off-site or colocated specialty behavioral health provider to an in-clinic consultant working directly with patients in the exam room (Robinson & Reiter, 2007; Strosahl, 1996).

Behavioral consultation, another type of integrated modality, has gained prominence in integrated care literature and professional practice (Robinson & Reiter, 2007; Robinson & Strosahl, 2009; Strosahl, 1996, 2001). This method of care involves not only colocating BHPs in primary care settings, but also fostering their close involvement with issues that are considered more behaviorally based (e.g., weight management, smoking cessation, and medical adherence). In these systems of care, the BHP's expertise includes treating psychological distress, as well as facilitating patient adherence to provider-prescribed treatment regimens. The professional practice of onsite BHPs differs from that of traditionally trained behavioral healthcare practitioners (Strosahl, 2001) in terms of the nature of the health concerns that prompt referrals (i.e., not just for behavioral health assessment, diagnosis, and treatment), the timeframe available to work with patients (i.e., 15–30 min therapy encounters), and the dissemination of information among providers, patients, and BHPs (via exam room consults, curbside consults [impromptu conversations between healthcare providers], and a shared electronic health record [EHR]).

A major difference between BHPs and traditional mental health providers lies in the types of health-related issues that prompt physicians' referrals. The role of BHPs has been extended to include fostering patients' compliance with and adherence to medically prescribed treatments, as well as other issues that may impact patient care (Adler et al., 2009; Robinson & Reiter, 2007) such as adjustment to a new diagnosis or relational stressors that are a part of the patient's inability to follow the prescribed treatment. Treating traditional behavioral health issues such as depression and anxiety, while still part of the repertoire of patient concerns that BHPs address, is no longer their sole focus (Robinson & Strosahl, 2009).

Another ideological shift regarding healthcare provision has to do with the duration of time BHPs spend with patients. Due to the fast pace of primary care and the likelihood that a physician may see as many as 28 patients a day, the typical 50-min session that BHPs have traditionally been trained to provide is unrealistic (Robinson & Reiter, 2007; Robinson & Strosahl, 2009). In an IPC context, BHPs often work with patients in an examination room setting for an estimated 15–30 min (Gunn & Blount, 2009; Robinson & Reiter, 2007; Robinson & Strosahl, 2009; Strosahl, 1996). This shift in location of sessions allows BHPs to reach a greater number of patients in the course of a day, and briefer visits with those patients help to refrain from slowing down the healthcare team's workflow.

The final shift in a consultation model involves how patient information is shared between BHP and PCP. In this model of care both the BHP and primary care provider (PCP) write progress notes within the same medical record (Blount, 2003; Doherty et al., 1996; Robinson & Reiter, 2007), as well as curbside consults about patients of mutual concern (Robinson & Strosahl, 2009; Strosahl, 1996). Curbside consultations may occur in hallways, providers' offices, or other locations within healthcare settings where pertinent information is delivered in vivo (i.e., concurrent) with the patient's visit (Peek, Baird, & Coleman, 2009; Robinson & Strosahl, 2009). Thus, information dissemination practices in the consultant model are continuous and instantaneous, and ensure frequent interactions among PCPs, BHPs, and other members of the healthcare team.

Contemporary literature on models of IPC outline their use in addressing specific behavioral health concerns or disease states such as depression (e.g., Reiss-Brennan et al., 2006; Rollman et al., 2006), anxiety (e.g., Price et al., 2000), substance abuse (e.g., Gerada et al., 2000), HIV (e.g., Zaller, Gillani, & Rich, 2007), diabetes (e.g., Meulepas et al., 2007; Phelps et al., 2009), genetic disease (e.g., Rolland & Williams, 2005; Smith & Harkness, 2003), and infertility (e.g., Burns, 1999). In addition, these models have also been used to target specific populations such as Latinos (e.g., Manoleas, 2008; Phelps et al., 2009; Willerton, Dankoski, & Martir, 2008), the elderly (e.g., Hegel et al., 2002), rural populations (e.g., Judd et al., 2004; Phelps et al., 2009), and children (e.g., Pratt et al., 2009; Valleley et al., 2007). However, these models do not specifically address the continuum of diverse patient populations, diagnoses, and other issues that providers typically experience while working in a primary care environment (Peek et al., 2009; Robinson & Strosahl, 2009). Also, the degree of specialization reflected in these models may hinder their application when attempting to address the myriad of biopsychosocial (BPS) issues and diverse populations that present in primary care (Peek et al., 2009; Robinson & Strosahl, 2009). Keeping the aforementioned limitations of contemporary IPC literature in mind, the framework presented below is applicable regardless of the targeted disease, the population receiving care, and/or the trajectory of the disease process/outcome.

MedFT-IPC Framework

Identified through use of a qualitative field-based study design, The *Medical Family Therapy in Integrated Primary Care Framework* (*MedFT-IPCF*) was developed using a method of inquiry known as ethnography of communication. This method is used to analyze, categorize, and describe patterns of interaction/communication within cultural, ethnic, and professional groups (Hymes, 1972; Saville-Troike, 2003). Although an in-depth discussion of the study itself is beyond the scope of this chapter (see Marlowe et al., 2012), a brief description is offered to contextualize the environment from which the MedFT-IPCF emerged.

Background

The MedFT-IPCF was created through direct observation and analysis of the MedFT's interactions with the PCPs (e.g., physicians, physician assistants, nurse practitioners), direct care staff (e.g., nurses, medical assistants, nursing assistants), and patients of the clinic; the aggregate of these observed interactions formed what is called the "act sequence" and served as the basic unit of analysis. The act sequence was broken down into three *Patient States*. The three *Patient States* were used to categorize the type of patient care visit and each one included slightly different interactional act sequences. For each *Patient State*, the MedFT's provision of care was then broken down into five different interactional phases (i.e., steps) whose sequence and inclusion were impacted by the preceding *Patient State*. Appendix is used to concisely present a description of each *Patient State*, followed by the interactional phases, and finally, a description of how a conjoint session (i.e., one where both MedFT and primary care provider are present at the same) alters those phases. It also outlines the rules for interaction and norms of interpretation that impact how each act sequence is framed. A detailed description of the MedFT-IPCF is defined and described in more detail below.

The Framework

Patient state: Framing the initial context of the encounter. Based on the analysis, three different *Patient States* were identified as providing the initial context for encounter between patient, MedFT, and provider: (a) *New Patient*, (b) *Return Visit—Worsening or No Change in Condition*, and (c) *Return Visit—Improving Condition*. These three states are primarily understood in context of the patient's degree/length/kind of relationship with the healthcare team and their presenting concern. As the first state would imply, these are first time patients to the center and know little if anything about IPC, as well as the role of the MedFT as a member of the healthcare team. Therefore, this initial interaction is not contingent on the patient's chief complaint, but focuses on joining (i.e., building rapport), educating/acclimating the patient to the IC model used by the healthcare team, and obtaining an initial psychosocial assessment. The psychosocial assessment includes gathering baseline data about depression and anxiety symptoms experienced in the past 2 weeks, relational issues/stress that the patient identifies as most troubling, behavioral health concerns such as smoking or weight loss, along with strengths which include patient-identified coping skills and support persons.

The second *Patient State* involves returning patients, where they come to learn more about the etiology and trajectory of their recently diagnosed and/or chronic medical condition and are reporting "no change" or "worsening" in their symptoms. Understandably, many patients whose medical condition has not changed or has worsened since their last visit may present with a degree of frustration, anger, and/or anxiousness. It is also during these kinds of visits that patient–provider–staff relationships have the potential to become strained and acrimonious. Given the potential volatility of the patient–provider encounter, the MedFT's overall interaction primarily focuses on joining with the patient in their frustration as a means by which to validate their experience, as well as an attempt to explore the origins of the patient's frustration.

The third *Patient State* deals again with a returning patient, but one whose medical condition has improved since their last medical visit. This last type of encounter elicits a focus by the MedFT on the successes of the patient–provider dyad over the course of treatment, as well as how to maintain those successes in the future. This *Patient State*, as with the others, includes specific interactional sequences that were commonly observed between the MedFTs, providers, and patients. These interactional sequences will be explained in greater detail to provide a richer description of what one may observe or do in each state.

Interactional **p**hases/**s**teps. In each *Patient State*, the MedFT's actual engagement with the patient is comprised of five *steps*, with the specifics of each step determined by the preceding *Patient State*. For example, what happens in a returning visit is impacted by the interactions that took place at the patient's previous visit. It is important to mention at this point that steps 1 through 4 (as outlined below) typically only involve the MedFT and patient; however, conjoint sessions (i.e., sessions where the MedFT and PCP meet with the patient at the same time) are also discussed.

Step 1: Patient briefing. During this step, the MedFT gathers an initial understanding of whether they have seen this patient before, as well as the patient's presenting medical and/or behavioral health issue. The information is usually obtained from a "face sheet" which is a sheet containing basic information about the patient including name, age, primary language, active medications, vitals (e.g., blood glucose level [BGL], weight, blood pressure [BP], temperature), possibly the outcome of an alcohol or substance abuse screen, and his or her chief complaint. This sheet is typically printed directly from the patient's medical record and is attached to the outside of the exam room door. It is essential that the MedFT be able to read, understand, and synthesize the patient's detailed medication list and biomarker information (e.g., blood pressure, blood glucose levels, oxygenation of blood). This information serves as a way of ascertaining what medical/behavioral health conditions the patient may be undergoing current treatment for, along with how well the patient is or is not managing said conditions. This information is ultimately used to check on the psychosocial health of the patient in relation to his or her biological health status, as well as alert the MedFT to precautions that may need to be taken if a patient is contagious or immunocompromised. This particular step, regardless of whether or not the patient is newly established as a patient of the clinic, sets the stage for the rest of the encounter since it helps the MedFT prepare for issues that may be placed higher on the agenda by the patient or PCP for the visit (e.g., a high BGL, HTN, positive test result for a sexually transmitted infection, or dramatic change in weight). In this case, the MedFT may help the patient to focus on an agenda that is realistic for the visit given the list of health issues and matters being presented for follow-up, as well as those identified by the PCP as primary concerns. While the MedFT would never reveal findings of test results to the patient prior to the PCP, he or she may use this information later in the encounter to help get the patient prepared psychosocially for the visit.

Step 2: Introduction. The second step marks the beginning of direct patient contact between the MedFT and the patient/members of his or her support system. It serves as a focal point orienting those in the exam room to the integrated model being practiced at the clinic. The introduction typically only takes place with new patients but is ultimately determined by whether or not the patient has had interactions with the MedFT in the past (i.e., a returning patient who have not yet met the MedFT). The MedFT enters the room and introduces him or herself by name prior to describing their professional role as a member of the healthcare team. He or she then asks the patient to introduce anyone who has accompanied them to their medical appointment and confirms that the patient would like for that support person to remain present for the interview. After the greeting has taken place, a standard introduction is relayed to the patient that incorporates three overarching ideas: (a) the role of the MedFT as part of the healthcare team, (b) the importance and purpose of the psychosocial assessment process, and (c) that the MedFT meets with all patients and is not merely involved because the medical provider and/or staff believe there is emergent and/or underlying pathology, or bad news to report.

It is important to make sure that the introduction incorporates these three aspects since its intention is to orient and relax the patient to the MedFT's inclusion in his care and the IPC model being practiced there. It is also important for the MedFT to cover how information discussed will be shared with the patient's provider and the limits of confidentiality (e.g., harm to self or others) prior to assessing and intervening. All of this helps to establish trust and build the relationship with the patient, and any accompanying support persons, for future interactions.

Step 3: Elicitation of the illness story. The MedFT typically begins this part of the interaction by inquiring about the reason for the patient's visit and, if the patient is new to the center, gathers the biopsychosocial history (e.g., length of diagnosis, family history, past/current treatment, psychosocial stressors accompanying illness, and/or treatment history) relevant to the presenting concern/reason for visit. It is important to mention that the MedFT's interview differs from that of the PCP's since the focus is mainly on the psychosocial experiences related to the medical concern and not only the medical concern itself. In order to be effective at this kind of interview, the MedFT must familiarize oneself over time with the literature (particularly for the more common health issues seen in primary care) on how the patient's biological and medical history may put her at risk or buffer her from certain psychosocial issues. It is also worth mentioning that the majority of psychosocial assessment takes place during this part of the interaction (i.e., assessment of emergent behavioral health issues, relational issues, and/or psychosocial factors impacting physical functioning). Based on the preferences of the medical provider, the MedFT assesses for other medical/psychosocial aspects of functioning, as well (e.g., medication/treatment compliance, medication side-effects, appetite, sleeping habits). A common mistake among newer MedFTs is to only screen for behavioral health issues and not attend to establish or support behavioral health goals. All patients have something they are working on, or wanting to work on, to improve their health (i.e., diet, weight, exercise, sleep, smoking, alcohol/drug use, relationship satisfaction, sexual intimacy, stress management). A MedFT can be particularly helpful to a busy PCP by taking these conversations on and working collaboratively with the patient, accompanying support persons, and PCP to set realistic health goals and action steps.

If the appointment is for a return visit where the patient's condition has worsened, the MedFT's conversation primarily revolves around dealing with any anger/frustration the patient may be experiencing, as well as attempting to ascertain where and to whom that anger and/or frustration is directed. As stated earlier, these kinds of visits present the greatest possibility for acrimony between the patient and the rest of the healthcare team, and the assessment portion of this step focuses on exploring and addressing this tension if it exists. Also, as a patient's medical condition worsens, other psychosocial issues might develop and/or become exacerbated (e.g., a patient whose congestive heart failure continues to worsen may become depressed), which the MedFT needs to assess for. In order to intervene effectively in these types of encounters, the MedFT must take care to validate the patient's anger and/or frustration without increasing their discontent. Instead, the MedFT must focus on letting the patient know his or her concerns are being taken seriously. This is an important and difficult position for the MedFT to take, especially if the source of the patient's anger is directed toward the rest of healthcare team. The goal here is to create a sense of acknowledgement of the patient's anger without necessarily expressing agreement. It is this position that allows the MedFT to connect with the patient while simultaneously staying connected to the rest of healthcare team (Marlowe, 2013).

During a return visit in which a patient's condition is improving, the MedFT focuses on assessing what actions the patient has taken to help facilitate the recovery process (i.e., agency), and reinforces the teamwork between themselves and the PCP/healthcare team. The MedFT also discusses any difficulties the patient has encountered during their attempt to comply with treatment, as well as any anticipated issues they might encounter as they move forward (e.g., a diabetic patient who is trying to change their eating habits but lives with family members who still maintain an unhealthy diet).

Step 4: Intervention. One can conceptualize Steps 3 and 4 as different sides of the same interactional coin; the elicitation of the illness story itself can be considered an intervention, while the subsequent interventions that arise from it further elicit the patient's illness experience (i.e., illness story). With this idea of interdependence in mind, interventions during this step can vary depending on whether or not the patient is new to the practice, the way in which the illness story is elicited, and what is shared with the MedFT once he initiates a conversation with the patient. However, four general types of intervention make up the majority of the MedFT's toolkit.

The first type of intervention, *brief problem solving/supportive therapy*, involves joining patients where they are emotionally regarding their psychosocial stressors, as well as exploring concrete ways they might deal with those stressors (e.g., discussing how a patient with diabetes might talk with his or her family members about not feeling supported as she attempts to make dietary/lifestyle changes). This type of intervention also includes relaxation techniques (e.g., breathing/mindfulness) and/or brief hypnotherapy depending on the patient issue (e.g., needle or blood phobia), along with the skillset of the MedFT. The second type of intervention, *planting seeds*, has to do with issues and/or concerns the patient relays during Step 3 (elicitation of the illness story) but have not yet been brought to the PCP's attention. The MedFT will encourage the patient to discuss these with his or her PCP during his medical visit, as well as teach the patient how to bring up difficult issues with the provider (e.g., a patient is not taking his medication as prescribed). This may also include germinating an idea for a resource, service, intervention, or health behavior change that may help the patient to accomplish his or her health goal(s). MedFTs may also use *psychoeducation and/or behavioral education*, the third intervention type, to address a presenting concern (e.g., sleep hygiene education/anxiety-reducing strategies for insomnia). The final type of intervention involves *referring the patient for additional services* (i.e., on site or in the community based on patient's expressed needs and readiness), which includes applying for Medicaid, dental services, substance abuse treatment, traditional psychotherapy, etc. Referrals are either internal or external and based on the patient's needs and/or the services offered by the clinic; patients who only require brief short term psychotherapy (less than six sessions) are typically referred internally to the MedFT (if the provider has availability) and those with more complex or specialized needs (e.g., intensive/specialized/long term therapy or couples therapy) are referred to the appropriate specialty behavioral health provider in the community.

Step 5: Relaying information. As the MedFT winds down their interaction with the patient, they recap their discussion as well as any "seeds" (mentioned in Step 4) planted during the conversation, and/or confirmation or provision of any outside referrals. Also, prior to exiting the room, the MedFT typically asks if the patient would like him or her to return once patient's medical visit begins to talk collaboratively with the PCP. This conjoint visit is offered regardless of the patient's presenting issue but is primarily relegated to times when anger/frustration, sadness, and/or suicidality exist. Once the MedFT ends their patient interaction (whether it is prior to the PCP seeing the patient or after the PCP exists the room), they then need to relay any pertinent information (e.g., changes in behavioral health status, suitable resources, strategies for treatment plan adherence) concisely to the PCP. Of course, the MedFT should always keep the patient/support persons' well-being in mind (e.g., safety) when leaving them alone in the exam room to talk to the PCP, as well as the overall logistics/flow of the clinic when deciding how to share information (i.e., working and communicating efficiently).

In most instances, once the MedFT ends the session and leaves the room, two modes of information relay become possible: (a) the MedFT seeks out the provider and relays any pertinent information, or (b) the BHP may attach pertinent information to the patient's face sheet (e.g., depression/anxiety score). The way information is relayed is dictated by the availability of the provider and the importance/severity of the information obtained. Of the two conditions described, severity supersedes availability, since ethically and legally information regarding suicidality, planned violence against staff, and/or any type of abuse needs to be communicated directly to the PCP immediately. Again, it is important to remember that the consultations between MedFT and medical provider should remain brief (anywhere from 30 s to 2 min), and are primarily dictated by the importance/biopsychosocial complexity of the information and the availability of the medical provider.

Another means of relaying information is the insertion of a MedFT note into the EHR system for each patient encounter. Ideally, the MedFT and PCP have already communicated the main elements of the note's content before the patient has even left the building. However, at times it is not possible or necessary given the PCP's familiarity with the particular patient and a prior shared agreement with the MedFT on treatment or lack of severity, to warrant interrupting the PCP during another patient visit in order to share information face to face. One exception to how information is shared has to do with any emergent behavioral health issues like suicidality or child abuse that might arise during the MedFT's assessment. In these instances, the MedFT shares with the patient the need to relay the entire assessment to the PCP in-person, and the MedFT may even go out of his way to request that the PCP step out of an exam room with another patient to discuss his findings. This degree of action by the MedFT is necessary given the level of risk and potential ramifications for the patient, bystanders, the healthcare team, and MedFT. Also, one must remember that assessing the severity and likelihood of patient or PCP follow-through regarding emergent behavioral health issues is a nuanced practice, and by sharing that assessment in its entirety with the PCP the MedFT better contextualizes their concerns for the PCP. Findings reported by the MedFT may be subsequently moved higher up on the PCP's list of issues to address at that visit.

Conjoint Sessions

Unlike the session format described above which takes place prior to the PCP entering the room, during conjoint sessions the MedFT typically assumes a more observational role for the encounter and the PCP takes the lead in the room. The MedFTs take on a more active role during the conjoint clinical interview if (a) the MedFT and provider have a good working rapport and predominantly see patients together, and/or (b) the presenting medical concern is more psychosocial or behavioral in nature (e.g., depression, anxiety, treatment adherence, adjustment to a medical diagnosis). Also, during these joint sessions the MedFT typically stands while the PCP takes the seat closest to the patient on the rolling stool. This positioning is done with the intent of allowing the PCP unfettered access to the patient (for the physical exam) and the EHR (i.e., computer) to enter biomarker information and generate patient prescriptions.

In conjoint sessions in which the MedFT has had no prior contact with the patient, the introduction of the MedFT and her role on the healthcare team is typically done by the PCP, although the MedFT may expand upon and/or clarify any portion of the introduction. However, during conjoint sessions that begin as solo interviews (i.e., a session in which the PCP entered the room during the MedFT's BPS assessment), the MedFT initially acquiesces to the PCP once she enters the exam room. However, the MedFT can still adopt a more active role through the relaying of pertinent information gained during the BPS assessment as the PCP performs her clinical interview. Step 5, relaying of information, does not typically take place during conjoint sessions, although both MedFT and PCP might confer outside the room to discuss a shared treatment plan or otherwise coordinate care.

Conclusion

Although MedFTs' use and utility has been outlined in multiple venues with specific disease states and populations (e.g., Anderson, Huff, & Hodgson, 2008; Davey, Foster, Milton, & Duncan, 2009; McDaniel, Harkness, & Epstein, 2001; Phelps et al., 2009; Pratt et al., 2009; Tyndall, Hodgson, Lamson, White, & Knight, 2012a, 2012b; Willerton et al., 2008), until now, no primary care model utilizing

MedFTs in an integrated and/or consultant capacity has been described in contemporary literature. The unique contributions of this framework are threefold: (a) it outlines how the provision of IPC services to nonspecific and nontargeted populations might look, (b) it describes how a MedFT might specifically function in providing those services, and (c) it breaks down the interactional sequence of events from initial patient contact to coordination of treatment to a degree of specificity not previously seen in the literature.

The point of constructing this framework is not meant to presuppose, as Doherty and colleagues (1996) warned against, that it or the interactional sequence it outlines is the optimal way for all IPC programs to function. It is instead meant to provide one way of organizing behavioral health services in integrated settings and is put forth here to elicit a broader conversation about what is and is not useful and in regard to working as a relationally based BHP in an IPC setting. Another hope inherent in this work is that, through studying and describing the actual practice of MedFT/MFTs in these venues, competencies can later be developed in regard to the training of student professionals who hope to work in this area (Tyndall et al., 2012a).

Discussion Questions

1. What do you think are the main differences between how a MedFT and another behavioral health provider (e.g., health psychologist, medical social worker, professional counselor) might engage in this model? Is there any difference?
2. How applicable is this model of care to your current work setting? Why or why not?
3. How do you think patients might benefit from BHP's utilizing this model of care?
4. What are some strengths to outlining the interactional sequence of the MedFT in an integrated care setting? What could be some drawbacks?
5. How do you think the hierarchical structure of a medical setting could support the function of this model of IPC?

Acknowledgement A special acknowledgement to Sharon Knight, Ph.D., from East Carolina University who provided invaluable feedback in the development of this chapter.

Appendix: Framework

FUNCTION/PURPOSE: To assess patient's psychosocial functioning, along with how said functioning impacts/is impacted by presenting biological concerns.

PARTICIPANTS:

P1—Patient

P2—MedFT
P3—Medical Provider

ACT SEQUENCE:

Condition A: New Patient

Phase One—"Patient Briefing"

P2—Gathers an overview of P1 presenting concern.
P2—Either retrieves patient encounter sheet from exam room door, which provides a description of the presenting concern and other information (e.g., initial or return visit, medication list, weight, height, age), or accesses information through EHR on nearby computer.

Phase Two—"Introduction"

P2—Enters room, greets P1 and takes seat at P1's eye level.
P2—Introduces self and presents service as standard of care for all patients while emphasizing that P2's inclusion is not indicative of any concerns by P3 or staff (i.e., P2 is not speaking with P1 because they are "crazy" or to cushion impending "bad" news).

Phase Three—"Elicitation of Illness Story"

P2—Asks P1 about presenting concerns as they relate to medical visit.
P2's elicitation encompasses both biological and psychosocial aspects.
P1—Relays illness story.

Phase Four—"Intervention"

Based on nature of illness story, P2 engages P1 in brief intervention based on presenting needs.

Phase Five—"Relaying of Information"

P2—Makes transition from sitting/leaning to standing—readying exit.
P2—Thanks P1 for participating in their exchange and if able, gives P1 timeframe for when P3 will enter room.
P2—Exits room and either seeks out P3 for "curbside" consultation regarding P1, or places pertinent information on sticky note and places it on encounter sheet in exam room door.

Condition B: Return Visit—Worsening or No Change in Condition

Phase One, Two, and Three are the same with the exception of no introduction by P2 during Phase Two.
Phase Four—"Intervention"

P2—Joins P1 in frustration over condition then assesses P1's level of satisfaction with P3 and medical staff.

P2—Engages P1 in conversation about difficulties of treatment. (compliance/ adherence) or relationship with P3.

If compliance/adherence or relationship issues between P1 and P3 are found, P2 focuses encounter to specifically address these.
Phase Five—"Relaying of Information"

P2—Thanks P1 for participating in their exchange and also inquires about returning for P1's encounter with P3.
P1—Either agrees or denies, which P2 then honors.
P2—Depending on if discord between P1 and P3 exists, and the extent, P2 will seek out P3 for "curbside" consultation; if little or no discord exists, P2 will leave information on sticky note on patient information sheet.

Condition C: Return Visit—Improving Condition

Phase One, Two, and Three are the same with the exception of no introduction by P2 during Phase Two.
Phase Four—"Intervention"

P2—Encourages and reinforces life choices made by P1 and treatment choices by P3.
P2—Engages P1 in conversation regarding strategies used to comply with treatment, as well as strategies that will be used in the future, and discusses any difficulties P1 may be encountering or expected to encounter.

Phase Five is the same as in *Condition A*.

RULES FOR INTERACTION:

Phase One–Phase Four:

If P2 accompanies P3 during medical visit, P2 takes on a more observational role, which includes offering pertinent information when appropriate (i.e., psychosocial, behavioral, adherence), but medical visit is primarily run by P3; the introduction of P2 to P1 will be done by P3.
If P2 is interacting with P1 when P3 enters room, P3 will ask P2 if they should "move on" to the next patient and return when P2 is finished; this decision is made by both P2 and P1, and is based on patient load of P3.
If P3 enters room during P2 and P1 interaction and stays, P2 will transition to standing/leaning position to allow P1 access to the seat and computer in the room. P2 will then adopt a more observational positioning during remainder of encounter.

Phase Five:

Information presented to P3 during curbside consultation and/or placed on sticky note deals primarily with psychosocial issues as they relate to presenting medical concern.
Consultations should not last more than 30 s to 2 min based on relevance/ importance of information.

If emergent issues are present (i.e., suicidal ideation, abuse, neglect, substance abuse) this requires immediate consultation.

NORMS OF INTERPRETATION:

The introduction by P2 during Phase Two combines elements of educating the patient about the psychosocial assessment process, role of the therapist as part of the medical team, services offered by the therapist (i.e., consultation and/or traditional psychotherapy), and humor.

During Phase Three, the elicitation primarily encompasses history of presenting medical concern (i.e., length of dx, family hx, past/current tx, psychosocial stressors accompanying illness, and/or tx history).

Based on P3's preference, Phase Three may also include other assessments (e.g., medication side effects, sleep, diet).

Interventions during Phase Four can include the following: brief problem solving/ supportive therapy, "planting seeds" (i.e., encouraging P1 to bring up certain issues during medical visit), psychoeducation, and/or psychosocial referral (i.e., social work referral for concrete services, referral to either P2 or outside provider for traditional psychotherapy).

During Phase Four/Condition B, "joining" does not entail agreeing with P1's frustration, particularly if it involves denigrating P3 or medical staff. Joining entails acknowledging P1's frustration while at the same time exploring possible reasons for relational discord.

If P2 either returns for medical visit after meeting with P1 or remains in exam room after P3 enters, their role may also include relaying pertinent information from their initial session to P3 during clinical interview.

If P2 and P3 conduct a conjoint session, Phase Five may or may not take place based on amount of information shared during session; if Phase Five does occur, it is typically done outside the exam room, and revolves around coordination of services (e.g., P3 prescribes an antidepressant for P1, and P2 conducts traditional psychotherapy).

Based on degree of rapport between P2 and P3 and nature of the presenting issue, P2 may take a larger role during conjoint sessions.

References[1]

Adler, L., Shaw, D., Sitt, D., Maya, E., & Morrill, M. I. (2009). Issues in diagnosis and treatment of adults ADHA by primary care physicians. *Primary Psychiatry, 16*(5), 57–63.

[1] An asterisk has been use to note references that the chapter authors recommend for further reading.

Anderson, R. J., Huff, N. L., & Hodgson, J. L. (2008). Medical family therapy in an inpatient psychiatric setting: A qualitative study. *Families, Systems & Health, 26*, 164–180. doi:10.1037/1091-7572.26.2.164.

Baird, M. A. (1998). Integrated primary care at HealthPartners of Minneapolis: A view from the deck. *Families, Systems & Health, 16*, 159–164. doi:10.1037/h0089066.

Blount, A. (2003). Integrated primary care: Organizing the evidence. *Families, Systems & Health, 21*, 121–133. doi:10.1037/1091-7527.21.2.121.

Blount, A., & Bayona, J. (1994). Toward a system of integrated primary care. *Families, Systems & Health, 12*, 171–182. doi:10.1037/h0089151.

Bodenheimer, T. (2006). Primary care—Will it survive? *New England Journal of Medicine, 355*, 861–864.

Burns, L. H. (1999). Genetics and infertility: Psychosocial issues in reproductive counseling. *Families, Systems & Health, 21*, 121–133.

Davey, M. P., Foster, J., Milton, K., & Duncan, T. M. (2009). Collaborative approaches to increasing family support for HIV positive youth. *Families, Systems & Health, 27*, 39–52. doi:10.1037/a0014910.

Doherty, W. J., McDaniel, S. H., & Baird, M. A. (1996). Five levels of primary care/behavioral healthcare collaboration. *Behavioral Healthcare Tomorrow, 5*(5), 25–28.

Gerada, C., Barrett, C., Betterton, J., & Tighe, J. (2000). The consultancy liaison addiction service: The first 5 years of an integrated, primary care-based community drug and alcohol team. *Drugs: Education, Prevention and Policy, 7*, 251–256.

Gunn, W. B., Jr., & Blount, A. (2009). Primary care mental health: A new frontier for psychology. *Journal of Clinical Psychology, 65*, 235–252. doi:10.1002/jclp.20499.

Heath, B., Wise Romero, P., & Reynolds, K. (2013). *A review of and proposed standard framework for levels of integrated healthcare.* SAMHA-HRSA Center for Integrated Care Solutions. Retrieved from http://www.cihslive.browsermedia.com/integrated-care-models/CIHS_Framework_Final_charts.pdf

Hegel, M. T., Imming, J., Cyr-Provost, M., Noel, P. H., Arean, P. A., & Unutzer, J. (2002). Role of behavioral health professionals in a collaborative stepped care treatment model for depression in primary care: Project IMPACT. *Families, Systems & Health, 20*, 265–277.

Hymes, D. (1972). Models of the interaction of language and social life. In J. J. Gumperz & D. Hymes (Eds.), *Directions in sociolinguistics: The ethnography of communication* (pp. 36–71). New York, NY: Holt, Rinehard and Winston.

Institute of Medicine. (1996). *Primary care: America's health in a new era*. Washington, DC: National Academy Press.

Judd, F., Davis, J., Hodgins, G., Scopellti, J., Biliana, A., & Hulbert, C. (2004). Psychiatry programme: A systems approach to education, training and service integration. *Australasian Psychiatry, 12*, 42–47. doi:10.1046/j.1039-8562.2003.02058.x.

Manoleas, P. (2008). Integrated primary care and behavioral health services for Latinos: A blueprint and research agenda. *Social Work in Health Care, 47*, 438–454. doi:10.1080/00981380802344480.

*Marlowe, D. (2013). Bridging conversations: Discussing the intra-professional relationship between medical family therapy and family therapy. *Journal of Family Therapy, 35*, 119–138. doi:10.1111/j.1467-6427.2011.00553.x.

*Marlowe, D., Hodgson, J., Lamson, A., White, M., & Irons, T. (2012). Medical family therapy in a primary care setting: A framework for integration. *Contemporary Family Therapy, 34*, 244–258. doi:10.1007/s10591-012-9195-5.

McDaniel, S. H. (1995). Collaboration between psychologists and family physicians: Implementing the biopsychosocial model. *Professional Psychology: Research and Practice, 26*, 117–122.

McDaniel, S., Harkness, J. L., & Epstein, R. (2001). Medical family therapy for a woman with end-stage Crohn's disease. *American Journal of Family Therapy, 29*, 375–395.

McDaniel, S. H., Hepworth, J., & Doherty, W. J. (1992). *Medical family therapy: A biopsychosocial approach to families with health problems*. New York, NY: Basic Books.
Meulepas, M. A., Braspenning, J. C. C., de Grauw, W. J., Lucas, A. E. M., Harms, L., Akkermans, R. P., & Grol, R. (2007). Logistic support service improves processes and outcomes of diabetes care in general practice. *Family Practice, 24*, 20–25. doi:10.1093/fampra/cml055
Miller, B., Mendenhall, T., & Malik, A. (2009). Integrated primary care: An inclusive three-world view through process metrics and empirical discrimination. *Journal of Clinical Psychology in Medical Settings, 16*, 21–30. doi:10.1007/s10880-008-9137-4.
Oakley, C., Moore, D., Burford, D., Fahrenwald, R., & Woodard, K. (2005). The Montana model: Integrated primary care and behavioral health in a family practice residency program. *The Journal of Rural Health, 21*, 351–354. doi:10.1111/j.1748-0361.2005.tb00106.x.
O'Connor, P. J., Solberg, L. I., & Baird, M. (1998). The future of primary care: The enhanced primary care model. *The Journal of Family Practice, 47*, 62–67.
Ostbye, T., Yarnall, K. S., Pollak, K. I., Gradison, M., & Michener, J. L. (2005). Is there time for management of patients with chronic diseases in primary care? *Annals of Family Medicine, 3*, 209–214. doi:10.1370/afm.310.
Peek, C. J. (2003). An evidence-based "elevator speech" for a practical world. *Families, Systems & Health, 21*, 135–140.
Peek, C. J., Baird, M. A., & Coleman, E. (2009). Primary care for patient complexity, not only disease. *Families, Systems & Health, 27*, 287–302. doi:10.1037/a0018048.
*Peek, C. J., & National Integration Academy Council. (2013). *Lexicon for behavioral health and primary care integration: Concepts and definitions developed by expert consensus* (AHRQ Publication No.13-IP001-EF). Retrieved from http://integrationacademy.ahrq.gov/sites/default/files/Lexicon.pdf
Phelps, K. W., Howell, C. D., Hill, S. G., Seeman, T. S., Lamson, A. L., Hodgson, J. L., & Smith, D. A. (2009). A collaborative care model for patients with type-2 diabetes. *Families, Systems, & Health, 27*, 131–140. doi:10.1037/a0015027
Pratt, K. J., Lamson, A. L., Collier, D. N., Crawford, Y. S., Harris, N., Gross, K., ... Soporito, M. (2009). Camp golden treasures: A multidisciplinary weight-loss and a healthy lifestyle camp for adolescent girls. *Families, Systems, & Health, 27*, 116–124. doi:10.1037/a0014912
Price, D., Beck, A., Nimmer, C., & Bensen, S. (2000). The treatment of anxiety disorders in a primary care HMO setting. *Psychiatric Quarterly, 71*, 31–45.
Reiss-Brennan, B., Briot, G., Daumit, G., & Ford, D. (2006). Evaluation of 'depression in primary care' innovations. *Administration and Policy in Mental Health and Mental Health Services Research, 33*, 86–91. doi:10.1007/s10488-005-4239-x.
Robinson, P. J., & Reiter, J. T. (2007). *Behavioral consultation and primary care: A guide to integrating services*. New York, NY: Springer.
Robinson, P. J., & Strosahl, K. D. (2009). Behavioral health consultation and primary care: Lessons learned. *Journal of Clinical Psychology in Medical Settings, 16*(1), 58–71. doi:10.1007/s10880-009-9145-z.
Rolland, J. S., & Williams, J. K. (2005). Toward a biopsychosocial model for the 21st century genetics. *Family Process, 44*, 3–24. doi:10.1007/s10488-005-4235-1.
Rollman, B. L., Weinreb, L., Korsen, N., & Schulberg, H. C. (2006). Implementation of guideline-based care for depression in primary care. *Administration and Policy in Mental Health and Mental Health Services Research, 33*, 43–53.
Samson, A. Y., Bensen, S., Beck, A., Price, D., & Nimmer, C. (1999). Posttraumatic stress disorder in primary care. *The Journal of Family Practice, 48*, 222–227.
Saville-Troike, M. (2003). *The ethnography of communication: An introduction*. Malden, MA: Blackwell.
Smith, A., & Harkness, J. (2003). Genetic counseling and family therapy: Exploring present and future possibilities. *Family Therapy Magazine, 2*, 22–25.
Strosahl, K. (1996). Confessions of a behavior therapist in primary care: The odyssey and the ecstasy. *Cognitive and Behavioral Practice, 3*, 1–28. doi:10.1080/13561820802338579.

Strosahl, K. (2001). The integration of primary care and behavioral health: Type II changes in the era of managed care. In V. Follette (Ed.), *Integrated behavioral healthcare: Positioning mental health practice with medical/surgical practice* (pp. 45–69). San Diego, CA: Academic Press.

*Tyndall, L., Hodgson, J., Lamson, A., White, M., & Knight, S. (2012a). Medical family therapy: Charting a course in competencies. *Contemporary Family Therapy, 34*, 171–186. doi:10.1007/s10591-012-9191-9.

*Tyndall, L., Hodgson, J., Lamson, A., White, M., & Knight, S. (2012b). Medical family therapy: A theoretical and empirical review [Special issue]. *Contemporary Family Therapy, 34*, 156–170. doi:10.1007/s10591-012-9183-9.

Valleley, R. J., Kosse, S., Schemm, A., Foster, N., Polaha, J., & Evans, J. H. (2007). Integrated primary care for children in rural communities: An examination of patient attendance at collaborative behavioral health services. *Families, Systems & Health, 25*, 323–332. doi:10.1037/1091-7572.25.3.323.

Willerton, E., Dankoski, M. E., & Martir, J. F. S. (2008). Medical family therapy: A model for addressing mental health disparities among Latinos. *Families, Systems & Health, 26*, 196–206. doi:10.1037/1091-7572.26.2.196.

Williams, J., Shore, S. E., & Foy, J. M. (2006). Co-location of mental health professionals in primary care settings: Three North Carolina models. *Clinical Pediatrics, 45*, 537–543. doi:10.1177/0009922806290608.

Zaller, N., Gillani, F. S., & Rich, J. D. (2007). A model of integrated primary care for HIV-positive patients with underlying substance use and mental illness. *AIDS Care, 19*, 1128–1133. doi:10.1080/09540120701335196.

Chapter 6
Building Relationships in Integrated Care

Dan Marlowe and Jennifer Hodgson

The USA is fast approaching a tipping point regarding behavioral health integration in primary care. With the unique confluence of changes to medical education, the movement by the medical community toward the patient-centered medical home, and a push by both governmental and international organizations for behavioral health integration (Agency for Healthcare Research and Quality, 2008; Evans, 2011; Institute of Medicine, 2001; World Health Organization, 2008), Medical Family Therapists (MedFTs) practicing in integrated care (IC) settings are reaping the benefits of the last 40 years of hard work by the progenitors of this care typology. This persistent push toward the inclusion of behavioral health professionals in healthcare settings has yielded increasingly sophisticated models and effectiveness research (e.g., AHRQ, 2008; Funderburk et al., 2010; Oakley, Moore, Burford, Fahrenwald, & Woodard, 2005; Phelps, Hodgson, Lamson, Swanson, & White, 2011; Robinson & Reiter, 2007; Strosahl, 2001, 2005; Unutzer et al., 2002; Valleley et al., 2007), as well as a burgeoning conversation regarding the academic and practice-based competencies required for IC practice (e.g., Blount & Miller, 2009; Gunn & Blount, 2009; Hunter & Goodie, 2010; O'Donohue, Cummings, & Cummings, 2009; Peek, Baird, & Coleman, 2009; Strosahl, 2005; Tyndall, Hodgson, Lamson, White, & Knight, 2012).

Contemporary contributions to the literature have dealt mainly with the science (e.g., efficacy/effectiveness, mechanisms of activation, and knowledge and practice based competencies) and business (e.g., model development and implementation, financial viability, and marketing) areas of IC. However, the literature so far has not included discussion and description of the relational components to the process of integration, that is, the therapeutic ways of relating to those within the healthcare system that makes the implementation, practice, and maintenance of IC possible. Through presenting the process and practice of integration as different yet complimentary and equally essential pieces of a larger whole, it can be argued that

D. Marlowe (✉)
Campbell University School of Osteopathic Medicine, Buies Creek, NC, USA
e-mail: marlowed@campbell.edu

J. Hodgson et al. (eds.), *Medical Family Therapy*, DOI 10.1007/978-3-319-03482-9_6,

integration has as much to do with how the MedFT accepts and acknowledges his or her healthcare counterparts by continuously joining, building, and maintaining rapport (process), as it does with competent, evidence-based clinical practice.

Process vs. Practice

While the discussion of competencies for behavioral health providers, specifically related to integrated care, is a relatively recent one in contemporary literature (e.g., APA, 2013; Bischoff, Springer, Reisbig, Lyons, & Likcani, 2012; NASW, 2005; Tyndall et al., 2012), the conversation surrounding competencies related to interprofessional education and integrated health care has a more established foothold. Especially noteworthy is the Interprofessional Education Collaborative Expert Panel's (2011) report entitled *Core Competencies for Interprofessional Collaborative Practice*. This consortium from the American Associations of Nursing, Osteopathic Medicine, Colleges of Pharmacy, Dental Education, Medical Colleges, and Schools of Public Health describe five domains related to effective interprofessional collaboration: (a) Values/Ethics, Roles/Responsibilities, (b) Interprofessional Communication, and (c) Teams and Teamwork with a subsequent description of behaviors demonstrative of each (i.e., competencies). However, after reviewing their work and several of the base works, they cited (e.g., Blue, Zoller, Stratton, Elam, & Gilbert, 2010; Canadian Interprofessional Health Collaborative, 2010; D'Amour & Oandasan, 2005), their conclusions can be enhanced by: (a) addressing the distinction between intra- and inter-field collaboration (interprofessional vs. interdisciplinary vs. both) and (b) describing the process by which to achieve interprofessional and interdisciplinary collaborative practice.

Intra- vs. Inter-field Collaboration

Concern with the competencies as presented in the Interprofessional Education Collaborative Expert Panel's (2011) document and corresponding literature is the emphasis on interprofessional collaboration "within" rather than "between" fields. Professions within a field (e.g., medicine) share fundamental roots of pedagogy and taxonomy when it comes to training, practice, and ultimately, collaboration, although variations between professions within a field exist (e.g., allopathic vs. osteopathic physicians vs. nurses). However, as many authors have pointed out (e.g., Blount, 2003; Blount & Bayona, 1994; Doherty, 2007; Robinson & Reiter, 2007; Robinson & Strosahl, 2009; Seaburn, Lorenz, Gunn, Gawinski, & Mauksch, 1993; Strosahl, 1996, 2005), this is simply not the case when it comes to the behavioral health and healthcare fields in either taxonomy or pedagogical tradition. While a good point of reference, the use of these competencies as an isomorphic framework for integrated behavioral/medical healthcare education and/or practice is cautioned against since the major differences between the two are rooted in the behavioral health and healthcare fields (i.e., interdisciplinary), and not in our constituent professions only (i.e., interprofessional).

Competencies as Outcome

Another perhaps more fundamental concern is the discussion of competencies as behavioral "endpoints" with little to no conversation regarding the process by which those endpoints are reached. As has been discussed by academicians from both the health sciences and medical fields (e.g., Grant, 1999; Huddle & Heudebert, 2007), this presents a major concern since it produces professionals that "have a large repertoire of behavioral skills but [do] not have the tools necessary to place these skills within a wider social, humanistic, or scientific context. . ." (Brooks, 2009, p. 99), which creates an inability to apply that knowledge. Brooks (2009) further noted that highly skilled professionals not only know "how" to do something, but more importantly, "know what to do, and when, and why, and especially, when not to do something" (p. 99). If competencies are meant to describe general behaviors indicative of competent practice, and in this instance behaviors indicative of competent IC professionals (Strosahl, 2005), providers should be able to describe general avenues (i.e., processes) for how those behaviors might be reached.

Common Factors and Integration

While the dominant view of the process of integration in the USA has mainly dealt with the reconciliation of the three organizational aspects of IC practice and overall model development (i.e., Three-World view; Peek, 2008), we see common factors as one way of expanding this description to include the relational/therapeutic aspects of that process (Hubble, Duncan, & Miller, 1999; Lambert, 1992, Lambert & Cattani-Thompson, 1996). Especially relevant to this discussion are the systemic common factors outlined by Sprenkle and Blow (2004): (a) relational conceptualization of issues/solutions, (b) expansion of the treatment system, and (c) expansion of the therapeutic alliance. Taken together, these factors provide for how to conceptualize the multiple parts of the system (i.e., the three worlds) and how they work together. While working with any singular part, it is important to take a positive/strength-based disposition toward all parts of the system, even in the face of seemingly divergent goals. The ability of the MedFT to simultaneously form alliances with each individual member, subsystem, and entire system is critical to building a healthy system. It is the relational synergy provided by these factors that allows for reconciling these worlds and the ultimate functioning of any model. After all, if one applies Peek's (2008) Three-World view metaphor in its entirety, the goal of creating IC models that satisfy the requirements of each world is not to make the model relatable/translatable across the worlds themselves but for each world's constituent population.

Utilizing this relational approach to common factors, we view Peek's three worlds (2008) as interlocking gears comprising the internal structure of a system (i.e., an IC model) whose output is collaborative, biopsychosocial care. However, borrowing from the field of engineering (Kohara Gear Industry, internet), an odd number of touching gears will never turn due to the fact that each moves those connected to it in the opposite direction, which creates a *locked* system that cannot function. Only by the addition of a forth gear can the others move in sync with one another, thereby creating a sustainable set of relationships. This fourth gear that ultimately provides the connection between the others and allows for functionality is how we conceptualize the relational components of integration.

Components of Integration

Doherty, McDaniel, and Baird's (1996) description of integration alluded to these components through the description of how both healthcare providers and MedFTs "appreciate the importance of each other's roles" (p. 25), as well as develop an "understanding and appreciation for each other's...cultures" (p. 27). The importance of these concepts still endures today and is referenced in contemporary integrated care literature. Peek (2011, Fig. 6.1) pointed out that integrated systems are characterized as those having a *shared culture*., The assertion is that these general constructs are considered the *active ingredients* of interprofessional collaboration (Suter et al., 2009). Given their stated significance then, what does it mean to appreciate and understand, and more importantly, what is it about our ability to appreciate and understand one another as professionals and as people in a profession that facilitates integration?

Competency 1: Conceptual flexibility. Engel's (1977, 1980) biopsychosocial model begins the conversation regarding this conceptual flexibility by juxtaposing biomedical and psychosocial issues as simultaneously lived "human experiences as well as disease abstraction" (1977, p. 131). His assertion is not necessarily to do away with the medical model but instead "to broaden the approach to disease to include the psychosocial without sacrificing the enormous advantages of the biomedical approach" (p. 131). Although directed toward the medical profession, these ideas can be stretched to include the capacity of a MedFT to conceptualize psychosocial and biomedical issues as both "disease and problems of living," (p. 133) as well. To achieve this type of double description (Keeney, 1983), MedFTs must, as Doherty (2007) stated, "care about the patient's diabetes and headaches, not just the patient's depression and anxiety" (p. 128).

If we take Engel's (1977) position to heart, then whether we view depression as a pathophysiologic condition or as an attachment injury, we know that neither description captures the "trueness" or "rightness" of the condition (Bateson,

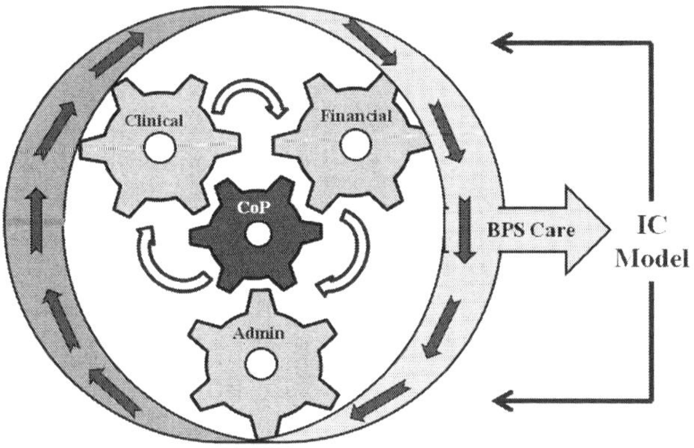

Fig. 6.1 A relational expansion of Peek's Three-World view

1972; Keeney, 1983). What these different descriptions do provide is a context for the coordinated conceptualization and treatment of the condition by healthcare provider, MedFT, and patient/family as a team (Shotter, 2008). The ability to integrate multiple descriptions of a problem is a proposed practice-based competency of IC as it relates to patient care (Strosahl, 2005). So this then begs the question how can a MedFT invite and integrate patients' descriptions while simultaneously dismissing the descriptions of their healthcare colleagues. From a more pragmatic standpoint, whether the MedFT does or does not wish to think from a pathophysiological perspective, the reimbursement system that allows for IC models to be financially sustainable in the USA requires providers to list a diagnosis (medical or mental) for payment to be disseminated.

Ultimately, it is this type of conceptual flexibility that allows us to forego, as Engel described, the "caste system…concerning what constitute appropriate areas for medical concern and care…" (1977, p. 135), whether that caste is medical or psychosocial in nature. The goal related to this component, then, is not to give up the underpinnings that inform how MedFTs understand therapeutic relationships and change (i.e., systemic/cybernetic/social constructionist). Instead, flexibility implies the inherent struggle to expand and connect the varying ways in which different parts of the team describe problems (i.e., biological or psychosocial), in order to provide more complete care for shared patients. Aside from MedFTs delivering psychotherapeutic interventions, common factors researchers imply that a therapist's fundamental skill is helping facilitate contexts and relationships in which change can occur (Blow, Sprenkle, & Davis, 2007; Keeney, 1987) regardless of the number of participants. So, while the MedFT may not be administering psychotherapeutic interventions to the healthcare professionals they work with, the way they relate to and engage healthcare providers, as psychotherapists, can in and of itself be considered a therapeutic act.

Competency 2: Understanding and acceptance. We cannot "not" communicate (Watzlawick, Beavin-Bavelas, & Jackson, 1967), and communication of any kind carries multiple messages embedded in the act itself. Adopting medical language, description of patient issues, and certain organizational customs demonstrates to the system the willingness of the newcomer (i.e., the MedFT) to acculturate (understand) and become a part of that system (acceptance). The importance of this component rests not only in what they offer their healthcare colleagues, but also recursively speaks to what they themselves want from those same professionals.

It is easy to misconstrue a healthcare provider as uncaring or apathetic to a patient's wants/needs when conflict arises (refusal of treatment by the patient, non-adherence, non-compliance, etc.), and/or when there is apprehension toward proposed changes in workflow resulting from the implementation of IC (e.g., introduction of psychosocial or substance abuse screening). Understanding, as a component, implies that MedFTs have extended themselves to see how an oncologist that pushes chemotherapy on a patient even when the patient declines, as well as a primary care provider who adamantly refuses to implement depression screening or behavioral consultation does so for good reason, even if that reason is not readily apparent.

What this means is that regardless of the concerns a healthcare provider might express towards implementing integrated care, little can be done to address those concerns if the MedFT makes an assumption about the motivations behind them (e.g., the healthcare team member is being difficult, she thinks she is better/smarter/more capable). However, while important, understanding is only one part of this competency, and ultimately means little without accepting the legitimacy of those expressed concerns. Acceptance in this vein does not necessarily mean agreement (Anderson, 1996), but that those concerns have been understood well enough within the contexts of those that voiced them (Marlowe, 2013). Only by demonstrating an openness to understanding why such actions are taken or not taken and the acceptance of their legitimacy, can the work then begin to move past the barriers to interprofessional collaboration.

If a healthcare provider refuses to screen for depression, stating that a lack of access to behavioral health services as one of the reasons for that refusal, and the MedFT in response leverages the argument that depression screening is a vital sign like blood pressure or "only" takes 2 min to complete, can that MedFT truly argue that he or she understands and accepts the validity of the concerns expressed by the provider? Rather than arguing their point on why a depression screen should be given, a MedFT who engages those same healthcare providers in a conversation regarding what would have to happen (practically and logistically) for screening to make sense for them to implement, will not only find mutually agreeable solutions but also demonstrate understanding and acceptance of the healthcare provider's concerns. A fundamental error that MedFTs often make when entering into a new healthcare setting is to assume all healthcare providers will see the extension of new services (i.e., behavioral health) as necessary, beneficial, and/or both. In addition, while one provider or administrator may be ready to adopt an integrated paradigm, all the providers in that setting may not buy into its implementation equally or at all. This requires that the

MedFT understand and accept each provider's position on integrated care prior to implementation of even the best evidence-based models. It is this attempt to not only understand, but accept the validity of stated concerns, that facilitates entrance into a system relationally and respectfully.

Competency 3: Acknowledgement and appreciation. Acknowledgement relates to one's ability as a MedFT to understand the inherent differences between themselves and their healthcare colleagues, as well as the reflexive professional and personal appraisal of the essential and nonessential differences separating the two fields. What this means is that as MedFTs acculturate to healthcare contexts, and by doing so shift their own thinking and practice, they must remember that even though they might walk, talk, and to some degree act like healthcare providers (e.g., wear a white coat, carry a pager, chart in the electronic health record) they are not healthcare providers trained in medicine.

This may seem like a self-defeating outlook given the hard work that has gone into alignment with healthcare professionals; however, while the attempt to tone down differences may lead to understanding of and acceptance by a healthcare system, it is their essential differences that ultimately make integration a meaningful endeavor. As alluded to by Doherty and colleagues (1996), it is this act of acknowledging difference that allows behavioral health and healthcare providers to find utility in working together. In knowing and acknowledging differences and the concomitant strengths and limitations of each discipline and profession, each is better able to appreciate what unique contribution the other makes to patient care. Ultimately, it is this appreciation for one another that allows for the "conscious [effort] to balance power and influence among the professionals according to their roles and areas of expertise," (p. 28) as well as the creation of a system of care in which "all professionals are committed to a biopsychosocial/systems paradigm and have developed an in-depth understanding of each other's roles and cultures" (p. 28). This is when and where the practice of IC, as envisioned, can actually occur.

In practice this may look like asking patients, patient support systems (e.g., families, friends), and members of the healthcare team how a transition to providing IC would best look like for them. Appreciating the existing workflow model, professional habits, and patient expectations with their visits may help MedFTs find a way to coexist that is both less threatening and more sustaining, and acknowledging the culture of and around that system may subsequently open pathways to change not otherwise available. Balancing strength-based observation with a *wondering and curious* approach to change (Anderson & Gehert, 2007) may reflect a way to help transform a practice that recognizes and respects the existing hierarchy and organizational/professional traditions already in place.

Conclusion

Ultimately, the importance of any set of IC competencies lies in the distinction between the practice of IC and the on-going relationships needed to help facilitate it. Even though IC has gained traction over the last ten years through the proliferation of programs that engage in some form of IC practice, it is far from being the standard of care. As such, many MedFTs (either experienced or new) looking to move into this area will more than likely find that the they have to help build these sites from the ground up, or as so aptly put, that they will *build the ship as they sail it* (Baird, 1995). Integrated care is not simply about placing MedFTs in healthcare settings, as many authors have previously noted, nor is it only about the evidence-based models they use.

If one is to take a closer look at the literature detailing the conceptual frameworks informing how these settings are constructed (e.g., Blount, 2003; Doherty et al., 1996), the determinants of difference center on how both MedFTs and healthcare providers relate to and with one another, which is implicitly couched in how they practice. These components speak to the idea that the relationships between MedFT, healthcare provider, patient, and the healthcare system are the vehicles through which the practice of integrated care is actualized, and is not solely contingent on nor determined by the specific ways in which the MedFT engages in psychotherapeutic intervention. Relating this to a ship metaphor, if the practice of integrated care is the ship itself, then these relational components provide the buoyancy necessary to help navigate the sometimes-turbulent waters of interprofessional care.

Discussion Questions

1. Name one way the author achieves explanation of each one of the competencies stated in the introduction.
2. Provide an example of how a MedFT might join, build, and maintain rapport with the healthcare team.
3. Brooks (2009) stated that it is just as important to "know what to do, and when, and why, and especially, when not do to something" (p. 99). Discuss this statement and instances in which you have found it true during training, practice, or research.
4. Give an example of points that you may make to a healthcare provider that refuses to screen a patient for depression using the example in competency 2 as your guide.
5. As stated in the chapter, it is important to have a *wondering and curious approach* to change. Discuss your interpretation of this statement, explaining why this is important.

References

Agency for Healthcare Research and Quality. (2008). *Integration of mental health/substance abuse and primary care (No. 173)*. Rockville, MD: AHRQ.

American Psychological Association Interorganizational Work Group on Competencies for Primary Care Psychology. (2013). *Competencies for psychology practice in primary care*. Retrieved from http://www.apa.org/ed/resources/competencies-practice.pdf.

Anderson, H. (1996). A reflection on client-professional collaboration. *Family, Systems, & Health, 14*, 193–206. doi:10.1037/h0089814.

Anderson, H., & Gehert, D. (2007). *Collaborative therapy: Relationships and conversations that make a difference*. New York, NY: Routledge.

Baird, M. (1995). Building the ship as we sail it. *Family Systems Medicine, 13*, 269–273. doi:10.1037/h0089066.

Bateson, G. (1972). *Steps to an ecology of mind*. Northvale, NJ: Jason Aronson.

Bischoff, R. J., Springer, P. R., Reisbig, A. M. J., Lyons, S., & Likcani, A. (2012). Training for collaboration: Collaborative practice skills for mental health professionals. *Journal of Marital and Family Therapy, 38*, 199–210. doi:10.1111/j.1752-0606.2012.00299.x.

Blount, A. (2003). Integrated primary care: Organizing the evidence. *Families, Systems, & Health, 21*, 121–133.

Blount, A., & Bayona, J. (1994). Toward a system of integrated primary care. *Families, Systems, & Health, 12*, 171–182. doi:10.1037/h0089151.

Blount, A., & Miller, B. (2009). Addressing the workforce crisis in integrated primary care. *Journal of Clinical Psychology in Medical Settings, 16*, 113–119. doi:10.1007/s10880-008-9142-7.

Blow, A. J., Sprenkle, D. H., & Davis, S. D. (2007). Is who delivers the treatment more important than the treatment itself? The role of the therapist in common facts. *Journal of Marital and Family Therapy, 33*(3), 298–317. doi:10.1111/j.1467-6427.2007.00375.x.

Blue, A. V., Zoller, J., Stratton, T. D., Elam, C. L., & Gilbert, J. (2010). Interprofessional education in US medical schools. *Journal of Interprofessional Care, 24*, 204–206. doi:10.3109/13561820903442887.

Brooks, M. A. (2009). Medical education and the tyranny of competency. *Perspectives in Biology and Medicine, 52*, 90–102. doi:10.1353/pbm.0.0068.

Canadian Interprofessional Health Collaborative. (2010, February). *A national interprofessional competency framework*. Retrieved April 3, 2012 from http://www.cihc.ca/resources/publications.

D'Amour, D., & Oandasan, I. (2005). Interprofessionality as the field of interprofessional practice and interprofessional education: An emerging concept. *Journal of Interprofessional Care, 19* (Suppl 1), 8–20. doi:10.1080/13561820500081604.

Doherty, W. (2007). Fixing health care: What role will therapists play? *Psychotherapy Networker, 31*(3), 24–60.

Doherty, W. J., McDaniel, S. H., & Baird, M. A. (1996). Five levels of primary care/behavioral healthcare collaboration. *Behavioral Healthcare Tomorrow, 5*(5), 25–28.

Engel, G. L. (1977). The need for a new medical model: A challenge for biomedicine. *Science, 196*, 129–136. doi:10.1126/science.847460.

Engel, G. L. (1980). The clinical application of the biopsychosocial model. *American Journal of Psychiatry, 137*, 535–544.

Evans, D. (2011). The patient-centered medical home as a curricular model: Medical students need an "educational home". *Academic Medicine, 86*, e2. doi:10.1097/ACM.0b013e318232df7f.

Funderburk, J. S., Sugarman, D. E., Maisto, S. A., Ouimette, P., Schohn, M., Lantinga, L., … & Strutynski, K. (2010). The description and evaluation of the implementation of an integrated healthcare model. *Families, Systems, & Health, 28*, 146–160. doi: 10.1037/a0020223.

Grant, J. (1999). The incapacitating effects of competence: A critique. *Advances in Health Sciences Education, 4*, 271–277.

Gunn, W. B., Jr., & Blount, A. (2009). Primary care mental health: A new frontier for psychology. *Journal of Clinical Psychology, 65*, 235–252. doi:10.1002/jclp.20499.

Hubble, M. A., Duncan, B. L., & Miller, S. D. (1999). *The heart and soul of change: What works in therapy*. Washington, DC: American Psychological Association.

Huddle, T. S., & Heudebert, G. R. (2007). Taking apart the art: The risk of anatomizing clinical competence. Viewpoint. *Academic Mecicine, 82*, 536–541. doi:10.1097/ACM.0b013e3180555935.

Hunter, C. L., & Goodie, J. L. (2010). Operational and clinical components for integrated-collaborative behavioral healthcare in the patient-centered medical home. *Families, Systems, & Health, 28*, 308–321. doi:10.1037/a0021761.

Institute of Medicine. (2001). *Crossing the quality chasm: A new health system for the 21st century*. Washington, DC: National Academy Press.

Interprofessional Education Collaborative Expert Panel. (2011). *Core competencies for interprofessional collaborative practice: Report of an expert panel*. Washington, DC: Interprofessional Education Collaborative.

Keeney, B. P. (1983). *Aesthetics of change*. New York, NY: The Guilford Press.

Keeney, B. P. (1987). The construction of therapeutic realities. *Psychotherapy, 24*, 469–476. doi:10.1037/h0085744.

Kohara Gear Industry. (internet). *Practial information on gears*. Retrived from http://www.khkgears.co.jp/en/gear_technology/pdf/gear_guide2.pdf.

Lambert, M. J. (1992). Psychotherapy outcome research: Implications for integrative and eclectic therapists. In J. C. Norcross & M. R. Goldfried (Eds.), *Handbook of psychotherapy integration* (pp. 94–129). New York, NY: Basic Books.

Lambert, M. J., & Cattani-Thompson, K. (1996). Current findings regarding the effectiveness of counseling: Implications for practice. *Journal of Counseling and Development, 74*, 601–608. doi:10.002/j.1556-6676.1996.tb02299.x.

Marlowe, D. (2013). Bridging conversations: Discussing the intra-professional relationship between medical family therapy and family therapy. *Journal of Family Therapy, 35*, 119–138. doi:10.1111/j.1467-6427.2011.00553.x.

National Association of Social Workers. (2005). *NASW standards for social work practice in health care settings*. Retrieved from http://www.socialworkers.org/practice/standards/NASWHealthCareStandards.pdf.

O'Donohue, W. T., Cummings, N. A., & Cummings, J. L. (2009). The unmet educational agenda in integrated care. *Journal of Clinical Psychology in Medical Settings, 16*, 94–100. doi:10.1007/s10880-008-9138-3.

Oakley, C., Moore, D., Burford, D., Fahrenwald, R., & Woodard, K. (2005). The Montana model: Integrated primary care and behavioral health in a family practice residency program. *The Journal of Rural Health, 21*, 351–354. doi:10.1111/j.1748-0361.2005.tb00106.x.

Peek, C. J. (2008). Planning care in the clinical, operational, and financial worlds. In R. Kessler & D. Stafford (Eds.), *Collaborative medicine case studies: Evidence in practice*. New York, NY: Springer.

Peek, C. J. (2011). A collaborative care lexicon for asking practice and research development questions. In C. Mullican (Ed.), *A national agenda for research in collaborative care: Papers from the collaborative care research network research development conference* (pp. 25–41). Rockville, MD: Agency for Healthcare Research and Quality.

Peek, C. J., Baird, M. A., & Coleman, E. (2009). Primary care for patient complexity, not only disease. *Families, Systems, & Health, 27*, 287–302. doi:10.1037/a0018048.

Phelps, K., Hodgson, J., Lamson, A., Swanson, M., & White, M. (2011). Satisfaction with life and psychosocial factors among ethnic minorities with type 2 diabetes. *Social Indicators Research, 106*, 359–370. doi:10.1007/s11205-011-9811-z.

Robinson, P. J., & Reiter, J. T. (2007). *Behavioral consultation and primary care: A guide to integrating services*. New York, NY: Springer.

Robinson, P. J., & Strosahl, K. D. (2009). Behavioral health consultation and primary care: Lessons learned. *Journal of Clinical Psychology in Medical Settings, 16*, 58–71. doi:10.1007/s10880-009-9145-z.
Seaburn, D. B., Lorenz, A. D., Gunn, W. B., Gawinski, B. A., & Mauksch, L. B. (1993). *Models of collaboration: A guide for mental health professionals working with health care practitioners*. Oakland, CA: Basic Books.
Shotter, R. G. (2008). *Conversational realities revisited: Life, language, body and world*. Chagrin Falls, OH: Taos Institute Publications.
Sprenkle, D. H., & Blow, A. J. (2004). Common factors and our sacred models. *Journal of Marital and Family Therapy, 30*, 113–129. doi:10.1111/j.1752-0606.2004.tb01228.x.
Strosahl, K. (1996). Confessions of a behavior therapist in primary care: The odyssey and the ecstasy. *Cognitive and Behavioral Practice, 3*, 1–28. doi:10.1016/S1077-7229(96)80028-9.
Strosahl, K. (2001). The integration of primary care and behavioral health: Type II changes in the era of managed care. In V. Follette (Ed.), *Integrated behavioral healthcare: Positioning mental health practice with medical/surgical practice* (pp. 45–69). San Diego, CA: Academic.
Strosahl, K. (2005). Training behavioral health and medical providers for integrated care: A core competencies approach. In W. O'Donohoe, N. Cummings, M. Byrd, & D. Henderson (Eds.), *Behavioral integrative care: Treatments that work in the primary care setting*. New York, NY: BrunnerRoutledge.
Suter, E., Arndt, J., Arthur, N., Parboosingh, J., Taylor, E., & Deutschlander, S. (2009). Role understanding and effective communication as core competencies of collaborative practice. *Journal of Interprofessional Care, 23*, 41–51. doi:10.1080/13561820802338579.
Tyndall, L., Hodgson, J., Lamson, A., White, M., & Knight, S. (2012). Medical family therapy: Charting a course in competencies. *Contemporary Family Therapy*. doi:10.1007/s10591-012-9191-9.
Unützer, J., Katon, W., Callahan, C. M., Williams, J. W. Jr., Hunkeler, E., Harpole, L., ... & Langston, C. (2002). Collaborative care management of late-life depression in the primary care setting: A randomized controlled trial. *Journal of the American Medical Association*. 288:2836–2845. doi: 10.1001/jama.288.22.2836.
Valleley, R. J., Kosse, S., Schemm, A., Foster, N., Polaha, J., & Evans, J. H. (2007). Integrated primary care for children in rural communities: An examination of patient attendance at collaborative behavioral health services. *Families, Systems, & Health, 25*, 323–332. doi:10.1037/1091-7527.25.3.323.
Watzlawick, P., Beavin-Bavelas, J., & Jackson, D. (1967). *Pragmatics of human communication: A study of interactional patterns, pathologies and paradoxes*. New York, NY: W. W. Norton.
World Health Organization. (2008). *Integrating mental health into primary care a global perspective*. Geneva: World Health Organization.

Chapter 7
Working with Providers and Healthcare Systems Experiencing Compassion Fatigue and Burnout

Angela Lamson, Patrick Meadors, and Tai Mendenhall

> In 'caring for the carers,' the challenge for health care organizations lies in developing respect and care for their employees in the same way that they require their employees to care for patients.—Wright (2004).

Over the last two decades, there has been a marked increase in the number of researchers who have focused on the operational definitions and prevalence of terms related to personal and professional trauma (e.g., Abendroth & Flannery, 2006; Brosche, 2003; Collins & Long, 2003; Figley, 2013; Lynch & Lobo, 2012; Maytum, Heiman, & Garwick, 2004; Meadors & Lamson, 2008; Meadors, Lamson, & Sira, 2010; Meadors, Lamson, Swanson, White, & Sira, 2009; Morse, Salyers, Rollins, Monroe-DeVita, & Pfahler, 2012; Paris & Hoge, 2010; Pfifferling & Gilley, 2000; Sabo, 2006; Schwam, 1998). With this increased volume of research, there has also been an increase in conceptual ambiguity in terms such as compassion fatigue and burnout.

Compassion fatigue has traditionally been associated with familial caregivers (Day & Anderson, 2011; Lynch & Lobo, 2012), and burnout has been the subject of publications ranging from retail (e.g., Cho, Rutherford, & Park, 2013; Chung, Rutherford, & Park, 2012; Rutherford et al., 2011) to behavioral health (e.g., Acker, 2012; Lim, Kim, Kim, Yang, & Lee, 2010; Morse et al., 2012; Paris & Hoge, 2010). Regardless, compassion fatigue and burnout can impact the well-being of both providers and the patients and families that they serve. It is up to all professionals to further develop an understanding of these terms to ensure the greatest level of awareness (Figley, 2002; Meadors et al., 2010; Meadors et al., 2009) and, thus, utilization of best practices toward self-care and sustainability in one's profession. If medical family therapists (MedFTs) fail in raising this awareness, many valuable providers could suffer from physical or emotional health problems, be involved with increased practice-related errors and ethical breaches, or hurt patients. This occupational hazard is especially risky among providers who

A. Lamson (✉)
East Carolina University, Greenville, NC, USA
e-mail: lamsona@ecu.edu

J. Hodgson et al. (eds.), *Medical Family Therapy*, DOI 10.1007/978-3-319-03482-9_7,

work with traumatized patients (Figley, 2013; Meadors & Lamson, 2008; Meadors et al., 2010).

The purpose of this chapter is to provide operational definitions for compassion fatigue (CF) and burnout (BRN) in a healthcare context based on research conducted with diverse medical and behavioral health providers (e.g., Meadors & Lamson, 2008; Meadors et al., 2009, 2010). In addition, the authors delineate research initiatives and outcomes from different healthcare contexts that may help training programs and MedFTs implement proactive approaches to prevent these debilitating professional hazards. Without a clear understanding of these concepts, and the systemic consequences associated with CF and BRN, it is likely that presenteeism (e.g., likelihood for practice-related errors, decreased productivity) and absenteeism (e.g., increased sick days, greater staff turnover) will emerge or be sustained in the providers' lives (Pfifferling & Gilley, 2000). These issues are especially important given the long work hours in health care. In addition, there are high demands in caring for others' lives, in particular, for those who are served in emergency departments, intensive care, wounded warrior units, or in fieldwork (natural and/or human-caused disaster areas) where providers are even more likely to encounter individuals in crisis or who experience a traumatic event (Peckham, 2013; Spickard, Gabbe, & Christensen, 2002). This chapter concludes with personal and professional recommendations that promote self-care in MedFTs and that can also be taught to other healthcare staff and providers faced with traumatic experiences and/or struggling in their professional contexts.

Compassion Fatigue and Burnout in Health Care

A majority of the US population will experience trauma within their lifetime and some will experience multiple traumas firsthand (Bride, 2007). More specifically, trauma exposure rates range from 40 to 81 %, with close to 20 % of males and 12 % of females exposed to multiple traumas in their lifetime (Breslau, Davis, Peterson, & Schultz, 1997; Kessler, Sonnega, Bromet, Hughes & Nelson, 1995; Stein, Walker, Hazen, & Forde, 1997). While women tend to be exposed to fewer traumas, researchers indicate that women are slightly more likely to report post-traumatic stress disorder (PTSD), depression, or suicidal thoughts when compared with men (24 % compared to 19 %) (Hoge, Auchterlonie, & Milliken, 2006). Certainly, these figures increase for those in military health contexts. Several researchers have focused on the effect of *direct* exposure to a traumatic event (i.e., primary traumatization) on an individual's well-being (Bride, Robinson, Yegidis, & Figley, 2004). However, as the field of traumatology has grown, it has become apparent that those who experience *indirect* exposure to a traumatic event (i.e., secondary trauma) endure similar distress and grief as those who experienced the event directly (Figley, 1999).

The incidence of indirect exposure to trauma may be most significant and heightened for behavioral health providers (such as MedFTs) and healthcare professionals (such as emergency department physicians or extenders, chaplains, and emergency medical technicians) who provide care for emotionally, physically, and sexually traumatized individuals.

It is particularly important in healthcare contexts to have clarity in trauma-related symptom development and management given the degree to which providers and extenders are inundated with direct and indirect exposure and coping strategies of traumatized patients. After all, healthcare providers are expected to overcome symptoms related to trauma, given real or pseudo beliefs about healthcare providers' ability to go from patient to patient with little or no emotional connection (Clark & Gioro, 1998; Rossler, 2012; Salyers et al., 2011; Showalter, 2010). Clark and Gioro (1998) maintained, however, that nurses and other providers are not immune from feelings associated with direct and indirect exposure to trauma. All healthcare professionals must recognize these feelings (e.g., that it is acceptable to grieve the loss of a patient) and develop a support network to help them cope. Unfortunately, many healthcare professionals have stated that lack of time to recover from trauma or loss experiences (e.g., repeated deaths and non-accidental traumas on a unit) has made it difficult to cope with caring for the traumatized (Figley, 2013; Pfifferling & Gilley, 2000), often leading them to be the hidden grievers in their patients' lives. While not every provider may go on to experience post-traumatic stress (PTS) or PTSD, some may recognize that their ability to care for patients is altered due to the complex interactions between their energy and empathy for patients (Figley, 1995, 2013).

Compassion Fatigue

Compassion fatigue (CF) was first introduced by Joinson (1992) in reference to nurses who were challenged by the everyday rigors of their emergency room duties. Valent (2002) interpreted CF as a specific form of secondary trauma that resulted from "deep involvement with a primarily traumatized person" (p. 19). This interpretation closely aligns with Figley's description (1995, 2013), whereby CF is suggested to be the consequence of working with traumatized individuals in combination with a strong empathic orientation. Compassion fatigue is also associated with a caregiver's reduced capacity to be empathic for a suffering individual (Adams, Boscarino, & Figley, 2006). By including the word "compassion" in the name for CF, the term takes on a different connotation than "secondary traumatization" or "vicarious traumatization" (Figley, 2013; McCann & Pearlman, 1990). Sabo (2006) argued that empathy is an essential component in a helping relationship, and at the core of a helping relationship is the ability to empathize with someone in need while still being able to provide help in a time of crisis. Healthcare providers must find the appropriate balance of empathy and compassion while working with a traumatized population.

Healthcare providers are expected to care for multiple patients, and the death of one patient may be followed at any time by another demanding or traumatized patient. Sabo (2006) and Hooper, Craig, Janvrin, Wetsel, and Reimels (2010), for example, found that nurses suffer from CF due to their consistent care for traumatized patients. Consistent and prolonged exposure to traumatized populations creates a cumulative effect for providers who have little time to grieve the loss or trauma of the first patient before caring for the next one. In an attempt to compensate for this lack of time, physicians and other medical and behavioral health professionals multitask and thereby decrease the perceived need for utilization of coping strategies that would allow them to overcome symptoms of CF (Pfifferling & Gilley, 2000). Figley's (2002, 2013) conceptual model identified ten key components that influence an individual's empathic response and residual compassion stress that ultimately drives toward the development of CF. In general, Figley suggests that prolonged exposure to trauma along with our natural empathic ability and life stressors can potentially lead providers to develop CF. While CF is one dimension of concern for providers' care of patients, the majority of research on the emotional well-being of healthcare providers has been related more to burnout (Grandey, Foo, Groth, & Goodwin, 2012; Salyers et al., 2011).

Burnout

"Burnout has been conceptualized as a defensive response to prolonged occupational exposure to demanding interpersonal situations that produce psychological strain and provide inadequate support" (Jenkins & Baird, 2002, p. 424). Demerouti, Bakker, Nachreiner, and Ebbinghaus (2002) further defined this phenomenon as prolonged exposure to mental strain that can be attributed to inadequate job design. According to Veninga and Spradley (1981), there are five stages of BRN, from stage one (honeymoon stage marked by high job satisfaction and commitment) through stage five (enmeshment whereby the symptoms of burnout are embedded into the person's life and she is more likely to be labeled as having something physically or emotionally wrong with her rather than being attributed to burnout).

Burnout has been found to have significant overlap with compassion fatigue (Baird & Kracen, 2006; Figley, 2002; Jenkins & Baird, 2002; Meadors et al., 2009) while at the same time having its own unique features. Someone who is experiencing BRN may have psychophysiological arousal symptoms (e.g., sleep disturbance, aggression, irritability) and exhibit mental and physical exhaustion resulting in lack of productivity and increased problems in work relationships, whether exposed to a traumatized patient or not (Valent, 2002). Much of the mental strain from jobs associated with BRN has been found to be organizationally related (e.g., administration, supervision, and paperwork) rather than operationally related (e.g., caring for victims, danger, trauma) (Brief & Weiss, 2002). Thus, it can be inferred that

BRN does not require the presence of a trauma or an empathic response. After all, BRN exists among a variety of professions such as banking, retail, and office work (Cho et al., 2013; Chung et al., 2012; Rutherford et al., 2011). Valent's (2002) definition further differentiates BRN from CF by stating that burnout is the result of frustration and an inability to achieve work goals, typically based on work stressors or management pressures. More specifically, Maslach and Leiter (2008) suggested that that there are six systemic sources of burnout, consisting of work overload, lack of control, insufficient rewards, unfairness, breakdown in a sense of community, and conflicts in values.

While the negative attributes of burnout have been widely researched, literature also exists on the buffering factors that may prevent it (e.g., support in the workplace, number of years on the unit, and workload) (Chang et al., 2006). Maytum and colleagues (2004) highlighted many of the personal (e.g., self-care activities, sense of humor, supportive relationships) and professional (e.g., time away from work, attending in-services, developing awareness of personal triggers) coping strategies that nurses have employed to deal with symptoms of BRN. Interestingly, nurses have been a focal point in research with very little attention given to the role of burnout in the lives of behavioral health providers, such as MedFTs. Thus, the following section will attend to projects that have been completed by MedFTs. The authors clarify roles that MedFTs can take to reduce CF and BRN for patients, providers, and self via training, technology, research, and projects within unique clinical contexts.

MedFTs Incorporating Education and Training

The licensure, certification, and professional training for MedFTs and most healthcare professionals emphasize the importance of continuing education to provide the best patient care. This continual learning process is essential in staying current with best practices and the ever-changing landscape of the healthcare system. Using continuing education modules as a mechanism to raise provider awareness and proactively identify symptoms and self-care strategies for CF and BRN is one way that training programs and healthcare systems can address this occupational hazard. Continuing education seminars have increased awareness of compassion fatigue symptoms and prevention/management strategies (Meadors & Lamson, 2008).

One example of using continuing education to proactively address symptoms of provider CF and BRN occurred in North Carolina. After an inpatient pediatric healthcare team experienced a difficult patient loss, the unit's management team realized the importance of addressing staff needs related to this child's death. With the existing research on the effectiveness of continuing education, the nurse managers, pharmacists, nurse educators, and MedFTs proposed a series of educational seminars that would focus on provider self-care and grief-work strategies. Through the interdisciplinary collaboration between the MedFT and nurse management teams, an educational module was developed around Figley's compassion fatigue and compassion stress model (Figley, 1995, 1997, 2002). The MedFTs provided the training over a 3-week period in five separate presentations to over 200 pediatric and neonatal healthcare providers and staff (Meadors et al., 2010).

The educational module objectives were (a) explore the interaction between personal and professional stressors, (b) understand the biopsychosocial symptoms associated with compassion fatigue and burnout, (c) gain knowledge about factors associated with grief as it pertains to compassion fatigue, (d) acquire and practice techniques to manage grief and compassion fatigue, and (e) learn about the purpose of a comfort team and personal/professional resources. In conjunction with the education module/training, the MedFTs organized and implemented a "comfort team" as a debriefing/forum for providers and staff to process their own grief in healthy ways. These comfort teams were incorporated into the Pediatric, Pediatric Intensive Care, and Neonatal Intensive Care Units, as well as into new policies and procedures for the management of patient deaths on those units.

As MedFTs, we can assist healthcare organizations in initiating more educational opportunities on the care of providers that include continuing education credits toward professional development. This educational module increased awareness of the symptoms of CF and reduced self-reported clinical stress levels (Meadors & Lamson, 2008; see Meadors et al., 2010 for a full description of training program). This module is one example of how continuing education can effectively address short-term implications of CF or BRN.

MedFTs Incorporating Technology

Healthcare researchers, educators, and providers are working to advance best practices in integrated care. At the University of Minnesota, for example, professionals across several departments and health organizations have responded to the need for targeted attention to CF prevention by developing an interactive cell phone app (available for iPhone, iPad, and Android) that engages healthcare workers (behavioral health + biomedical) in a variety of ways outside of and during care provision. This self-care app is purposefully biopsychosocial-spiritual in its scope; it includes personalizable checklists, prompts, record keeping, and tracking mechanisms to help providers tend to their physical needs (e.g., hydration, eating, exercise, relaxation, sleep), emotional health (e.g., reflections, debriefings, processing), and relational and social support (e.g., group sequences, family reminders). It includes close-ended and open-ended platforms to process personal functioning and workplace experiences, alongside links to empirically grounded online assessments of deployment readiness and ongoing provider well-being. Stimulating and interesting tips explain why certain aspects of self-care are vital. The app is currently undergoing final pilot testing and refinement and will be available to the public in 2014. For more information (and to access the app), go to http://www.sph.umn.edu/ce/perl/mobile/.

MedFTs Incorporating Research

After a series of meetings over the course of a year with diverse medical and behavioral health providers, a team of MedFTs from East Carolina University started working to better understand concepts associated with secondary trauma in an effort to develop more effective methods of addressing provider symptoms. This team of researchers conducted a study with pediatric providers nationwide to explore the overlap and differences between the terms related to secondary traumatization: PTSD, secondary traumatic stress (STS), CF, and BRN (Meadors et al., 2009). The primary aims for this research included: (a) How do the concepts of PTSD, STS, CF, and BRN differ? and (b) Are BRN symptoms correlated to higher symptom levels of STS and/or CF? Secondary aims included: (a) Which of these trauma-related issues are most prevalent in pediatric healthcare providers? (b) Do individuals within different disciplines suffer more from PTSD, STS, CF, and/or BRN? (c) Are hours of direct patient care correlated to higher levels of PTSD, STS, BRN, and/or CF? and (d) Are demographic factors, experiences with trauma, STS, PTSD, or BRN predictive of higher levels of CF?

Researchers assessed 167 providers and extenders (physicians, nurses, chaplains, child life specialists, and other healthcare professionals) located nationwide who were currently employed by a pediatric intensive care unit, neonatal intensive care unit, and/or pediatric unit or had been employed in one of these units within the year of assessment. The participant pool was predominantly female ($n = 137$). Five questions in the survey related to the type of traumatizing events that participants' experienced: (a) When was the last time that you were involved with a pediatric or neonatal patient death? (b) When have you directly cared for a patient who was traumatized? (c) How many traumatized patients have you cared for in the past month? (d) How many hours of direct patient care do you have in a typical day? and (e) What is the acuity level of the patients that you directly care for? The Secondary Traumatic Stress Scale (Bride et al., 2004) (to assess secondary traumatic stress), the Professional Quality of Life Scale (Stamm, 2002) (to assess compassion fatigue and burnout), and the Impact of Events Scale-Revised (Weiss & Marmar, 1997) (to assess post-traumatic stress) were also utilized to capture these unique overlapping concepts.

Providers who reported higher levels of BRN also reported higher levels of CF; however, this does not suggest a causal relationship between BRN and CF. In addition, chaplains were found to have a higher prevalence of CF than any of the other professions. Thus, there may be something unique within the chaplaincy profession or prevalence by which chaplains interface with traumatized patients (e.g., higher empathic ability or response) that may put chaplains at greater risk for CF. This study was one of the first known studies to attempt to quantitatively differentiate between the terms associated with secondary trauma. The findings suggested that each of the terms of BRN, CF, and STS was conceptually different from one another, which may alter the way that healthcare organizations or training programs recognize and manage them. These conceptual delineations have the potential to influence the unique manners in which MedFTs care for themselves (i.e., trauma-based symptoms versus work overload) and also how MedFTs approach the management, educational, or clinical techniques related to occupational risks to healthcare providers and staff. Furthermore, conceptual clarity strengthens the rigor for future research conducted by MedFTs in these areas.

MedFTs in Unique Contexts

Natural and Human-Caused Disasters

MedFTs represent a relatively new addition to the larger field of traumatology. They bring with them a worldview that is comfortable with the systemic complexities of overlapping human and relationship systems. This worldview also makes valuable contributions to the way in which fieldwork is conducted and the manner in which interdisciplinary teams function on the ground (Mendenhall & Berge, 2010). However, MedFTs working at disaster sites are arguably at greater risk for CF and BRN than their clinic- or hospital-based (only) colleagues, as they are doing potentially dangerous fieldwork in addition to the complex work that matches what they already do in clinics or hospitals.

The heartbreaking nature of surviving victims' stories, from their content alone to the repeated exposure of verbalized or similar content, can wear down MedFTs and other providers serving within behavioral health capacities. Simultaneously, the providers' experiences of sitting with surviving victims as they continue to endure the loss, ambiguity, and pain of trauma poses great risk for CF or BRN. For example, when the third author (Mendenhall) deployed with a team following a tsunami that devastated an entire coastal region, providers heard over and over again stories of how parents fleeing from the waves had to choose at the last moment which one of the two children they were running with (whose hands they were holding) to let go of so that they could grab hold of a tree or street sign in hopes of saving one. Hearing a single story like this could be difficult, but team members heard different versions of this story hundreds of times. Others sat with families and perused thousands of pictures of dead bodies that had been taken shortly before they were buried in mass graves, crying with families when they finally found a picture of a loved one (confirming death) or when they did not (prolonging their ambiguous loss). In human-caused disasters, many of the same types of sequences can follow, alongside a more difficult element of meaning-making (i.e., while someone can potentially narrate a natural disaster to an "act of God" or nature's randomness, this is difficult to do with airplanes flying into buildings or bombs exploding at a public sporting event) (Mendenhall, 2006a, 2006b; Mendenhall & Berge, 2010).

Compassion fatigue and BRN symptoms that MedFTs see most commonly in fieldwork cut across our own biopsychosocial-spiritual systems, just as the effects of trauma and disaster do with the patients and families we serve. Physically, insomnia is one of the most concerning culprits, alongside fatigue, headaches, and gastrointestinal distress. Behaviorally, providers sometimes find themselves abusing alcohol or drugs (often in an attempt to combat their insomnia), being irritable with colleagues, or avoiding the principal roles of fieldwork they are assigned to (e.g., wandering over to offer logistic support in a supply tent instead of talking with people who are suffering). Psychologically, providers oftentimes find themselves feeling depressed or angry, struggle with concentration or memory, or experience emotional numbing or unresponsive to the stories they are hearing. Institutionally, clinical performance declines, paperwork goes undone (or is done poorly), and ethical violations increase (e.g., pressuring a physician colleague for sleep medications from the pharmacy truck or offering a business card to a surviving victim who may never be a formal patient). Socially, providers' irritability with colleagues can extend to family and friends. So, too, does their declining capacities for empathy (e.g., a provider finding him or herself unable to support a spouse who is struggling with workplace stress because their stress is so much "less than" fieldwork stress). Isolation from said family members and friends can soon follow (Everly & Mitchell, 2003; Figley, 2002; Mendenhall & Berge, 2010; Sabin-Farrell & Turpin, 2003; Wright, 2004).

In addition to the basic strategies for avoiding CF and BRN outlined in the following section, specific and additional strategies utilized in fieldwork can vary from one deployment to the next according to the unique attributes of each site and situation. Common practices include structuring deployments so that no team (within the larger response organization) is in the field longer than 2 weeks at a time. While in the field, responders are generally only allowed to work for 2–3 days at a time, followed by a day of rest (because days working are often very long days). During work days, responders work in pairs of two and, therefore, have "buddies" with whom they directly work and can frequently check in and process with. Larger group processing and support is offered, as well (e.g., at the end of a shift). Workers are encouraged to monitor their own health and functioning and are immediately accommodated when they ask for a break to reground themselves in whatever manner they need (Figley, 2002; Mendenhall, 2006a; Mendenhall & Berge, 2010).

Military Contexts

MedFTs function in a variety of primary, secondary, or tertiary healthcare settings. When these settings are grounded within a military or veteran healthcare context, trauma, compassion fatigue, or burnout may be even more common for providers. Certainly, military personnel are always mission ready, but what is not often thought about are the medical and behavioral health providers in a military health system that are on active duty and may be deployed at any time. Furthermore, these providers may be at risk for multiple layers of exposure to trauma, given their own likelihood for deployment to war zones (with the potential for personal injury), while also caring for patients with common medical traumas (e.g., broken bones from accidents when the patient is not deployed or in combat), treating those who were injured during deployments (e.g., amputations), and managing complex medical plans for veterans (e.g., treating PTSD simultaneous to chronic pain).

Compassion fatigue and BRN can be potential outcomes for these providers, especially because military personnel have experienced more traumatic injuries and combat exposure during Operation Iraqi Freedom and Operation Enduring Freedom than any other time in US history (Gawande, 2004; Hoge et al., 2008; United States Army Surgeon General, 2005). Providers are commonly treating military and veteran families who have faced significant injuries (National Archives and Records Administration, 2013) and mourning with those who faced casualties (Department of Defense, 2012). In comparison to previous wars, providers are caring for more wounded warriors who are now surviving their injuries. With the increased exposure to patient traumas comes an increase in the likelihood for CF.

Given the importance of caring for providers in much the same way that providers care for their patients, a study was initiated in the southeastern United States in which healthcare providers (in a primary care setting on a military base) were assessed for CF and BRN. Through the initial results from the assessments, it appeared that providers are resilient (i.e., did not seem to have high prevalence of CF or BRN). Despite being resilient, the MedFT research team did learn more about some of the unique concerns that are most prevalent among providers (e.g., lack of sleep and high turnover due to deployment of providers or permanent change of station).

Some keys to recognizing and minimizing CF or BRN within the military contexts include (a) ensuring that providers have the chance to attend to relationships with patients and also with the other providers (e.g., staff lunches, networking opportunities), (b) creating collaborative plans on how to best advocate for resources that can reduce overtime or work overload, (c) promoting supervision and peer mentorship time that addresses professional and personal development, (d) having a way to debrief (individually or as a team) following potentially traumatic cases on the unit, and (e) constructing an environment that facilitates conversations about healthy ways to manage stress, exhaustion, and relational challenges.

Perhaps the most important to remember is that providers, while trained very well in biological and/or psychosocial health and illness, are human and are not without risk of developing CF or BRN. Keeping these concerns silent hurts the person with the symptoms and can be detrimental to those surrounding that provider (e.g., the provider's family and friends). It is thereby essential that teams look out for one another and make the well-being of each provider a key focal point on the unit. Finding several ways to manage symptoms of CF and BRN as they arise can only improve personal quality of life and sustainability in one's profession.

Strategies for Self- and Other Preservation

Given the long work hours and the need to be efficient, safe, and effective, providers must maintain a high level of self-care to sustain their careers. The intent of this section is to (a) offer straightforward strategies to reduce the likelihood for BRN and CF in MedFTs and (b) provide ways for MedFTs to better care for or work with providers who may be struggling with CF or BRN. The authors conclude this section with specific questions that MedFTs can ask themselves or other providers who may be experiencing symptoms of CF or BRN.

Many of the best ways to ensure one's own health and functioning include following what we already tell our own patients to do (Mendenhall, 2012). As MedFTs work to practice what they preach within the contexts of the care provided, it is important to honor the biopsychosocial-spiritual continuum of good (baseline/general) care with particular attention given to perceived BRN or CF and to keep an eye out for colleagues who may be at risk.

Take time for yourself. As trite or cliché as it may sound, this is one of the first things that providers who eventually burnout or experience CF have stopped doing. Time for self can encompass any variety of things but usually involves doing things that are not work-related. Self-time outside of work may include participating in hobbies (e.g., music, art, motorcycling, home remodeling) and/or church or community activities, exercise (light or intensive), reading for pleasure, or even just taking a few moments with your morning coffee and newspaper. These things represent the "little" things in life that can enrich and reenergize us. Within work contexts, endeavor to practice self-care in exact or modified forms (e.g., take power walks by one's self or with a colleague, meditate, practice relaxation sequences during downtimes while on call, journal during breaks).

Consult with colleagues and friends. Supervision and consultation should not stop once formal training as a MedFT is complete. Supervision with someone who has served as a mentor or via a collegial peer group can be a useful way to process difficult cases and debrief about ways to be accountable to self-care practices. While supervision must be done in a confidential manner, it can still be done over lunch and/or can include practices that may help providers better care for themselves while also helping them to learn new techniques for working with patients, such as diaphragmatic breathing or stress management exercises.

Attend to your own physical health. MedFTs should know the drill, because they discuss it nearly every day with their patients! In practice, ask yourself, "Am I living on coffee and candy bars?" or "Am I drinking plenty of water and eating nutritious foods? Am I getting into bed at night with the television still turned on, or am I following what I know to be good patterns of sleep hygiene?" Within the busy contexts of health care, it can be easy to work so hard that one suddenly realizes it has been several hours since drinking a glass of water, taking a break to rest, or even eating something. If it is too difficult to remember these practices, set up a peer reminder plan (or set cell phone alarms or self-care apps to get your periodic attention), to ensure that the most basic needs are attended to along the way.

Be social. In everyday lives and in the care provided by MedFTs, the social support that other people offer (and that we offer them) is an important resource in protecting against any host of behavioral health struggles. People are social creatures that need relationships with others. Talk with colleagues around the water cooler; go out with them for lunch or for happy hour at the end of the day. Connect with people in ways that engender and promote friendship, fun, and laughter. Even within the fast-paced contexts of health care, this is not very hard to do if there is a conscious effort to do it. Also, try to have some friends that are not in your profession or when talking with colleagues after work, try not to talk with them only about things that happened at work.

Be intentional about your personal relationships. So often spouses or partners, children, and other family members are at the bottom of to-do lists, taken almost entirely for granted. Providers may presume that spouses and family members will still be there after work and other "important" things are attended to. But personal relationships are more important than work, and attending to them (going out on dates, saying "I love you" with words and actions) is not something that should occur only in the contexts of courtship, holidays, birthdays, or on deathbeds! After work, talk about things other than just a rundown of the day's events. Embrace, literally and figuratively, the people who mean the most in life.

Set and be firm with your boundaries. From early socialization as graduate students, many MedFTs want to be liked by all colleagues, bosses, and friends. MedFTs may therefore find it difficult to say "no" or decline the multitude of opportunities that exist. However, it is okay to say "no" when feeling overextended. It is better to do ten things well than it is to do 11 things poorly. And contrary to what many may think, people will usually have greater respect for a provider who can say "no" gracefully than a provider who says "yes" and does the job poorly.

If you are hurting, seek help. MedFTs need to pause and reflect, if he is feeling overwhelmed and it is not getting better, is feeling anxious or depressed but cannot shake it, is feeling burned out, is emotionally fragile and/or irritable, is chronically unable to sleep and exhausted, or anything else that is deteriorating overall well-being or effectiveness in work. All providers – whether they are MDs, MedFTs, Social Workers, or from any other healthcare discipline – are bound by respective ethical codes to do this. The MedFT should talk to a supervisor or mentor about what is going on or go to see a therapist or a physician. There is nothing shameful about seeking help when it is needed. Just like the patients and families that MedFTs care for, providers, too, are human. If a MedFT needs help, it is important that he reach out for it. While most people may intuitively know that it is not healthy to only focus on work, sometimes it takes a colleague or friend to point out the truth (i.e., observation of emotional or physical exhaustion or other concerns). The following paragraphs include a list of questions to discern if a MedFT or someone that a MedFT works with is at risk for CF or BRN.

Ask yourself whether you are still thinking about ways you can help your patient (s) even after you have left work for the day. While thinking about some patients on an infrequent basis after work hours is typical, those who struggle with CF experience this on a frequent basis and, thus, have difficulty taking time for self-care practices.

Do you feel like you unplug from your emotions once you get home from work? Empathic ability and response is part of what increases the likelihood for CF and, thus, may make it difficult to maintain empathy in relationships at home or in one's personal life or further propel CF in more than one aspect of life (i.e., personal and professional), so it is important to maintain boundaries of self-care and relationships that fuel us. At work, it is important to recognize that empathic exhaustion includes spending unproductive time with patients that is no longer benefitting their health care.

Ask yourself whether you are trying to work harder and longer to get "caught up." Those facing BRN often compromise time for self by extending work hours beyond the typical work week. Unfortunately, and even paradoxically, this may result in lower overall productivity and compromised quality.

Part of BRN is being isolated from others in your profession, so make it a point to stay engaged in a supervision group with "like" professionals. We should always be working to improve the quality, effectiveness, and humanness of our efforts. Regular support, supervision, and consultation with/from colleagues (e.g., through formally arranged group meetings, spontaneous hallway conversations, etc.) will help to allay the sense of professional isolation that can sometimes contribute to BRN. Doing this can also provide a context and forum in which we can call on each other to engage in more purposeful self-care sequences if/when the need to do so is evident to others before it is evident to us.

Conclusions

Operationalized concepts of CF and BRN allow researchers, clinicians, and administrators to effectively assess, prevent, and buffer the effects of providers' reactions to trauma. Compassion fatigue and BRN significantly impact the healthcare system, but healthcare systems can utilize MedFTs and promote proactive approaches to addressing these concerns and help providers protect themselves from the daily and chronic implications of experiencing trauma. Compassion fatigue and BRN have received a great deal of attention within the last decade, and it has become increasingly important that MedFTs develop evidence-based practice strategies to combat BRN (e.g., better work conditions, maximize potential autonomy) and CF (e.g., debriefing, support groups, psychoeducation training on how to manage trauma events or crises).

Discussion Questions

1. Describe five ways that MedFTs could address CF or BRN with healthcare colleagues in a way that enhances self-care and patient productivity for the entire team.
2. What are some technologies or applications that exist or should be developed to help MedFTs and other providers be more accountable to self-care practices?
3. Develop a strategic plan that could be implemented into a unique healthcare context that would reduce the likelihood for CF and BRN for medical and behavioral health providers.

References[1]

Abendroth, M., & Flannery, J. (2006). Predicting the risk of compassion fatigue. *Journal of Hospice and Palliative Nursing, 8*, 346–356. doi:10.1097/00129191-200611000-00007.

Acker, G. M. (2012). Burnout among mental health care providers. *Journal of Social Work, 12*, 475–490. doi:10.1177/1468017310392418.

Adams, R., Boscarino, J., & Figley, C. (2006). Compassion fatigue and psychological distress among social workers: A validation study. *American Journal of Orthopsychiatry, 76*, 103–108. doi:10.1037/0002-9432.76.1.103.

Baird, K., & Kracen, A. (2006). Vicarious traumatization and secondary traumatic stress: A research synthesis. *Counseling Psychology Quarterly, 19*, 181–188. doi:10.1080/09515070600811899.

Breslau, N., Davis, G., Peterson, E., & Schultz, L. (1997). Psychiatric sequelae of posttraumatic stress disorder in women. *Archives of General Psychiatry, 54*, 81–87. doi:10.1001/archpsyc.1997.01830130087016.

*Bride, B. (2007). Prevalence of secondary traumatic stress among social workers. *Social Work, 52*, 63–70. doi:10.1093/sw/52.1.63.

*Bride, B., Robinson, M., Yegidis, B., & Figley, C. (2004). Development and validation of the secondary traumatic stress scale. *Research on Social Work Practice, 14*, 27–35. doi:10.1177/1049731503254106.

Brief, A., & Weiss, H. (2002). Organizational behavior: Affect in the workplace. *Annual Review in Psychology, 53*, 279–307. doi:10.1146/annurev.psych.53.100901.135156.

Brosche, T. (2003). Death, dying, and the ICU nurse. *Dimensions of Critical Care Nursing, 22*, 173–179. doi:10.1097/00003465-200307000-00006.

Chang, E. M., Daly, J., Hancock, K. M., Bidewell, J. W., Johnson, A., Lambert, V. A., & Lambert, C. E. (2006). The relationships among workplace stressors, coping methods, demographic characteristics, and health in Australian nurses. *Journal of Professional Nursing, 22*, 30–38. doi: 10.1016/j.profnurs.2005.12.002.

Cho, Y.-N., Rutherford, B. N., & Park, J. (2013). The impact of emotional labor in a retail environment. *Journal of Business Research, 66*, 670–677. doi:10.1016/j.jbusres.2012.04.001.

Chung, T., Rutherford, B., & Park, J. (2012). Understanding multifaceted job satisfaction of retail employees. *International Journal of Retail & Distribution Management, 40*, 699–716. doi:10.1108/09590551211255974.

Clark, M., & Gioro, S. (1998). Nurses, indirect trauma, and prevention. *Image, 30*, 85–87. doi:10.1111/j.1547-5069.1998.tb01242.x.

[1] An asterisk has been used to note references that the chapter authors recommend for further reading.

Collins, S., & Long, A. (2003). Working with the psychological effects of trauma: Consequences for mental health-care workers – A literature review. *Journal of Psychiatric and Mental Health Nursing, 10*, 417–424. doi:10.1046/j.1365-2850.2003.00620.x.

Day, J. R., & Anderson, R. A. (2011). Compassion fatigue: An application of the concept to informal caregivers of family members with dementia. *Nursing Research and Practice*. doi:10.1155/2011/408024.

Demerouti, E., Bakker, A., Nachreiner, F., & Ebbinghaus, M. (2002). From mental strain to burnout. *European Journal of Work and Organizational Psychology, 11*, 423–441. doi:10.1080/13594320244000274.

Department of Defense. (2012). DoD101: An introductory overview of the Department of Defense. Retrieved from http://www.defense.gov/pubs/dod101/index.html#evolved.

Everly, G., & Mitchell, J. (2003). *Critical incident stress management (CISM): Individual crisis intervention and peer support* (2nd ed.). Ellicott City, MD: International Critical Stress Incident Foundation.

Figley, C. (1995). *Compassion fatigue: Coping with secondary traumatic stress disorder*. New York, NY: Brunner/Mazel.

Figley, C. R. (1997). *Burnout in families: The systemic costs of caring*. Boca Raton, FL: CRC Press.

Figley, C. (1999). Compassion fatigue: Toward a new understanding of the costs of caring. In B. H. Stamm (Ed.), *Secondary traumatic stress: Self-care issues for clinicians, researchers, and educators* (2nd ed., pp. 3–28). Luthersville, MD: Sidran Press.

Figley, C. (2002). Compassion fatigue: Psychotherapists' chronic lack of self-care. *Journal of Clinical Psychology/In Session: Psychotherapy in Practice, 58*, 1433–1441. doi:10.1002/jclp.10090.

*Figley, C. (Ed.). (2013). *Treating compassion fatigue*. New York, NY: Brunner-Routledge.

Gawande, A. (2004). Casualties of war: Military care for the wounded from Iraq and Afghanistan. *New England Journal of Medicine, 351*, 2471–2475. doi:10.1056/NEJMp048317.

Grandey, A., Foo, S. C., Groth, M., & Goodwin, R. E. (2012). Free to be you and me: A climate of authenticity alleviates burnout from emotional labor. *Journal of Occupational Health Psychology, 17*, 1–14. doi:10.1037/a0025102.

*Hoge, C. W., Auchterlonie, J. L., & Milliken, C. S. (2006). Mental health problems, use of mental health services, and attrition from military service after returning from deployment to Iraq or Afghanistan. *Journal of Medical Association, 295*, 1023–1032. doi:10.1001/jama.295.9.1023.

Hoge, W., Castro, A., Messer, C., McGurk, D., Cotting, I., & Koffman, L. (2008). Combat duty in Iraq and Afghanistan, mental health problems and barriers to care. *U.S. Army Medical Department Journal*, 7–17. Retrieved from http://search.ebscohost.com/login.aspx?direct=true&db=mth&AN=35600233&site=ehost-live.

Hooper, C., Craig, J., Janvrin, D. R., Wetsel, M. A., & Reimels, E. (2010). Compassion satisfaction, burnout, and compassion fatigue among emergency nurses compared with nurses in other selected inpatient specialties. *Journal of Emergency Nursing, 36*, 420–427. doi:10.1016/j.jen.2009.11.027.

Jenkins, S., & Baird, S. (2002). Secondary traumatic stress and vicarious trauma: A validational study. *Journal of Traumatic Stress, 15*, 423–432. doi:10.1023/A:1020193526843.

Joinson, C. (1992). Coping with compassion fatigue. *Nursing, 22*, 116–122.

Kessler, R. C., Sonnega, A., Bromet, E., Hughes, M., & Nelson, C. B. (1995). Posttraumatic stress disorder in the national comorbidity survey. *Archives of General Psychiatry, 52*, 1048–1060. doi:10.1001/archpsyc.1995.03950240066012.

Lim, N., Kim, E. K., Kim, H., Yang, E., & Lee, S. M. (2010). Individual and work-related factors influencing burnout of mental health professionals: A meta-analysis. *Journal of Employment Counseling, 47*, 86–96. doi:10.1002/j.2161-1920.2010.tb00093.x.

Lynch, S. H., & Lobo, M. L. (2012). Compassion fatigue in family caregivers: A Wilsonian concept analysis. *Journal of Advanced Nursing, 68*, 2125–2134. doi:10.1111/j.1365-2648.2012.05985.x.

Maslach, C., & Leiter, M. P. (2008). Early predictors of job burnout and engagement. *Journal of Applied Psychology, 93*, 498–512. doi:10.1037/0021-9010.93.3.498.

Maytum, J., Heiman, M., & Garwick, A. (2004). Compassion fatigue and burnout in nurses who work with children with chronic conditions and their families. *Journal of Pediatric Health Care, 18*, 171–179. doi:10.1016/j.pedhc.2003.12.005.

*McCann, L., & Pearlman, L. (1990). Vicarious traumatization: A framework for understanding the psychological effects of working with victims. *Journal of Traumatic Stress, 3*, 131–149. doi:10.1007/BF00975140.

*Meadors, P., & Lamson, A. (2008). Compassion fatigue and secondary traumatization: Provider self-care on intensive care units for children. *Journal of Pediatric Healthcare, 22*, 24–34. doi:10.1016/j.pedhc.2007.01.006.

*Meadors, P., Lamson, A., & Sira, N. (2010). Development of an educational module on provider self-care. *Journal of Nurses in Staff Development, 26*, 152–158. doi:10.1097/NND.0b013e3181b1b9e4.

*Meadors, P., Lamson, A., Swanson, M., White, M., & Sira, N. (2009). Secondary traumatization in pediatric healthcare providers and staff: Compassion fatigue, burnout, and secondary traumatic stress. *Journal of Death and Dying, 60*, 103–128. doi:10.2190/OM.60.2.a.

*Mendenhall, T. (2006a). Trauma-response teams: Inherent challenges and practical strategies in interdisciplinary fieldwork. *Families, Systems, & Health, 24*, 357–362. doi:10.1037/1091-7527.24.3.357.

Mendenhall, T. (2006b). Reflections from the field: With Green Cross in Sri Lanka. *Traumatology, 11*, 141–142. doi:10.1177/153476560501100207.

*Mendenhall, T. (2012). Practicing what we preach: Answering the call for responder self care and resiliency. *The Dialogue (SAMHSA/DTAC), 8*(3), 2–4. http://www.samhsa.gov/dtac/dialogue/Dialogue_vol8_issue3_Final.pdf.

*Mendenhall, T., & Berge, J. (2010). Family therapists in trauma-response teams: Bringing systems thinking into interdisciplinary fieldwork. *Journal of Family Therapy, 32*, 40–54. doi:10.1111/j.1467-6427.2009.00482.x.

*Morse, G., Salyers, M. P., Rollins, A. L., Monroe-DeVita, M., & Pfahler, C. (2012). Burnout in mental health services: A review of the problem and its remediation. *Administration and Policy in Mental Health, 39*, 341–352. doi:10.1007/s10488-011-0352-1.

National Archives and Records Administration. (2013). *Statistical information about casualties of the Vietnam War: Electronic and special media records services division reference report.* College Park, MD: National Archives and Records Administration. Retrieved from http://www.archives.gov/research/military/vietnam-war/casualty-statistics.html.

Paris, M., & Hoge, M. A. (2010). Burnout in the mental health workforce: A review. *The Journal of Behavioral Health Services and Research, 37*, 519–528. doi:10.1007/s11414-009-9202-2.

Peckham, C. (2013). Physician lifestyles linking to burnout: A Medscape survey. *Medscape.* Retrieved from http://www.medscape.com/features/slideshow/lifestyle/2013/public#1.

Pfifferling, J., & Gilley, K. (2000). Overcoming compassion fatigue. *Family Practice Management, 7*, 39–45. http://www.aafp.org/fpm/2000/0400/p39.html.

*Rossler, W. (2012). Stress, burnout, and job dissatisfaction in mental health workers. *European Archives of Psychiatry and Clinical Neuroscience, 262*(2), 65–69. doi:10.1007/s00406-012-0353-4.

Rutherford, B. N., Hamwi, G. A., Friend, S. B., & Hartmann, N. N. (2011). Measuring salesperson burnout: A reduced Maslach burnout inventory for sales researchers. *Journal of Personal Selling and Sales Management, 31*, 429–440. doi:10.2753/PSS0885-3134310405.

Sabin-Farrell, R., & Turpin, G. (2003). Vicarious traumatization: Implications for mental health of health workers? *Clinical Psychology Review, 23*, 449–480. doi:10.1016/S0272-7358(03)00030-8.

Sabo, B. (2006). Compassion fatigue and nursing work: Can we accurately capture the consequences of caring work? *International Journal of Nursing Practice, 12*, 136–142. doi:10.1111/j.1440-172X.2006.00562.x.

Salyers, M. P., Hudson, C., Morse, G., Rollins, A. L., Monroe-DeVita, M., Wilson, C., & Freeland, L. (2011). BREATHE: A pilot study of a one-day retreat to reduce burnout among mental health professionals. *Psychiatric Services, 62*, 214–217. doi: 10.1176/appi.ps.62.2.214.

Schwam, K. (1998). The phenomenon of compassion fatigue in perioperative nursing. *Association of Operating Room Nurses Journal, 68*, 642–645. doi:10.1016/S0001-2092(06)62569-6.

Showalter, S. E. (2010). Compassion fatigue: What is it? Why does it matter? Recognizing the symptoms, acknowledging the impact, developing the tools to prevent compassion fatigue, and strengthen the professional already suffering from the effects. *American Journal of Hospice & Palliative Medicine, 27*, 239–242. doi:10.1177/1049909109354096.

Spickard, A., Gabbe, S., & Christensen, J. (2002). Mid-career burnout in generalist and specialist physicians. *Journal of the American Medical Association, 288*, 1447–1450. doi:10.1001/jama.288.12.1447.

*Stamm, B. H. (2002). Measuring compassion satisfaction as well as fatigue: Developmental history of the compassion fatigue and satisfaction and fatigue test. In C. R. Figley (Ed.), *Treating compassion fatigue* (pp. 107–119). New York, NY: Brunner/Mazel.-Routledge.

Stein, M., Walker, J., Hazen, A., & Forde, A. (1997). Full and partial posttraumatic stress disorder: Findings from a community survey. *American Journal of Psychiatry, 154*, 1114–1119. http://www.cme.psychiatryonline.org/data/Journals/AJP/3679/1114.pdf.

United States Army Surgeon General. (2005). Mental Health Advisory Team (MHAT-II): Report (pp. 1–30). Washington, DC: Department of the Army, Office of the Surgeon General.

Valent, P. (2002). Diagnosis and treatment of helper stresses, traumas, and illnesses. In C. Figley (Ed.), *Treating compassion fatigue* (pp. 13–37). New York, NY: Brunner/Routledge.

Veninga, R. L., & Spradley, J. P. (1981). *The work stress connection: How to cope with job burnout*. Boston, MA: Little, Brown.

Weiss, D. S., & Marmar, C. R. (1997). The impact of event scale – revised. In J. P. Wilson & T. M. Keane (Eds.), *Assessing psychological trauma and PTSD: A handbook for practitioners* (pp. 399–411). New York, NY: Guilford Press.

Wright, B. (2004). Compassion fatigue: How to avoid it. *Palliative Medicine, 18*, 3–4. doi:10.1191/0269216304pm866ed.

Chapter 8
MedFT Supervision in Context

Angela Lamson, Keeley Pratt, Jennifer Hodgson, and Aubry Koehler

While clinicians have been identifying as Medical Family Therapists (MedFTs) since 1992 (McDaniel, Hepworth, & Doherty, 1992), there has been relatively little published about providing supervision to them in healthcare settings. The first article written on this topic was by Gawinski, Edwards, and Speice in 1999. In it, they focused on the personal and professional experiences of two doctoral-level interns working in a healthcare setting, as well as their supervisor's experiences overseeing them in their clinical roles. The second publication was written by Edwards and Patterson in 2006 and focused on the essential skills needed to provide effective supervision to MedFT trainees in primary care settings. Since 2006, there has been a growth in opportunities for the integration of MedFTs in a variety of healthcare contexts (Hodgson, Lamson, Mendenhall, & Crane, 2012), and as a result three more publications have been released in recent years to help supervisors gain competency as more trainees secure work in primary, secondary, and tertiary care settings (Hodgson, Rambo, Boyd, Koehler, & Lamson, 2013; Pratt & Lamson, 2011, 2012).

There are many unique complexities associated with the supervision of systemic therapists and MedFTs in healthcare contexts (Hodgson et al., 2013). While MedFTs may herald from a diversity of professional homes or disciplines (e.g., Counseling, Marriage and Family Therapy, Medicine, Nursing, Psychology, and Social Work), supervisors need to be aware of how to navigate both the clinician's primary discipline (in relation to code of ethics and scope of practice), as well as her skill set in MedFT (Hodgson et al., 2013; Pratt & Lamson, 2011, 2012). Unfortunately, with so little guidance in the literature, it is unclear if supervisors' perceptions about the necessary skills of a MedFT are (a) directed by their own personal biases regarding what they believe MedFTs should be able to do, (b) based on recommendations and evaluations from research studies on MedFT competencies (Bischoff, Springer, Reisbig, Lyons, & Likcani, 2012; Tyndall, Hodgson, Lamson,

A. Lamson (✉)
East Carolina University, Greenville, NC, USA
e-mail: lamsona@ecu.edu

J. Hodgson et al. (eds.), *Medical Family Therapy*, DOI 10.1007/978-3-319-03482-9_8,

White, & Knight, 2012a), or (c) grounded in current MedFT literature (e.g., Marlowe, Hodgson, Lamson, White, & Irons, 2012; McDaniel, Doherty, & Hepworth, 2014; Tyndall et al. 2012a, 2012b). Furthermore, supervisors have had little guidance on how to bridge the medical and behavioral health worlds in order to provide a direction that is appropriate for supervisees' skill level, respectful of the work culture and context, and sensitive to the complexity of the healthcare setting.

The purpose of this chapter is to help both supervisors and supervisees understand the navigation process into the healthcare culture, provide necessary steps for choosing a MedFT supervisor, offer elements that should be considered when developing a supervision contract, present developmental trajectories of MedFTs in training, describe ways to assess one's practice as a supervisor and maximize consistency and productivity in the supervision process via the three-world view (Peek, 2008), and detail the potential supervision dynamics and challenges across a continuum.

Navigating Healthcare Culture

In contrast to 50-min traditional therapy settings (e.g., commonly done in behavioral health agencies, private practices, and some co-located healthcare practice locations), healthcare settings are moving toward briefer, fast-paced patient behavioral health encounters. In these more contemporary settings, multiple providers oftentimes function in different and overlapping roles, sometimes serving the same patient at the same time in the same room. Additionally, healthcare providers that were not trained in traditional behavioral health programs may use jargon unfamiliar to most behavioral health providers (BHPs) and often operate within implicit role hierarchies (e.g., physician, nurse, medical office assistant, check-in/out staff). MedFTs, who have been acculturated to this setting, its language, and the assumed norms, are well equipped to collaborate and function as part of a healthcare team and participate in the provision of a systemically based model of patient care.

By no means are supervisors required to become experts in all areas of health care; however, they should take time to familiarize themselves with the culture. For example, Edwards and Patterson (2006) recommended that supervisors new to overseeing clinicians in a healthcare setting may want to shadow one or more members of the healthcare team to orient themselves to the context, culture, workflow patterns, and available resources. Supervisors might also consider orienting themselves to supervision via a biopsychosocial-spiritual (BPSS) framework (Engel, 1977, 1980; Wright, Watson, & Bell, 1996) and educating themselves and their supervisees on conducting BPSS interviews (Hodgson, Lamson, & Reese, 2007) that provide vital data to the healthcare team (which includes the patient and accompanying members of the patient's support system).

It is also important that supervisors support supervisees by encouraging them to reflect on their experiences as BHPs in a healthcare setting. Supervisees may be the only BHP at their site and are often challenged by non-collaborating colleagues or may be confronted with issues of illness and death for which they may have received only minimal training while in their degree programs (Edwards & Patterson, 2006). Learning to navigate the healthcare culture is more than knowing how to intervene, enter the workflow, and document one's work. Supervisors need to work with supervisees to debrief existing illness stories and process biases about health care that may influence patient care.

Selecting a MedFT Supervisor

Ideally, a MedFT supervisor should have firsthand knowledge of and experience in the differences between traditional 50-min and brief 5–15-min integrated care therapy models. Specifically, the supervisor should be familiar with MedFT, how a healthcare practice works, and how a MedFT supervisor operates within a healthcare system to further develop the supervisee's skills. A supervisor's experience with MedFT and health care should be considered as the supervisee takes the step of selecting a supervisor and constructing a supervision contract. The following considerations are provided for supervisees before embarking on the MedFT supervision process.

Know Your State's Criteria for Supervision

The supervisor's credentials are oftentimes critical for meeting the requirements of a discipline-specific license. Regardless of the discipline in which a MedFT is trained, supervision is a key element toward achieving competency. For example, Marriage and Family Therapy students, or new professionals, are required to find an American Association for Marriage and Family Therapy (AAMFT) Approved Supervisor near their location of practice (note: some states only require a state-approved supervisor instead of a AAMFT approved supervisor).

The licensing requirements for Psychology students and new professionals can vary state by state, with certain states requiring that one's supervisor be a Licensed Clinical Psychologist co-located at the site in which the supervisee is practicing. Other states require that the Psychology supervisor meet the criteria set by the state licensure board in order to provide supervision to the supervisee outside of their employment site. Social Work students and new professionals should check with their state supervision requirements pertaining to the level and type of license needed for qualified supervisors. Supervision requirements for counselors differ from state to state; thus, students and new professionals need to check with their state-specific requirements to determine if a Licensed Professional Counselor or a Licensed Professional Counselor with a supervisor designation (LPC-S) is required for supervision.

Know the Credibility of the Supervisor

Before selecting a supervisor, it is important that MedFT supervisees do the following basic checks: (a) verify via a supervisor's license that she can provide the proper level or type of supervision, (b) ensure that there are no ethical violations against the potential supervisor, and (c) review state-specific supervision requirements prior to seeking a supervisor and signing a contract. Some additional questions a supervisee will want to pose to a possible supervisor are:

1. What is your experience collaborating with healthcare providers via research, teaching, and/or clinical/supervisory activities, and what is your supervisory role, philosophy, and expectations?

   Tip: Supervisees will want to listen for integrated care models that the supervisor has tried within healthcare contexts. The supervisor may be able to show you some writing samples that she has completed for the local hospital or healthcare setting websites or newsletters. The supervisor should be known by at least some of the providers or supervisors within the healthcare context where the practice will take place.

2. What levels of integrated care do you feel most comfortable supervising a supervisee within?

   Tip: The supervisor should be knowledgeable about the differences between collaboration from a distance, co-located, and fully integrated models of care. The supervisor should be able to assist supervisees in building a model that fits the uniqueness of each provider, as well as the needs of the healthcare system.

3. What evidence-based models are you most confident supervising for those who are working in a healthcare setting where sessions may be limited to 15 min or less?

   Tip: Supervisors should be able to cite current work that is published on integrated care or brief interventions in healthcare contexts and then have a critical lens on the value of the research and its fit with the supervisee's healthcare context.

4. What experience do you have providing systemic and relationally based care in a healthcare setting?

   Tip: Supervisors should be able to describe, process, and analyze cases and supervision through a systemic and relational lens. Supervision should include questions that expand the patient or supervisee's system to include supportive peers, colleagues, or family members, optimal resources, and recognition that the health of the supervisee will influence the health of her patients.

Supervisees should be prepared to engage potential supervisors on these topics of discussion before signing a supervision contract to make sure there is a good fit between the supervisor, supervisee, and the supervisee's work setting.

Developing a Supervision Contract

After goodness of fit has been confirmed and both parties are ready to sign a contract, the details of supervision should be negotiated. This contract should minimally detail the logistics of supervision such as contact information for the supervisor and supervisee, length of supervision (e.g., 6-month or 1-year term), location and time of supervision, payment, cancelation/no-show policy, emergency procedures, and frequency of contact (e.g., once a week, once a month). Some supervisors may expand on this and describe their supervision style or philosophy of supervision. In addition, contracts can include supervision goals that will become the focal point for supervisees' growth and the metrics that will be used to conduct evaluations on progress.

With an increased use of electronic documentation in healthcare settings, the supervision contract should clearly state the ways in which electronic information may be shared between patient and MedFT, MedFT and other providers, and between MedFT and supervisor. This would include content that can be shared via secured encrypted e-mail, electronic health record (EHR), and telehealth systems and should indicate who has access and signing privileges on clinical notes. Most BHPs have been trained to document in charts viewed only by them. In contrast, with a shared EHR, notes documented by one provider are typically viewable by all other providers and staff who have access to that patient's chart. MedFTs and their supervisors should meet with the site's administrative staff, prior to signing the contract, to discuss who has rights for viewing and documenting in charts. For example, in some EHRs, phone notes are viewable to front desk staff as well as healthcare providers. If this is the case, notes written by the MedFT should be carefully completed with attention to process, but without specific clinical content that can damage the patient's confidentiality.

Another important issue that should be addressed within the contract is whether there are particular crises that must be communicated to supervisors and how these crises should be communicated to members of the healthcare team and the provider responsible for care management that day. MedFTs should be aware that access to a patient's chart does not guarantee providers will read all the notes within the electronic file or that a patient who has received integrated care has shared the same information with all providers included in the visit. With this in mind, MedFTs should make efforts to communicate any "red flag issues" directly to involved providers and collaborate with supervisors to ensure that the proper action and follow-up plans are made and delegated accordingly.

Specifically, the supervision contract should indicate what constitutes red flag issues that the supervisor feels are important for the supervisee to instantly communicate to the supervisor on-site and involved providers at the time of occurrence. These topics may include, but are not limited to, suicidal ideations, homicidal ideations, child or elder abuse and/or neglect, and intimate partner violence. The contract may also include a backup plan of who the supervisee should consult if the supervisor is not available during the time of emergency. Both supervisor and supervisee should be aware of the site's protocol on red flag issues prior to signing the supervision contract so that a step-by-step plan can be included in the contract for the supervisee.

If the MedFT will have both an on-site and off-site supervisor (common to those still enrolled in training programs), the contract should also detail the roles of multiple supervisors. It is best if a meeting is set in which all supervisors and the supervisee will be in attendance to discuss the procedures for supervision and protocol on what information must be shared with each supervisor. The communication between both the on-site and off-site supervisors should be detailed, for example, both supervisors could provide a joint annual evaluation. Finally, both the on-site and off-site supervisors should be aware of the patient information that will be disclosed by the supervisee to each supervisor.

Another necessary component of the contract is the evaluation process for the supervisee and supervisor. Evaluation is an important part of tracking supervisees' progress and making sure supervisors are not becoming focused on only a few skills/competencies. It is common for supervisors to ask supervisees to construct several goals they would like to work on over the course of supervision or to document a list of competencies they would like to acquire in order to ensure continuity in the supervision process. However, evaluation metrics must then be relevant and coincide with the goals or competencies developed. Examples of general (non-MedFT specific) supervisor–supervisee evaluations include the Supervisory Styles Index (Long, Lawless, & Dotson, 1996) and the Basic Skills Evaluation Device (Nelson & Johnson, 1999). The evaluation metrics (e.g., a self-report evaluation conducted by the supervisee; a measure completed by the supervisor of the supervisee's skills and vice versa) should be determined and included as part of the contract so that both supervisors and supervisees are aware of what is being evaluated and how to gauge success and overall functioning in the given healthcare setting. If supervisors have difficulty adjusting one of the published evaluations to meet their MedFT supervision needs, it may be more suitable to construct an action plan based on the list of MedFT core competencies (see Chap. 3; Tyndall, Hodgson, Lamson, White, & Knight, 2014). Select competencies could be added into a contract along with an action plan to guide progress (see Table 8.1 for a sample template developed by Lamson for use in graduate training).

Finally, the supervision contract should detail elements that may constitute grounds for terminating the supervision contract. For example, some circumstances may naturally present a reason for termination, such as a supervisee or supervisor relocating to a different state or a supervisee graduating. However, there may be other reasons for terminating a contract, such as the supervisor or supervisee engaging in unethical practices, not attending supervision meetings, or the supervisor–supervisee relationship lacking optimal fit. To ensure protection of the

Table 8.1 Sample plan of action for obtaining MedFT competency

Competency	Describe specific training you received regarding this competency	How were you evaluated for this competency
Sample:		
MedFT Competency #8 Demonstrate awareness of and sensitivity to cultural and contextual variables pertaining to health, illness, loss, and trauma	MedFT (a) attended grand rounds with BHPs and other healthcare providers on cultural beliefs pertaining to illness, death, and dying; (b) read a text that focused on treating culturally diverse patients; and (c) completed a rotation on the trauma and end of life units within the healthcare setting	MedFT was evaluated by (a) a pre- and posttest associated with the grand rounds, (b) completing an assessment on diversity awareness and then discussing the outcome from the assessment and (c) receiving positive clinical evaluations from patients and supervisors while on rotation in trauma and end of life units

The supervisee is charged with reviewing this plan of action with his site supervisor and MedFT supervisor. A copy of progress toward the plan of action should be turned in to both supervisors at predetermined times throughout the duration of the supervision contract

supervisor's license and supervisee's professional future, termination details should be stated in the contract explicitly.

Based on the information above, it would appear that a supervision contract is the length of a book. However, a typical contract is 3–4 pages long. It should be signed and dated by all parties, copies should be provided to the supervisor and supervisee, and a copy should be kept at the site of the supervisee's placement. The contract is a first step toward entering into a new supervisorial relationship. Once this step has been completed, it is time for the supervisor to engage the supervisee in supervision based on his or her developmental skill level.

The Developmental Trajectory of MedFT Supervisees

Developmentally, each supervisee has different access to and involvement in healthcare settings based on the vision of his or her current or past graduate program/training, scope of practice, and strengths or challenges associated with billing systems. In addition, all behavioral health learners enter the workforce with different levels of systemic training and healthcare experience. Mechanisms for helping the supervisor to determine what type, style, and level of integration is present in a healthcare setting will help them to tailor supervision so it is both contextually sensitive and relevant.

Different levels of behavioral health integration in healthcare settings require different levels of supervision. For example, Pratt and Lamson (2011, 2012) adapted Doherty, McDaniel, and Baird's (1996) five levels of Primary Care/Behavioral Healthcare Collaboration (PCBHC) when developing their systemic supervision framework. These levels ranged from minimal collaboration at a distance (level 1) to close collaboration in a fully integrated site (level 5). In 2013, there was an introduction of two other mechanisms for determining ways in which integrated behavioral health services have been incorporated into a healthcare system (Heath, Wise Romero, & Reynolds, 2013; Peek & National Integration Academy Council, 2013). Supervisors may want to review all three mechanisms and choose the one that best fits their situation; however, for the purposes of providing an example, Doherty and colleagues' (1996) model will be applied in this chapter.

Each level of integrated care has unique challenges related to collaboration, such as learning protocols, documentation, emergency procedures, and ethical standards. Pratt and Lamson (2011, 2012) adapted Doherty and colleagues' (1996) model to include the role of the supervisor and provided sample supervisee and supervisor questions based on the level of collaboration between supervisee and healthcare providers. Supervisors should note that the level of collaboration may also differ by provider within a context, whereby some relationships may reflect a level 3 collaboration (basic collaboration on-site), while other relationships within a context may be at a level 5 (fully integrated system) (Doherty et al., 1996). Overall, supervisors and supervisees need to consider the context, as well as the relationship dynamics, within the context.

Therapists with relational and systemic training also typically align with one of the five levels identified on the Medical Family Therapy in Healthcare Continuum (MedFT-HCC) (Hodgson, Lamson, Mendenhall, & Tyndall, 2013; See Chap. 1; Hodgson, Lamson, & Mendenhall, 2014). Supervisors must be prepared to tailor their method and practices based on the BHP's skill level in relational and systemic therapies, the BHP's healthcare experience and training, and the level of integrated care being practiced at the healthcare site. For example, those who are not systemically trained may have acquired other healthcare experience and training and may interface and provide integrated care in a healthcare context at any of Doherty and colleagues' (1996) five levels on the PCBHC model. However, the intent for this segment is to showcase ways in which supervisors can be most helpful in guiding the development of MedFTs (with and without prior formal or relational or BPSS training) via the MedFT-HCC (Hodgson et al., 2013; See Preface; Hodgson et al., 2014) in relationship to the PCBHC model (see Fig. 8.1).

An Interface of the MedFT-HCC and PCBHC Models for Supervision

As previously mentioned, any level of skill within the MedFT-HCC (Hodgson et al., 2013; See Preface; Hodgson et al., 2014) can interface with almost all of Doherty and colleagues' (1996) levels. The following describes ways in which

	Primary Care/Behavioral Healthcare Collaboration (Doherty, McDaniel, and Baird, 1996)				
Medical Family Therapy Healthcare Continuum (Hodgson, Lamson, Mendenhall & Tyndall, 2013)	Level 1 Minimal collaboration with other providers (separate systems, separate facilities, rare communication with HCP)	Level 2 Basic collaboration from a distance (separate systems, separate facilities, periodic letter and phone contact with HCP)	Level 3 Basic collaboration on-site (consult model only; regular communication-occasionally face-to-face with HCP)	Level 4 Close collaboration in a partly IC system (some shared systems; same facilities; face to face consultation with HCP; collaborative routines difficult)	Level 5 Close collaboration in a fully IC system (shared systems and facilities; all HCPs function face-to-face as a team; regularly collaborate)
Level 1 *Rarely…* 1) Applies a relational and/or biopsychosocial-spiritual (BPSS) lens in practice, research, and/or policy/advocacy work. 2) Conducts research on healthcare topics including relational and/or BPSS aspects of health, and writes in collaboration with other healthcare researchers. 3) Includes individuals, couples, families, AND healthcare professionals into their work. 4) Advocates and advances clinical models and policies that promote relational or BPSS health and well-being.	Able to apply a relational and BPSS lens; rarely includes support persons in therapy or applies the BPSS framework; collaborate only as needed	**Skill applies to PCBHC Level 1 and 2**	This interaction is not possible; Level 1 MedFT-HCC collaborates only as perceived it is needed	**Not Possible in PCBHC Levels 3-5**	
Level 2 *Occasionally….* 1) Applies a relational and/or biopsychosocial-spiritual (BPSS) lens in practice, research, and/or policy/advocacy work. 2) Conducts research on healthcare topics including relational and/or BPSS aspects of health, and writes in collaboration with other healthcare researchers. 3) Includes individuals, couples, families, AND healthcare professionals into their work. 4) Advocates and advances clinical models and policies that promote relational or BPSS health and well-being.	Trained to use a relational and BPSS lens although only occasionally invites support persons into tx; providers communicate on less than 50% of patient care cases	**Skill 5 applies to PCBHC Levels 1-3**		This interaction is not possible; Level 2 MedFT-HCC occurs when providers communicate on less than 50% of patient care cases	**Not Possible in PCBHC Level 4 and 5**
Level 3 *Usually…* 1) Applies a relational and/or biopsychosocial-spiritual (BPSS) lens in practice, research, and/or policy/advocacy work. 2) Conducts research on healthcare topics including relational and/or BPSS aspects of health, and writes in collaboration with other healthcare researchers. 3) Includes individuals, couples, families, AND healthcare professionals into their work. 4) Advocates and advances clinical models and policies that promote relational or BPSS health and well-being. 5) Trained to apply a broad range of family therapy and BPSS interventions and conduct family therapy.	Some family therapy training; treatment provided through relational and BPSS lens; minimal collaboration	Some family therapy training; treatment provided through relational & BPSS lens -periodic consultation with larger system; at a distance	Some family therapy training; treatment through relational & BPSS lens -occasional to regular consultation with larger system, but on less than 75% of patient care cases	**Skill applies to PCBHC Level 3 and 4**	This interaction is not possible; Level 3 MedFT-HCC occurs when providers with family therapy training communicate on less than 75% of patient care cases
Level 4 *Consistently…* 1) Applies a relational and/or biopsychosocial-spiritual (BPSS) lens in practice, research, and/or policy/advocacy work. 2) Conducts research on healthcare topics including relational and/or BPSS aspects of health, and writes in collaboration with other healthcare researchers. 3) Includes individuals, couples, families, AND healthcare professionals into their work.	This interaction is not possible; Level 4 MedFT-HCC occurs only in contexts in which collaboration is possible at each patient encounter	**Not Possible in PCBHC Level 1 and 2**	Trained family therapist; consistent in including family or healthcare professionals in most visits using relational family therapy theories and interventions	**Skill applies to PCBHC Level 3-5**	

Fig. 8.1 (continued)

4) Advocates and advances clinical models and policies that promote relational or BPSS health and well-being. 5) Trained to apply a broad range of family therapy and BPSS interventions and conduct family therapy. 6) Experienced in conducting BPSS research across traditional and integrated care practice contexts. 7) Integrated in outpatient and/or inpatient healthcare teams, attends to the needs of healthcare team members, is a part of healthcare team meetings, and/or practices conjointly with diverse healthcare professionals. 8) Identified as a MedFT clinician or MedFT researcher and integrates in/with healthcare contexts/ professionals into most of their work.					
<u>Level 5</u> *Proficiently…* 1) Applies a relational and/or biopsychosocial-spiritual (BPSS) lens in practice, research, and/or policy/advocacy work. 2) Conducts research on healthcare topics including relational and/or BPSS aspects of health, and writes in collaboration with other healthcare researchers. 3) Includes individuals, couples, families, AND healthcare professionals into their work. 4) Advocates and advances clinical models and policies that promote relational or BPSS health and well-being. 5) Trained to apply a broad range of family therapy and BPSS interventions and conduct family therapy. 6) Experienced in conducting BPSS research across traditional and integrated care practice contexts. 7) Integrated in outpatient and/or inpatient healthcare teams, attends to the needs of healthcare team members, is a part of healthcare team meetings, and/or practices conjointly with diverse healthcare professionals. 8) Identified as a MedFT clinician or MedFT researcher and integrates in/with healthcare contexts/ professionals into most of their work. 9) Experienced at administrating, supervising in diverse medical contexts (i.e., primary, secondary, and tertiary care systems) incorporating both traditional and integrated care models. 10) Experienced in training healthcare professionals in family therapy and MedFT practice, research, policy, and/or administration.	This interaction is not possible; Level 5 MedFT-HCC occurs only in contexts offering IC on site	**Not Possible in PCBHC Levels 1-3**		Trained family therapy educator; proficient at traditional & IC tx via relational theories and interventions, with ability to train or supervise others	**Skill applies to PCBHC Level 4 and 5**

Key: **Tx** = treatment; **BPSS** = biopsychosocial-spiritual model; **IC** = integrated care; HC = healthcare

NOTE: The arrow represents the continuation of the same description from the previous level.

Fig. 8.1 Primary care/behavioral healthcare collaboration (Doherty et al. 1996)

supervisors may respond based on the supervisee's skill level within the MedFT-HCC.

Level 1 MedFT-HCC

- Relational and/or lens is used in practice.
- Supervisee accepts referrals from healthcare professionals.
- Collaboration with healthcare professionals or spiritual advisors is carried out on an "as needed" basis.

Role of Supervisor. Supervisors at this skill level should be trainers in systemic therapy, family therapy theories, and the BPSS approach and have experience collaborating with healthcare providers. Supervisors may also benefit from learning the conscious-competence model (Burch, 1970) to support the developmental progress of supervisees interested in the full continuum of skills within the MedFT-HCC (Hodgson et al., 2013; See Preface; Hodgson et al., 2014) and PCBHC (Doherty et al., 1996).

Level 2 MedFT-HCC

- Relational and/or BPSS lens is used in practice.
- Supervisee accepts referrals from healthcare professionals.
- Supervisee occasionally includes couple, family, and/or healthcare professionals in work context.
- Supervisee has learned and uses BPSS or a relational approach to practice, but only occasionally consults with healthcare colleagues and is not typically in a setting other than her own private practice/work setting.

Role of Supervisor. Supervisors at this skill level should be trainers in systemic therapy, family therapy theories, and the BPSS approach and have experience collaborating with healthcare providers. For MedFTs working in settings where there is only occasional inclusion of family systems or healthcare professionals, supervision should focus on the concerns of the patient population. At this level, clinical care and supervision likely follows a more traditional behavioral health format (e.g., 50-min sessions) whereby sessions are typically conducted in a separate office located off-site from the healthcare context or away from other healthcare providers. The supervisor may need to assess what the supervisee knows about systemic interventions involving BPSS symptoms or use of larger collaborative teams in healthcare management. Time talking about team dynamics is likely to be limited because at this level the MedFT is often isolated from other healthcare providers. If collaboration is brought up, it would be in the context of how to obtain appropriate releases of information.

Level 3 MedFT-HCC

- Family therapy practice is provided via a relational and BPSS lens.
- Supervisee functions primarily in a healthcare context and regularly seeks out consultation from healthcare colleagues.

- Supervisee uses MedFT techniques and family therapy interventions, usually incorporates family/support system members into treatment plans, and attends to relationships among healthcare team members.

Role of Supervisor. Supervisors at this skill level should be trainers in systemic therapy, family therapy theories, and the BPSS approach and have experience working in a healthcare setting interfacing regularly with healthcare providers. One of the first aims of MedFT supervision should be to assist the supervisee in understanding the healthcare culture of which they are to be a part (Edwards & Patterson, 2006). The healthcare culture should include site-specific considerations including the BPSS issues and concerns that patients present within their given setting, and the supervisee's role on the healthcare team. The supervisor should provide the supervisee with resources to further develop the supervisee's understanding of a patient's presenting health concerns and the subsequent BPSS symptoms that could arise as a result of an identified health condition. The supervisor should also help the supervisee practice ways to concisely and consistently communicate BPSS and relational information with the treatment team.

In addition, at this level the supervisor can facilitate the conceptualization of health conditions through a systemic and relational lens to explore the influence of BPSS health on the family and other important figures in a patient's life. Finally, a MedFT supervisor should encourage the supervisee to think about his own experiences with illness and the potential influence of these experiences in his interactions with patients. In these cases, the supervisee must learn to recognize transference and countertransference in the healthcare setting with supervision pertaining to the supervisee's own beliefs, values, culture, and past experiences with illness.

Level 4 MedFT-HCC

- Family therapy is provided via traditional and integrated care practice contexts.
- Supervisee is part of collaborative rounds, team meetings, or sessions with diverse healthcare professionals.
- Supervisee consistently includes family members and/or healthcare professionals in most aspects of work.
- Supervisee works in/with healthcare contexts/professionals and incorporates others into their work.

Role of Supervisor. Supervisors at this skill level should be trainers in systemic therapy, family therapy theories, and the BPSS approach and have experience collaborating with healthcare providers in a partly integrated care system. Supervisors may focus on MedFT techniques and relational family therapy theories, models, and interventions that occur within traditional and integrated care visits; assess the preparation and documentation of treatment plans to ensure that a relational task/intervention is included; assess health or an intervention from the perspective of the patients and families; attend to relationships among healthcare team members; and determine whether the MedFT is exploring the need for a curriculum or support system for maintaining wellness among the healthcare team.

Level 5 MedFT-HCC

- Supervisee is proficient at using and training others to provide traditional and integrated care using relational family therapy theories, models, and interventions in diverse healthcare contexts (i.e., primary, secondary, and tertiary care systems).

Role of Supervisor. Supervisors at this skill level should be trainers in systemic therapy, family therapy theories, and the BPSS approach and have experience collaborating with healthcare providers in a fully integrated care system. At this level, the supervisor is commonly in a role of training the trainer. The hope is that the supervisee has been trained well enough to then teach others what he does and thereby replicate a successful model. One way to ensure the sustainability of the model is through Peek's (2008) three-world view. Peek posited that providers face three simultaneous challenges or "world views": (a) the clinical challenge to provide exceptional patient care; (b) the operational challenge to employ efficient, well-integrated, and patient-friendly systems of care; and (c) the financial challenge of staying financially feasible and utilizing healthcare resources (Patterson, Peek, Heinrich, Bischoff, & Scherger, 2002). In the Three-World view, it is important to look at each world in relation to the others. It is thought that one world cannot function independently. Similarly, no one world is considered more important than another, so supervisees must be clear on how these worlds function independently and interdependently.

Assessing One's Role as a Supervisor

For many supervisors venturing into health care for the first time, there is limited knowledge of its clinical, organizational, or financial systems (Peek, 2008). The way documentation, billing, and collaboration are done in healthcare settings is significantly different from the specialty behavioral health settings in which most supervisees, and their supervisors, were trained to function. For example, most BHPs were trained to document therapy sessions in a paper chart or EHR that is maintained and viewed only by them. However, more and more healthcare systems are implementing a shared EHR that all providers housed in the same setting are expected to use. This method of open communication may pose ethical challenges or call for changes to policies and protocol due to differences in the ways that behavioral health and medical providers seek consent and engage in treatment. Supervisors will need to learn how and when to make recommendations for revisions to patient consent forms to ensure the healthcare system is being transparent with patients about healthcare team collaboration and the exchange of and access to protected health information (Hodgson, Mendenhall, & Lamson, 2013; Hudgins, Rose, Fifield, & Arnault, 2013).

Furthermore, supervisors will need to understand the differences in treatment policies and reimbursement procedures that may influence patient care and

Table 8.2 A guide of the Three-World view for MedFT supervisors and supervisees

	Clinical World	Operational World	Financial World
Questions for the supervisee pertaining to the Three-World view	• Can the supervisee assess and intervene using a BPSS approach with patients, families, and providers? • Does the supervisee understand the levels of collaboration and can she identify which one(s) is practiced on-site accurately (Doherty et al., 1996)? • Does the supervisee understand how to diagnose behavioral health issues, as well as assist in providing evidence-based interventions (e.g., smoking cessation, insomnia, weight loss)? • Does the supervisee understand how on/off-site supervisors communicate? • Is the supervisee able to recognize self of the therapist concerns and does she demonstrate the ability to manage them effectively?	• Where is supervision conducted and how often? • How are MedFTs documenting time with patients and for supervision? • How are charts/notes shared and who is signing off on the supervisee's work? • What are the emergency supervision procedures? • What is the feedback from the healthcare team on how the supervisee is fitting into the workflow of the healthcare system? • What is the data extraction process that may be used to track and report on the integrated care model? • Where does therapy take place when sessions need to go past 15 min so the workflow does not get backed up? • What are the collaboratively agreed upon protocols for managing challenging patients or crises? • Does the supervisee know all the healthcare team administrators' and members', names and roles?	• How are MedFTs reimbursed for their time? • What diagnoses or codes are used for reimbursement? • What time increments are used in billing? • What insurance panels cover services? • What metrics or benchmarks are being used to determine integrated care program/position sustainability? • How are the merits of integration being captured if MedFT services are not being billed (i.e., provider productivity, patient improvement in health outcomes, changes in claims data for medical services)

supervisee practices. For example, if supervisees are expected to meet a clinical quota to offset a portion of their salary, reimbursement mechanisms may determine if more or less traditional care should be done to meet the criteria. In some states, reimbursement for IC is much harder to achieve, although this is beginning to change. The following is a guide that represents a series of questions that supervisors may want to consider in relation to Peek's Three-World view (see Table 8.2) when working with supervisees in healthcare contexts.

Common MedFT Challenges

On-Site–Off-Site Supervision

If the MedFT has both an on-site and off-site supervisor, the roles of multiple supervisors may get confusing. Regularly scheduled supervision meetings with all supervisors and the supervisee may be helpful to evaluate the supervision process and to make sure messages delivered to the supervisee are consistent across supervisors. Depending on the length of the supervisee's placement and developmental skill level, such meetings may need to be conducted every other month or biannually.

Generalist and Specialist Considerations

An additional challenge for the supervision of MedFTs is that sites will differ based on the healthcare setting and the type and intensity of care delivered. For example, in primary care settings, MedFTs need to develop competency in understanding the biopsychosocial and sometimes spiritual implications of treatment and consult a wide variety of conditions, diseases, and preventative health concerns. Thus, MedFTs in primary care settings are expected to be generalists and to have a breadth of knowledge regarding their patients' presenting concerns and treatment options. However, in secondary (e.g., dermatology or cardiology) and tertiary care (diabetology and endocrinology) settings, MedFTs treat and consult with patients and collaborate with providers about the psychosocial and spiritual meaning of acute or specialized conditions, and this work may even occur while patients are hospitalized.

MedFTs in secondary and tertiary care need to be specialists in patients' presenting concerns and have an in-depth knowledge about specific health complications relative to the primary diagnosis. The MedFT supervisor will need to tailor the content of supervision to the type of care offered at the location of the supervisee's placement and to know whether the MedFT is expected to function as a generalist or a specialist. The supervisor will also want to ensure that as the supervisee gains competency in understanding the health conditions common to his setting, his scope of practice is appropriate to his level of training, code of ethics, and licensure law and not extending beyond.

Collaborating with Other BHPs

Before a supervisee begins his or her work within a healthcare setting, it is important that both supervisor and supervisee acquaint themselves with any other BHPs already employed at that setting. While some settings may have multiple BHPs, others may have none. Larger care facilities (i.e., hospitals) may have psychiatric, chaplaincy, or other behavioral health consult services available that are mainly accessed when a problem is identified that falls outside of the treating physician's scope of practice or comfort zone. If there are occasions where the MedFT supervisee is expected to consult with or share care alongside other BHPs directly or indirectly, collaboration and mutual respect of overlapping and distinct roles will be instrumental in facilitating a successful placement experience. Other BHPs, from similar or different disciplines and orientations, can be vital resources for supervisees in case conceptualization, crisis management, and treatment planning. Also, they may be able to give valuable feedback to the supervisor on the supervisee's ability to collaborate with others, respond to consults appropriately, and follow organization protocols.

In the case where a supervisee is the only BHP affiliated with the setting, special provisions must be made to ensure she has access to clinical support when the supervisor is not on-site or available. For example, the medical director may be requested to provide auxiliary support and backup supervision for the supervisee. Supervisors who need to be on-site in any capacity, especially due to a limited availability of experienced BHPs, should be certain that they have completed the necessary steps (e.g., certification and/or orientation) to be able to access the supervisee's work. Supervisors should avoid agreeing to supervise anyone at a placement that blocks the supervisor's access to observing the supervisee's live or video-recorded work (with appropriate patient and site-written permissions).

The following fictitious case study was written to apply many of the ideas presented thus far in this chapter. Any similarity to a real supervisory situation or clinical case is strictly coincidental. Corresponding discussion questions have been developed to incite thoughtful reflection and discussion relative to it.

Case Study

A MedFT doctoral-level intern is working at a primary care context that is currently operating at a level 3 on both the PCBHC and the MedFT-HCC (Hodgson et al., 2013; see Preface; Hodgson et al., 2014). After conducting a routine depression screening using the Patient Health Questionnaire (PHQ-9, Kroenke, Spitzer, & Williams, 2001) with a 58-year-old male Spanish-speaking patient, the MedFT learns that the patient is severely depressed (PHQ-9 score of 21) and has suicidal ideation. The patient reports having both access and a plan, but only moderate-level intent (identified as a 5 on a scale of 0–10, with 0 indicating the patient fully intends to attempt suicide and 10 indicating the patient does not intend to attempt suicide). The patient reports experiencing chronic unmanaged back pain most days of the week and that the pain has increased his desire to end his life.

The patient is presenting today to his primary care provider for pain management. Although he is receiving financial assistance, he expressed concern during the check-in process regarding his ability to pay the reduced fee for his appointment today or his outstanding balance that has accumulated from previous appointments. The patient lives alone and has some extended family in the area. His immediate family lives in Mexico. The patient's friend has dropped him off for his appointment today and will be picking him up afterwards.

Reflection Points

In thinking about the how to approach the case study, supervisors and supervisees should first consider safety issues to ensure that proper precautions are taken, such as developing a safety contract with the patient and family members present (if any), not leaving the patient unattended, and consulting with the provider of record for that visit to develop and implement a treatment plan (i.e., hospitalization or discharge). Each location will have or need to develop protocol for extreme cases (e.g., suicidal ideations, homicidal ideations, child or elder abuse and/or neglect, and intimate partner violence). Ideally, these protocols have been put into place before a crisis occurs. Protocol must take into account federal and state laws, the ethical codes of the involved providers, and potentially complicating factors from each of Peek's (2008) Three-Worlds—clinical, operational, and financial—and the intersection of these worlds.

Clinically, supervisors must guide supervisees in administering assessments and intervening appropriately, in accordance with the results of the clinical assessments. Assessments are of little use if their results do not inform treatment. Supervisors and supervisees should discuss the type of evidence-based interventions that correspond with different assessment outcomes. For example, patients with a subclinical or "mild" score on the PHQ-9 may be offered basic behavioral or relational coping strategies during the encounter, whereas patients with a "moderate" or "severe" score may be offered behavioral coping strategies, possibly psychopharmaceuticals by his primary care provider, and a referral for traditional psychotherapy and/or a psychiatric evaluation (Kroenke et al., 2001).

In the above case study, it will be important for supervisors and supervisees to navigate the particular needs of a Spanish-speaking patient presenting with safety issues. The availability of healthcare interpreters, forms and assessments in the patient's first language, and referral sources that are linguistically and culturally accessible to the patient are paramount. Without planning and careful consideration, safety issues may be tragically missed or misunderstood.

Operationally, supervisors and supervisees should consider workflow patterns, provider roles, systems of documentation, and the current levels of collaboration on both the PCBHC and the MedFT-HCC (Hodgson et al., 2013; see Preface; Hodgson et al., 2014) models. For example, a supervisee working in a healthcare context at level 4 on both the PCBHC and the MedFT-HCC will likely have less resistance when seeking provider collaboration on safety issues than a supervisee working in a level 2 system. Supervisors and supervisees working in a lower-level system (Doherty, McDaniel, & Baird, 1996) will need to compensate for operational barriers by discussing with providers preferred methods of collaboration. Notably, preferences will likely vary for each provider so individual discussion should be pursued. It is also judicious to have these types of planning discussions prior to crisis situations.

Financially, it is important that supervisors and supervisees are aware both of reimbursement procedures related to their roles and also the general procedures of the location, specifically with regard to how these impact patient care and expectations for provider productivity. For example, does the patient's financial status (e.g., an outstanding bill discovered by the front desk staff before the appointment) affect his access to care? How do expectations for provider productivity limit time spent in the room with patients? Supervisors and supervisees are by no means expected to single-handedly remove systemic barriers but are encouraged to think through potential barriers as much as possible, so these do not compromise patient care and provider collaboration, especially in the event of safety issues.

The following questions may be useful in guiding a thought process or discussion regarding the development and implementation of protocol for the above case study (and others like it) that takes into account the impact and intersection of the clinical, operation, and financial worlds:

1. What supervision/clinical protocols should follow the identification of suicidal/homicidal, child maltreatment, or domestic violence issues to ensure patient safety (e.g., MedFT leaves the room, calls/retrieves supervisor, etc.)?
2. Who should be involved in the resolution of the crisis situation discussed in the case study (e.g., providers, support staff, family, community members)? How can the supervisor(s) and supervisee best facilitate the involvement of providers and staff in a way that is constructive to the situation and also mindful of patient consent and confidentiality?
3. How can the PCBHC and MedFT-HCC level influence the way in which the MedFT navigates a course of action? Collaborates with providers and staff? Documents the encounter?
4. What are the potential barriers to patient care and collaboration in this case study, and how might the supervisor(s) and supervisees shift or navigate around these barriers?

Conclusion

MedFTs must be prepared to work in diverse healthcare settings, and, thus, MedFT supervisors must be accountable to training and overseeing the next generation of systemic and collaborative providers. By bridging mental, behavioral, and medical systems of care through relational and collaborative interventions, patients can truly receive care that encompasses their BPSS needs. MedFTs serve a great need in primary and specialty care systems, whereby health, illness, death, and trauma are experienced within the family and healthcare contexts. It is through an attentive, involved, and supportive supervisory relationship that MedFTs can build and sustain a career. The supervision relationship is one that can last a professional lifetime, so make the journey all it can be.

Discussion Questions

1. What core competencies and supervision/clinical theories do you believe are vital for success when working with a MedFT supervisee?
2. What is the role of a supervisor who is working with a supervisee who is trying to initiate an integrated care model at a new site?
3. What are some steps that a supervisor can take to strengthen the relational lens used by a supervisee and his healthcare team?

Resources for Supervisors

While not all supervisors have been trained in relationally based and/or integrated care services, some may find the following educational and training materials beneficial (see Chap. 3; Tyndall et al., 2014):

- Agency for Healthcare Research and Quality's Academy for Integrating Behavioral Health and Primary Care (www.integrationacademy.ahrq.gov/).
- East Carolina University (for a reading list pertaining to MedFT) (http://www.ecu.edu/che/cdfr/phdmft.html).
- Collaborative Family Healthcare Association (www.CFHA.net).
- Integrated Behavioral Health Project (www.ibhp.org).
- National Council for Behavioral Health (www.thenaitonalcouncil.org/).
- SAMSHA-HRSA Center for Integrated Health Solutions (www.integration.samhsa.gov).

References[1]

Bischoff, R., Springer, P., Reisbig, A., Lyons, S., & Likcani, A. (2012). Training for collaboration: Practice skills for mental health professionals. *Journal of Marital and Family Therapy, 38*, 199–210.

Burch, N. (1970). Teacher effectiveness training instructor guide.

*Doherty, W. J., McDaniel, S. H., & Baird, M. A. (1996). Five levels of primary care/behavioral healthcare collaboration. *Behavioral Healthcare Tomorrow, 5*, 25–28.

*Edwards, T. M., & Patterson, J. E. (2006). Supervising family therapy trainees in primary medical settings: Context matters. *Journal of Marital and Family Therapy, 32*, 33–43. doi:10.1111/j.1752-0606.2006.tb01586.x.

Engel, G. L. (1977). The need for a new medical model: A challenge for biomedicine. *Science, 196*, 129–136. doi:10.1126/science.847460.

Engel, G. L. (1980). The clinical application of the biopsychosocial model. *American Journal of Psychiatry, 137*, 535–544. http://ajp.psychiatryonline.org/.

*Gawinski, B. A., Edwards, T. M., & Speice, J. (1999). A family therapy internship in a multidisciplinary healthcare setting: Trainees' and supervisors' reflections. *Journal of Marital and Family Therapy, 25*, 469–484. doi:10.1111/j.1752-0606.1999.tb00263.x.

Heath, B., Wise Romero, P., & Reynolds, K. (2013). *A standard framework for levels of integrated care*. Washington, DC: SAMSHA-HRSA Center for Integrated Health Solutions. http://www.integration.samhsa.gov/resource/standard-framework-for-levels-of-integrated-healthcare.

Hodgson, J., Lamson, A., Mendenhall, T. (2014). Preface. In J. Hodgson, A. Lamson, T. Mendenhall, & R. Crane (Eds.), *Medical family therapy: Advanced applications*. New York, NY: Springer.

Hodgson, J., Lamson, A., Mendenhall, T., & Crane, R. (2012). Medical family therapy: Opportunity for workforce development in healthcare. *Contemporary Family Therapy, 34*, 143–146. doi:10.1007/s10591-012-9199-1.

Hodgson, J., Lamson, A., Mendenhall, T., & Tyndall, L. (2013, October). *Medical family therapy health care continuum*. Poster presented at the American Association for Marriage and Family Therapy Annual Conference, Portland, OR.

*Hodgson, J., Lamson, A. L., & Reese, L. (2007). The biopsychosocial-spiritual interview method. In D. Linville, D. Lusterman, & K. Hertlein (Eds.), *Therapist notebook for family healthcare* (pp. 3–12). New York, NY: Hayworth Press.

*Hodgson, J., Mendenhall, T., & Lamson, A. (2013). Patient and provider relationships: Consent, confidentiality, and managing mistakes in integrated primary care settings. *Families, Systems, & Health, 31*, 28–40. doi:10.1037/a0031771.

Hodgson, J., Rambo, A., Boyd, T., Koehler, A., & Lamson, A. (2013). Supervision in evolving contexts. In T. Todd & C. Storm (Eds.), *The complete systemic supervisor: Context, philosophy, and pragmatics* (2nd ed.). Bloomington, IN: iUniverse.

Hudgins, C., Rose, A., Fifield, P. Y., & Arnault, S. (2013). Navigating the legal and ethical foundations of informed consent and confidentiality in integrated primary care. *Families, Systems, & Health, 31*, 9–19. doi:10.1037/a0031974.

Kroenke, K., Spitzer, R. L., & Williams, J. B. (2001). The PHQ-9: Validity of a brief depression severity measure. *Journal of General Internal Medicine, 16*(9), 606.

Long, J. K., Lawless, J. J., & Dotson, D. R. (1996). Supervisory styles index: Examining supervisees' perceptions of supervisory style. *Contemporary Family Therapy, 18*(4), 191–201. doi:10.1007/BF02195719.

[1] An asterisk has been used to note references that the chapter authors recommend for further reading.

Marlowe, D., Hodgson, J., Lamson, A., White, M., & Irons, T. (2012). Medical family therapy in a primary care setting: A framework for integration. *Contemporary Family Therapy, 34*(2), 244–258. doi:10.1007/s10591-012-9195-5.

McDaniel, S. H., Doherty, W. J., & Hepworth, J. (Eds.). (2014). *Medical family therapy and integrated care* (2nd ed.). Washington, DC: American Psychological Association.

McDaniel, S. H., Hepworth, J., & Doherty, W. J. (Eds.). (1992). *Medical family therapy*. New York, NY: Basic Books.

Nelson, T. S., & Johnson, L. N. (1999). The basic skills evaluation device. *Journal of Marital and Family Therapy, 25*(1), 15–30.

Patterson, J. E., Peek, C. J., Heinrich, R. L., Bischoff, R. J., & Scherger, J. (2002). *Mental health professionals in medical settings: A primer*. New York, NY: W.W. Norton & Company.

Peek, C. J. (2008). Planning care in the clinical, operational, and financial worlds. In R. Kessler & D. Stafford (Eds.), *Collaborative medicine case studies: Evidence in practice* (pp. 25–38). New York, NY: Springer.

Peek, C.J., & National Integration Academy Council. (2013). *Lexicon for behavioral health and primary care integration: Concepts and definitions developed by expert consensus*. (AHRQ Publication No.13-IP001-EF). Retrieved from http://integrationacademy.ahrq.gov/sites/default/files/Lexicon.pdf.

*Pratt, K., & Lamson, A. L. (2011). Supervision for the integrated behavioral health provider. In R. Curtis & E. Christian (Eds.), *Integrated care: Creating a thriving practice*. New York, NY: Haworth Press.

*Pratt, K., & Lamson, A. L. (2012). Supervision in behavioral health: Implications for students, interns and new professionals. *The Journal of Behavioral Health Services & Research, 39*(3), 285–294. doi:10.1007/s11414-011-9267-6.

*Tyndall, L. E., Hodgson, J. L., Lamson, A. L., White, M., & Knight, S. M. (2012a). Medical family therapy: Charting a course in competencies. *Contemporary Family Therapy, 34*(2), 171–186. doi:10.1007/s10591-012-9191-9.

Tyndall, L., Hodgson, J., Lamson, A. L., White, M., & Knight, S. (2012b). Medical family therapy: A theoretical and empirical review. *Contemporary Family Therapy, 34*(2), 156–170. doi:10.1007/s10591-012-9183-9.

Tyndall, L., Hodgson, J., Lamson, A., White, M., & Knight, S. (2014). Charting a course in competencies. In J. Hodgson, A. Lamson, T. Mendenhall, & R. Crane (Eds.), *Medical family therapy: Advanced applications* (pp. 33–54). New York, NY: Springer.

Wright, L. M., Watson, W. L., & Bell, J. M. (1996). *Beliefs: The heart of healing in families and illness*. New York, NY: Basic Books.

Chapter 9
Preparing for Leadership Roles in Healthcare Settings

Kenneth Phelps, Katherine Kueny, Barry Jacobs, Tommie Boyd, John Rolland, Macaran Baird, and James Zubatsky

Introduction

Medical Family Therapy (MedFT), like most fields and specialties, started with a vision. Over the last few decades, pioneers have been training the next generation to carry this vision into an ever-changing community and healthcare landscape. Over time, it has become increasingly clear that the spirit of MedFT cannot just be carried in the minds of those professionals. MedFTs have to turn that vision into reality. Considerable work has advanced in this vein, including the development of multiple degree and certificate programs, greater presence in healthcare environments, and advocacy for collaboratively oriented care. None of this progress could have occurred without the steady leadership of MedFTs. As we look to our future, it is important to visit the experiences of some MedFTs, new and seasoned, to gain a sense of where we have been and where we are going.

Each professional included in this chapter documented their personal journey in leadership, including the theories they drew upon to advance our field and lessons they have learned along the way. Contributors are from diverse contexts and backgrounds, representing both medicine and behavioral health. As they speak about leadership, examples are provided from the micro-level of clinical interaction to the macro-level of cultural change. Each writer's section begins with a brief introduction of his or her current work to provide the reader with a sense of the varied contexts and roles inhabited by MedFTs. The chapter ends with a personal interview with Mac Baird, M. D., where he provides a personal take on leadership and professional development.

K. Phelps (✉)
Department of Neuropsychiatry and Behavioral Science, University of South Carolina School of Medicine, Columbia, SC, USA
e-mail: Kenneth.phelps@uscmed.sc.edu

J. Hodgson et al. (eds.), *Medical Family Therapy*, DOI 10.1007/978-3-319-03482-9_9,

Kenneth W. Phelps, Ph.D., Assistant Clinical Professor, Outpatient Clinic Director, Department of Neuropsychiatry and Behavioral Science, University of South Carolina School of Medicine

Dr. Phelps is an LMFT- and AAMFT-Approved Supervisor who specializes in the treatment of couples with co-occurring physical, relational, and sexual difficulties. He leads educational efforts in the department on various therapies, including couple, sex, family, and group therapy. He also works closely with the Faculty Development Office to deliver conflict management presentations to various clinical departments. He is a member and past committee chair of the Collaborative Family Healthcare Association (CFHA) as well as a member of the American Association for Marriage and Family Therapy (AAMFT) and the American Association of Sexuality Educators, Counselors, and Therapists (AASECT). Past grants and publications involve the impacts of diabetes, cancer, and sleep apnea on personal and relational health. Dr. Phelps earned his undergraduate in Psychology as well as graduate degrees in Marriage and Family Therapy (MFT) and MedFT from East Carolina University. He completed a doctoral internship in Behavioral Medicine at Concord Hospital, Dartmouth Family Practice Residency Program.

Self of Leadership

More than a decade ago, I sat fearful on a cold gym bleacher as I heard my name announced: "Mr. Phelps won vice president of the student body." I had never thought of myself as a leader but internally hoped that I would one day have the skill set to engender change and build connection among a larger group. As I ponder my internal emotions during this period in my life, I am reminded that I had great doubt in my ability. I had purposefully selected vice president instead of president of the student body because it seemed less risky at the time. Fifteen years later, I have made substantial gains in my confidence as a leader. From my philanthropic leadership in my college fraternity to organizational leadership as membership chair in the CFHA, my leadership roles along the way have provided valuable professional development.

There have been many pivotal moments during my journey. During my undergraduate coursework, I found myself studying the nonverbal and verbal behavior of leaders that surrounded me. I learned a great deal from how they addressed others and found myself particularly captivated by leaders who could calmly de-escalate conflict situations among a group. Raised in a family with few verbal spats, I lacked experience or skills in understanding the dynamics of interpersonal conflict. Thus, my introduction to systems theory in an early MFT course sparked intrigue into group functioning. Eventually, my interest in systems theory, in-home work with the Autism Society, hospital-based work with families of children admitted to the intensive care unit, and personal experiences with a family member's stroke felt like a natural fit for MedFT. Fortunately, I was accepted. When I sat holding the acceptance letter to the MedFT program, it meant much more to me than a degree that could teach me to be a better researcher or an advanced collaborative clinician. Deep down, I felt that following the MedFT path in training might provide me with an experience that would build my leadership capability to engender change among larger groups as I had once hoped, whether a system of health care or community of need.

I am blessed to say that years later I have been able to fulfill that original hope. Currently, I spend much of my time in an administrative role as the Director of the Psychiatric Outpatient Clinic within the Department of Neuropsychiatry and Behavioral Science at the University of South Carolina School of Medicine. In this capacity, I am responsible for instituting policies and procedures for clinical care, ensuring effective workflow between office staffs and medical providers, and hiring of new staffs or faculty who contribute to our clinic. Additionally, I assist with troubleshooting our referrals and communication channels for providers referring into our facility. As a faculty member, I spend time seeing my own patients and leading a rotation where a multidisciplinary team (psychiatrists, pediatricians, rotating medical students, MedFTs, and psychologists) evaluate complex children and families in our outpatient context. While wearing my administrative and faculty hats, I have learned to draw on specific approaches that bolster my competence and provide a framework for effective leadership.

Theory of Leadership

In my development, I have used concepts from therapeutic theories and the organizational behavior field. As a relational based researcher, I have always respected and admired the contributions of Dr. John Gottman (1999, 2011). While Gottman's theories have considerable relevance to my work with couples navigating an illness, I also find his work to be applicable in the delivery of multidisciplinary, team-based care. For instance, Gottman (1999) writes in his comprehensive text *The Marriage Clinic* about responding to bids for connection. While we do not seek an intimate bond with our work colleagues, we do seek relational approachability and respect. Thus, ensuring that we acknowledge and respond adequately to everyone on a healthcare team can be important to create a safe environment. Gottman's notable conceptualization of the Four Horsemen of the Apocalypse can be quite pertinent to the work of a MedFT. The occurrence of defensiveness, stonewalling, criticism, and contempt not only erodes relational satisfaction in a marriage but also detracts from effective patient care on a team. I find myself quite often using the "antidotes" to these four horsemen as a leader and team member:

- Criticism: move from you to I
- Defensiveness: take responsibility for part of the problem
- Stonewalling: self-soothing to reduce physiological reactivity and enhance engagement
- Contempt: increase respect

While I find the principles outlined by Gottman to be helpful when someone is leading others from a position of equality, often a MedFT might be leading in a hierarchical system. An example of this might include supervising medical students, residents, or staffs in an outpatient clinic. In this scenario, the MedFT must outline specific objectives or expectations for those in the system. This is not too dissimilar to how structural family therapists place parents in the role of ensuring that youth in the family are aware of hierarchy and expectations (Minuchin & Fishman, 1981). A MedFT might be ideally suited for such a position due to the foundational appreciation for systems theory (von Bertalanffy, 1968). As we know, a change in one part of the system reverberates through other parts of the system. Forecasting those impacted by a new policy and procedure or workflow change can be crucial to ensure that the appropriate stakeholders are involved along the way.

Unfortunately, within every system there will be times when individuals do not meet the outlined expectations of administration. In these circumstances, I have found it helpful to address a few questions from the stance of a leader: (a) Was the expectation clearly communicated? (b) Did the individual have the resources or the internal capability to achieve this expectation given his or her current work demands? (c) Has this been an acute or a chronic problem for this person? (d) Is anything specific in the system influencing the person's ability to achieve the expectation? These questions can help guide discussions about unmet expectations. I have found the books *Crucial Conversations* and *Crucial Confrontations* particularly helpful (Patterson, Grenny, McMillan, & Switzler, 2002, 2005). These authors offer practical tips for having difficult dialogues within many occupational environments. Armed with these techniques (e.g., master the stories you are saying in your mind; decide if you are addressing content, pattern, or relationship; look for silence or violence), I have found myself confidently approaching instead of avoiding conversations that could lead to conflict. Given my history of non-confrontation, I truly appreciated these authors' comments about how avoiding an issue that needs to be addressed is like sitting on a block of stinky cheese and expecting it to just stop smelling. Just as we arm our patients and families with skills in treatment, I have found the acquisition of leadership skills as necessary on the journey toward becoming an effective MedFT.

Lessons Learned

As a therapist who often practices cognitive behavioral therapy (Beck, 1995), I have to ever remind myself to identify and work with the affect in the room, not just thoughts and behaviors. This is isomorphic to my biggest lesson as a leader. Early on, I often paid particular attention to the specifics of how our newest procedure was going while missing the important, broader questions as follows: How is this change going for everyone? How are they feeling about this change? What is the emotional temperature of the group? Over time, I have come to appreciate that the most perfect policy or procedure will miserably fail if individuals in the system do not feel acknowledged and heard throughout the process. In reflecting upon this, I am reminded of a wise quotation from American poet Maya Angelou: "I've learned that people will forget what you said, people will forget what you did, but people will never forget how you made them feel" (Kelly, 2003, p. 263). The importance of making people feel valued during a difficult change was illuminated for me early in my role as clinic director. Soon after assuming this role, our system decided to convert to a new electronic medical record, which undoubtedly is a frustrating change in a busy clinical practice. It was through this change that I came to appreciate validating the experiences of those in our system while problem-solving their concerns simultaneously.

After recognizing the importance of people feeling valued in any system, I quickly began to include multiple stakeholders in committees to address clinic policies, workflow, and staffing concerns. Just as in group therapy, a sizable committee (>10) can become unmanageable (Bieling, McCabe, & Antony, 2009). I quickly learned another lesson: it is important to be thoughtful and purposeful with who is involved in creating change. Throughout this process, I turned again to the work of Patterson et al. (2002). They cite four types of decision making: (1) command, (2) consult, (3) vote, and (4) consensus. As a MedFT, I often prided myself on collaboration; thus, I would try to reach consensus on all topics as a leader. Over time, it has become clear that this approach is not always the answer. Consensus can be time intensive and inefficient for some areas of practice. Thus, the second lesson I have come to appreciate involves the selective use of all four strategies outlined by Patterson and colleagues when in a leadership role.

A final lesson I would highlight as important for MedFTs is to remember what you are doing and why you are doing it. I have found that it is easy to take off the clinician hat when we put on the administrative or the research hat. Our work as clinicians gives us the honor of being close to the stories of a patient, couple, or family traversing the complex, frightening journey of an illness. It is helpful to utilize these stories to advocate for improved, family-oriented care. For instance, I typically send an e-mail to our front office staffs during the holidays thanking them for all their hard work and reminding them that their pleasant greetings can help brighten the day of the patient grappling with terminal illness, individual coping with severe depression, or couple attempting to recover from the interpersonal trauma of infidelity. I believe that reminding myself and others about the valuable work we are privileged to do can generate a system of compassion.

Katherine J. Kueny, Ph.D., Assistant Professor and the Director of Behavioral Medicine, General Internal Medicine Division, University of Nebraska Medical Center

Dr. Kueny holds her LIMHP and LMFT in the state of Nebraska and is an AAMFT-Approved Supervisor. She earned her master's degree from East Carolina University and her Ph.D. from Kansas State University, both in MFT. She has been working at UNMC since completing her doctoral internship in the Family Medicine department. As the first behavioral medicine provider in the General Internal Medicine department, Dr. Kueny has since built a behavioral medicine program for its residents. She conducts therapy and research as part of a patient-centered medical home model and is the director of the MedFT Certificate Program at UNMC.

Self of Leadership

Throughout the course of my graduate training in MFT, I encountered professional and personal experiences that sparked my interest in providing clinical care and education focused on the biopsychosocial (BPS) model of care (Engel, 1977). To explore this interest, I selected a MedFT doctoral internship. During my internship, I learned from my mentor that entering the field of MedFT was about paving your own path and seeking opportunities to expand collaborative health care, education, and research. He connected me with the division leader of General Internal Medicine, who expressed interest in adding a behavioral medicine component to his department. After a long interview process, I was offered the opportunity to emerge as a leader and fulfill a gap that has strengthened the residency program and overall patient care that we provide.

Prior to joining the department, General Internal Medicine was lacking a behavioral health curriculum as well as behavioral health providers. I was fortunate to have a division leader who believed in the BPS model of care (Engel, 1977). My division leader shared an investment in my vision and provided the support and space for me to develop as a leader. Throughout this process, I received support and guidance from my mentors in MedFT and my colleagues in Internal Medicine. I was patient and carefully observed clinic and departmental processes. During this time, I was also faced with a cluster of personal experiences that opened my eyes to further need for MedFTs. Soon after I married my husband, we endured two family losses due to illnesses, followed by my husband being diagnosed with lymphoma just shy of our first wedding anniversary. After almost 3 years of providing patient care, surveying needs, networking, establishing relationships, gaining buy-in, and providing informal education to residents and staffs, I had a renewed spark and personal investment to move forward and implement curriculum components, including new collaborative and integrative care protocols. I always valued integrated care, but I witnessed firsthand the need for more BPS training and care in healthcare settings and was committed to doing everything I could to help meet this need.

As our clinic worked toward implementing a patient-centered medical home (PCMH) model, my role evolved. I gradually incorporated behavioral health education into the residency program, which later became a formal behavioral medicine curriculum to address educational gaps. In addition, I implemented several new protocols, including one for depression screening in the residency clinic. Collaboration with other physicians, nurse practitioners, physician assistants, and nurses occurred throughout the development and implementation process. This was instrumental in being able to model the interdisciplinary care and education I passionately valued.

While my journey was not easy, it did lead me to where I am today. As the Director of Behavioral Medicine, I have a formal behavioral medicine curriculum for residents, which includes a monthly seminar for three to four residents each month, video reviews, and monthly noon conferences. I also now serve on the

PCMH board and have helped implement new protocols and research projects to further enhance the growth of our PCMH. A few of these projects include a new BPS chronic pain protocol and a research study on shared medical visits for patients with type 2 diabetes.

Recently, I was named the Director for the MedFT Certificate Program, which consists of teaching MedFT courses and supervising master's MFT interns in my clinic. I also recently created a doctoral level MedFT internship which would prepare a doctoral MFT student for a career as a behavioral medicine faculty member. This position has helped fulfill the need for another behavioral medicine position in my department, despite funding constraints. Although the journey is not complete, my leadership in MedFT emerged as part of an organic, reflective, and continuous process of personal, professional, and system growth.

Theory of Leadership

During the early stages of my faculty development, my leadership guidance came from past mentors and supervisors, in addition to current leaders and stakeholders in the General Internal Medicine Division. I sought a formal behavioral medicine consultation from a current leader in the field, who also built a behavioral medicine program in Internal Medicine. This consultation provided a vehicle for our department to come together to identify resources and barriers in order to develop a direction for the integration of behavioral medicine curriculum into our specific residency program. Simultaneously, I immersed myself, not only in the literature but also in practice and conversations. Leadership evolved through a process of integrating my vision for the future, collaboration, practice, theory, consultation, and core concepts driving my work.

Most of my leadership process has been rooted in the BPS model of care (Engel, 1977). The core concepts of the BPS model not only influence my clinical practice but also provide a foundation for my leadership style, curriculum content, approaches to curriculum development, and research. The BPS model is more than an approach to working with patients and collaborating with physicians and extenders; it is how I engage people and various systems. The more I incorporate this model into my tasks as Director of Behavioral Medicine, the more I recognize the entire clinic incorporating it into patient care, education, and research.

Beyond the BPS model, it became clear to me that in order to engage physicians and residents in enhancing their behavioral medicine skills and knowledge, I had to first understand how to develop a new curriculum. When searching for tools and models of curriculum development, I was directed to a curriculum development for medical education book by Kern, Thomas, Howard, and Bass (1998). These authors provided a structure that allowed me to pay attention to the framework of curriculum development, prior to prematurely implementing curriculum components. Throughout my leadership journey, I have followed their step-by-step approach to curriculum development: (a) problem identification and general needs assessment, (b) needs assessment of targeted learners, (c) goals and objectives, (d) educational strategies, (e) implementation, and (f) evaluation and feedback. This approach allowed me to slow down and adequately address the needs, goals, barriers, and most effective strategies specific to my department.

Lessons Learned

Every 2 years, I have the opportunity to teach and mentor a new group of first-year medical students as part of their Integrated Clinical Experience course. After a few months of medical school, the students address how overwhelming the experience can be. Every year, we tell our students that medical school is like trying to eat an elephant. You have to take it one bite at a time. My leadership journey also required that I take "one bite at a time." Though I learned many lessons along the way, the following themes emerged that are critical to my ability to lead and create change: (a) integrating yourself into a new system takes time, willingness to learn, and willingness to teach; (b) systems change is a process that requires the involvement of the system, collaboration, and relationship building; (c) MedFTs can play an integral role in initiating research opportunities; and (d) for sustainable change, a sturdy infrastructure is important.

When I started my position in the General Internal Medicine Division, I felt like a visitor in another country for the first time. Although I knew I was the first behavioral health provider and behavioral faculty member the department had ever had, I did not account for the staffs being unfamiliar and uncomfortable with me. I realized I had to learn their language and culture and allow them to learn my role, as well. I went to lunch with nurses, diabetes educators, social workers, and physicians whenever I had the chance. I took the initiative to ask questions and share my input. During brief consultations with medical providers, I would share pieces of my training, background, and experiences. I limited my assumptions and kept a curious mind. With time, and willingness to learn and teach, successful integration into new systems can occur.

The second theme that emerged for me had to do with system change. I was entering this new setting, full of ideas for enhancing patient care, residency education, and research opportunities. I pursued change in a system that had been functioning for many years without me. It was unrealistic to expect this change to be received with open arms, without first establishing strong, collaborative relationships with various stakeholders. I needed to first become a part of the system, prior to recommending any change. When asked to participate in any collaborative project or meeting, I said yes. When I heard of opportunities, like the PCMH board, I took initiative in expressing my interest in becoming involved. Opportunities did not come to me at first. I had to create space for them. I embraced the system and allowed the system to embrace me. Throughout this slow, evolving process, growth occurred.

As my relationships in the department grew stronger, opportunities for collaborating and developing new protocols or curriculum changes became more frequent. I recognized innovative pieces of our curriculum that were not getting researched or published. I learned that this was a role I could play. Recently, I was asked to be on a team to implement shared medical visits for patients with type 2 diabetes. The team was ready to implement immediately, and I requested that we take some extra time to conduct research. Although I am not an expert, I have now taken on the role of initiating research and have learned that becoming a leader in the field is more than doing great things. It is about sharing the great things that you are doing in order to push the field to continue to grow. During my training, I was taught that it was not enough to be doing collaborative work but that it was important to take advantage of research opportunities to show why the work was important. This is a role that I believe MedFTs are equipped to initiate, as a result of their systemic training and ability to elicit and respect multiple viewpoints.

Furthermore, I have learned not to underestimate the importance of administrative responsibilities and tasks. I have kept in mind Peek's Three-World view, which recognizes that healthcare systems function simultaneously in clinical, operational, and financial worlds (Peek, 2008). I have continued to ask myself what change in health care is needed (clinical), what it will take for this need to be met (operational), and what resources will be required to meet this need (financial). This includes having an understanding of billing, being aware of financial barriers, participating in staff and board meetings, effectively triaging referrals, and assisting in the management of team conflict and communication. I worked closely with the biller, receptionists, clinic director, and nursing staff to help develop processes that would be efficient for the team as a whole. I had several meetings with administration trying to make sure that we were following the rules of the hospital and handling my patient care and administrative tasks appropriately. I also led staff development trainings as needed. In general, these steps provided a sturdy infrastructure, which is necessary for sustainable change.

Barry J. Jacobs, Psy.D., Director of Behavioral Sciences, Crozer-Keystone Family Medicine Residency Program

Dr. Jacobs is a clinical psychologist, MedFT, and author of the book, *The Emotional Survival Guide for Caregivers: Looking After Yourself and Your Family While Helping an Aging Parent* (2006). Dr. Jacobs earned his bachelor's degree from Brown University and his doctorate in clinical psychology from Widener University. As a clinician, he specializes in helping families cope with serious and chronic medical illnesses. As an educator, he works as the Director of Behavioral Sciences for the Crozer-Keystone Family Medicine Residency Program in Springfield, PA, and has held adjunct faculty positions with the Temple University School of Medicine, University of Pennsylvania School of Nursing, and the Institute for Clinical Psychology of Widener University. He is the national spokesperson on family caregiving for the American Heart Association and a member of the American Association of Retired Persons (AARP) Caregivers Advisory Panel. He was a member of the American Psychological Association (APA) Presidential Task

Force on Caregiving that produced the Caregiver Briefcase website. A former journalist, he writes an advice column for *Take Care*!, the newsletter of the National Family Caregivers Association, and was the long-time editor of the "In Sickness & Health" column for the APA journal *Families, Systems, & Health*. He is a past board member of the CFHA and contributes frequently to its "Families and Health" blog. He is also an honorary board member of the Well Spouse Association and is on the expert panel for the Caregiving Crisis Great Challenge for TEDMED.com.

Self of Leadership

The primary care team is angry. At our weekly "huddle," family physicians fume, the social worker frets, and the pharmacist frowns. I am trying to explain the behavior of Ella, a caustic, depressed woman who out of deeply rooted fear that no one will ever care enough to meet her needs lambasts her clinicians at nearly every interaction. The team members, however, are having none of it. They eye me skeptically and continually grouse about her bracing manner. As this team's leader, I am left with a common dilemma: Do I push my point to try to help them become more empathetic and effective, or do I risk losing my credibility and authority with them?

Such multidisciplinary teams have become more prevalent in primary care since 2007 when four major medical organizations signed the "Joint Principles of the Patient-Centered Medical Home" (Patient Centered Primary Care Collaborative, 2007). Among the key principles of this new model of primary care is "physician-directed medical practice" in which physicians lead teams of healthcare professionals housed in primary care offices to address the full range of patients' BPS problems. My family medicine center—the Crozer-Keystone Center for Family Health in Springfield, PA, in suburban Philadelphia and the primary outpatient training site for the Crozer-Keystone Family Medicine Residency Program—became a certified PCMH by 2008 and began developing team-based care, especially for our most complex, chronically ill patients. We immediately confronted the many questions of operating a high-caliber team: Who comprises the team? How do members develop common, interdisciplinary goals and coordinate their clinical interventions? How do they communicate quickly and efficiently with one another as well as with patients and family members? And, of course, who leads and how?

I came to team leadership relatively late in my career. As a clinical psychologist and MedFT working for over two decades in a range of settings, including physical medicine rehabilitation centers, subacute rehabs, skilled nursing homes, retirement communities, acute care hospitals, and family medicine offices, I had served as the psychosocial expert on many clinical teams. In that capacity, I offered observations about and treatment recommendations for the psychiatric and psychological sequelae of patients' medical illnesses as well as suggestions for partnering with and supporting their often overtaxed family caregivers. It was only a year ago that I took the helm of my family medicine center's new "Super-Utilizer team," based on the work of family physician Jeff Brenner with the highest utilizers of medical services (see Gawande, 2011, for a description), after the physician-leader suddenly stepped aside at the program's inception. It has taken all my clinical wisdom and gumption to try to create effective team processes and clinical strategies for these challenging patients.

Take Ella, for instance. Though only 56 years old, she looks 15 years older because of her morbid obesity, grayish pallor, and poor grooming. Her persistent impoverishment and depression have undermined her ability to properly care for her diabetes, emphysema, knee pain, and other chronic conditions. Because her problems are so multifarious, I had to help devise means for the multidisciplinary team members to each assess her and develop their own clinical perspectives but then blend those perspectives into a coherent and cohesive treatment plan. That meant creating from scratch weekly treatment planning meetings in addition to monthly gatherings to revise and revise again our team processes. Because her stance towards the team was one of hostile dependency, I had to create a safe forum for team members to process their countertransference toward her as the best means to prevent all of us from feeling demoralized or developing an adversarial us-vs.-her approach. That meant modeling turn-the-other-cheek calm in the face of her hostility while still demonstrating understanding of the hurt feelings of our well-meaning but beleaguered team members.

Theory of Leadership

I have drawn on influences from three different parts of my career in order to create a set of standards with which I measure myself today as a leader. In graduate school in the 1980s, I was intensely interested in psychoanalytic concepts of how unconscious processes, especially anger, affect relational systems through mechanisms such as projective identification. From the early works of Ivan Boszormenyi-Nagy (1965)—a psychoanalytically oriented, family psychiatrist and family therapy pioneer who devised contextual therapy (and who taught at Hahnemann at the time)—I learned how small groups, such as families, might develop a sense of cohesion through prejudicial scapegoating of outsiders. I have been keenly aware since then of the propensities of anxious and overwhelmed healthcare professionals to sometimes denigrate the patients they are serving (e.g., "she's manipulative"). I understand the need for healthcare team leaders to firmly limit such scapegoating and find other means to bolster professional morale. From the writings of the British psychoanalyst Wilfred Bion (1959), I learned that it is normal and expectable for group members to become critical of their leader (much as teenagers turn on their parents) as a phase during their development to become effective working teams. I have been cognizant since then that I need to tolerate my team members' criticism because doing so creates a safer emotional space for the group to develop greater self-sufficiency and confidence.

After graduate school, I worked for 5 years in a physical medicine rehabilitation hospital where I participated in hundreds of clinical team meetings chaired by seasoned physiatrists and neurologists. What I learned from them is that the team leader must be attuned and flexible, tightening and loosening the reins in response to team members' changing needs. Specifically, I saw firsthand that when team members were feeling very anxious, it behooved the physician-leader to firmly direct the clinical plan. But when team members were feeling confident about their approaches to a given case, it was essential for the leader to step back and let the members devise their own plan, the better to foster their sense of mastery and competence.

Nowadays, as a team leader myself, I have also benefited from recent articles within the Family Medicine literature on training primary care physicians to assume PCMH team leadership (e.g., Saba, Villela, Chen, Hammer, & Bodenheimer, 2012; Safford & Manning, 2012). In particular, Perry Dickinson, Professor of Family Medicine at the University of Colorado-Denver, has developed training materials (Perry Dickinson et al. 2011) that spell out team leader competencies, e.g., setting expectations for team performance and system change; sharing information and being receptive to others' ideas; and managing team members' interpersonal issues.

Lessons Learned

The prime lesson I have learned thus far is that the team leader needs to constantly gauge and manage the affective life of the group—what happens among team members, between team members and patients, and between team members and the leader. The clinical outcomes of decreased medical symptoms, utilization, and costs are predicated upon whether or not trust is established and maintained and effective working partnerships are formed. The anxious reactions, heated arguments, and angry outbursts that sometimes punctuate the clinical course can undermine all progress. As a MedFT, I am trained to detect how roiling emotions ripple through our systems of health care and affect our success. But, as a leader, I also have to be willing to use that knowledge to intervene—to offer firm guidance when needed, kind words when feelings are ruffled, and broad tolerance for uncertainty and conflict. It is too easy for us to take umbrage at the Ellas in our practice; I need to nudge team members toward joining with these desperate patients as the best means for meeting their goals and ours.

This appreciation for emotion is paired with respect for a cognitive axiom: Know what you do not know and be willing to change. I have learned that there is no perfect team process or plan; different patients place different demands upon us, and I have to direct team members to adjust what we do to meet those idiosyncratic needs. What those specific adjustments should be is decided through concerted team engagement and communication via our regularly scheduled meetings, daily informal hallway conversations, and frequent e-mail and electronic medical record messages. We deliberate and debate and then talk some more. We honor everyone's viewpoint. We admit our clinical miscues (I take the lead in that, too). We push one another to learn, refine our approaches, and hopefully get better at what we do.

Tommie V. Boyd, Ph.D., Chair of the Department of Family Therapy and Director of the Medical Family Therapy/Family Systems Health Care program, Nova Southeastern University

Dr. Boyd is Chair of the Department of Family Therapy for Nova Southeastern University (NSU), Director of the Medical Family Therapy/Family Systems Health Care program, and Director of Collaboration with NSU health clinics. As an LMFT- and an AAMFT-Approved Supervisor with over 30 years of experience, Dr. Boyd provides supervision to students and interns in the areas of clinical theory and practice of MedFT. She collaborates with the NSU Health Professional Division in clinical services, overseeing direct training and supervision of MedFT students and interns. Over the past 10 years, Dr. Boyd has served as Program Director for the family therapy graduate programs at NSU. As an educator, Dr. Boyd collaborates, trains, and supervises students to focus on caring for the patient, the family, and support systems. She recently co-edited a book, *Family Therapy in Review: Contrasting Contemporary Models* (Rambo, West, Schooley, & Boyd, 2012), that is widely used as a family therapy textbook. Dr. Boyd has presented widely on topics of aging, grief and loss, geriatric issues, Parkinson's disease, diabetes support groups, mechanical ventilation withdrawal and family support systems, and autism as well as conducted research on these same topics.

Self of Leadership

Practicing MedFT has been an integral part of my professional experience for the past 30 years. In the early 1990s, I became a trainer for a large OB-GYN clinic with over 70 physicians, nurses, practitioners, and frontline staff. This training included engagement of professionals not only in the life of the patient but also in the family network. The training expanded to other medical practices and teams of professionals in a variety of community service agencies. From the beginning, the importance of a multidisciplinary team was apparent to me.

Later, I served on a team of medical and behavioral health professionals in a hospital setting which provided an integral approach to treatment of chronic pain patients. These patients, referred by their physicians, had undergone multiple treatments and yet continued to experience chronic pain with little hope for relief. Our multidisciplinary team evaluated the patient as a group. As a MedFT, I led the evaluation of relational aspects of the patients' lives, including family and friends. I observed the BPS issues that emerged from being a patient for quite some time. Couple relationships as influenced by chronic pain symptoms became the topic of my dissertation research.

My leadership in the MedFT field now includes serving as department chair of the family therapy programs at NSU (COAMFTE-accredited master's and doctoral level programs). I serve on NSU medical school committees and on the boards of various clinics. I am involved with the pediatric clinic, family medicine clinic, geriatric clinic, and internal medicine clinic as well as with our own family therapy clinic. Our department is involved with training interns and residents about the integration of psychological, relational, and medical issues. We teach and train how to integrate partners, children, and extended family input into successful treatment.

In this capacity, I develop and supervise master's and doctoral family therapy internships at NSU's Health Professions Division (HPD) (which includes a medical school, a nursing program, and an array of other allied health programs) and at other medical locations throughout the South Florida community. I also advise HPD faculty and provide a referral source for their patients and families. We strive for a collaborative team approach; our family therapy interns enter the treatment room together with residents, supervising physicians, nursing students, physician's assistant students, and so on. We are an integral part of the treatment team and outreach services at other area medical centers. We are also a resource to the community as a whole, and I train area physicians on a wide range of psychosocial issues.

In addition, my leadership role has extended into the development of interdisciplinary groups of professionals connected to look at various needs of the aging population in South Florida, including groups focused on geriatrics, diabetes, and Parkinson's disease, and in hospice settings. These larger groups of medical and behavioral health professionals have expanded teaching and training for one another and the community. Engagement in these communities provides integral conversations and a focus on the needs of others; thus, from a MedFT perspective, I can train interns and expand their involvement into community settings. Affiliations with the American Society of Aging, National Society of Aging, and Gerontology have provided opportunities to present and broaden the relevance of MedFT for seniors and their families.

In addition to my leadership role in the department, course offerings for the MedFT/Family Systems Healthcare courses promote an integral understanding of the issues families encounter during an illness and the grief and loss they experience when patients do not survive. Families continue to need a supportive environment which promotes health and wellness. As part of the coursework and internship, student interns complete their clinical requirements in a healthcare setting at the NSU clinics or an outside medical facility. These experiences provide hands-on training in a variety of settings and medical issues. These students work alongside physicians, nurse practitioners, physician assistants, their staff, and other professionals in a collaborative, interactive manner.

Medical issues and how families cope are integral to better understand how MedFTs can integrate into a healthcare setting. My research has included how patients with Parkinson's disease and their caregivers cope with the multiple issues of this illness, returning veterans and their families who experience major health changes, end-of-life issues, and training of residents in MedFT. Leading these research studies has solidified in my mind the need for understanding the unique nature of medical situations experienced by our patients and their families. The more we know, the better equipped we are to serve and train, direct programs, and educate future MedFTs.

Theory of Leadership

A systemic framework guides my thinking and practice, as I believe a relational lens promotes a deeper understanding of how individuals operate in family systems and how families and professionals can best work together. My relational understandings relate to the work of Gregory Bateson (2000). In addition, I am resource and solution oriented, operating on the assumption that patients and families are integral in the solutions to the issues they identify (Greenberg, Fanshorn, & Danilkewich, 2001). Engel's (1977) ideas regarding the connection between the biological, psychological, and social aspects of individuals and their extended families continue to serve as a basis for understanding how families integrate these areas of their lives. Along with the relational, solution-oriented, and BPS understandings that influence my work, I am sensitive to gender, race, class, and cultural issues and how they influence the ways in which families identify their interactions with medical professionals (McGoldrick & Hardy, 2008).

Putting it all together, I teach and train others to respect BPS individuality; look at behaviors and symptoms in context and from a relational perspective; and look for the patient's and family's own resources with the assumption that they have keys to their own solutions. This three-part model of practice informs and guides my work.

Lessons Learned

Over the years I have experienced, learned, and grown from the ideas of the populations I teach, train, and serve. They have taught me to sit back and intensely listen—listen to their stories, the stories that are important to them and that provide a depth of knowledge and understanding of who they are. Patience with the process of finding solutions is important, especially from a systemic perspective. Families, when allowed to tell their stories and in their own way, will find the solutions that fit with their own systems and their family traditions. An example that clearly identifies this concept occurred in a training hospital, when a physician shared with an obese patient the need to take better care of himself, specifically by giving up his four packs of cigarettes and eight sugared colas per day, which the patient stated he would not do. A MedFT, trained in a systemic, relational manner, asked the patient what he might be willing to do to take care of himself. He thought for a moment, reflecting on what he could do, and responded that he could smoke two less cigarettes and drink one less soda per day. The MedFT responded that this was interesting, asked if he actually thought he could do that so quickly, and made an appointment to see him at the next doctor's visit in 2 weeks. At the follow-up appointment, the patient had reduced his smoking to one pack per day and one cola per day. This was the patient's way of remaining in control and taking care of his health in a way that seemed possible to him. The learned and reinforced lesson was to listen to what the patient identified as a solution. This was much more effective than the unilateral demand the patient had initially envisioned. This is a small example of how to engage, collaborate, and listen to patients and their families. They possess the key to develop self-management skills of their own, those that fit and are possible for them. In addition to this basic, central lesson, so important to all that I do, I have learned some context-specific lessons over the years.

Lessons learned from patients:

- Patient responses directly reflect the relationship/rapport established through the medical/MedFT involvement.
- Asking patients/families what will work for them is crucial; this provides a basis for the patients themselves to select options that fit their philosophy of change.
- Attempting to take control and over-advising promote resistance.
- Collaboration with patients, families, and caregivers is essential in treatment and improvement in healing.
- So is including the family and caregivers.
- Overwhelmed patients lose focus and are less likely to remember suggestions/directions, so be patient and go slow.

Lessons learned from family therapy interns:

- Modeling is essential; show, rather than just tell, when interns are entering healthcare settings for the first time.
- Patience is as important for interns as it is for patients and families.
- Positive and strength-based interventions promote collaborative solutions with patients.
- Positive and strength-based supervision promotes collaborative training and helps develop enthusiastic, dedicated interns.

Becoming a leader in MedFT, I think, hinges on being oneself, being compassionate and responsive to others, and taking every opportunity to listen, learn, and pass those skills along to future MedFTs. I continue to look for novel ways to teach and train professionals and students. Being a director in a clinic or an educational setting requires the same skills. In every setting, I have learned to listen intently to the patient, to my colleagues, and to my students.

John S. Rolland, M.D., M.P.H., Executive Co-Director of the Chicago Center for Family Health and Professor of Psychiatry and Behavioral Neuroscience, University of Chicago Pritzker School of Medicine

Dr. Rolland is a Professor of Psychiatry and Behavioral Neuroscience at the University of Chicago Pritzker School of Medicine and Executive Co-Director of its affiliate postgraduate training institute, the Chicago Center for Family Health. He pursued his training in Medicine and Psychiatry at the University of Michigan and Yale University and earned a master's degree from the Harvard School of Public Health. He was the Founding Director of the Center for Illness in Families affiliated with Yale University. Widely recognized for his conceptual model and clinical work with families facing serious physical disorders, his publications include his landmark book, *Families, Illness, and Disability: An Integrative Treatment Model* (Rolland, 1994), and he is the coauthor of *Individuals, Families, and the New Era of Genetics: BPS Perspectives* (Miller, McDaniel, Rolland, & Feetham, 2006). From 2000 to 2003, he co-led a multi-year international project in Kosovo, the Kosovar Family Professional Education Collaborative, addressing family-centered training and service delivery needs in the aftermath of trauma, genocide, and loss. He is a Distinguished Fellow of the American Psychiatric Association and a former Fellow of the Institute for Social and Policy Studies at Yale. Past-President of the American Family Therapy Academy (AFTA), his professional honors include AFTA's Innovative Contributions to Family Therapy Award. He serves on the editorial boards of a number of journals including *Families, Systems, & Health* and has been active and served on the Boards of the CFHA, Physicians for Social Responsibility (PSR) and Physicians for a National Health Program (PNHP).

Self of Leadership

Near the end of medical school, I debated between Family Medicine and Psychiatry and ultimately decided to go into Community Psychiatry and Public Health. There have been both personal and professional experiences that have influenced my development as a family-focused practitioner. Personally, I was influenced by two experiences during my psychiatric residency. First, my mom had a stroke, which became one of my first close encounters with how families and the healthcare system interacted. Later in my residency, my first wife developed and later died of cancer. I remember there being no advice or support provided to me or our family in these experiences. I saw how marginalized the family was and that there was little effort to reach out to those outside of the "patient," who were also suffering. As I reached out to the providers and my professors for insight and understanding, I began to realize that there was no road map given to help individuals, couples, and families navigate these situations. No one had anything to offer to me in the situation. Almost everything was pathologizing. There was no guidance on whether what I and we as a family were experiencing was normal or dysfunctional. I remembered how I felt during these experiences and knew I wanted to help families not go through what I went through. I also wanted to help providers do a better job of understanding the importance of family and how illness impacts the entire family system.

My training in Community Psychiatry and Public Health taught me about behavioral health services design and delivery developed for larger community and regional populations. Long before I learned family systems theory, I was taught about systems theory at a community level and mindfulness to the complementary and competing interests and needs of multiple stakeholders. This went from the individual and family level through community health, behavioral health, and educational levels to larger system public sector and government budgetary priorities. Issues of social justice and equitable access to care were foundational to my training and thinking. Leadership always meant working collaboratively with the community and, in particular, consumers of health care and organizations that advocated for their needs. Theories of community organization and organizing and activism were important in forging my own leadership style. Over the years, I have found others with this common purpose through PSR and PNHP.

After completion of my training, my first job was as a director of a community mental health center affiliated with a community-based hospital during the time of deinstitutionalization of the chronically mentally ill. In this situation, a local state mental hospital was closed and 300 patients were discharged to the community with funds for staffing to develop community-based programs. During this time, in my role as a consultant to medical services and the emergency room in the hospital, I learned out of necessity to include available family members in my assessment of patients' behavioral health crises. To no surprise, I learned that this was far more clinically effective and time efficient.

Later, I returned to Yale for a postdoctoral fellowship at the Center for Health Studies at the Institute for Social and Policy Studies. My focus was family-centered approaches to behavioral health care with major illness. During this time, I travelled to New York for formal training in family therapy with Betty Carter and Peggy Papp. This time allowed me to combine my training and experience as a community psychiatrist with family therapy as applied to families facing chronic illness and disability. Upon completion, I founded with colleagues the Center for Illness in Families, an independent center affiliated with Yale. I learned that families in these situations are typically in desperate need for guidance and support. Healthcare providers, healthcare systems, and illness-based consumer organizations were very interested. We emphasized prevention, resilience, psychoeducation, and initial and periodic consultation to families, alongside emphasizing to healthcare professionals our expertise with complex cases. Emphasis on both is essential to a broad-based service that appeals to consumers and healthcare professionals.

After remarriage, I moved to Chicago and co-founded the Chicago Center for Family Health with Dr. Froma Walsh. We created the center as an independent affiliate of the University of Chicago, jointly sponsored by the Medical School and the School of Social Service Administration (Social Work). This center and its specialized programs in families, illness, and collaborative health care has been my professional base for the past 20 years. My Family Systems Illness Model and Dr. Walsh's Family Resilience Framework have provided a conceptual base for clinical practice, service delivery, and professional training (Rolland & Walsh, 2005). MedFT doctoral fellows have been based on-site both in family medicine and tertiary care settings, such as the University of Chicago Kovler Diabetes Center. Opportunities to train and consult to both international healthcare systems/services and some innovative national ones have provided me with a sustaining vision of what is possible on a broader scale. Over the years, I have continued to direct family training within the Department of Psychiatry.

Theory of Leadership

A theme of my way of leadership is to create your own system, but be affiliated with a larger healthcare system/university-based medical center. The advantage of this approach is autonomy to develop one's own ideology. Its challenge is that funding, growth, and sustainability are always your responsibility as a leader. Personally, I prefer the independence. In this regard, my credentials as a physician and psychiatrist are very useful. For me, the fact that my thinking did not fit mainstream Psychiatry (technically, my professional/discipline home) was significant in needing to create my own professional systems.

Professionally, in addition to my personal family experiences with illness and readings, I was strongly influenced by my primary mentors, Betty Carter in multigenerational family life cycle and Dan Levinson in individual life cycle development. They informed and inspired my conceptual thinking about how illness, family systems, and individual family members' development interact across time. Their writings (McGoldrick, Carter, & Garcia-Preto, 2010) and use of my conceptual model (*Families, Illness, & Disability: An Integrative Treatment Model*, 1994) and Dr. Walsh's *Strengthening Family Resilience* (2006) guide our overall training of MedFTs. To name a few of the other valuable texts that are used in our training Drs. Walsh and McGoldrick's *Living Beyond Loss: Death in the Family* (2004) provides a systemic base to work with life-threatening illness and palliative/hospice care. *Medical Family Therapy and Integrated Care* (McDaniel, Doherty, & Hepworth, 2013) and the *Shared Experience of Illness* (McDaniel, Hepworth, & Doherty, 1997), as well as the work of Wright and Bell (2009) on belief systems in illness, are very valuable. Doherty and Baird's (1986) formulation of developmental levels in family-centered medical care provides an excellent conceptual base for clinical models of care and the role of MedFTs. Also, I find Seaburn and colleagues' *Models of Collaboration: A Guide for Mental Health Professionals Working with Physicians and Health Care Professionals* (1996) very beneficial. The writings of medical anthropology and leaders in the role of culture, such as Arthur Kleinman (1988) and Laurence Kirmayer (2012), are also incorporated.

Lessons Learned

Personally, in healthcare settings, I have learned to identify myself as a "family-oriented behavioral health consultant." Certainly as a psychiatrist, this is more acceptable to patients and their families, who have no prior exposure to behavioral health professionals. Outside of my practice or a mental behavioral health clinic setting, I have always found the term "consultant" an easier entry point to a relationship with patients/families, program development, and leadership.

In recent years, I have become increasingly interested in funding for family-centered prevention models of integrated behavioral health care. This means both providing family-oriented behavioral health care to individuals/families at high risk for a condition, such as diabetes, and families entering the world of chronic illness, such as cancer, cardiovascular disease, or dementia. I have had most success implementing brief family psychoeducation consultations that can be incorporated as a family-oriented behavioral consultation in routine intake protocols or multi-family group psychoeducational "modules" (e.g., four evening sessions or a week-end skill-building format). The latter is very cost effective, identifies higher risk families, and networks families facing the same disease. I have found prevention-based models of integrated behavioral health care to be more challenging in terms of getting the buy-in needed to access the financial and administrative resources to establish an effective program. Ultimately, I think that these types of prevention-oriented initiatives would need support at the government and policy levels if any real impact is going to be made for a long term.

Repeatedly, I have learned that the first step to effective collaboration is to help other healthcare professionals understand both what MedFTs do and how these providers can add value in their particular healthcare setting. It is important to be able to concisely describe how this benefits the organization in the short and long term, thereby getting buy-in. Often, to gain initial access to a clinical service or organization, it is useful to provide services at a lower cost and intervene with complex cases to demonstrate effectiveness.

Macaran A. Baird, M.D., M.S., Head of the Department of Family Medicine and Community Health, University of Minnesota with James M. Zubatsky, Ph.D., Postdoctoral Fellow, University of Chicago Center for Family Health

Dr. Baird is the Head of the Department of Family Medicine and Community Health at the University of Minnesota. This large department with over 150 residents and multiple practice locations sponsors eight family medicine residencies in both rural and urban locations. Dr. Baird began his medical career in 1978 as a rural physician and therapist. He and Bill Doherty coauthored *Family Therapy and Family Medicine* in 1983, which launched his academic and leadership career. Since his rural days, Dr. Baird has held a number of leadership positions, including Family Medicine Residency Director at the University of Oklahoma; Professor and Chair of Family Medicine at Upstate Medical University at Syracuse, New York; Associate Medical Director for HealthPartners (where he helped integrate behavioral health services into 24 primary care clinics); and Medical Director of Mayo Medical Services (now MMSI) for Mayo Clinic, Rochester, Minnesota. Since 2002, he has been in his current position at the University of Minnesota Medical School. He was a coauthor for the Institute of Medicine's 2001 *Health and Behavior Report* and has been a member of advisory panels for the Robert Wood Johnson Foundation and the MacArthur Foundation as well as for other organizations. His current research and clinical focus are in the integration between behavioral medicine and primary care and identifying the social and care system factors that inhibit positive outcomes for patients and families.

Dr. Zubatsky is an LMFT with specific interest in the impact of medical illness on couples and families. He earned his master's degree from the University of San Diego in MFT and his doctoral degree from the University of Minnesota in Family Social Science, specializing in MedFT. He is currently pursuing a postdoctoral fellowship at the University of Chicago-affiliated Center for Family Health, with clinical responsibilities at the Illinois Masonic Medical Center Family Practice. His clinical interests include chronic illness in families, dementia, end-of-life issues, and couples therapy. Dr. Zubatsky has authored several peer-reviewed journal and media articles and received the Minnesota Association of Marriage and Family Therapy's Student of the Year award while attending the University of Minnesota.

The following are excerpts from an interview conducted between Dr. Zubatsky and Dr. Baird regarding leadership roles in MedFT. An interview format allowed both professionals from different generations of MedFT to engage in a conversation on past, present, and future topics of leadership in the field.

Zubatsky: How did you first become interested working in MedFT?

Baird: When I was a resident in training here at the University of Minnesota, I wanted to learn what at that time I called "office counseling." It had to do with seeing patients with supervision during my routine office or hospital visits and learning what some people call "the rest of the story." Some of my supervisors in my family medicine residency were AAMFT Approved Supervisors. During my residency from 1975 to 1978, I was heavily seeking supervision and qualified as a family therapist by the end of my program. I also earned a master's degree in Family Practice with a minor in Counseling. This qualified as an advanced degree in a related field. My supervisors introduced me to family therapy, family systems, and general systems theory. As a resident, I was almost always in a healthcare setting. We did not call it MedFT yet. Many years later this term was coined by Bill Doherty, Susan McDaniel and Jeri Hepworth.

Zubatsky: Were there any mentors or people that helped you along the way, that got you started in the field or helped you to work your way up towards a leadership position?

Baird: I have had many mentors. Locally, several of the behavioral health faculty would either see patients with me in my family medicine residency clinics almost every week or in the hospital. Jack Kelly, MD, Jerry Ronning, MD and Gus (Elof) Nelson, MA of Divinity, were my most active mentors and supervisors. Several others joined from time to time. When they could not be with me directly, I would videotape family interviews and we would review them later in the week. Several of them introduced me to MFT as a whole field of behavioral health that grew out of Psychiatry, Psychology, and Social Work. At the time, it never occurred to me that this was a relatively new field. However, at that time you could put the entire literature for family therapy on one table. So I read much of the foundational literature created by the pioneers of the field, many of whom I soon met at national meetings.

Soon after, I started a rural group practice in Wabasha, Minnesota. I met Bill Doherty and we became fast friends and collaborators. We were invited to write a book about the interface of Family Therapy and Family Medicine—called *Family Therapy and Family Medicine* (Doherty & Baird, 1983)—which took several years to complete and publish. I also started teaching locally and nationally about the high value of engaging families during key points of medical care. At that time, there were about 10–12 other family physicians who were similarly interested and writing/teaching nationally. In the early 1980s, we connected with both the academic forces of family therapy/family social science and family medicine academic departments and thought leaders. During that time, I had contact with many of the early pioneers from both fields and adopted some as mentors. We would have extended discussions at national meetings, and intermittent phone calls from these mentors commonly interrupted my rural practice time. Before long, I was giving workshops on these topics for academic departments in both fields. Don Bloch connected me with many pioneers of family therapy when I was writing the book with Bill Doherty. Thereafter, among my mentors, were Rabbi Ed Freidman, Salvador Minuchin, and Carl Whitaker. It was a great privilege for me to have such contacts. Several are deceased now, but I still consider them all as my mentors. During those years, I also hired an AAMFT consultant to drive 75 miles once per month from Minneapolis to Wabasha to see my most challenging families/patients as a co-therapist. If I was too busy or did not plan well enough to be available for those joint sessions, I still owed him a full half-day's pay! So, I learned to be organized and usually saw the families. This helped me continue to grow as a therapist.

Zubatsky: So what were some of your experiences along the way as you worked in this integration between behavioral health and medicine in becoming a leader in the field? Can you take us through the journey a little bit?

Baird: It was always a mystery to me how anyone could separate the behavioral health from the medical health or overall health. Having been trained as both a family physician and family therapist, it didn't make sense to me. So I never did make the mind/body split. Since I was trained to interview families, it was natural for me in my routine rural Minnesota medical practice to presume that the social and family context of the patient was quite often relevant and sometimes critical to manage something that was complicated. This was especially true when things did not quite add up. That is when I would enjoy engaging a wider group, most often the family. Sometimes it was the employer. It could have been a social agency, but I would engage the most relevant wider group with patients' permission. Such a strategy seemed natural to me and would often lead to a whole different set of questions and, therefore, more varied opportunities for more satisfactory outcomes. Soon after, I started practicing and teaching locally.

Following this, I was invited to national meetings to make presentations or workshops. Almost once per month I was invited as a guest faculty to visit departments of family medicine and some family therapy training programs. I would interview their families and cases that did not make sense or were troubling them. I would insist that we get family members involved in the interview that we would do live. This is what Carl Whitaker called the "battle for structure" (Whitaker & Malone, 1953). I enjoyed those consultations and academic visits very much. Most often, those difficult cases had all kinds of systems issues wrapped around them.

Zubatsky: What led you to working your way up to an administrative or leadership position? What did it take for you to "climb the ladder?"

Baird: I do not know if I have wisdom on that. I ended up in my first administrative leadership roles after I was vocal about systemic changes that I thought would help us do a better job wherever I was working. I left an intimate and rewarding rural practice to join other very smart people also committed to exploring family systems issues at the University of Oklahoma, Department of Family Medicine. We all wanted to learn more about engaging families in health care. Bill Doherty, PhD, Howard Stein, PhD, Joanne Patterson, PhD, and Steve Spann, MD, Richard Clover, MD and others had come together to explore this family/medical territory in the Department of Family Medicine, then chaired by Christian Ramsey, MD.

My intellectual transition away from rural practice and into a robust academic environment was quite painful. In 1983, my family and I moved to Oklahoma after much discussion. I made this move for two reasons. First, I wanted to learn more at a faster rate, because I was bridging these two fields of family medicine and family therapy. As a physician in a rural practice, I did not think I could keep up with both fields. I know it may sound odd, but my second reason was that after the book, *Family Therapy and Family Medicine* (1983), I had a problem with too much local credibility. Trainees in family therapy or family medicine spending rotations with me in the practice or other members of the local behavioral health and nursing teams started to express unquestioned confidence in my clinical approach. I would often raise the question, "What if I'm completely wrong on this hypothesis for this patient/family? If that were the case, what should we do as a next step?" Literally, they would say to me, "You can't raise that question because you're the expert here." I knew I wasn't an expert and still had much to learn.

Zubatsky: So in a leadership position, more of a collaborative capacity, what kind of personal characteristics do you feel have helped you in your role as a leader?

Baird: One of the things I believe comes from systems thinking, and maybe it is a personality quirk, is that if you're really thinking this way (systemically), you have to keep looking beyond the immediate presenting complaint or problem to find a better approach to any problem, whether it's administrative or clinical. Often this permits the whole group to raise the larger questions, often a level or two above the presenting issue. If one does that, whether in a small environment or larger institution, often one will raise questions that can challenge the integrity of the larger system. The group may have been avoiding a difficult issue for a long time. This was often a way to avoid short-term conflict but that avoidance could be undermining the function of the group.

To clarify the similarities and differences between work systems and families, I have often referred to the McMaster Model of Family Functioning (Epstein, Bishop, & Levin, 1978). In this model there are six dimensions of healthy functioning: problem solving, communications, roles, affective responsiveness, affective involvement, and behavior control. Each has a most effective method of functioning. For example, clear and direct communication is the most effective while unclear and indirect communication is the least effective. For all six dimensions, one can list the ways business organizations may be parallel. I have often referred to this model to help me set administrative direction.

Another systems theory I have found useful is the Fundamental Interpersonal Relations Orientation (FIRO) Model of group interaction first published in the 1950s to describe how small groups of 6–8 people function as they come to action on a topic (Schutz, 1958). Doherty and Colangelo adapted this model to describe the various schools of family therapy in 1984. In the original model, the hypothesis was that in order to function well, a group must move in linear order through the following issues:

- Inclusion: Who is included (membership) and what behaviors are included as normal in the group? If the group solves these related topics reasonably then the group can move successfully to manage:
- Control: Who is in charge, and of what? If they settle this, then the people involved can move to into planning and strategy. This may be an ongoing process but reasonable stability about roles is needed to move to:
- Intimacy (for business purposes, consider this as a Shared Philosophy): What are the shared values and assumptions that can be expressed and are noticeable/visible in the work system; i.e., mission/vision.

I have used the FIRO model explicitly in my several administrative roles. I have found that the most common dilemmas in work systems commonly follow these small group dynamics. First, who is the group? If the working group does not have consistent membership or attendance, the leader must retrace decisions, revisit past discussions and morale fades as time is wasted. Therefore, first one must define the group with whom one is working. Very commonly in administrative roles, there was no defined boundary on who you were dealing with. There would be people absent or wouldn't be there, or people who wondered through and wouldn't be serious participants. It would undermine the whole process by not defining the boundaries around the whole conversation.

One of the things that I did differently early in my administrative career was that I was fairly tough on defining boundaries. Then I could define who was in charge of what. Only then, could the group delegate and not otherwise undermine someone. Then the group talked productively about a shared philosophy. The FIRO model used the term "intimacy." At an administrative level, I use "shared philosophy" as more appropriate. Frequently, groups avoid defining the inclusion and control issues and can talk endlessly about mission and vision. It can easily become meaningless, because they hadn't done any of the earlier steps. This breeds cynicism on the part of many workers.

Zubatsky: In MedFT, what particular skill sets do you believe are important in assuming a leadership role or position?

Baird: Well, a characteristic more than a skill set is humility. Humility goes a long way to improve leadership. Arrogance is just toxic to leadership. It really ruins things. And so, whatever expert knowledge base we have, if we aspire to leadership responsibility with a projected arrogance we will be unlikely to succeed. Few people trust arrogant leaders. So number one is humility.

Number two is to be courageous enough to engage the full group that is in conflict to most effectively work toward resolution of the conflict. No matter what theories we champion, it is important to engage those who are in conflict. When I see things around me that just don't work, it is often because we're not directly interacting with those most relevant to the problem.

Number three, a leader must help develop and/or provide direction for a group. General direction may be declared such as we will be honest and respectful. So direction setting of that type is critical to leadership and is parallel to how a therapist providers ground rules for the therapy sessions.

Number four, relieve pressure on the most pressured member of the team, if possible. Avoid creating a "hot seat" which can foster the creation of scapegoats rather than solve real problems. Understand who the most vulnerable person in the room is and develop a strategy to help that person, shift the vulnerability, or share it. In business or administration it is common for the most vulnerable person to be the person who has the biggest administrative title or, alternatively, the one closest to the problem being discussed but with no perceived authority. Commonly, my goal is to find out who's on the hot seat. The goal would not to be to skewer that person, but to interrupt the process of scapegoating.

Zubatsky: Looking back, are there a couple of valuable lessons that you have learned in your wealth of experience and years of being in this position?

Baird: Well one, given my recent illness that I have learned is that I have probably overcommitted to work over the years. You are in a newer generation that may do better with that balance. Working 60 or 70 h per week was our pattern. I think you may find a more reasonable way to get work done!

Zubatsky: We're still working on that!

Baird: The second thing is that your generation may be less naïve than I was in my early years. I used to assume the integrity of the layers above me. Although that is commonly a safe assumption, it is not universally valid. Now I stay alert for signs of trouble at all administrative layers and seek ways to ensure integrity in my own unit and in those with whom I work. By respectfully raising awkward questions, I gain either reassurance or expose nonsense as early as possible. It is usually something that can be corrected. By doing this, I believe I have helped institutions to do things that they aren't very eager to do but must do to stay healthy.

Zubatsky: What is it like in a healthcare setting as far as the supervisor-supervisee relationship that may be similar or different to that of traditional mental health?

Baird: First, the pace of the clinical interactions is much quicker than they are in family therapy or psychotherapy settings. So there's less time to contemplate the next step and less time for moment by moment supervision or feedback to trainees. Therefore, the coaching is a bit truncated compared to a therapist's training.

Second, creating change in families, structural or systematic, is not often done via one interaction. That type of change usually takes several or many interactions. Therapy is often much more strategic than medical interactions which are often focused on near-term treatment or diagnostic issues.

Third, in healthcare settings, there are more operational and logistical things to consider. Not only are the topics more concrete, such as there are certain medications to use, etc., there are more space and privacy complications in healthcare settings. Where the two fields are parallel is when medical clinicians are recommending lifestyle changes or more fundamental change on the part of patients and treatment is increasingly seen in the context of families. Those parallels exist.

Finally, there is a difference in the perceived need for a high degree of self-awareness. A therapist is properly trained to be self-aware and understand one's reaction to a patient and family, while a physician may not have such training. In my mind, a good therapist assumes that if therapy is "stuck" or stalled, the therapist him or herself is part of what is "stuck." In other words, the therapist can be part of the problem; it is not unusual. Then a supervisor, including for experienced therapists, can assist the therapist to change prior to expecting the patient or family to change. I still assume that is valid for me whether as an administrative leader trying to solve a "stuck" problem or as a therapist. If I'm stuck in some way and nothing is happening, I automatically assume that I'm part of the problem.

Zubatsky: What advice would you give a future professional who is considering a leadership position?

Baird: There is no substitute for just gaining experience in leadership roles to learn the ins and outs of managing or leading people. So that includes managing personnel issues, budget issues and helping a group set a strategic direction. It is a continuous learning experience. Sometimes because of academic titles or other things, any of us can be put into leadership roles without what we would desire as preparation. Training as a MedFT offers part of the background that can be extremely helpful as preparation for such leadership.

Future Directions

Given recent shifts in the healthcare landscape, it is fertile ground for MedFTs in leadership roles. Our training in systems theory is ideally suited for working alongside varied colleagues, whether on research projects, clinical or educational teams, or administrative committees. In order to move us forward, we need to be visible. MedFTs have traditionally practiced within the primary care environment where family physicians often think systemically, as well. The PCMH is but one example of the multidisciplinary team-based approaches that are being developed and implemented to better address our society's complex healthcare problems. Others include the emerging care transition programs that are designed to decrease hospital readmissions (for an overview, see Peikes et al., 2012) and disease management programs for specific conditions such as diabetes and chronic heart failure. While all of these programs are geared toward reducing medical morbidity, they are not always led by physicians. In many instances, nurses have taken the administrative and clinical lead to address BPS goals and systemic change. MedFTs, experts in the relational consequences of illness, knowledgeable about systems and change, and advocates for interprofessional collaboration, are ideally situated to take up the cudgel, as well. We can only do so, though, if we accomplish the following:

- Create and run broad-based, interdisciplinary, clinical programs, not just the ones that focus on narrower behavioral or relational goals.

- Nurture and empower collaborators from all disciplines, not just like-minded, systemically oriented therapists in education and practice.
- Conduct research to link the use of team-based treatment approaches and particular team processes to patients' clinical outcomes.

MedFTs' continued visibility as leaders in the primary care context will be important as well as moving into specialty contexts. Partnering with general practitioners and specialists allows for our skill sets to be employed in new, expanding ways. The next step for MedFT educators is curriculum expansion to incorporate the skills needed for integration into tertiary and home/community healthcare environments. There is enormous opportunity for MedFTs to design and provide services in chronic illness-based and specialty medicine (e.g., Oncology, Cardiology, Rehabilitative Medicine, Pediatrics, Obstetrics and Gynecology, Palliative Care/Hospice). Since it is by definition family based, the burgeoning field of genomics is particularly well suited to the relational/systemic skills of a MedFT. Greater access to medical in-patient services would also be an area of exploration. It is typically a crisis point in health care, where patients and their families are vulnerable, biomedical providers often need behavioral healthcare support, and all are usually brought into closer physical proximity. Many of these settings have a collaborative team ethos and structure that is just not family oriented enough; a leader with advanced family-oriented behavioral health skills would bring a powerful set of skills needed to bring together the patient, family/support system, and healthcare team.

For emerging MedFT leaders, it is important to identify healthcare settings that would be appropriate and begin inquiring about needs and opportunities within those settings early in one's career. Doctoral internships often provide an opportunity for networking and possibly creating new jobs to expand the field. Established MedFTs can contribute to the enhanced training and future growth of the field by developing internship opportunities for master's and doctoral level students. Not only do internships provide opportunities for students, but they also help to expand the collaboration and services offered within the healthcare setting.

As MedFTs merge into new practice settings or create new training environments, specific attention should be paid to the executive team, such as medical directors, administrative leadership of healthcare systems, and benefit directors. These are the individuals who have or know how to access financial resources to support our services. Forging an effective relationship with a clinical service's/center's medical and nursing directors greatly benefits overall development and implementation of family-sensitive service delivery models. Finally, increased exposure to and opportunities for training in organizational development and management skills would help promote greater MedFT leadership.

At this point of the field's research development, MedFTs need to lead collaborative research and program evaluation teams in collaboration with other healthcare disciplines to demonstrate how we fit into a broad range of healthcare contexts. Academically, products of this work can be presented at professional conferences both within and outside of the MedFTs' core discipline area(s).

MedFTs should join non-guild organizations, such as the National Council on Family Relations (NCFR), AFTA, and the CFHA where relational and systemic thinkers are moving to advance health care in this direction. Additionally, assuming learner and leadership positions in organizations that value family-based healthcare approaches (e.g., National Family Caregivers Association (NFCA), Well-Spouse Foundation) and illness-oriented, consumer-based organizations (e.g., MS Society, American Diabetes Association) is important in increasing awareness and further developing MedFT.

Another means of dissemination includes publishing in diverse healthcare journals, emphasizing the application and benefits of a systems perspective and the role of MedFTs within various healthcare contexts and illnesses. Indeed, MedFT's leaders need to continue their efforts at increasing visibility and presence in the literature. Leading research teams on collaboration and behavioral health integration can help pave the way for students and new professionals' future jobs and training opportunities. Established MedFT researchers offering mentorship and support to young professionals are invaluable, thereby creating the MedFT researchers of tomorrow. For sustainability of MedFT leaders in this changing healthcare climate, ongoing research and advocacy will be needed to show the value of our systemic and BPS lenses.

Conclusion

MedFTs have the opportunity to understand illness and wellness in unique ways; they have the systemic education and experience to work in settings outside the therapy room, where they are constantly learning from—and training—other medical professionals. This network of relationships will extend to and enhance all healthcare settings. The future of health care will depend on therapists and other professionals learning to deliver care from a BPS, relationally, economically, and culturally sensitive perspective. Imbedding systemic training into healthcare education, political, and larger healthcare systems will be required if MedFT is to flourish as a field. Larger system issues such as reimbursement and access must be considered as well as individual family and treatment systems. Serving as leaders, voicing our concerns for medical treatment, and advocating for the best medical care possible, MedFTs play an important role in the changing healthcare system. Our message for burgeoning leaders is to look beyond the individual patient and family system, to the treatment system, and to the larger healthcare system. Our relational, sensitive perspective is needed at all levels.

The professionals in this chapter reflect the wide-ranging work of MedFTs. Across care settings, from primary to specialty care, each is working to move forward the mission and spirit of MedFT. While each individual has a distinct approach to leadership, common themes run through all the narratives, including creating opportunities for the next generation, seeking mentorship, viewing problems and creating solutions systemically, listening to important stakeholders, and including consumers in our decisions. As a collective unit, the importance of systems or relational thinking was repeatedly mentioned as well as drawing on existing theoretical knowledge to improve our aptitude as leaders.

Discussion Questions

- How would you define an effective leader?
- Which theoretical approaches align with your own view of effective leadership?
- What concepts beyond systems theory seem common among the MedFT leaders?
- Given the various future directions, what path would best fit with your clinical, research, or administrative goals?

References[1]

Bateson, G. (2000). *Ecology of mind.* Chicago, IL: University of Chicago Press.
Beck, J. S. (1995). *Cognitive therapy: Basics and beyond.* New York, NY: The Guilford Press.
Bieling, P., McCabe, R., & Antony, M. (2009). *Cognitive-behavioral therapy in groups.* New York, NY: The Guilford Press.
Bion, W. (1959). *Experiences in groups.* New York, NY: Basic Books.
Boszormenyi-Nagy, I. (1965). A theory of relationships: Experience and transaction. In I. -Boszormenyi-Nagy & J. L. Framo (Eds.), *Intensive family therapy* (pp. 33–86). New York, NY: Harper & Row.
Dickinson, P., Deaner, N., Jortberg, B., & O'Neill, C. (2011). *Building PCMH sustainability through training internal quality improvement leaders* [PowerPoint slides]. Retrieved on March 31, 2013, from http://www.fmdrl.org/index.cfm?event=c.beginBrowseD&clearSelections=1&criteria=dickinson#3627
Doherty, W. J., & Baird, M. A. (1983). *Family therapy and family medicine.* New York, NY: Guilford.
Doherty, W., & Baird, M. (1986). Developmental levels in family centered medical care. *Family Medicine, 18*, 153–156.
*Doherty, W. J., & Colangelo, N. (1984). The family FIRO model: A modest proposal for organizing family treatment. *Journal of Marital and Family Therapy, 10*, 19–29.
*Engel, G. (1977). The need for a new medical model: A challenge for biomedicine. *Science, 196*, 129–136. doi:10.1126/science.847460.
Epstein, N. B., Bishop, D. S., & Levin, S. (1978). The McMaster model of family functioning. *Journal of Marital and Family Therapy, 4*(4), 19–31. doi:10.1111/j.1752-0606.1978.tb00537.
Gawande, A. (2011, January 24). The hot spotters – Can we lower medical costs by giving the neediest patients better care? *The New Yorker*, pp. 41–51.
Gottman, J. (1999). *The marriage clinic: A scientifically based marital therapy.* New York, NY: W. W. Norton & Company.
Gottman, J. (2011). *The science of trust: Emotional attunement for couples.* New York, NY: W. W. Norton & Company.

[1] An asterisk has been used to note references that the chapter authors recommend for further reading.

Greenberg, G., Fanshorn, K., & Danilkewich, A. (2001). Solution focused therapy: Counseling model for busy family physicians. *Canadian Family Physician, 47*, 2289–2295.

Kelly, B. (2003). *Worth repeating: More than 5,000 classic and contemporary quotes*. Grand Rapids, MI: Kregel Academic & Professional.

Kern, D. E., Thomas, P. A., Howard, D. M., & Bass, E. B. (1998). *Curriculum development for medical education: A six-step approach*. Baltimore, MD: The Johns Hopkins University Press.

Kirmayer, L. (2012). Cultural competence and evidence-based practice in mental health: Epistemic communities and the politics of pluralism. *Social Science & Medicine, 75*, 249–256. doi:10.1016/j.socscimed.2012.03.018.

Kleinman, A. M. (1988). *The illness narratives: Suffering, healing, and the human condition*. New York, NY: Basic Books.

*McDaniel, S., Doherty, W., & Hepworth, J. (Eds.). (2013). *Medical family therapy and integrated care* (2nd ed.). Washington, DC: APA Press.

McDaniel, S., Hepworth, J., & Doherty, W. (Eds.). (1997). *The shared experience of illness: Stories of patients, families, and their therapists*. New York, NY: Basic Books.

McGoldrick, M., Carter, E. A., & Garcia-Preto, N. (Eds.). (2010). *The evolving family life cycle: Individual, family, and social perspectives* (4th ed.). New York, NY: Allyn & Bacon.

McGoldrick, M., & Hardy, K. (Eds.). (2008). *Revisioning family therapy: Race, class, culture, and gender in clinical practice* (2nd ed.). New York, NY: Guilford.

Miller, S., McDaniel, S., Rolland, J., & Feetham, S. (Eds.). (2006). *Individuals, families, and the new era of genetics: BPS perspectives*. New York, NY: WW Norton.

Minuchin, S., & Fishman, H. C. (1981). *Family therapy techniques*. Cambridge, MA: Harvard University Press.

Patient Centered Primary Care Collaborative. (2007). Joint principles of the patient-centered medical home. Retrieved on March 31, 2013, from www.aap.org/en-us.professional-resources/practice-support/quality-improvement/Documents/Joint-Principles-Patient-Centered-Medical-Home.pdf

Patterson, K., Grenny, J., McMillan, R., & Switzler, A. (2002). *Crucial conversations: Tools for talking when the stakes are high*. New York, NY: McGraw Hill.

Patterson, K., Grenny, J., McMillan, R., & Switzler, A. (2005). *Crucial confrontations: Tools for resolving broken promises, violated expectations, and bad behavior*. New York, NY: McGraw Hill.

*Peek, C. J. (2008). Planning care in the clinical, operational, and financial worlds. In R. Kessler & D. Stafford (Eds.), *Collaborative medicine case studies: Evidence in practice* (pp. 25–38). New York, NY: Springer.

Peikes, D., Zutshi, A., Genevro, J., Smith, K., Parchman, M., & Meyers, D. (2012). *Early evidence on the patient-centered medical home (Agency for Healthcare Research and Quality Publication No. 12-0020-EF)*. Princeton, NJ: Mathematica Policy Research.

Rambo, A., West, C., Schooley, A. L., & Boyd, T. V. (2012). *Family therapy review: Contrasting contemporary models*. New York, NY: Routledge.

*Rolland, J. S. (1994). *Families, illness, and disability: An integrative treatment model*. New York, NY: Basic Books.

Rolland, J. S., & Walsh, F. W. (2005). Systemic training for healthcare professionals: The Chicago Center for Family Health Approach. *Family Process, 44*, 283–301. doi:10.1111/j.1545-5300.2005.00060.x.

Saba, G. W., Villela, T. J., Chen, E., Hammer, H., & Bodenheimer, T. (2012). The myth of the lone physician: Toward a collaborative alternative. *Annals of Family Medicine, 10*, 169–173. doi:10.1370/afm.1353.

Safford, B. & Manning, C. A. (2012, May/June). Six characteristics of effective practice teams. *Family Practice Management, 19*(3): 26–30.

Schutz, W. C. (1958). *FIRO: A three dimensional theory of interpersonal behavior*. New York, NY: Rinehart.

*Seaburn, D., Gunn, W., Mauksch, L., Gawinski, B., & Lorenz, A. (1996). *Models of collaboration: A guide for mental health professionals working with health care practitioners*. New York, NY: Basic Books.

von Bertalanffy, L. (1968). *General system theory*. New York, NY: George Braziller.
*Walsh, F. (2006). *Strengthening family resilience* (2nd ed.). New York, NY: Guilford.
*Walsh, F., & McGoldrick, M. (Eds.). (2004). *Living beyond loss: Death in the family* (2nd ed.). New York, NY: Norton.
Whitaker, C. A., & Malone, T. P. (1953). *The roots of psychotherapy*. New York, NY: Blakiston.
*Wright, L. M., & Bell, J. M. (2009). *Beliefs and illness: A model for healing*. Calgary: 4th Floor Press Inc.

Chapter 10
The Medical Family Therapist as Transdisciplinary Trainer

Randall Reitz and Laura Sudano

The healthcare system in the United States is in transformation. Many of the recent and pending changes represent unprecedented opportunities for MedFTs and other systemic clinicians. As documented in other chapters in this book, patient-centered medical homes and accountable care organizations place a high premium on outcome-based health care where the family and healing relationships are at the core of health interventions (see Chap. 19; Hodgson, Fox, & Lamson, 2014). Clinicians of all disciplines are increasingly required to approach health care from a relational perspective (DeGruy & McDaniel, 2013; Talen & Valeras, 2013). While MedFTs excel in this skill set and knowledge base, others can learn much of what we do. For example, two models have been proposed to describe different levels of family involvement in care (Doherty & Baird, 1986 and Heru, Keitner, & Glick, 2012). The required skill set for different disciplines can be mapped across these levels:

R. Reitz (✉)
St Mary's Family Medicine Residency, Grand Junction, CO, USA
e-mail: reitz.randall@gmail.com

J. Hodgson et al. (eds.), *Medical Family Therapy*, DOI 10.1007/978-3-319-03482-9_10,

Heru et al. (2012)	Level 1: Family Inclusion		Level 2: Family Psychoeducation		Level 3: Family Therapy
Doherty and Baird (1986)	Level 1: Minimal emphasis on family	Level 2: Ongoing medical information and advice	Level 3: Feelings and support	Level 4: Systematic assessment and planned intervention	Level 5: Family therapy
Radiologist, pathologist	XXX				
Medical assistant	XXX	XXX			
Registered nurse, internist, oncologist, sports medicine	XXX	XXX	XXX		
Psychologist, social worker, psychiatrist, family physician, pediatrician (all subspecialties)	XXX	XXX	XXX	XXX	
Couple and family therapist, medical family therapist	XXX	XXX	XXX	XXX	XXX

Using this nonscientific stratification, family therapists are unique in their ability to practice the full breadth of family interventions, but most Counseling professions and primary care clinicians should be skilled at assessing families and conducting brief interventions. And, while healthcare professionals who provide little direct patient interaction (e.g., radiologists, pathologists) can get by with little emphasis on family, other professionals require the ability to support families in distress and manage their interactions (e.g., registered nurses, internists, oncologists).

Similarly, most healthcare disciplines are moving toward a competency-based system for assessing skill and readiness for independent practice. For example, healthcare disciplines such as Pediatrics, Family Medicine, Psychiatry, Primary Care Psychology, Clinical Social Work, and Nursing provide a list of competencies that a trainee should meet before graduation or licensure. There is now a transdisciplinary list of competencies for behavioral health clinicians practicing in collaborative settings (Bischoff, Springer, Reisbig, Lyons, & Likcani, 2012). Similarly, leaders in the field of MedFT have created a list of important training points (Tyndall, Hodgson, Lamson, White, & Knight, 2012). In the table below, we present a crosswalk between the competencies of six healthcare disciplines and related competencies from the MedFT standards.

	Competencies from other disciplines[b]					
Medical Family Therapy Competencies[a]	Pedi atrics	Family Med	Psych iatry	P.C. Psych	L.C.S.W.	R.N.
1. Develop sufficient understanding of the relevant biomedical issues, language, culture, and providers in primary, secondary, and tertiary healthcare systems	7 13	PC1 MK1 PROF1	2A 3B/C	2B 3B 5A/C	1 3 5 18	2 5 8 9
2. Apply Marriage and Family Therapy (MFT) evidence-based models to Medical Family Therapy (MedFT) cases		PC3/4 C1/2 PBL1	2B	1A 5C		9
3. Demonstrate skills in helping families manage the demands of acute and chronic illnesses	12 13	PC1/2/3 C1/2	2B 3A	5C		7
4. Demonstrate skills in providing integrated care	7	SBP4 C3	3A	5A/D	11	6 9
6. Demonstrate the ability to empower patients to advocate for themselves in the healthcare system	8	PC3 SBP2/3	3A	2B 5D	2 8 9	5 6 8
7. Demonstrate the ability to motivate health-related behavior change	12 13	PC2/3 C1	2B	5C	10	7 9
8. Demonstrate awareness of and sensitivity to cultural and contextual variables pertaining to health, illness, loss, and trauma	14	PC3 PROF3	1A/B 2B	3B 5C	2 3	7 9
10. Facilitate communication between patients, families, and healthcare providers and invite coordination of services		PC3 SBP4 C1/2/3	3A/B/C	2A 4B 5C/D	8 11	4 6 9
11. Demonstrate the ability to refer, document, and communicate with healthcare professionals	5	PC3 SBP4 C3/4	3A/B/C	2B 4B	4 13	4 6
14. Understand the clinical, operational, and financial elements of healthcare systems	6 10 11	PC4 SBP1	2A	2A/B 5A		2 4 5 9
16. Understand the bidirectional relationships between health and wellness on mental health functioning	12	PC2/3/4	2A/B	1A 5B	6	3 7
17. Understand psychopharmacology and its systemic effects	4		2B			7
18. Understand disease processes and developmentally appropriate treatments	3	PC3/4	1A/B 2B	5B		7 9
20. Apply systems theory and the biopsychosocial-spiritual (BPSS) approach to research, education, clinical, supervision, and/or consultation services	11	MK2 PBL3		1A/B 2A	5 17 19	2
21. Evaluate and design intervention and program research associated with BPSS health issues and collaborative care models	7	PBLI1/3		1A/B	14 15	2 3

(continued)

Medical Family Therapy Competencies[a]	Competencies from other disciplines[b] Pediatrics	Family Med	Psychiatry	P.C. Psych	L.C.S.W.	R.N.
22. Demonstrate the ability to conduct a BPSS assessment	1 2 3	MK1/2	1A/B	5B	6	7 9
25. Integrate BPSS elements into treatment plans and other clinical documents	3	PC2	2A	1A 5C	7 13	7 9
26. Evidence skills in designing and building transdisciplinary collaborative care teams	10 11	PC5 PROF2 SBP4 C3	3A/B/C	2A/B 4B 5D	11	6

[a]Selected from Tyndall et al., 2012
[b]The codes in the cells reflect the numbering system from the cited competency documents: Pediatrics: Accreditation Council for Graduate Medical Education (2013), Family Medicine: Accreditation Council for Graduate Medical Education and American Board of Family Medicine (2013), Psychiatry: American Board of Psychiatry and Neurology (2011), Primary Care Psychology: American Psychological Association (in press), Social Work (LCSW): National Association of Social Workers (2005), Nursing (RN): American Association of Colleges of Nursing (2008)

This table demonstrates two key points: (a) there is significant overlap between the competencies of each of the professions, and (b) a professional trained in MedFT competencies will have mastered competencies similar to other healthcare professions. To demonstrate the depth of this overlap, it is helpful to examine the competencies of one of the other professions more closely. The Family Medicine Milestones Project (2013) is a joint initiative of the American Board of Family Medicine (ABFM) and the American Council on Graduate Medical Education (ACGME). As currently constituted, the competencies that were listed in the crosswalk table are as follows:

Patient Care

PC1—Cares for acutely ill or injured patients in urgent and emergent situations and in all settings
PC2—Cares for patients with chronic illnesses
PC3—Partners with the patient, family, and community to improve health through disease prevention and health promotion
PC4—Partners with the patient to address issues of ongoing signs, symptoms, and health concerns that remain over time without clear diagnosis despite evaluation and treatment, in a patient-centered, cost-effective manner
PC5—Performs specialty appropriate procedures to meet the healthcare needs of individual patients, families, and communities and is knowledgeable about procedures performed by other specialists to guide their patients' care

Medical Knowledge

MK1—Demonstrates medical knowledge of sufficient breadth and depth to practice Family Medicine
MK2—Applies critical thinking skills in patient care

Professionalism

PROF1—Completes a process of professionalization
PROF2—Displays professional conduct and accountability
PROF3—Demonstrates humanism and cultural proficiency
PROF4—Maintains emotional, physical, and mental health and pursues continual personal and professional growth

System-Based Practice

SBP1—Provides cost-conscious medical care
SBP2—Emphasizes patient safety
SBP3—Advocates for individual and community health
SBP4—Coordinates team-based care

Practice-Based Learning and Improvement

PBLI1—Locates, appraises, and assimilates evidence from scientific studies related to their patients' health problems
PBLI2—Demonstrates self-directed learning
PBLI3—Improves systems in which the physician provides care

Communication

C1—Develops meaningful, therapeutic relationships with patients and families
C2—Communicates effectively with patients, families, and the public
C3—Develops relationships and effectively communicates with physicians, other health professionals, and healthcare teams
C4—Utilizes technology to optimize communication

A close reading of the Family Medicine competencies makes it clear why all residencies within this specialization are required to include a designated Behavioral Science faculty member (ACGME, 2007) and why many residency programs choose a MedFT for this role. For example, one intent behind the Family Medicine competencies is to train physicians who can effectively communicate with families and provide care at both individual and family levels. The competencies assert that family physicians should be able to promote improvement in health behaviors and manage diseases without a clear medical etiology. They reinforce team-based care skills, such as those required for integrated care and medical homes. They require training to promote the emotional and behavioral health of family physicians and cultural competency. And, they require critical evaluation and application of scientific literature.

In considering the skill set of a MedFT as described in our own competencies—especially a MedFT with the advanced scientific training of a PhD program—the overlap in training ability clearly supports a central role for MedFTs in training family physicians. For while many behavioral health disciplines bring expertise in counseling and integrated care and MFTs bring expertise in family-based care, only MedFTs integrate these skill sets.

A similar close analysis of the competencies of other professions is equally supportive role of MedFTs in their training. That being said, there are obviously other competencies for these professions that are best taught by the members of that profession. For example, while a MedFT could be helpful in training a family physician in the cognitive aspects of MK2 (i.e., "Applies critical thinking skills in patient care"), a MedFT would be much less capable than a Family Physician faculty at addressing the medical basis of a patient's care decisions. MedFTs could extrapolate from our training to theirs, but the Family Physician faculty can draw upon years of experience in making the same decisions.

Perspective from Nursing Education
Courtney Kasun, MNSc, RN
Nursing Faculty at Colorado Mesa University
Doctoral Candidate

The Behavioral Sciences were almost completely absent from my master's program. I will have a class in family dynamics at the doctoral level, but it will be taught by nursing faculty, as was related content in my bachelor's (BSN). In this program, our biggest focus in the Behavioral Sciences was a course called "Mental Health." Outside of that, bits and pieces were threaded throughout the curriculum. Mental Health was an overwhelming class, focusing on psychiatric diagnoses and meds, rather than psychosocial support and interventions applicable to all patients.

At all levels of nursing, students would benefit from thorough education on working with patients, couples, and families. I would argue that this knowledge is more important, especially for those being prepared to work at the "bedside," than in-depth knowledge of the characteristics of various psychiatric diagnoses. All nurses will need to work with patients and their families to teach, promote change, and provide support.

(continued)

I have not had a designated Behavioral Science faculty at any level of my training. In fact, finding nursing faculty to teach mental health is difficult. The proportion of nurses practicing full time in mental health settings is low when compared with the number of nurses in the profession. Furthermore, the experience of these nurses can vary greatly. Many professions, nursing included, are still fairly siloed when it comes to education, for a variety of reasons. I think engaging professionals from other disciplines to teach their content of expertise (e.g., MedFTs teaching the Behavioral Sciences to Nursing students) has great value. However, the nursing faculty would still need to fill the role of helping students translate the knowledge gained from experts to the professional frame of nursing.

Other Supporting Recommendations

Moving beyond narrowly defined competencies, there is rich literature that supports MedFT involvement in training other disciplines. For example, with Pediatrics, the ACGME recommends that Pediatrician education include "understanding the complex developmental processes of infants, children, adolescents and young adults, in the context of their families and communities" and "understanding the biological, psychological, and social influences on development in the emotional, social, motor, language, and cognitive domains" (ACGME, 2009, p. 30). Similarly, the American Academy of Pediatrics (AAP) has adopted the ecobiodevelopmental (EBD) framework (Shonkoff et al., 2011), which seeks to understand the promotion of health and prevention of disease across the life-span that builds on advances in neuroscience, molecular biology, genomics, and social sciences (Shonkoff, Boyce, & McEwen, 2009). Taken together, these Pediatric models converge on inextricable interactions among the personal experiences (e.g., family and social relationships), environmental influences (e.g., exposures to toxic chemicals and inappropriate electronic media), and genetic predispositions that affect learning, behavior, and health across the life-span.

Regarding Psychiatry, the ACGME (2008) states that core competencies for residents include their need to communicate with families, provide psychoeducation, and have exposure to couple, family, group, and other therapies. Families, as acknowledged within the core competencies for Psychiatry residents, are an important part of treatment. Much research supports the incorporation of family skills and family intervention into the Psychiatry curriculum of residency training programs (Berman et al., 2006; Heru, 2004; Heru et al., 2012; Josephson, 2008; Rait & Glick, 2008a, 2008b; Stubbe et al., 2008). Further, research within the field of psychiatry suggests that family-based interventions and family involvement are beneficial for those patients who are in treatment (Landsman, Groza, Tyler, & Malone, 2001; Wood, Piacentini, Southam-Gerow, Chu, & Sigman, 2006). When looking at Child and Adolescent Psychiatry, parental involvement helps maintain treatment gains and facilitates children's transition home (Cafferty & Leichtman, 2001; Nickerson, Salamone, Brooks, & Colby, 2004). From a clinical perspective, researchers highlight that psychiatric family skills are especially vital in a residential setting. For example, Nickerson, Brooks, Colby, Rickert, and Salamone (2006) discovered that nearly 100 % of respondents from adolescent treatment centers agreed that "adolescents were placed in residential treatment to learn how to get along better with family" (p. 691) and that approximately half of parents have face-to-face contact with residential staff at least once every 2 weeks.

In Family Medicine, researchers suggest that a variety of family interviewing techniques are useful with individual patients, with family members accompanying patients, and in family conferences (Campbell, McDaniel, Cole-Kelly, Hepworth, & Lorenz, 2002). One study suggests that 39 % of patients came to an office appointment with a family member or friend (Botelho, Lue, & Fiscella, 1996). Older adults who attend their routine medical visits are more likely to have a family member with them (Wolff & Roter, 2011). Specifically, patients who were accompanied by a family member were more likely to be older, be less educated, and have extensive physical and behavioral health needs than unaccompanied patients.

Perspective from Family Medicine Education
Kyle Leonard, MD
Family Medicine Resident
St Mary's Family Medicine Residency

"I'm so sorry. Her liver isn't working and I can't stop the bleeding. I have given her over 20 units of blood but she continues to bleed to death," I said to a room full of many tearful, angry, and scared family members. The patient was a 36-year-old mother and a faithful wife who unfortunately had a serious alcohol problem which led to cirrhosis. She fell and suffered a large hematoma, which her body was unable to clot. Questions of miracles, anger at medicine's shortcomings, wails of her children, and a silent stare from her husband are etched in my mind. As a Family Medicine resident, I am forever thankful for the support of the MedFT in that difficult conversation. She coordinated grief counseling, supported me in mediating the conversation, and provided feedback after the patient encounter was finished.

This is just one of the countless interactions in which a MedFT and other behavioral science team members are essential in learning and providing high-quality family medicine. It is a huge asset at my residency program to have a longitudinal behavioral science curriculum in which we work closely with MedFTs. During outpatient precepting, they are readily available and

(continued)

eager to discuss or see patients. They provide quick counseling techniques to help navigate situations beyond the expertise of the MD faculty. In addition, MedFTs participate in hospital rounds to help with conversations about a new diagnosis, family meetings for end-of-life care, supporting patients with drug abuse, and a variety of other common situations we face.

We also have designated "psych days" in which we practice family systems and counseling skills with the MedFTs and coordinate both office and home visits with their assistance. The family therapist on faculty provides teaching for patient care, alongside personal support. He or she coordinates the resident support group in which the residents discuss hopes and dreams, set goals for the future, and are empowered through personal struggles. He or she meets with us individually several times a year to check in. Without a doubt, the MedFTs here are a huge and needed component to Family Medicine training.

Training for the Patient-Centered Medical Home

The patient-centered medical home (PCMH) provides excellent clinical opportunities for MedFTs and for transdisciplinary training. The PCMH movement was started by Pediatricians and is endorsed by the AAP as a way to promote health and prevent disease across the life-span (Sia, Tonniges, Osterhus, & Taba, 2004). The AAP cites research that early environments play an important role in health outcomes in adulthood (Johnson, Riley, Granger, & Riis, 2013). That is, maladaptive environments or toxic stress characterized by early childhood adversities impact a number of health outcomes in adulthood such as cardiovascular disease, cancers, asthma, and depression (Araújo et al., 2009; Berasain et al., 2009; Chen & Miller, 2007; Danese et al., 2008). As such, the AAP has called on Pediatricians to "become leaders in science-based strategies to build strong foundations for children's life-long health" (Johnson et al., 2013, p. 319). Patient- and family-centered care has been a preferred approach in Family Medicine training and education. The Institute for Patient- and Family-Centered Care (IPFCC) emphasizes the "planning, delivery, and evaluation of health care that is grounded in mutually beneficial partnerships among healthcare providers, patients, and families" (IPFCC, 2010). In sum, this approach recognizes the importance of families in the role of a patient's health and well-being.

Advocates for the PCMH model transcend the primary care disciplines. Consensus for PCMH standards was first achieved in 2007 with the creation of the document, Joint Principles of the Patient-Centered Medical Home, which was endorsed by the principal professional associations for family physicians, pediatricians, internists, and osteopathic physicians. This document calls for "robust partnership between physicians, patients, and the patient's family" (American Academy of Family Physicians, American Academy of Pediatrics, American College of Physicians, & American Osteopathic Association, 2007, p. 2). The Family Medicine Working Party, which consists of the major Family Medicine professional associations and research groups, released the Joint Principles for Integrating Behavioral Healthcare into the Patient-Centered Medical Home (2012). This document updates the original Joint Principles standard, specifically calling for the integration of behavioral health- and family-oriented care in the PCMH: "The partnership around the care planning process between physicians, patients, and the patient's family must include behavioral health clinician. . .(and) understanding of the central role of the patient and family in articulating needs and developing a care plan" (pp. 3–4).

Perspective from Pediatrician Education

Patrice Whistler, MD, MPH, FAAP
Pediatrician
Western Colorado Pediatric Associates

As a pediatrician, each day my clinic schedule is filled with families that face distress and conflict despite their best efforts in parenting. Some of these families face a difficult pediatric diagnosis such as diabetes, ADHD, autism, or asthma. Others have parents who struggle with their own mental health and substance issues. Many of them face the day-to-day obstacles from living in poverty, as large percentages of my panel come from single-parent, divorced, and foster families.

My medical school and pediatric residency education were void of behavioral health staff available for training or consultation. There was minimal behavioral science education at all, with mandatory Psychiatry rotations only as medical students. If a patient revealed a serious concern (e.g., "Doc, I just don't want to hurt anymore."), we were in charge of communicating that patient's wishes and concerns to family and faculty without behavioral health support. Child Psychiatry was an elective that only a few of us participated in. In this rotation, child psychiatrists were the primary faculty, and their activities included assisting with groups and intake interviews and conducting psychosocial consultations.

As a result, most of my own behavioral health education has been through self-study and continuing medical education. Through integrated care training I have been able to create a robust integrated care and MedFT service in my large multidisciplinary private practice. The initial deficit in behavioral science and MedFT training has been time consuming and difficult to overcome.

I feel that having interaction and education from behavioral health faculty (ideally with the systemic perspective of a MedFT) is critical for residents in

(continued)

training. Much of the care provided by pediatricians and family physicians involves medical conditions that stem from family issues and mental health concerns or can be treated best with addressing those concerns. Integrating behavioral science staff into daily medical practice, in the outpatient and inpatient setting, ensures higher quality of care for all patients.

What Does Transdisciplinary Training Look Like?

D'Amour, Ferrada-Videla, Rodriguez, and Beaulieu (2005) explored core concepts and theoretical frameworks for interprofessional collaboration to improve understanding of frameworks used in health organizations. Through research, they suggest that there are three team concepts in the collaboration literature: (a) multidisciplinary team, (b) interdisciplinary team, and (c) transdisciplinary team. A transdisciplinary team refers to "a type of professional practice in which consensus-seeking and the opening up of professional territories play a major role" (D'Amour et al., 2005, p. 120). In other words, a transdisciplinary team shares knowledge, expertise, and skills that exceed discipline boundaries. People from different disciplines are committed to sharing expertise, knowledge, and skills so that information from their respective disciplines can be collected, evaluated, and discussed by other team members.

Furthermore, transdisciplinary training is a collaborative endeavor in which the expertise of one tradition is shared with another. The purpose of transdisciplinary training is to combine insights and work toward a common goal, specifically for human service delivery. Given the increasingly complicated world, science and healthcare disciplines strive to meet the needs of those families with whom they work.

For example, the field of Maternal and Child Health (MCH) has focused on collaborating with multiple disciplines to promote the well-being of children and families (Dodds et al., 2010). Researchers found that the effects of interdisciplinary training of MCH trainees help graduates (a) develop attitudes and beliefs in the value of interdisciplinary practice, (b) gain interdisciplinary skills, and (c) gain attitudes, beliefs, and skills to "improve outcomes for families and to effect change in MCH systems involving programs, organizations, partnerships, and policies" (Margolis, Rosenberg, Umble, & Chewning, 2012, p. 956).

Returning to the discussion of Family Medicine training, here are examples of potential roles and formats in which a MedFT in the position of Behavioral Science faculty at a Family Medicine residency, can train other disciplines and maximize their skill set as system thinkers and family-oriented clinicians.

Clinical precepting. Physicians call their outpatient supervision "precepting." During the first 6 months of a resident's training, a preceptor is required to meet all patients and replicate some aspect of care (Department of Health and Human Services: Centers for Medicare & Medicaid Services, 2011). Unlike behavioral health supervision, physicians usually discuss cases that were not observed live or audio/video-recorded. Residents see a patient sufficiently to make an assessment, come out to report their findings to the preceptor, and finalize a plan of action together, and then the resident (with or without the preceptor) returns to the exam room to finish the appointment. Precepting often follows the Socratic method (i.e., the faculty member asks questions to gauge the resident's knowledge base and plan for treatment, rather than spoon-feeding supervision).

Only another physician (preferably of the same specialty) can serve as the preceptor of record for a case. So, the behavioral science faculty member's presence in the precepting room is often a luxury. As with all teaching that occurs during clinic hours, the MedFT needs to ensure that he or she minimizes the impact on the flow of the clinic and the physician teaching. However, MedFTs have a lot to offer in this setting. Here are some best practices:

- Review the patient list for the "clinic half-day," and seek out residents scheduled with cases that are familiar to you or who have presenting problems related to relationship distress, potential phase-of-life challenges (e.g., new mothers, sexually active adolescents, older adults providing care for a loved one), behavioral health, chronic illness, or addiction. Discuss the resident's strategy for the appointment with a focus on building a therapeutic relationship, assessment techniques, and short behavioral interventions.
- Listen in on the many precepting discussions occurring concurrently, and roll over to join cases that could benefit from your expertise. With a high-performing resident, the MedFT's involvement might be limited to concurring on the assessment and plan. With a novice resident, there is a rich opportunity to highlight family system principles or recommend a behavioral health intervention. These discussions will often carry over to the exam room, with the MedFT finishing the appointment with the resident or receiving a personal introduction from the resident.

Perspective from Psychiatry Education

Kenneth W. Phelps, PhD, LMFT
Assistant Clinical Professor, Department of Neuropsychiatry and Behavioral Science
University of South Carolina School of Medicine

Exhausted parents seek help for their preschooler's hour-long tantrums. A maternal grandmother of a teen with obsessive compulsive disorder finds herself desperate for help due to entanglement with many compulsive behaviors. A husband expresses fear of how to support his wife with anorexia and alcohol abuse. A sibling of an adult with nonepileptic seizures presents with

(continued)

confusion about how to respond to these conversion episodes. A son is worried about his mother's worsening depression after a recent diagnosis of multiple sclerosis. As a MedFT faculty member in a Department of Neuropsychiatry, I am tasked to provide psychiatric residents with family-based skills to improve the efficacy of their current treatment modalities (e.g., psychopharmacology, cognitive behavioral therapy, psychodynamic therapy).

Family skills are gained through an array of teaching modalities. During the week, live sessions are conducted via a two-way mirror where a transdisciplinary team (psychiatry, psychology, pediatrics, MedFT) discuss the biopsychosocial and spiritual aspects of the case. Residents also complete their personal genogram early in training to better identify their own relational biases. After this experience, residents and fellows engage in co-therapy sessions with the MedFT faculty to treat a variety of common couple and family issues. Didactics also enrich the experience, focusing on systems theory, development during the life course, and accrual of family skills that can be integrated into psychopharmacology visits (e.g., tracking, seeking exceptions, externalization, enactment). Throughout these educational endeavors, learning is fostered through discussion and active learning with the hope of developing systemically minded early-career physicians.

Hospital attending and rounding. Teaching that occurs in the hospital is referred to as rounding and attending. The hospital environment is fast paced, complex, and expensive. The MedFT trainer needs to clearly define his or her role in this vast, dynamic 24/7 operation.

In a teaching hospital, "rounding" has many formats and connotations. Typically, all the residents on the inpatient service visit all the patients on their list first thing in the morning. They review nursing notes from the evening and check in on the patient's health status. After this, residents and the attending faculty meet together to review the cases. In a previous era, this occurred in "walking rounds" or "bedside rounds," but it more commonly now occurs in a conference room where the physicians can talk freely about cases and use the hospital's electronic health record to efficiently review important patient data. After these "seated rounds," residents will frequently make a follow-up visit to their patients to implement any indicated revisions to the treatment plan and/or to prepare for discharge.

Each of these rounding moments provides excellent opportunities for a MedFT to train residents. The hospital setting is typically a bastion for the biomedical aspects of health where labs, imaging, bandages, and pharmaceuticals are the focus. However, psychosocial dynamics are oftentimes contributory to medical admissions, and attempting to navigate the inpatient process can be a source of acute family distress (Schmidt & Azoulay, 2012). The inpatient MedFT should continually raise awareness of patients' underlying psychosocial issues. For while psychosocial issues are ubiquitous, it is common for young physicians to feel helpless to treat them and frustrated when they repeatedly impede care.

When in walking rounds, the MedFT can shadow the resident and facilitate a pre-visit discussion. Questions may include the following: What is the patient's psychosocial context? What are his or her resources and obstacles to care? What family dynamics affect care? How can the family be better engaged in treatment during and after the hospitalization? What do you like most and least about this patient and family? What behavioral interventions and skills would be appropriate to try today? What role, if any, do you want me (the MedFT trainer) to play?

During bedside visits, the MedFT trainer should introduce himself or herself and participate as planned. It is helpful to take detailed notes of the resident's performance, ideally on a pre-made form. This form can be based on established resident competencies (see Family Medicine competencies described earlier) or other popular forms; the most commonly used is Patient Centered Observation Form (Mauksch, 2011). It is not uncommon for a bedside visit to include misunderstandings and differences of opinion. Similarly, a resident will often struggle when attempting new skills. In these moments, the MedFT should balance the need for the resident to learn through overcoming adversity with the need for adequate and safe patient care. The severity of the breakdown in communication and the medical risk (e.g., suicidal ideation, resident inattention to important details, challenging family dynamics around a life support/organ donation decision) increase the need for MedFT intervention. Time permitting, the MedFT will facilitate a post-visit discussion and present his or her notes from the visit. Or alternatively, the notes can be batched for a cumulative feedback session at the end of walking rounds.

During seated rounds, the role of the MedFT is to act as the voice for the patient, family, and BPSS model (Engel, 1977, 1980; Wright, Watson, & Bell, 1996). This role divides between teaching and care consulting. Coordinating these efforts with the attending physicians and the chief resident is vital. The MedFT can offer a running commentary on cases, can use the Socratic method to draw out a resident's thinking on a case, or can have designated time for feedback and a teaching moment during the seated rounds. The work time after seated rounds provides an excellent opportunity for joint appointments and family case conferences with residents.

Formal didactics. Residencies typically offer multiple classroom-like formats. Some prefer "noon conferences" that occur between the scheduled rotations of a resident's day. Others block out several hours on a dedicated day of the week. Some do a mixture of both. These curricular elements are more like workshops and seminars than like graduate school classes. Some are short and narrowly focused (e.g., a 20-min EKG reading workshop), and others are coordinated as a themed series (e.g., a "Pediatric Day" that includes a rotating series of stations that teach vaccinations, treating ear infections, counseling parents on healthy eating, and interpreting developmental screening). Except for the most biomedical among the topics, most clearly involve education within the purview of MedFT. Examples include the following:

- A monthly series that covers common psychiatric diagnoses in primary care settings: Ideally this would be multidisciplinary (e.g., including the MedFT, a Family Physician faculty, psychiatrist, and/or pharmacist) and case based (i.e.,

residents present their cases or a teaching case is presented that serves as the focus of the various presentations).
- Presenting a BPSS perspective to a medical presentation: Possibilities are innumerable, including obesity, diabetes, asthma, chronic pain, child development difficulties, and tobacco cessation.
- Partnering with a physician to teach bedside manner and basic counseling skills relevant to difficult patient encounters, such as managing an out-of-control pediatric visit, apologizing for a mistake, delivering bad news, or redirecting a tangential or an angry patient.

In each of these settings, it is important to focus closely on the needs and learning style of the residents. That is, while it would be ideal if all residents were keyed up to learn Family Therapy skills equivalent to a master's-level trained clinician, this is rarely the case. Rather, residents need to be able to interact with families with respect and skill, assess basic family dynamics, recommend changes in behavior, and know when/how to refer to a MedFT or other behavioral health clinicians. Similarly, residents frequently prefer small, manageable interventions for specific situations (e.g., "Here is my 5-min intervention for smoking cessation...") rather than broad theoretical discussions.

With the ascension of the Internet and readily available medical informatics, the focus of medical didactics is evolving away from memorizing and regurgitating reams of knowledge and toward understanding how to look up information on the fly, to make decisions, to work as a team, and to collaborate with patients and families. Each of these changes has a strong behavioral and systemic overlay that is ideal for MedFT involvement.

Support and insight. Residency is an incredibly demanding time that occurs concurrently with a young physician's exploration of values, independence, and professional priorities. The long hours, sleep deprivation, fast pace, and life-or-death decision making can take a toll on even the most dedicated learner (Thomas, 2004). For these reasons, Family Medicine residencies are required by the ACGME (2007) to offer some form of emotional support services for trainees. Much of this will occur informally through colleagues and mentors. To formalize the process, many residencies offer support groups. While some residencies contract for services from a group therapist, others rely on faculty members for this role. Other formalized types of support include scheduled meetings with the behavioral science faculty and retreats for team building between faculty and residents.

The behavioral science faculty members are often central to these programs but can also require a delicate balance and ethical discernment. Providing support to trainees requires the MedFT to wear multiple hats simultaneously: supporter, health advisor, evaluator, and teacher. While some models have been created to guide this process (e.g., Reitz, Simmons, Runyan, Hodgson, & Carter-Henry, 2013), the MedFT needs to ensure that the core faculty roles of teaching and evaluating are not undermined by supportive roles. Care needs to be maintained so that providing support does not evolve into providing therapy.

Professional Identity

By choosing to assume the role of a trainer of other disciplines (especially if this is a major portion of a person's professional activity), the MedFT chooses to split his or her professional identity between these professions. One is no longer purely a MedFT but is also a trainer of nurses, family physicians, psychologists, etc. One's loyalty naturally extends to the profession of the trainees and one's fellow faculty members. This represents a broadening of one's perspective and influence but also a weakening of the connection to one's primary discipline.

For example, one of the authors (RR) trains family physicians at a Family Medicine residency. As a MedFT, his primary professional home has been the Collaborative Family Healthcare Association (CFHA). Once he became a Behavioral Science faculty, he joined the Society of Teachers of Family Medicine (STFM) and started attending their conference. He also attends the Behavioral Science Forum whenever possible. This leaves a much reduced opportunity to attend Family Therapy-specific conferences, resulting in increased obstacles to the remaining abreast of contemporary research and theories or of building a professional network with other family therapists. Over time, his professional identity has shifted away from solely MFT and toward Family Medicine education.

Conclusion

Using a transdisciplinary approach, the MedFT teaches skills and knowledge that are essential to most healthcare professions and in most healthcare settings: family-oriented care, integrated care, diagnostics, developing healing relationships, and psychotherapy. Given that the field of MedFT spans both Family Therapy and integrated care, MedFTs offer a unique and highly valuable skill set for training most healthcare disciplines and particularly Primary Care, Nursing, and other professions with direct patient care.

Reflection Questions

1. What types of settings and disciplines would benefit most from transdisciplinary training from a MedFT?
2. What are the key skills and knowledge areas in which a MedFT could offer training to a: (a) Family physician? (b) Pediatrician? (c) Registered nurse? (d) Social worker?
3. In what ways is a MedFT an essential trainer for other disciplines? In what ways are MedFTs insufficient in the training of other professions?

4. How can a transdisciplinary trainer maintain his or her core identity as a MedFT while working in isolation from other MedFTs and alongside professionals and trainees of different disciplines?

References

Accreditation Council for Graduate Medical Education. (2007, July 1). *ACGME program requirements for graduate medical education in family medicine*. Retrieved from http://www.acgme.org/acgmeweb/Portals/0/PFAssets/ProgramRequirements/120pr07012007.pdf

Accreditation Council for Graduate Medical Education. (2008, April 12). *ACGME program requirements for graduate medical education in psychiatry*. Retrieved from http://www.acgme.org/acgmeweb/Portals/0/PFAssets/ProgramRequirements/400_psychiatry_07012007_u04122008.pdf

Accreditation Council for Graduate Medical Education. (2009, July 1). *ACGME program requirements for graduate medical education in developmental-behavioral pediatrics*. Retrieved from http://www.acgme.org/acgmeweb/Portals/0/PFAssets/2013-PR-FAQ-PIF/336_developmental_behavioral_peds_07012013.pdf

Accreditation Council for Graduate Medical Education. (2013). *The family medicine milestone project. Joint initiative of ACGME and The American Board of Family Medicine*. Chicago, IL: Accreditation Council for Graduate Medical Education.

American Psychological Association (in press). *Competencies for primary care psychology practice*. Washington, DC: American Psychologist.

American Academy of Family Physicians, American Academy of Pediatrics, American College of Physicians, & American Osteopathic Association. (2007, March). *Joint principles of the patient-centered medical home*. Retrieved from http://www.aap.org/en-us/professional-resources/practice-support/quality-improvement/Documents/Joint-Principles-Patient-Centered-Medical-Home.pdf

American Association of Colleges of Nurses. (2008, October). *The essentials of baccalaureate education for professional nursing practice*. Retrieved from http://www.aacn.nche.edu/education-resources/baccessentials08.pdf

American Board of Psychiatry and Neurology (2011). *American Board of Psychiatry & Neurology Psychiatry and Neurology Core Competencies, Version 4.1*. Approved by the ABPN Board of Directors in February 22, 2009. Buffalo Grove, IL.

Araújo, J. P., Lourenço, P., Azevedo, A., Friões, F., Rocha-Gonçalves, F., Ferreira, A., et al. (2009). Prognostic value of high-sensitivity C-reactive protein in heart failure: A systematic review. *Journal of Cardiac Failure, 15*, 256–266. doi:10.1016/j.cardfail.2008.10.030.

Berasain, C., Castillo, J., Perugorria, M. J., Latasa, M. U., Prieto, J., & Avila, M. A. (2009). Inflammation and liver cancer: New molecular links. *Annals of the New York Academy of Sciences, 1155*, 206–221. doi:10.1111/j.1749-6632.2009.03704.x.

Berman, E. M., Heru, A. M., Grunebaum, H., Rolland, R., Wood, B., & Bruty, H. (2006). Family skills for general psychiatry residents: Meeting ACGME core competency requirements. *Academic Psychiatry, 30*, 69–78. doi:10.1176/appi.30.1.69.

Bischoff, R. J., Springer, P. R., Reisbig, A. M. J., Lyons, S., & Likcani, A. (2012). Training for collaboration: Collaborative practice skills for mental health professionals. *Journal of Marital and Family Therapy, 38*, 199–210. doi:10.1111/j.1752-0606.2012.00299.x.

Botelho, R. J., Lue, B. H., & Fiscella, K. (1996). Family involvement in routine health care: A survey of patients' behaviors and preferences. *The Journal of Family Practice, 42*, 572–576.

Cafferty, H., & Leichtman, M. (2001). Facilitating the transition from residential treatment into the community: II. Changing social work roles. *Residential Treatment for Children and Youth, 19*, 25. doi:10.1300/J007v19n02_02.

Campbell, T. L., McDaniel, S. H., Cole-Kelly, K., Hepworth, J., & Lorenz, A. (2002). Family interviewing: A review of the literature in primary care. *Family Medicine, 34*, 312–318.

Chen, E., & Miller, G. E. (2007). Stress and inflammation in exacerbations of asthma. *Brain, Behavior, and Immunity, 21*, 993–999. doi:10.1016/j.bbi.2007.03.009.

D'Amour, D., Ferrada-Videla, M., Rodriguez, L. S. M., & Beaulieu, M. D. (2005). The conceptual basis for interprofessional collaboration: Core concepts and theoretical frameworks. *Journal of Interprofessional Care, 1*, 116–131. doi:10.1080/13561820500082529.

Danese, A., Moffitt, T. E., Pariante, C. M., Ambler, A., Poulton, R., & Caspi, A. (2008). Elevated inflammation levels in depressed adults with a history of childhood maltreatment. *Archives of General Psychiatry, 65*, 409–415. doi:10.1001/archpsyc.65.4.409.

DeGruy, F., & McDaniel, S. (2013). The landscape of integrated behavioral health care initiatives. In M. Talen & A. Valeras (Eds.), *Integrated behavioral health in primary care: Evaluating the evidence, identifying the essentials* (pp. vii–ix). New York, NY: Springer.

Department of Health and Human Services: Centers for Medicare & Medicaid Services. (2011, December). *Fact sheet: Guidelines for teaching physicians, interns, and residents.* Retrieved from http://www.cms.gov/Outreach-and-Education/Medicare-Learning-Network-MLN/MLNProducts/downloads/gdelinesteachgresfctsht.pdf

Dodds, J., Vann, W., Lee, J., Rosenberg, A., Rounds, K., Roth, M., . . . Margolis, L. H. (2010). The UNC-CH MCH leadership training consortium: Building the capacity to develop interdisciplinary MCH leaders. *Maternal and Child Health Journal, 14*, 642–648. doi: 10.1007//s10995-009-0483-0.

Doherty, W. J., & Baird, M. A. (1986). Levels of physician involvement with families. *Family Medicine, 18*, 153–156.

Engel, G. L. (1977). The need for a new medical model: A challenge for biomedicine. *Science, 196*, 129–136. doi:10.1126/science.847460.

Engel, G. L. (1980). The clinical application of the biopsychosocial model. *American Journal of Psychiatry, 137*, 535–544. Retrieved from http://ajp.psychiatryonline.org/

Family Medicine Working Party. (2012, July 11). *Joint principles: Integrating behavioral healthcare into the patient-centered medical home.* Retrieved from http://www.advancingcaretogether.org/pdfs/BH-PCMH%20Joint%20Principles.pdf

Heru, A. M. (2004). Basic family skills for an inpatient psychiatrist: Meeting accreditation council for graduate medical education core competency requirements. *Families, Systems & Health, 22*, 216–227. doi:10.1037/1091-7527.22.2.216.

Heru, A. M., Keitner, G. I., & Glick, I. D. (2012). Family therapy: The neglected core competency. *Academic Psychiatry, 36*, 433–435. doi:10.1176/appi.ap.11090160.

Hodgson, J., Fox, M., & Lamson, A. (2014). Family therapists in primary care settings: Opportunities for integration through advocacy. In J. Hodgson, A. Lamson, T. Mendenhall, & R. Crane (Eds.), *Medical family therapy: Advanced applications* (pp. 357–380). New York, NY: Springer.

Institute for Patient- and Family-Centered Care. (2010, December 29). *Frequently asked questions [What is patient- and family-centered health care]*. Retrieved from http://www.ipfcc.org/faq.html

Johnson, S. B., Riley, A. W., Granger, D. A., & Riis, J. (2013). The science of early life toxic stress for pediatric practice and advocacy. *Pediatrics, 131*, 319–327. doi:10.1542/peds.2012-0469.

Josephson, A. M. (2008). Reinventing family therapy: Teaching family intervention as a new treatment modality. *Academic Psychiatry, 32*, 405–413. doi:10.1176/appi.ap.32.5.405.

Landsman, M., Groza, V., Tyler, M., & Malone, K. (2001). Outcomes of family centered residential treatment. *Child Welfare League of America, 80*, 351–378.

Margolis, L. H., Rosenberg, A., Umble, K., & Chewning, L. (2012). Effects of interdisciplinary training on MCH professionals, organizations, and systems. *Maternal and Child Health Journal, 17*, 949–958. doi:10.1007/s10995-012-1078-8.

Mauksch, L. (2011, May). *Patient centered observation form.* Retrieved from http://oafp.org/assets/Family-Medicine-PCO-Form.pdf

National Association of Social Workers. (2005). *Clinical social work in social work practice*. Washington, DC: National Association of Social Workers.
Nickerson, A. B., Brooks, J. L., Colby, S. A., Rickert, J. M., & Salamone, F. J. (2006). Family involvement in residential treatment: Staff, parent, and adolescent perspectives. *Journal of Child and Family Studies, 15*, 681–694. doi:10.1007//s10826-006-9041-1.
Nickerson, A. B., Salamone, F., Brooks, J. L., & Colby, S. (2004). Promising approaches to engaging families and building strengths in residential treatment. *Residential Treatment for Children and Youth, 22*, 1–18. doi:10.1300/J007v22n01_01.
Rait, D., & Glick, I. (2008a). Reintegrating family therapy training in psychiatric residency programs: Making the case. *Academic Psychiatry, 32*, 76–80. doi:10.1176/appi.ap.32.2.76.
Rait, D., & Glick, I. (2008b). A model for reintegrating family therapy training in psychiatric residency programs. *Academic Psychiatry, 32*, 81–86. doi:10.1176/appi.ap.32.2.81.
Reitz, R., Simmons, P., Runyan, T., Hodgson, J., & Carter-Henry, S. (2013). Multiple role relationships in healthcare education. *Families, Systems & Health, 31*, 96–107. doi:10.1037/a0031862.
Schmidt, M., & Azoulay, E. (2012). Having a loved one in the ICU: The forgotten family. *Current Opinion in Critical Care, 18*, 540–547. doi:10.1097/MCC.0b013e328357f141.
Shonkoff, J. P., Boyce, W. T., & McEwen, B. S. (2009). Neuroscience, molecular biology, and the childhood roots of health disparities: Building a new framework for health promotion and disease prevention. *The Journal of the American Medical Association, 301*, 2252–2259. doi:10.1001/jama.2009.754.
Shonkoff, J. P., Garner, A. S., Siegel, B. S., Dobbins, M. L., Earls, M. F., Garner, A. S., McGuinn, L., Pascoe, J., & Wood, D. L. (2011). The lifelong effects of early childhood adversity and toxic stress. *Pediatrics, 129*, 232–246. doi:10.1542/peds.2011-2663.
Sia, C., Tonniges, T. F., Osterhus, E., & Taba, S. (2004). History of the medical home concept. *Pediatrics, 113*, 1473–1478. doi:10.1542/peds.113.5.S1.1473.
Stubbe, D., Martin, A., Block, M., Belitsky, R., Carter, D., Ebert, M., . . . Leckman, J. F. (2008). Model curriculum for academic child and adolescent psychiatry training. *Academic Psychiatry, 32*, 366–376. doi: 10.1176/appi.ap.32.5.366.
Talen, M., & Valeras, A. (2013). Introduction and overview of integrated behavioral health in primary care. In M. Talen & A. Valeras (Eds.), *Integrated behavioral health in primary care: Evaluating the evidence, identifying the essentials* (pp. 3–8). New York, NY: Springer.
Thomas, N. K. (2004). Resident burnout. *Journal of the American Medical Association, 292*, 2880–2889. doi:10.1001/jama.292.23.2880.
Tyndall, L. E., Hodgson, J. L., Lamson, A. L., White, M., & Knight, S. M. (2012). Medical family therapy: Charting a course in competencies. *Contemporary Family Therapy, 34*, 171–186. doi:10.1007/s10591-012-9191-9.
Wolff, J. L., & Roter, D. L. (2011). Family presence in routine medical visits: A meta-analytical review. *Social Science & Medicine, 72*, 823–831. doi:10.1016/j.socscimed.2011.01.015.
Wood, J. J., Piacentini, J. C., Southam-Gerow, M., Chu, B. C., & Sigman, M. (2006). Family cognitive behavioral therapy for child anxiety disorders. *Journal of the American Academy of Child and Adolescent Psychiatry, 45*, 314–321. doi:10.1097/01.chi.0000196425.88341.b0.
Wright, L. M., Watson, W. L., & Bell, J. M. (1996). *Beliefs: The heart of healing in families and illness*. New York, NY: Basic Books.

Chapter 11
Honoring the "Spiritual" in Biopsychosocial-Spiritual Health Care: Medical Family Therapists on the Front Lines of Graduate Education, Clinical Practice, and Research

Emilee Delbridge, Janie Taylor, and Carrie Hanson

Sally quickly fired off her questions, all of which came unsolicited: "How can a loving God do such a thing? What purpose does life have anyway? Why am I here? Who am I? My life doesn't matter! Why shouldn't I just end it all?" Dr. Jones, the attending resident, continued his assessment, asking Sally about pain in her abdomen. It was easy to see that she was annoyed as she stared back at Dr. Jones, silent at first, and then replied, "You're not listening, are you? You are all fakes, you and all of my Bible-thumping friends." She gathered her purse and walked out of the exam room.

Across town, David, a provisionally licensed clinician was meeting Bruce, a patient who had just told his biomedical healthcare provider that he was feeling hopeless. David began to assess the situation and quickly learned that Bruce's wife of 57 years had died six weeks earlier. According to Bruce's self-report, he and his wife had spent all of their time together. Now alone, the widower was struggling with his grief. In spite of his emotional pain, Bruce assured David, "I know that God has a plan. I just miss my Sarah."

Regardless of the healthcare setting, what Sally and Bruce are doing is common. They are both trying to make sense of and to find meaning in their respective situations. In both direct and indirect ways, patients offer insights into how they find meaning in their lives (Pargament, 2007). Meaning-making has roots in an individual's personal beliefs. Some patients find meaning in their spiritual or religious beliefs; others do not embrace such beliefs. All are equally valid. When they present for treatment, patients have often reached a point at which their existing philosophies do not align with their present experiences or they may be questioning their own abilities to navigate their present realities. Patients' "stuckness" may lead to a call and the subsequent medical and/or therapeutic appointment (Barrett, 2009).

E. Delbridge (✉)
Indiana University Purdue University-Indianapolis, Indianapolis, IN, USA
e-mail: edelbrid@iupui.edu

J. Hodgson et al. (eds.), *Medical Family Therapy*, DOI 10.1007/978-3-319-03482-9_11,

The word "spirituality" encompasses a broader focus than "religion." Spirituality refers to life principles that permeate and give life to an individual's or a group's entire being (Astrow, Puchalski, & Sulmasy, 2001; Dombeck & Karl, 1987); it is "the human experience of discovering meaning, purpose, and values, which may or may not include the concept of a God or transcendent being" (Prest, Russel, & D'Souza, 1999, p. 64). These foundational beliefs are developed throughout the life-span and serve to inform daily activities and interpretations of morals, faith, love, suffering, God, or higher power (Beusher & Beck, 2008; McSherry, 2006). Religion, in contrast, is a set of organized beliefs, practices, rituals, and/or language that is characteristic of a community searching for transcendent meaning, generally organized around the belief in a deity, or that which is existential (Koenig, McCullough, & Larson, 2001; Sulmasy, 2002).

Healing the Whole Person

Healthcare workers put themselves on the front lines where they are regularly exposed to difficult health situations and scenarios. Multiple times a day, they work with patients and family members of those who are suffering and dying (McClung, Grossoehme, & Jacobson, 2006). VandeCreek and Burton (2001) believed that during such times patients try to juxtapose their respective belief systems (or lack thereof) with the health decisions, triumphs, tragedies, and losses that are occurring. Thus, it becomes helpful to assist patients and their families as they wrestle with matters that cause existential distress in their search(es) for meaning and purpose (Puchalski, Lunsford, Harris, & Miller, 2006). Healthcare provision has embraced this premise at various times throughout history.

Prior to the Renaissance, hospitals functioned as religious and charitable organizations that housed the chronically ill and poor. In the years that followed, however, medical science and religion were divided, and matters of the body were separated from those of the mind and spirit (Mauceri, 1986; Taylor, Hodgson, Lamson, Sira, & Musick, in press). A courtship of sorts between medical science and theological training and practice began in the 1920s, when the Rev. Anton Boisen recommended that ministerial students study patients in mental institutions to learn about the human soul, as he believed that difficult times encouraged individuals to embrace fresh starts (Cabot & Dicks, 1953).

Engel (1977, 1980), appreciative of systems theory, offered an alternative to Western practices of biomedical care by expanding the framework to aspects of patients' experiences not addressed by the contemporary and prevailing scientific approaches. He noted that "Nothing exists in isolation ... every system is influenced by the configuration of the systems of which each is a part" (1980, p. 537). This viewpoint helped to expand the medical lenses of the time. Patients were recognized to be made up of multiple cells and organs, which in turn are organized into ever-increasingly large and complex parts (e.g., the patient's body) and contexts (e.g., relationships, environment). Engel coined this perspective the "biopsychosocial" (BPS) approach.

Watson, Bell, and Wright (1992) and Wright, Watson, and Bell (1996) later encouraged the expansion of the BPS model to include spirituality—thus, a "biopsychosocial-spiritual" (BPSS) approach—on the grounds that an individual's or a family's belief systems can impact treatment and healthcare outcomes. VandeCreek and Burton (2001) concurred and related that the spiritual component of a person's being must be considered, especially if the patient sees it as being important in his or her life. Addressing spiritual concerns can be even more important for individuals who see sickness as being part of a divine plan or what their higher power (however defined) desires to occur in their lives (Koenig, Moberg, & Kvale, 1988). Pargament (1997) amplified this thought, as he found that people view their spiritualities as resources that provide strength during difficult situations.

The challenge to offer holistic care beckons for healthcare disciplines and spirituality to integrate once more. Multiple reasons exist for doing so. First, spirituality has been identified as a critical component of patients' and families' health care and well-being (Chapman & Grossoehme, 2002), especially during times of crisis (Fogg, Weaver, Flannelly, & Handzo, 2004). Multiple researchers have linked spirituality with physical well-being and behavioral health (e.g., George, Ellison, & Larson, 2002; Hill & Pargament, 2003; Koenig et al., 2001; Larson, Swyers, & McCullough, 1998; Seybold & Hill, 2001; Thorensen, 1999; Thorensen, Harris, & Onan, 2001). Likeminded researchers are beginning to gain insight into how spirituality contributes to positive coping in patients who suffer with severe, chronic, and terminal conditions (e.g., Brady, Peterman, Fitchett, Mod, & Cella, 1999; Carey, 1985; Cotton, Larkin, Hoopes, Cromer, & Rosenthal, 2005; Koenig et al., 2001; Phelps et al., 2009; Post, Puchalski, & Larson, 2000; VandeCreek, Pargament, Belavich, Cowell, & Friedel, 1999).

A second reason for integrating spirituality into care rests in patients' desire for their spiritual needs to be addressed (Bienenfeld & Yager, 2007). While the BPSS aspects of an individual are recognized, it is not surprising to learn that between 33 and 94 % of patients want their spiritual concerns addressed by healthcare team members (Carey, 1985; Daaleman & Nease, 1994; Ehman, Ott, Short, Ciampa, & Hansen-Flaschen, 1999; Fitchett, Meyer, & Burton, 2000; King & Bushwick, 1994; Koenig et al., 2001). Seen to be part of the patients' "core selves," spirituality is recognized to "promote [patient] resiliency" (Barrett, 2009, p. 5).

Bienenfeld and Yager (2007) found that an individual's religious community may serve as a resource to treatment, often offering important social support. There are times, however, when a religious community holds beliefs which cause an individual to resist a treatment protocol. For example, some religious groups do not believe in blood transfusions (Singelenberg, 1990). Such a belief may prevent a patient from receiving treatment which has been deemed necessary, even life saving, by the healthcare community. The role of system-oriented healthcare providers is to consider all aspects of a patient's context (i.e., biological, psychological, social/relational, and spiritual). In a situation like this, it would be appropriate for providers to fully understand the patient's spiritual and religious beliefs and to provide the patient with all the medical information related to treatment recommendations and options.

Finally, the need to make health care more patient centered has been recognized by many. The Patient Protection and Affordable Care Act (ACA, 2010) was signed into law in March 2010. The purpose of the ACA is to increase both the quality and affordability of health care in the United States. Reiner (2011), who works within the Veterans Affairs Maryland Health Care System (VAMHCS), offers performance metrics which can be customized to help design treatment plans that are cost effective, safe, and patient specific. The protocols recommended by ACA and VAMHCS reinforce mandates of the Institute of Medicine (IOM) set forth in 2001. While a patient-centered care model is used to assure physical comfort, healthcare team members strive to address and honor each patient's cultural, spiritual, and individual needs (IOM, 2001). For example, emotional support is provided to help eliminate both fear and anxiety, and this help extends to patients' families and friends. The IOM model for healing environments is also aided by strong interdisciplinary collaboration. Biological components are complemented by integrated care which is psychological, social, and spiritual in nature. A patient's treatment team may include his or her medical doctor, a psychiatrist and/or psychotherapist, a medical social worker, and a chaplain or a minister, with each member contributing to the patient's care according to his or her respective area of expertise.

Spirituality: The Least Attended to Component of Patients' and Families' Lives

In spite of findings that have shown that patients desire holistic approaches and that their health is advanced when providers widen their respective lenses to include spirituality, it remains the least addressed dimension of the BPSS approach. Clinical practitioners have been slow to integrate spirituality in healthcare provision. Many educators offer little to no instruction in it. Research to guide these pursuits, while burgeoning, is still underdeveloped.

Multiple reasons contribute to this disparity. Providers often cite personal discomfort and lack of training regarding how to talk about spirituality. The lack of existing curriculum options or an agreed-upon set of spirituality competencies can give educators pause. Cultural and political contexts can also act as barriers. While questions have long existed in many circles about how to measure that which is existential in nature, researchers who have examined the healthcare benefits of integrating spirituality have lagged behind those whose research may be more easily quantified and recognized as beneficial.

A Call to Advance Spirituality across Education, Practice, and Research

The IOM's 2001 mandate for healthcare providers to address patients' needs includes those which are spiritual in nature. While extensively addressing spirituality during healthcare treatment may require additional training as well as one's willingness to adopt a posture of curiosity, doing so can reduce unnecessary treatment and costs (IOM, 2001). It also serves to advance the patient's healthcare outcomes when the provider widens his or her care provision lens to include spirituality. Not only can the patient's physical and mental well-being improve, but the inclusion of spirituality can also offer the patient a resource when dealing with a chronic or a terminal condition. A call has been issued; it must not go unheeded. It is, indeed, imperative that the field includes spirituality education, clinical practice, and research.

Spirituality in Graduate Education

The collaborative and systemic nature of Medical Family Therapy (MedFT) training, coupled with its emphasis on relationships and self of the therapist, makes graduate training the ideal place to cultivate spirituality-sensitive clinicians. However, the current lack of curriculum consensus regarding spirituality across and within graduate training programs has led to a fragmentation of the information taught to MedFT trainees. Trainees are often prepared in settings wherein sensitive topics are separated into special courses, lectures, or weekend intensives. This style of instruction may encourage new professionals to think that compartmentalizing topics like spirituality from other facets of their learning is necessary. However, this perpetuates biases and hierarchies that hinder the practice of integrated BPSS care. In a field that strives to be holistic, interdisciplinary courses will be essential in moving healthcare integration forward.

Teaching spirituality within a politically correct culture brings unique challenges. Many people equate spirituality with religion and thereby fear bringing it into the classroom. This nation's separation of "church" and "state" has made it difficult for people to talk about and express their spiritual views. This approach has left some providers unprepared to address patients', trainees', and oftentimes their own spiritual issues. People may be concerned about offending others; therefore, they remain silent and perpetuate the chasm between spirituality and integrated care. It is imperative that MedFTs are trained in how to discuss spirituality in a non-offensive (at worst) and enriching (at best) manner. Developing ways to have open and frank discussions requires practitioners to demonstrate patience as well as to possess a clear model for how to train learners. Some of the essential skills for future practitioners would be to demonstrate understanding, respect, and tolerance regarding the human experience of spirituality.

In the absence of MedFT core spiritual competencies, it can be challenging for trainers to integrate spirituality into training and supervision. Borrowing from the fields of Hospice, Nursing, Psychology, Social Work, and Chaplaincy, one can formulate or add to a class these basic tenets of spiritual competence: spiritual self-awareness, awareness of others' spirituality, discussing spirituality, and assessing and evaluating providers' attention to spirituality. This first section provides an overview of some of the basic elements of teaching and incorporating spirituality into course curriculum. Ideas for topics, lesson plans, class activities, exercises, and additional resources are discussed.

Teaching Strategies and Resources

Trainees using the BPSS model are taught the importance of healing the whole person (McKee & Chappel, 1992; Sulmasy, 2002). Readings and class lectures contain discussions about the differences between religion and spirituality as well as a historical overview of medicine's and behavioral health's inclusion and exclusion of spiritual components in healing. Meaningful elements that can assist trainees in understanding spirituality may include an open dialogue about the complexities of including and discussing spirituality with colleagues, patients, and/or patients' families. Another important topic to discuss includes the relationships between different faiths and religions as well as how these belief systems intersect with science and medicine (Table 11.1).

Spiritual self-awareness. Across disciplines, the necessity for spiritual awareness of self and others is imperative to the learning process. Trainees can begin to understand how spirituality influences their clinical work by exploring their personal attitudes, beliefs, and values. The completion of a spiritual genogram can assist trainees in their own process of spiritual self-exploration. Some questions that trainees may reflect upon could include the following: What role did spirituality/religion (or the absence of) play in your life as a child? What role does spirituality/religion (or the absence of) play in your life now? How does your spirituality/religion (or the absence of) influence how you see illness, disease, health, and family support in times of need, dying, death, etc.? While working to identify and explore their own spiritual beliefs, trainees can begin to identify the limits of their own understandings, personal biases, and potential areas for growth (Table 11.2).

Others' spirituality. The process of increased awareness of others' spirituality is a journey that takes time, openness, and understanding. Instructors are encouraged to engage trainees in discussions and activities that expose them to different ways of being spiritual. Trainees can begin to engage in becoming aware of others by studying various spiritual beliefs and practices, agnosticism, and atheism. It may be helpful to show a video that explores different religions and spiritual beliefs and practices (see Table 11.3). Another approach to widening learners' understanding would be to encourage them to meet in small groups to engage in conversations around their own spiritual beliefs and practices. Then, the large group can

Table 11.1 Healing the whole person: resources

Readings	Author(s)	Description
Spirituality and the therapeutic process: A comprehensive resource from intake to termination	Aten and Leach (2009)	Offers practical strategies, techniques, and examples on how therapists can honor patients' spiritual experiences throughout the therapeutic process
Narrative medicine: Honoring the stories of illness	Charon (2006)	Discusses narrative medicine, which can be a reflective practice that draws on stories (at times, of illness) to aid providers and patients in making sense of illness and disease
Religion, spirituality, and marriage and family therapy: A study of family therapists' beliefs about the appropriateness of addressing religious and spiritual issues in therapy	Carlson, Kirkpatrick, Hecker, and Killmer (2002)	Explores family therapists' beliefs about the importance of spirituality in their personal and professional lives and their beliefs about addressing spiritual issues in therapy
Spiritual issues in family therapy: A graduate-level course	Patterson, Hayworth, and Turner (2000)	Describes a graduate-level seminar on spirituality and its place in family therapy
Religion and spirituality in psychotherapy: A practice-friendly review of research	Post and Wade (2009)	Reviews research on religion and spirituality in psychotherapy with a focus on religion/spirituality and therapists, religion/spirituality and patients, and religious/spiritual interventions
A biopsychosocial-spiritual model for the care of patients at the end of life	Sulmasy (2002)	Introduces a model that expands the biopsychosocial model to include the spiritual aspects of a patient's well-being
Spirituality and healing	Torosian and Biddle (2005)	Offers a brief historical review of spirituality and healing, talks about the multiple dimensions of cancer, and discusses the clinical impact of spirituality
Case studies		
Making sense of spirituality in nursing and healthcare practice	McSherry (2006)	Two short case studies with reflecting questions that illustrate the intersection of health care and spirituality

reconvene and discuss the content and process of the small group discussions. This process could include asking questions about the difficulty that participants may have experienced when sharing and listening to others talk about their spiritual beliefs and practices. It is important to note that these discussions may include difficult emotions, such as vulnerability, fear, or other feelings that can act as barriers to open dialogue(s).

Table 11.2 Spiritual self-awareness: resources

Readings	Author	Description
Religious and spiritual issues in psychotherapy practice: Training the trainer	Bartoli (2007)	Explores therapists' reluctance to address religious and spiritual issues in training programs and clinical practices; offers suggestions on how practitioners can enhance their spiritual and religious competencies
The spiritual genogram in family therapy	Frame (2000)	Describes how practitioners can utilize spiritual genograms, a multigenerational map of family members' religious and spiritual affiliations, events, and conflicts, during the course of therapy; includes practical information as well as a case illustration
Spirituality as a dimension of family therapists' clinical training	Haug (1998)	Discusses the crucial role the self of therapist plays in effective therapy; talks about the need to include a spiritual dimension in therapy training programs in order to increase therapists' spiritual understanding

Introducing trainees to spiritual elements of health and healing involves the conscious inclusion of spiritual and religious cultures. Class time can be enriched with guest speakers or a panel comprising spiritual and religious leaders, members of spiritual and religious communities, healthcare professionals who incorporate spirituality into their work, or patients who are willing to share their personal spiritual journeys through acute or chronic illness.

Whether there is an entire class dedicated to teaching MedFTs how to explore and discuss spirituality or whether the topic of spirituality is incorporated into courses on culture, ethics, theory, or practice, there are many resources available to address the spiritual dimension of the BPSS model. Case studies, role-plays, film, and literature can all be used in the process of teaching and discussing spirituality. Regardless of the methods used to teach and discuss spirituality, it is important to foster MedFTs' curiosity, humility, and respect as they explore spirituality with themselves and others in relation to understanding or conducting research and their own development of clinical skills and patient care.

Spirituality in Clinical Practice

Finding providers who integrate spirituality into the care they provide can be challenging. Research has shown that healthcare professionals, especially physicians and physician extenders, are often reluctant to address patients' spiritual concerns (Anandarajah & Hight, 2001; Hage, 2006). One reason for providers' reluctance includes, as outlined above, lack of training. Others report worries about having to disclose, and/or resistance toward, disclosing their personal beliefs

Table 11.3 Others' spirituality: resources

Readings	Author(s)	Description
Spiritual diversity: Multifaith perspectives in family therapy	Walsh (2010)	Addresses the diversity and complexity of spirituality in society and families
Spiritual resources in family therapy (2nd ed.)	Walsh (2009)	Explores the role of spirituality in couple and family relationships and illustrates ways practitioners can tap spiritual resources for coping, healing, and resilience
Talking about spirituality in healthcare practice: A resource for the multi-professional healthcare team	White (2006)	Offers a framework within which healthcare professionals can discuss spirituality and prepare themselves to discuss patient spirituality
Videos		
Alain de Botton: Atheism 2.0	de Botton (2012)	A TED talk about atheism that incorporates the human need for connection, ritual, and transcendence
The Smith family	Oldham and Wright (2002)	A documentary about a Mormon family's struggle with HIV, AIDS, and their journey to redefine family, faith, and forgiveness in the midst of illness
The wisdom of faith with Huston Smith: A Bill Moyers special	Smith (2010)	Discusses major religions, e.g., Hinduism, Buddhism, Confucianism, Christianity, Judaism, and Islam
Literature		
A Grief Observed	Lewis (1991)	Written after the author's wife's death as a way of surviving the "mad midnight moment," this text is an honest reflection on the fundamental issues of life, death, and faith in the midst of loss

(even though they may never be put in a position to do so). While Griffith and Griffith (2003) found that some healthcare providers, whether working in traditional therapy or in integrated settings, have a concern that their patients may have a deeper spiritual experience, it should be noted that some also indicated a failure to see how integrating spirituality into care would contribute to positive medical outcomes.

Regardless of one's belief system, Griffith and Griffith (2003) suggested that an attitude of curiosity on the part of providers can help create a climate of respect and openness. While it is not the healthcare provider's job to debate the truths of one's beliefs, he or she should seek to establish a conversation which allows an individual to share what he or she believes, what is real to him or her, and what gives meaning to his or her life. In order to do so, the healthcare provider steps aside from taking a position of knowledge and assumes a role of curiosity. He or she becomes a fellow sojourner with the individual, often asking questions as a means for acquiring additional information. A patient can speak fully of his or her spiritual or religious experience when he or she feels that his or her personhood is respected.

When entering into such a conversation, the provider can pose queries which invite the patient to share what he or she finds to hold value. Providers may ask the patient what brings meaning to his or her life. Information shared can offer the provider with a platform for additional comments and discussion. For example, if a person sees accomplishment as imperative, he or she may discount physical cues of exhaustion in order to work more hours. Those who place relationships as priorities may disregard their own needs so that children, for example, might have food, clothing, and designer-named footwear. It is suggested that the provider ask the patient to educate him or her about how his or her beliefs evolved and why they are held. Questions about what the patient believes to be valuable can also be helpful. A respectful and safe environment is essential for the patient in sharing his or her thoughts and beliefs.

Engaging in a conversation about religion and spirituality depends less on knowing what questions to ask and more on the provider's ability to listen carefully. In fact, Griffith and Griffith (2003) explained that religious discussions usually begin naturally. It is not uncommon for patients to make statements like "Only God can help me now." The expression of such a belief allows a provider the opportunity to ask for additional information to seek clarity. Conversations may also include metaphors (such as "God is my shepherd" [Psalm 23] or "He is my healer" [Psalm 103:3]) as well as patients' accounts of their participation in religious rituals, spiritual practices, and their respective faith communities. Patients may indicate that they cannot follow a prescribed food regimen because they are fasting or keeping a kosher diet. They may be hesitant to schedule a procedure on a day considered holy by their faith or indicate that it is imperative they make a trip out of the country because of a planned pilgrimage.

It is suggested that a platform for discussion be provided. When inquiring about the beliefs of the patient, the provider must also be aware of what he or she is experiencing and be willing to ask himself or herself why his or her feelings are so strong. It can be very difficult, for example, if a surgeon believes that a patient needs a surgical procedure but his or her patient refuses to entertain the procedure because it is contraindicated by existing religious beliefs. Various faith traditions, such as Jehovah's Witnesses, have resources available to aid healthcare providers in learning about possible options. (Jehovah's Witnesses also have a 24-h hotline where providers can receive case-specific consultation [718-560-4300].) If, after the discussion and treatment are completed, the provider continues to experience discomfort, it may be helpful for him or her to seek supervision.

Clinical Resources

Hodgson, Lamson, and Reese's (2007) work provided an instrument whereby a healthcare provider can develop a comprehensive profile of a patient. Their interview method helps the provider gather information about the individual's biomedical, psychological, social, and spiritual well-being. After acquiring insight into a patient's spiritual history and evolution, it becomes important for the healthcare provider to learn about the individual's beliefs. When contemplating treatments, it is imperative that interventions be both patient centered and respectful. When assessing a patient's spirituality, there are multiple measures that may be helpful (for examples, see Table 11.4).

The healthcare providers in the two examples put forth in the introduction to this chapter may find these measures useful. Insight into Sally's beliefs may be gained from her responses to the items included in the Brief Multidimensional Measure of Religiousness and Spirituality. Not only could information be gained about her beliefs, but the history of her faith could also provide great understanding into her comments about God. The Brief RCOPE could help David learn how Bruce's spirituality may assist and/or impact his grief experience, as the items provide a score that rates his coping with the stressors he is experiencing.

MedFTs are especially well equipped to engage in clinical practice that embraces spirituality. Their systemic orientation enables them to see and understand the interplay of each of the four components of the BPSS model. It enables them to integrate spirituality (the final "S") into excellent clinical work and to collaborate with others along the way and as indicated. A systemic orientation also opens discussions within training about how to integrate spirituality. MedFTs' skills in research can serve to further inform and advance spirituality in the very care MedFTs provide and use in training.

Spirituality in Healthcare Research

MedFTs are in a prime position to develop lines of research, insofar as they already approach care collaboratively (guided by their training in relationships, relational theories, and multi-method research designs). Investigators can join forces with other healthcare professionals to develop viable and robust research projects and interventions (Linville, Hertlein, & Prouty Lyness, 2007; Mendenhall, Pratt, Phelps, & Baird, 2012). Examples of these integrated partnerships can include collaborations between and across professionals representing fields within behavioral health, medicine, spirituality, and religion.

Potential challenges in addressing spirituality in healthcare research are similar to the challenges, described above, in addressing spirituality in graduate education and clinical practice. Questions may arise as follows: *How do we define or operationalize spirituality? Can we do this in a manner that is inclusive, respectful,*

Table 11.4 Assessment measures

Instrument	Developer(s)	Description
Spiritual Well-Being Scale (SWBS)	Ellison (1983)	A 20-item measure of dispositional religiousness/spirituality that assesses spiritual well-being on two subscales: existential and religious
Daily Spiritual Experience Scale (DSES)	Underwood and Teresi (2002)	A 16-item self-report measure of spiritual experience that specifically aims to gauge ordinary, or daily, spiritual experiences, not mystical experiences, and how they are a part of everyday life
Spiritual Experience Index—Revised	Genia (1991)	A 23-item scale that measures faith and spiritual journey, aiming not to impose any particular faith as part of the questions; this questionnaire includes two subscales: spiritual support and spiritual openness
Duke University Religion Index (DUREL)	Koenig and Bussing (2010)	A 5-item scale that measures organizational, non-organizational, and intrinsic dimensions of religiousness
Brief RCOPE	Pargament, Feuille, and Burdzy (2011)	A 14-item measure of religious coping with major life stressors. Two overarching forms are measured: positive and negative religious coping
Spiritual Assessment Inventory (SAI)	Hall and Edwards (1996)	A 49-item measure which assesses two dimensions of spiritual development: awareness of God and quality of relationship with God; five factors are measured (awareness, instability, grandiosity, realistic acceptance, defensiveness/disappointment)
Brief Multidimensional Measure of Religiousness and Spirituality (BMMRS)	Fetzer Institute (2003)	A 38-item instrument that measures religious and spiritual disposition as well as function; measures are obtained for daily spiritual experiences, meaning, values, beliefs, forgiveness, private religious practices, religious/spiritual coping, religious support, religious/spiritual history, commitment, organizational religiousness, and religious preference

and shared (enough) so that patients are engaged in participating? How do we gain access to patients? This requires those who have primary contact and/or gate-keeping power (often other healthcare providers) to buy-in to the importance of the research being proposed. It also requires buy-in from patients (and their families), which can circle back to whether investigators' definitions of spirituality and goal(s) of the study are meaningful or compelling.

Another matter to be addressed relates to gaining adequate funding to complete relevant and rigorous research. Most funding within health care favors the so-called hard sciences. However, more research has been conducted on spirituality in recent years (e.g., Ribaudo & Takahashi, 2008; Weaver, Flannely, Strock, Krause, & Flannelly, 2005), and this is encouraging. Funding lines are, indeed, available to support researchers' investigating spirituality. Examples of sources of funding include foundational, state, and federal organizations (e.g., Duke University's Center for Spirituality, Theology, and Health; the John Templeton Foundation; the National Network to Eliminate Disparities in Behavioral Health [NNED]; and the University of Minnesota's Center for Spirituality and Healing).

Research Resources and Strategies

Some of the approaches to conducting spirituality research within MedFT may take the form of various methodologies, some of which have been suggested by others. Other areas rich for research regarding spirituality revolve around training and education (as discussed earlier in this chapter).

Assessment tools. Some tools especially appropriate for relational and systemic researchers, like MedFTs, include the Spirituality Index of Well-Being (SIWB; Frey, Daaleman, & Peyton, 2005) and the HOPE questions for clinical encounters (Anandarajah & Hight, 2001; de Jager Meezenbroek et al., 2012; see Table 11.4 for further details). Researchers can incorporate these scales and measures into the clinical practice and care of patients in order to expand the constructs that are tracked. If MedFTs studied patients' levels of spiritual coping, for example, while also measuring patients' medical or behavioral health symptom reduction, the results could contribute to a better understanding of what spiritual and medical interventions and treatments affect positive patient outcomes.

Methodologies and designs. Mendenhall et al. (2012) identified research methods that are well aligned with the research goals and agendas of MedFTs (also see Chap. 13; Mendenhall, Pratt, Phelps, Baird, & Younkin, 2014). The authors provided comprehensive examples of potential quantitative and qualitative research ideas. Using a Three-World view of health care (Cohen & Crabtree, 2008; Peek, 2008), multiple research questions were offered regarding the clinical, operational, and financial worlds of MedFT. Such research could include spirituality by including spiritual assessment forms in the intake paperwork for behavioral health sessions. If demographic information is gathered that includes religious or spiritual affiliation, providers can also ask about (perhaps with a prompt from the electronic medical record system) the patient's use of their reported spiritual resources. If the patient reports barriers, rather than supports, then a behavioral health provider could be informed or the physician could inquire about viable options for increased support. Some examples of integrated care support might include family therapists, chaplaincy services, or accessing patients' religious or spiritual support systems or organizations.

These questions and conversations regarding spiritual coping or resources could then be documented by providers. If satisfaction surveys are provided to patients, results could be compared to patients whose providers did not have conversations with them about spiritual coping or religious resources. Additionally, the course of the symptoms or the disease could be compared and measured as well as the number of comorbid conditions or frequency of hospitalizations. In line with Campbell's (2003) suggestion to expand integrated care outcome research, spirituality or spiritual coping could be one of the outcomes that is identified and evaluated.

Mendenhall et al. (2012) outlined a few unique areas of research methodologies that could promote the field of MedFT and provide meaningful results for patients and their families. Community-based participatory research (CBPR) and practice-based research networks (PBRNs) are key examples of this. Partnering with patients and consumers in a particular area is an excellent way to understand what the needs and concerns of the community really are. Ensuring that interests, such as spiritual beliefs and practices, are welcomed as potential conversation topics and research agendas is important. Given that research indicates that patients desire that their physicians inquire about their beliefs and religious coping (Hebert, Jenckes, Ford, O'Connor, & Cooper, 2001), it would follow that these topics would show up on the agendas of collaborative, community-driven research plans. Researchers could invite multiple religious leaders to be a part of the research process as well as provide compelling reasons for integrating spirituality into health care.

Given that PBRNs include multiple professionals, treatment interventions that include spiritual or religious assessment and coping could be compared across various sites. The larger number of participants in the study, along with the similarities across sites, could increase the external validity of the results. If a patient's spiritual distress is recognized by the provider, a referral to an appropriate professional on-site could occur. Alternately, a follow-up phone call by a trained professional could be provided to the patient. The patient's satisfaction could be measured over time, and future levels of functioning (such as lower levels of anxiety or depression, higher compliance with medical appointment attendance, compliance with medication regimens) could also be determined. These outcome measures could then be compared to similar clinical sites in that same research network to determine the effectiveness of assessing and addressing spiritual distress in patients.

Opportunities for researchers to explore the relationships between health care and spirituality abound. Some of the potential barriers and the important contributions of such research have been highlighted here. Options exist for MedFT researchers to partner with other healthcare providers, focus on the health outcomes and functioning of patients and families, and conduct educational research regarding the teaching and supervision approaches of training MedFT and healthcare professionals.

Conclusion

The BPSS approach is integral to integrated health care. Spirituality was initially absent from this model (Engel, 1977; McKee & Chappel, 1992; Tyndall, Hodgson, Lamson, White, & Knight, 2012), but the dimension has been included more consistently in recent years. This chapter has included discussions about the challenges and the approaches related to actively including the spiritual dimension of the BPSS model in the education of healthcare professionals, the provision of clinical services, and research related to spirituality within integrated care. Each of these areas is connected to the other: research informs clinical practice, patient care informs how future professionals are best trained, and graduate education is best provided when it is recursively informed by patient outcomes.

Reflection Questions

Graduate Education:

1. With our contemporary cultural emphases separating church and state, alongside the potential legal ramifications of mingling the two, many healthcare professionals purposely avoid the topics of religion and spirituality. Thinking about your own experiences as a learner or a practitioner, what are some of your personal fears and assumptions that make it challenging to integrate spirituality into your work as a clinician, teacher, or researcher?
2. People can derive spirituality from a myriad of sources, including faith communities, nature, art, and meditation. What are some ways that you have developed your spiritual self? What about those around you? How can you incorporate examples of spiritual diversity into your curriculum?

Clinical Practice:

3. What questions could a provider ask that would help to uncover what a patient identifies as valuable in his or her life?
4. It can be difficult for healthcare providers when patients do not respect their beliefs. It can be equally difficult when patients adopt beliefs that conflict with those of the provider. How can such a chasm in beliefs be bridged?

Healthcare Research:

5. Identify a spiritual or a religious concern that a patient or a family has presented within your integrated care setting. How would you describe their concern(s) in terms of a quantitative research question? What would the independent and dependent variables be? How would you attempt to answer the research question(s)?
6. Based on this chapter's exploration of MedFT and spirituality, what is a research question you find interesting or challenging? What methodology would you use to explore the question? What resources might you need to start to conduct this qualitative study?

References[1]

Anandarajah, G., & Hight, E. (2001). Spirituality and medical practice: Using the HOPE questions as a practical tool for spiritual assessment. *American Family Physician, 63*, 81–88. Retrieved from http://www.aafp.org/afp/2001/0101/p81.pdf

Astrow, A. B., Puchalski, C. P., & Sulmasy, D. P. (2001). Religion, spirituality, and health care: Social, practical, and ethical considerations. *The American Journal of Medicine, 110*(4), 283–287.

Aten, J., & Leach, M. (2009). *Spirituality and the therapeutic process: A comprehensive resource from intake to termination*. Washington, DC: American Psychological Association. doi:10.1037/11853-000.

Barrett, T. C. (2009). Spirituality and psychotherapy. *Human Development, 30*(2), 5–11.

Bartoli, E. (2007). Religious and spiritual issues in psychotherapy practice: Training the trainer. *Psychotherapy: Theory, Research, Practice, Training, 44*(1), 54–65. doi:10.1037/0033-3204.44.1.54.

Beusher, L., & Beck, C. (2008). A literature review of spirituality in coping with early-stage Alzheimer's disease. *Journal of Clinical Nursing, 17*, 88–97. doi:10.1111/j.1365-2702.2007.02126.x.

Bienenfeld, D., & Yager, J. (2007). Issues of spirituality and religion in psychotherapy supervision. *Journal of Psychiatry Related Sciences, 44*(3), 178–186.

Brady, M. J., Peterman, A. H., Fitchett, G., Mod, M., & Cella, D. (1999). A case for including spirituality in quality of life measurement in oncology. *Psycho-Oncology, 8*, 417–428. doi:10.1002/(SICI)1099-1611(199909/10)8:5<417::AID-PON398>3.0.CO;2-4.

Cabot, R. C., & Dicks, R. L. (1953). *The art of ministering to the sick*. New York, NY: The MacMillan Company.

Campbell, T. L. (2003). The effectiveness of family interventions for physical disorders. *Journal of Marital and Family Therapy, 29*, 263–281. doi:10.1111/j.1752-0606.1995.tb00178.x.

Carey, R. G. (1985). Change in perceived need, value, and role of hospital chaplains. In L. E. Holst (Ed.), *Hospital ministry: The role of the chaplain today* (pp. 28–41). New York, NY: Crossroad Publishing Company.

*Carlson, T. D., Kirkpatrick, D., Hecker, L., & Killmer, M. (2002). Religion, spirituality, and marriage and family therapy: A study of family therapists' beliefs about the appropriateness of

[1] An asterisk has been used to note references that the chapter authors recommend for further reading.

addressing religious and spiritual issues in therapy. *The American Journal of Family Therapy, 30*, 157–171. doi:10.1080/019261802753573867.

Chapman, T. R., & Grossoehme, D. H. (2002). Adolescent patient and nurse referrals for pastoral care: A comparison of psychiatric vs. medical-surgical populations. *Journal of Child and Adolescent Psychiatric Nursing, 15*(3), 118–123. doi:10.1111/j.1744-6171.2002.tb00334.x.

Charon, R. (2006). *Narrative medicine: Stories that heal*. New York, NY: Oxford University Press.

Cohen, D., & Crabtree, B. (2008). Evaluative criteria for qualitative research in health care: Controversies and recommendations. *Annals of Family Medicine, 6*, 331–339. doi:10.1370/afm.818.

Cotton, S., Larkin, E., Hoopes, A., Cromer, B. A., & Rosenthal, S. L. (2005). The impact of adolescent spirituality on depressive symptoms and health risk behaviors. *The Journal of Adolescent Behaviors, 36*(6), 529. doi:10.1016/j.jadohealth.2004.07.017.

Daaleman, T. P., & Nease, D. E. (1994). Patient attitudes regarding physician inquiry into spiritual and religious issues. *The Journal of Family Practice, 39*(6), 564–568.

de Botton, A. (2012, January). *Alain de Botton: Atheism 2.0*. Retrieved from http://www.ted.com/talks/alain_de_botton_atheism_2_0.html

de Jager Meezenbroek, E., Garssen, B., van den Berg, M., van Dierendonck, D., Visser, A., & Schaufeli, W. B. (2012). Measuring spirituality as a universal human experience: A review of spirituality questionnaires. *Journal of Religion and Health, 51*, 336–354. doi:10.1007/s10943-010-9376-1.

Dombeck, M., & Karl, J. (1987). Spiritual issues in mental health care. *Journal of Religion and Health, 26*(3), 183–197.

Ehman, J. W., Ott, B. B., Short, T. H., Ciampa, R. C., & Hansen-Flaschen, J. (1999). Do patients want physicians to inquire about their spiritual or religious beliefs in they become gravely ill? *Archives of Internal Medicine, 159*, 1803–1806. doi:10.1001/archinte.159.15.1803.

Ellison, C. W. (1983). Spiritual well-being: Conceptualization and measurement. *Journal of Psychology and Theology, 11*(4), 330–340.

*Engel, G. L. (1977). The need for a new medical model: A challenge for biomedicine. *Science, 196*(4286), 129–136. doi:10.1126/science.847460.

*Engel, G. L. (1980). The clinical application of the biopsychosocial model. *American Journal of Psychiatry, 137*, 535–544.

Fetzer Institute. (2003). *Multidimensional measurement of religiousness/spirituality for use health research: A report of the Fetzer Institute/national institute on aging working group*. Kalamazoo, MI: Fetzer Institute.

Fitchett, G., Meyer, P. M., & Burton, L. A. (2000). Spiritual care in the hospital: Who requests it? Who needs it? *Journal of Pastoral Care, 54*(2), 173–186.

Fogg, S. L., Weaver, A. J., Flannelly, K. J., & Handzo, G. F. (2004). An analysis of referrals to chaplains in a community hospital in New York over a seven year period. *The Journal of Pastoral Care and Counseling, 58*(3), 225–235. Retrieved from: http://www.journals.sfu.ca/jcpc/index.php.jpcp

Frame, M. (2000). The spiritual genogram in family therapy. *Journal of Marital and Family Therapy, 26*(2), 211–215. doi:10.1111/j.1752-0606.2000.tb00290.x.

Frey, B. B., Daaleman, T. P., & Peyton, V. (2005). Measuring a dimension of spirituality for health research: Validity of the spirituality index of well-being. *Research on Aging, 27*, 56–577. doi:10.1177/0164027505277847.

Genia, V. (1991). The Spiritual Experience Index: A measure of spiritual maturity. *Journal of Religion and Health, 30*, 337–347.

George, L. K., Ellison, C. G., & Larson, D. B. (2002). Exploring the relationships between religious involvement and health. *Psychological Inquiry, 13*(3), 190–200. doi:10.1207/S15327965PLI1303_04.

*Griffith, J. L., & Griffith, M. E. (2003). *Encountering the sacred in psychotherapy: How to talk with people about their spirituality*. New York, NY: The Guilford Press.

Hage, S. M. (2006). A closer look at the role of spirituality in psychiatric training programs. *Professional Psychology Research and Practice, 37*(7), 303–310.
Hall, T. W., & Edwards, K. J. (1996). The initial development and factor analysis of the Spiritual Assessment Inventory. *Journal of Psychology & Theology, 24*(3), 233–246.
Haug, I. (1998). Spirituality as a dimension of family therapists' clinical training. *Contemporary Family Therapy, 20*(4), 471–483. doi:10.1023/A:1021628132514.
Hebert, R. S., Jenckes, M. W., Ford, D. E., O'Connor, D. R., & Cooper, L. A. (2001). Patient perspectives on spirituality and the patient-physician relationship. *Journal of General Internal Medicine, 16*, 685–692. doi:10.1111/j.1525-1497.2001.01034.x.
Hill, P. C., & Pargament, K. I. (2003). Advances in the conceptualization and measurement of religion and spirituality. *American Psychologist, 58*(1), 64–74.
Hodgson, J., Lamson, A. L., & Reese, L. (2007). The biopsychosocial-spiritual interview method. In D. Linville & K. M. Hertlein (Eds.), *The therapist's notebook for family health care: Homework, handouts, and activities for individuals, couples, and families coping with illness, loss, and disability* (pp. 3–12). Philadelphia, PA: Haworth Press.
Institute of Medicine. (2001). *Crossing the quality chasm*. Washington, DC: Institute of Medicine.
King, D. E., & Bushwick, B. (1994). Beliefs and attitudes of hospital inpatients about faith healing and prayer. *Journal of Family Practice, 39*, 349–352. doi:10.1093/fampra/11.1.3.
Koenig, H. G., & Bussing, A. (2010). The Duke University Religion Index (DUKE-L): A five-item measure for use in epidemiological studies. *Religions, 1*(1), 78–85. doi:10.3390/rel1010078.
*Koenig, H. G., McCullough, M. E., & Larson, D. B. (2001). *Handbook of religion and health*. New York, NY: Oxford University Press.
Koenig, H. G., Moberg, D. O., & Kvale, J. N. (1988). Religious activities and attitudes of older adults in a geriatric assessment clinic. *Journal of the American Geriatrics Society, 36*, 362–374.
Larson, D. B., Swyers, J. P., & McCullough, M. E. (1998). *Scientific research on spirituality and health: A report based on the scientific progress in spirituality conferences*. Bethesda, MD: National Institute for Healthcare Research.
Lewis, C. S. (1991). *A grief observed*. New York, NY: HarperCollins.
*Linville, D., Hertlein, K. M., & Prouty Lyness, A. M. (2007). Medical family therapy: Reflecting on the necessity of collaborative healthcare research. *Families, Systems & Health, 25*, 85–97. doi:10.1037/1091-7527.25.1.85.
Mauceri, J. (1986). *The great break: A short history of the separation of medical science from religion*. Barrytown, NY: P.U.L.S.E.
McClung, E., Grossoehme, D. H., & Jacobson, A. F. (2006). Collaborating with chaplains to meet spiritual needs. *Medsurg Nursing, 15*(3), 147–156. Retrieved from http://www.medsurgnursing.net/
McKee, D. D., & Chappel, J. N. (1992). Spirituality and medical practice. *Journal of Family Practice, 35*, 205–208.
McSherry, W. (2006). *Making sense of spirituality in nursing and health care practice*. London: Jessica Kingsley. Retrieved from http://www.rcn.org.uk/development/practice/spirituality/what_spirituality_is_and_is_not/spirituality_case_studies
*Mendenhall, T. J., Pratt, K. J., Phelps, K. W., & Baird, M. A. (2012). Advancing medical family therapy through research: A consideration of qualitative, quantitative, and mixed-methods designs. *Contemporary Family Therapy, 34*, 187–203. doi:10.1007/s10591-012-9186-6.
Mendenhall, T. J., Pratt, K. J., Phelps, K. W., Baird, M. A., & Younkin, F. L. (2014). Advancing medical family therapy through qualitative, quantitative, and mixed-methods research. In J. Hodgson, A. Lamson, T. Mendenhall, & R. Crane (Eds.), *Medical family therapy: Advanced applications* (pp. 241–258). New York, NY: Springer.
Oldham, T., & Wright, N. (Producers), & Oldham, T. (Director). (2002). *The Smith Family* [Documentary]. Retrieved from http://www.thesmithfamilyfilm.com/home.html
Pargament, K. I. (1997). *The psychology of religion and coping: Theory, research, and practice*. New York, NY: The Guilford Press.

*Pargament, K. I. (2007). *Spiritually integrated psychotherapy: Understanding and addressing the sacred*. New York, NY: The Guilford Press.

Pargament, K. I., Feuille, M., & Burdzy, D. (2011). The Brief RCOPE: Current psychometric status of a short measure of religious coping. *Religions, 2*(1), 51–76. doi:10.3390/rel2010051.

Patterson, J., Hayworth, M., & Turner, C. (2000). Spiritual issues in family therapy: A graduate-level course. *Journal of Marital and Family Therapy, 26*(2), 199–210. doi:10.1111/j.1752-0606.2000.tb00289.x.

*Peek, C. J. (2008). Planning care in the clinical, operational, and financial worlds. In R. Kessler & D. Stafford (Eds.), *Collaborative medicine case studies: Evidence in practice* (pp. 25–38). New York, NY: Springer.

Phelps, K. W., Howell, C. D., Hill, S. G., Seemann, T. S., Lamson, A. L., Hodgson, J. L., & Smith, D. A. (2009). A collaborative model for patients with Type-2 diabetes. *Families, Systems, and Health, 27*(2), 131–140.

Post, S. G., Puchalski, C. M., & Larson, D. B. (2000). Physicians and patient spirituality: Professional boundaries, competency, and ethics. *Annals of Internal Medicine, 132*, 578–583.

Post, B., & Wade, N. (2009). Religion and spirituality in psychotherapy: A practice friendly review of research. *Journal of Clinical Psychology, 65*(2), 131–146. doi:10.1002/jclp.20563.

Prest, L. A., Russel, R., & D'Souza, H. (1999). Spirituality and religion in training, practice and personal development. *Journal of Family Therapy, 21*, 60–77. doi:10.1111/1467-6427.00104.

Puchalski, C. M., Lunsford, B., Harris, M. H., & Miller, R. T. (2006). Interdisciplinary spiritual care for seriously ill and dying patients: A collaborative model. *The Cancer Journal, 12*(5), 398–416.

Reiner, B. I. (2011). Transforming health care service delivery and provider selection. *Journal of Digital Imaging, 24*(3), 373–377.

Ribaudo, A., & Takahashi, M. (2008). Temporal trends in spirituality research: A meta-analysis of journal abstracts between 1944 and 2003. *Journal of Religion, Spirituality, and Aging, 20*, 16–28. doi:10.1080/15528030801921972.

Seybold, K. S., & Hill, P. C. (2001). The role of religion and spirituality in mental and physical health. *Current Directions in Psychological Science, 10*, 21–24.

Singelenberg, R. (1990). The blood transfusion taboo of Jehovah's Witnesses: Origin, development, and function of a controversial doctrine. *Social Science & Medicine, 31*(4), 515–523.

Smith, H. (2010, February 16). *The wisdom of faith with Huston Smith: A Bill Moyers special: Confucianism*. Retrieved from http://www.youtube.com/watch?v=SAy4ug6PMM8

*Sulmasy, D. P. (2002). A biopsychosocial-spiritual model for the care of patients at the end of life. *The Gerontologist, 42*, 24–33. doi:10.1093/geront/42.suppl_3.24.

Taylor, J., Hodgson, J., Lamson, A. L., Sira, N., & Musick, D. (in press). A systemic review of literature on hospital chaplaincy. *Journal of Pastoral Counseling*.

The Patient Protection and Affordable Care Act. (2010). *Public Law 111-148*. Washington, DC: United States Government Printing Office.

Thorensen, C. E. (1999). Spirituality and health: Is there a relationship? *Journal of Health Psychology, 4*, 291–300.

Thorensen, C. E., Harris, A. H., & Onan, D. (2001). Spirituality, religion, and health: Evidence, issues, and concerns. In T. G. Plante & A. C. Sherman (Eds.), *Faith and health: Psychological perspectives* (pp. 15–52). New York, NY: The Guilford Press.

Torosian, M., & Biddle, V. (2005). Spirituality and healing. *Seminars in Oncology, 32*(2), 232–236. doi:10.1053/j.seminoncol.2004.11.017.

*Tyndall, L. E., Hodgson, J. L., Lamson, A. L., White, M., & Knight, S. M. (2012). Medical family therapy: Charting a course in competencies. *Contemporary Family Therapy, 34*, 171–186. doi:10.1007/s10591-012-9191-9.

Underwood, L. G., & Teresi, J. A. (2002). The daily spiritual experience scale: Development, theoretical description, reliability, exploratory factor analysis, and preliminary construct validity using health-related data. *Annals of Behavioral Medicine, 24*(1), 22–33. doi:10.1207/S15324796ABM2401_04.

VandeCreek, L., & Burton, L. (2001). A white paper—Professional chaplaincy: Its role and importance in healthcare. *Journal of Pastoral Care, 55*(1), 81–97. Retrieved from http:www.jpcp.org/
VandeCreek, L., Pargament, K., Belavich, T., Cowell, B., & Friedel, L. (1999). The unique benefits of religious support during cardiac bypass surgery. *The Journal of Pastoral Care, 53*(1), 19–29.
*Walsh, F. (2009). *Spiritual resources in family therapy* (2nd ed.). New York, NY: The Guilford Press.
Walsh, F. (2010). Spiritual diversity: Multifaith perspectives in family therapy. *Family Process, 49*(3), 330–348. doi:10.1111/j.1545-5300.2010.01326.x.
Watson, W. L., Bell, J. M., & Wright, L. M. (1992). The medical map is not the territory: Or, "Medical Family Therapy?"—Watch your language. *Family Systems Medicine, 10*(1), 35–39. doi:10.1037/h0089250.
Weaver, A. J., Flannely, L. T., Strock, A. L., Krause, N., & Flannelly, K. J. (2005). The quantity and quality of research on religion and spirituality in four major gerontology journals between 1985 and 2002. *Research on Aging, 27*(2), 119–135. doi:10.1177/0164027504270476.
White, G. (2006). *Talking about spirituality in health care practice: A resource for the multi-professional health care team*. Philadelphia, PA: Jessica Kingsley.
*Wright, L. M., Watson, W. L., & Bell, J. M. (1996). *Beliefs: The heart of healing in families and illness*. New York, NY: Basic Books.

Part II
Research

Chapter 12
Medical Family Therapy Scientist-Practitioners

Lisa Zak-Hunter, Jerica Berge, Zephon Lister, Maureen Davey, Laura Lynch, and Wayne Denton

The scientist-practitioner model of training and practice highlights the interconnected relationships between clinical practice and research. As described by Crane and Hafen (2002), the term "scientist-practitioner" is used to describe behavioral health providers and training programs that both utilize and produce clinical research. The model highlights three interrelated roles: a consumer of new research, evaluator of one's own clinical skills, and researcher who reports original work and findings (Crane, Wampler, Seprenkle, Sandberg, & Hovestadt, 2002). Therefore, scientist-practitioners may provide treatment, evaluate clinical research, and conduct research or perform any combination of these. Ultimately, they are united in their understanding, appreciation, and drive to connect the worlds of research and clinical practice.

The model dates to the late 1940s when the field of Psychology moved to propose a new method of education which included graduate-level training in both clinical and research skills (Raimy, 1950). Since the inception, its feasibility has been debated. Critics contend the model cannot adequately train students in both skill sets. Advocates disagree and argue that not only is this type of training and practice possible, it is imperative in order to move forward both our knowledge base and clinical practice (Crane et al., 2002). The establishment, and indeed survivability, of a field rests in its ability to provide evidence of its effectiveness.

In order to firmly establish Medical Family Therapy (MedFT) as a distinct and respectable field, it has become increasingly vital that MedFT produce its own empirical evidence (Mendenhall, Pratt, Phelps, & Baird, 2012). The use of a MedFT scientist-practitioner model is an integral part of meeting this need. MedFTs are present in a variety of research, training, and practice institutions (e.g., family therapy or health care, academic or clinical, private or public sector). Each of these environments has differing degrees of support for the integration of research and clinical work. How a scientist-practitioner is defined, supported, and

L. Zak-Hunter (✉)
Via Christi Family Medicine Residency, Wichita, KS, USA
e-mail: lisa.zak-hunter@viachristi.org

J. Hodgson et al. (eds.), *Medical Family Therapy*, DOI 10.1007/978-3-319-03482-9_12,

practiced varies accordingly. On one hand, this allows for diversity and richness in clinical research questions and skills evaluation, research methodologies, and collaboration with other healthcare disciplines. However, this variation may cause confusion or uncertainty about what a MedFT scientist-practitioner is and how to implement this model.

To address these concerns, this chapter illustrates four different settings in which MedFT research and training occurs. The authors offer these descriptions to help clarify and define the MedFT scientist-practitioner. The research questions, methodologies, opportunities, and training are diverse. Collaborators span across Family Therapy, Family Medicine, Psychiatry, Nursing, and Pharmacy. We begin by describing the experiences of two scientist-practitioners positioned within different medical training sites. We follow this with an example of MedFT clinical research in academia. We conclude with the experiences of an author who has worked in both types of arenas. Each author describes the scientist-practitioner model in their setting and offers examples of research projects and outcomes. Lessons learned and skills sets found to be most valuable are put forth in conclusion.

Family Medicine

Jerica Berge, PhD, MPH, LMFT,CFLE, Department of Family Medicine & Community Health, University of Minnesota

Scientist-Practitioner

The University of Minnesota is a top-ten research institution; as such, there is an expectation that research and clinical care inform each other and be evidence-based. This expectation helps to facilitate the scientist-practitioner model that I—and my students—use. The students that I supervise are couples and family therapy (CFT) students in the Family Social Science Program at the University of Minnesota who are specializing in MedFT and family medicine residents at the University of Minnesota Medical School.

Our program is structured so that MedFTs have clinical, teaching, and research experiences simultaneously. The research expectation for MedFT students is similar to the expectations set for our family medicine residents. They are allowed to choose among three research-based experiences; these include (a) participating in quality improvement (QI) projects (e.g., diabetes, asthma, or chronic pain committees that address improving patient care and clinic efficiency), (b) engaging in community-based participatory research (CBPR) initiatives (e.g., childhood and adolescent obesity prevention interventions via partnering with local partners such as the YMCA and community members), or (c) conducting or collaborating with a faculty member in traditional research projects.

QI projects focus on improving the quality of patient care or clinic efficiency. To this end, students learn how to conduct literature reviews to examine evidence-based practices and conduct and measure small pilot projects in a clinic. This research experience is useful for students who are planning on working primarily in clinical settings once they graduate. With the CBPR option, students become involved with carrying out research in collaboration with community members and organizations. This approach focuses heavily on local change and sustainability of projects. MedFT students who take a strong interest in this research approach are commonly looking for future occupations that include elements of outreach or clinical leadership. The traditional research option includes working with a faculty member who is a principal investigator on a grant. The student learns how to write grant proposals, how to conceptualize and carry out a study, and how to present and get published. These skills are essential for students who are looking for future positions in academic research settings.

Regardless of the research option they choose, students learn how to conceptualize a strong study design, formulate scientific hypotheses, and answer important research questions. Additionally, as students participate in research opportunities that match their interests, they inform their own clinical practice as they learn how to interpret study findings, weigh out inconsistencies in the literature, and identify evidence-based practices to inform their clinical decision making. Furthermore, as the scientist-practitioner faculty member, I am able to engage in all three levels of research and practice ongoing. This allows me to continually evolve in my own clinical skills and research efforts. This bidirectional informing process greatly improves the quality and quantity of my work. I also learn from the MedFT students and family medicine residents as they ask questions that I have not thought of before, discuss concepts that cross both clinical and research domains, or as they grow from an experience that, at first, they thought would be impossible.

Project Outcomes

Research opportunities in our program have led to many positive clinical, teaching, and scientific outcomes. One example is the UMatter study. The main aim of UMatter is to test a group visit format for teenage girls to target obesity prevention. MedFT students and family medicine residents participate at differing levels. MedFT students either participate in the evaluation side of the study or the intervention delivery. MedFTs who are involved in the evaluation component of the study assist in the study design, help with data collection, and participate in the analysis and dissemination of results. Other students are involved with the intervention delivery, or clinical care aspect of the study. They assist with teaching the group sessions focused on healthy eating, physical activity, mental health wellness, and body image (Berge, Law, Johnson, & Wells, 2010; Neumark-Sztainer, Story, Hannan, & Rex, 2003; Neumark-Sztainer et al., 2000).

Results of the UMatter study to date indicate that after participating in the group sessions, the girls' intake of fruits and vegetables increases and their level of physical activity increases. They also reported high satisfaction with the group sessions (Berge, Neumark Sztainer, & Prasad, 2013). From a clinical perspective, residents and MedFTs reported satisfaction (via self-report survey and focus groups) with the group session format and expressed feeling that their adolescent patients took more personal responsibility related to their health goals, including their mental health wellness. Additionally, clinic flow was not interrupted by the group format, and it was noted that girls' attendance in the group sessions was higher than their attendance at their previous well child checkups.

Another research example in our program is the Interprofessional Care Research Project (Moon, Lounsberry, Berge, Wootten, Prasad, & Abbott, 2012). This project aims to use integrated care (MedFTs, family medicine residents, pharmacy residents, social workers, care coordinators, nurses) approaches within the clinic to create "best models of care" for patients and as a cutting-edge educational model to teach MedFTs and family medicine residents the benefits of multiple providers collaborating in patient care. Students are involved in the research in multiple ways. Some are directly involved with the evaluation of the project (e.g., patient and provider satisfaction surveys, quantitative data collection such as BMI or electronic medical records data collection) while others take a leading role in the delivery of the project (e.g., collaborative patient care visits with medical residents, MedFT students, pharmacists, and nurses). Additionally, all MedFT students and family practice residents are expected to improve patient care by using the interprofessional model in their practice. Thus, research, clinical care, and education objectives are all met. One successful example that resulted from our Interprofessional Care Research Project was with a morbidly obese, homebound, patient who had multiple chronic conditions including diabetes, high blood pressure, kidney disease, and major depression. The MedFT student, family medicine resident, PharmD resident, and care coordinator created an interprofessional care plan for this patient that addressed the patient's biopsychosocial-spiritual needs. They conducted two home visits as an interprofessional care team and included other family members in the visit to increase patient compliance with the care plan. After the home visits, the interprofessional care team continued to meet as a team to discuss the care plan and meet individually or as dyads or triads with the patient to address patient concerns/needs. This patient lost a significant amount of weight and was able to come to clinic appointments instead of being homebound.

Lessons Learned

There have been several key lessons learned in developing a scientist-practitioner model at the University of Minnesota. First, it is important to have strong partnerships between MD/DO, PharmD, Nursing, and PhD MedFT faculty regarding a research agenda. Having a shared commitment to the importance of research among faculty with different specialties helps to promote and prioritize research in the midst of a busy outpatient clinical setting. For example, in UMatter, a PhD MedFT faculty member and an MD faculty member lead the research project. In the Interprofessional Care Research project, there are several key core faculty including a PhD MedFT, an MD/DO, a PharmD, and a Social Work faculty member. Otherwise, when only one faculty from a single discipline heads the research project, it is difficult for the project to be far-reaching or sustainable across MedFT students, family medicine residents, faculty, nursing staff, administration, and patients. Second, finding specific ways to support research in a clinical setting is important. One way we have accomplished this in our program is through a monthly meeting called "the Percolator Meeting" where MedFTs, family medicine residents, and faculty come to discuss or "percolate on" their research ideas. Having a monthly forum to focus specifically on research ideas and to check-in regarding progress on research projects elevates the importance of research and its connection to clinical practice. Third, having readily available research opportunities is central to promoting excitement and inspiring passion for research in students and residents. This entails having faculty continuously involved in research projects themselves. Whether it is QI projects (e.g., diabetes, asthma, pain), CBPR initiatives, or traditional research, faculty in our program are all involved with some type of research opportunity so residents can easily get involved with research opportunities while observing the faculty being excited and committed to research.

Important Skills

Our program has found that there are some key skills necessary to promote a scientist-practitioner model in MedFT settings. First, faculty members must have both a desire/passion regarding research, their own research agenda, and skills to carry out a research agenda. Knowledgeable scientist-practitioner faculty show excitement and passion about research that informs patient care and vice versa. This enthusiasm becomes contagious to MedFT students and family medicine residents.

One way we have been successful in promoting this atmosphere is that several of our faculty have dual degrees, one in their original training such as MD, DO, or PhD, but also a secondary degree in Public Health (e.g., MPH). In fact, these faculty hold joint appointments in other departments such as Public Health, Family Social Science, or Psychology. Having these connections in other departments widens the variety of research opportunities and resources that are readily available to our MedFT students and family practice residents. Additionally, these connections allow for generating or infusing research ideas within students and faculty because we allow ourselves to be influenced by other researchers' expertise and ideas.

Second, having faculty that have been trained in research methodologies is useful in helping MedFT students and medical residents feel less overwhelmed with having to attend to both clinical and research responsibilities. Additionally, faculty who have diverse expertise in QI, CBPR, and traditional research methods help to bolster and validate different types of research skills. This allows for all faculty to be tapped regarding their expertise, with faculty with an expertise in all three areas being able to fill in across research types.

Finally, involving multiple players in the research opportunities at our program helps increase the clinic-wide focus on research. For example, in our QI projects, front desk staff, nursing staff, administration, family medicine residents, MedFT students, MedFT faculty, MD/DO faculty, and PharmD faculty are involved in the project. This allows for a more comprehensive or "systemic" approach to identifying an issue, carrying out the change identified, and increasing the likelihood that the change will be sustainable.

Overall, the scientist-practitioner model in our program at the University of Minnesota is well accepted and successful for training both MedFT students and family medicine residents. In part, this is due to the fact that the faculty in the program support and model the dual scientist-practitioner role to students and students are eager to learn the scientist-practitioner role themselves.

Zephon Lister, PhD, LMFT, Department of Family and Preventive Medicine, University of California, San Diego

Scientist-Practitioner

Our collaborative care program in the Department of Family and Preventive Medicine at the University of California, San Diego, consists of 3 licensed behavioral health providers (2 MedFTs and 1 Clinical Health Psychologist), 12 marriage and family therapists in training, and 2 psychiatrists. Our marriage and family therapist trainees/interns come through collaboration with the Marriage and Family Therapy program at the University of San Diego where students can focus a portion of their training in MedFT. Our collaborative care program is housed within the department's three family medicine clinics and provides medical and behavioral health services to over 35,000 patients. The Patient-Centered Medical Home (Rosenthal, 2008) is the service delivery model for the clinics. One component of this is an integrated-collaborative care model that provides behavioral health services to patients. In addition to the behavioral health clinicians, other providers include faculty physicians, residents, pharmacists, nurses, and integrative medicine specialists.

Our family medicine department has a partially supported research division that has focused on two primary areas: integrating mental/behavioral health services into primary care and improving clinical care. One example of the integration of behavioral health services into primary care was the implementation of universal depression screening into all of the family medicine clinics (Lister, Sieber, & Kallenberg, 2012). A project developed within this larger frame served to improve clinical care through group medical visits. Behavioral health providers, physicians, pharmacists, nurses, and health educators collaborated together to develop a program focused on improving self-management behaviors in patients living with chronic illness. The providers evaluated the translation of patient self-management research into real world conditions and the challenges encountered in this effort (Sieber, Newsome, Fiorella, & Mantilla, 2012).

The research division is headed by one of the behavioral health faculty and was set up to help providers with questions and projects of interest. Meetings are scheduled once a month, wherein providers have an opportunity to learn more about conducting practice-based research, develop or identify research questions, and gain support for or receive guidance on particular research projects. However, with the majority of providers often having less than 2 hours a week to commit to research activities and many having no protected time at all, it is often challenging for providers to have the time and resources to develop research questions and projects.

As a MedFT working in this setting, there have been opportunities both created and provided to develop and conduct practice-based research. Because of limited resources and time restraints, being a scientist-practitioner or MedFT-researcher in this setting has required the ability to be focused, collaborative, and practical. In order to do this successfully, we have concentrated efforts in two areas: (a) setting up systems for systematic data collection and (b) focusing on questions that naturally arise out of our clinical service.

One way we have set up a system for organized data collection takes advantage of our electronic health record system (EHR) and uses standardized instruments across clinics, such as the PHQ-9. For example, although patient information is managed via EHR, the system is primarily designed for clinical practice. It is often not configured or captured in a way to easily extract information or conduct practice-based research. Therefore, we developed tools within the EHR that allowed us to better capture and track information that make data retrieval and analysis easier for future projects. For example, a form was created to collect and track patient PHQ-9 scores. Once this data was entered, scores could be tracked over time and compared with other clinical variables (HbA1c, clinic visits, medications, etc.)

A second effort has gone to support research questions that naturally arise out of clinical service. We have realized that questions always evolve from care. So during our monthly research meetings, providers often raise questions directly based on their experiences in patient care. For example, one provider asked "Because we know that mental health and psychosocial variables significantly influence patients' ability to follow through on treatment recommendations, what are ways we can better identify these variables within our clinic population?" Another question raised by providers was "What are ways we can improve the self-management behaviors of patients living with chronic illness?"

Project Outcomes

Our department has engaged in and collaborated on several projects in the past few years that have focused on integrating mental/behavioral health services into primary care and improving clinical care. We have learned useful lessons and insights from each of our projects. Here, I will focus on our universal depression screening program and diabetes management coaching study to illustrate the success and benefits of translational clinical research, the challenges and barriers experienced in this process, and the steps to address them.

Driven by both the 2011 National Committee on Quality Assurance (NCQA) PCMH standards and the 2009 US Preventive Services Task Force (USPSTF) recommendations for depression screening (NCQA, 2011; USPSTF, 2009), we developed and implemented an EHR-based office visit screening system for depression using the PHQ-2 and PHQ-9 on all patients. Those who screened positive on the PHQ-2 completed a PHQ-9. A score greater than 9 triggered an evidence-based depression management protocol, and a score greater than 15 prompted an assessment and follow-up by a MedFT prior to their encounter with the PCP. After the assessment, the MedFT and PCP would collaborate on a treatment plan to address the patient's depressive symptoms. In addition to the clinical utility of the EHR-based screening system, we have used the data from PHQ-9 scores to identify and address other clinical research questions. For example, it was found that patients with multiple medical comorbidities were screened least often, yet had the highest positive screen rates, and more often scored above 10 on the PHQ-9 ($p < 0.05$) (Lister et al., 2013). This finding led us to question how we could better identify these individuals as they came into the clinic and how to develop and evaluate ways to assist these patients in both their behavioral health symptoms and health behavior practices. This is the focus of a MedFT coaching model currently in development. Findings such as these can also provide the data for clinical improvement projects.

Our type 2 diabetes decision aid coaching study arose from physician frustration over patients with poor disease management and low adherence to treatment recommendations. We wanted to know how these patients could be better engaged in order to increase self-management behaviors. Twenty-two physicians were randomly assigned across our three family medicine clinics to either provide usual care or work with a MedFT who served as an outreach health coach for their patients with diabetes. Each MedFT health coach met with each physician in the intervention group to identify the patients most in need of intervention, then MedFTs sent these identified patients a video on diabetes management, called to encourage video viewing, and discussed any patient-perceived barriers to self-management. Initial markers of patient activation in self-management, patients' video-viewing behavior, and healthcare encounters in the subsequent 6 months were compared between groups. Results showed that patients targeted by a MedFT health coach were more likely to view the video, be seen by their primary care physician (PCP) within 6 months, and have disease-relevant laboratory tests performed than patients receiving usual care from their PCP (Sieber, Newsome, & Lillie, 2012). Findings from this study are now being taken, adapted, and expanded to address patients with depression, anxiety, obesity, hypertension, and dyslipidemia with the goals of increasing PCP and patient engagement as well as strengthening the collaborative team around the patient to support better health outcomes. Additionally, this new project has been expanded to include other health behavior researchers in the university with the goal of obtaining NIH funding for further research.

Lessons Learned

Before developing a research question or designing a study, it was important to identify and utilize existing evidence-based approaches. In our program there is an ongoing effort to stay current on evidence-based practices through administrative updates, journal clubs, clinic service meetings, and personal initiative. As mentioned, for the scientist-practitioner in an environment with limited research support, we have found that it is important to be focused, collaborative, and practical. This is best done by focusing on questions that naturally arise during patient care and that have immediate relevance and application to a specific clinical population. Focusing on these types of questions increases the likelihood of support and implementation of study findings into clinic practice once the research is completed.

One of the most important lessons we have learned in conducting practice-based research in our environment is to start with the end in mind. This means setting up the systems and protocols that will be needed to effectively provide the information needed for future projects. For example, when our EHR system was first installed, we encountered a situation where data that we had been collecting for a couple years could not be extracted because of how it was formatted. This experience has informed all of our later projects making sure that any information that we hoped to use was entered into the system in a format that could be extractable for future use. Clinically, we also explored the best ways to record encounters in the EHR to allow easy collaboration and tracking between behavioral health and medical providers and access to behavioral health patient data that is relevant to medical care.

Another lesson has been the benefit of developing collaborative opportunities with others of the same interest both in and outside of the department. Effective collaboration can often reduce some of the already limited time and resources of many scientist-practitioners. Some providers in our clinics have been able to collaborate with other researchers with existing projects and use the funding from these projects to get more protected time to do research.

Finally, it is important to receive funding to support research and provide more protected time. Although in our case the data are available, there is still a significant amount of time and resources needed for data management and analysis, interpretation, and writing up results. Searching for funding can be extremely time consuming, however, and often has a low yield for many scientist-practitioners who spend significant time on patient care. It is important to find a balance between looking for funding that fits into current projects and spending a lot of time shaping programs to fit funding opportunities. This is one area where active collaboration with others can provide the support and resources needed to develop a competitive proposal.

Important Skills

Skills we have found useful to be an effective MedFT scientist-practitioner in an environment that can only provide limited to moderate research support include (a) staying current on evidence-based practices and research, (b) managing resources, and (c) interdisciplinary collaboration. While many of the questions that have guided our research projects have come from issues related to our day-to-day clinical practice, it has been equally important that we keep up to date on relevant clinical research to ensure that the questions we are asking and researching have not already been addressed. With limited resources, it is important not to overextend what means are available. Ways to do this include asking answerable questions, garnering provider support, and maximizing the systems already in place. For example, in our clinics, pre-visit questionnaires are already given to every patient. Adding the PHQ-2 to this already existing process allowed us to enhance our clinical service while not significantly impacting the current workflow of the medical staff. A third set of skills that are often overlooked are interdisciplinary collaboration skills. As mentioned, one of the ongoing challenges for scientist-practitioners is achieving the balance between being both a scientist and a practitioner. Learning to effectively collaborate can ease some of the tension between these roles. Skills important for effective collaboration include having the ability to conceptualize and respect multiple view points, identify and utilize strengths of various disciplines, and have a systemic orientation to patient care. These important skills reinforce and illustrate how the systemic training of MedFT can play an essential role in effective collaboration as a scientist-practitioner.

Academia

Maureen Davey, Ph.D., LMFT and Laura Lynch, M.S., Department of Couple and Family Therapy, Drexel University

Scientist-Practitioner

Clinical research in our academic setting is being conducted in a Department of Couple and Family Therapy (CFT) that includes accredited Marriage and Family Therapy and Post-Masters programs and a CFT PhD program, which is housed within a College of Nursing and Health Professions at Drexel University. Our department's current goal is to implement the scientist-practitioner model by more tightly integrating our research and clinical training (Davey, Davey, Tubbs, Savla, & Anderson, 2012; Hodgson, Johnson, Ketring, Wampler, & Lamson, 2005). We have had the privilege of partnering and placing our students in many clinics in the community (e.g., oncology, HIV, primary care clinics) that serve diverse patient populations. We are committed to finding effective ways to increase culturally sensitive and interdisciplinary collaborative care. CFT graduate students and nursing faculty in our college regularly collaborate on projects focused on developing and evaluating MedFT intervention programs. In order to illustrate the scientist-practitioner model in our academic setting, we describe two recently completed clinical research studies that were conducted in a nurse-managed primary care interdisciplinary clinic (the Center) that serves a low-income minority patient population.

The Center was founded as a community partnership with residents from four public housing developments in North Philadelphia. Approximately 80 % of the patient population is African American and most are not married; 64 % are covered by Medicaid and nearly 20 % are uninsured. The Center anchors the revitalization of a community once considered an example of urban decay. The Center's director is dedicated to reviewing its program and clinical outcomes and developing innovative approaches to care. Therefore, staff are used to working in an environment of continuous quality improvement based on clinical research. This made our partnership and conducting the two clinical research studies acceptable and feasible. The Center had the following colocated interdisciplinary clinical services in place when the two studies were conducted from 2009 to 2010: (a) outpatient behavioral health department, (b) primary care department with two primary behavioral health therapists who are embedded in primary care (one pediatric behavior health therapist and one adult behavioral therapist), (c) part-time couple and family therapist who did trauma-informed family therapy (1 day a week, at the time of the two studies), and (d) creative arts therapies (art, music, movement, yoga). A nursing colleague contacted our department to collaboratively develop and work on two MedFT projects at the Center because of our shared focus on biopsychosocial approaches to care that more holistically treat patients at the Center. Together we planned and evaluated outcomes from two clinical studies that focus on collaboration at the Center and how childhood trauma affects adult health outcomes which are described below.

Project Outcomes

Our team, which included CFT doctoral students interested in MedFT, nursing faculty, and CFT faculty, first conducted a qualitative focus group (FG) study in 2009 to describe the Center's mental and physical healthcare team's collaboration (Bruner, Davey, & Waite, 2011; Bruner, Waite, & Davey, 2011). Thirty-nine providers out of 57 total staff participated in six different FGs. Content analysis revealed facilitators (communication systems, provider interactions, patient factors, structural/building issues, shared vision) and barriers to collaboration between the multidisciplinary staff at the Center (patient factors, provider interactions, volume of work, structural/building issues), provider demographics (patient treatment, demographics, provider overload, provider roles), patient demographic characteristics (cultural factors, underprivileged) that affect collaboration, and providers' perceptions of family and community involvement in patient care (patient centered, referrals, family as a tool). Staff described a more patient-centered approach to care at the Center, with serendipitous family and community involvement, an area of future growth. When patients at the Center asked, then staff reached out to family members to support patient outcomes and treatment adherence. However, this was not described as an intentional approach to care (which is the philosophy of MedFT). The director of the Center appreciated these findings and agrees that this is an area of future growth.

A second area of growth at the Center is the development of ongoing, cultural sensitivity training for staff while also hiring more providers who match the ethnic and racial minority patients that the Center currently serves. After we shared the project outcomes with upper administration and with all staff at their monthly meeting, the clinical director at the Center began taking active steps to address many of the potential areas for growth. For example, land adjacent to the Center was secured which will allow the Center to expand its current services and address many of the space and provider proximity issues. Noteworthy, the director is now collaborating with the CFT department to develop a MedFT clinical space (five clinical offices and administrative support) and is working towards becoming more family centered. Additionally, the director is now hiring more minority providers.

The second clinical research initiative was a replication of the Adverse Childhood Experiences (ACES) Centers for Disease Control and Prevention (CDC) study with a sample of the Center's low-income adult minority primary care patients ($n = 801$). A cross-sectional, retrospective, quantitative survey was conducted to examine the association between Center patients' reports of past childhood trauma and their current healthcare outcomes (Lynch, Waite, & Davey, 2013; Waite, Davey, & Lynch, 2013). Results suggested that the number of ACES in the Center's sample of adult patients were considerably higher than the original CDC ACES study, as almost 50 % of patients surveyed at the Center reported four or more ACEs, confirming that trauma is central in this urban primary care setting. The results of the cumulative ACEs score suggested that participants who cumulatively reported experiencing more childhood trauma were more likely to be diagnosed with type 2 diabetes in adulthood (Lynch et al., 2013) and to report poorer self-rated health in adulthood (Waite et al., 2013). Outcomes from our ACES replication study presented a convincing justification for a dramatic change in the delivery of primary care at the Center. Based on our findings, interventions to treat traumatized and ill patients at the Center are now being implemented by all staff including MedFTs, who are running trauma and mindfulness meditation support groups. For example, the Sanctuary Institute, which is a collaborative effort of Andrus Children's Center and Dr. Sandra L. Bloom, is now working with all staff at the Center. The primary mission of the Sanctuary Institute is to help organizations implement a trauma-informed, whole-system organizational approach known as the Sanctuary Model (Panzer & Bloom, 2003). All staff are now being trained in the Sanctuary Model and, after 3 years, will receive certification in this well-respected trauma-informed model. Using the scientist-practitioner approach, this ACES replication study helped the Center better understand the needs of the community and, based on the findings, begin to use more trauma-informed and systemic approaches to care.

Lessons Learned

We learned several lessons in the study that explored providers' perceptions of collaborative care (Bruner, Davey, et al., 2011; Bruner, Waite, et al., 2011). The first is that it is important to consider and address the existing power dynamics and privilege in the system in which clinical research is being conducted, as well as to examine one's own areas of power and privilege. These dynamics will inevitably impact the research and clinical processes. For example, many support staff who were racial minorities did not openly share their opinions during the focus groups and were quiet compared to other providers at the Center.

Second, it is important to ensure the "buy-in" of participants in which the research is being conducted. If providers do not appreciate the value of conducting a clinical research study, then they are less likely to participate. For example "several of the groups arrived substantially late to the FGs, which may have been a feasibility issue or may have indicated their level of investment in the process" (Bruner, Davey, et al., 2011, p. 168). Clinical researchers need to remember to partner with administrators or champions who can advocate for a clinical research initiative and with staff at all levels in order to communicate how it will directly benefit the patients they serve.

Third, researchers should consider the unique barriers faced by the populations they are studying. In this study, for example, providers' busy schedules (because of their heavy caseloads) compromised their ability to make it to focus groups on time, as well as our ability to follow-up with them (Bruner, Davey, et al., 2011). These types of barriers can affect the feasibility and acceptability of a study. If these barriers are identified earlier in the research process, clinical researchers can plan how to overcome them.

We also learned important lessons after conducting the ACES replication study at the Center (Lynch et al., 2013; Waite et al., 2013). First, we learned that secondary clinical data has limitations. In this study (Lynch et al., 2013), participants' type 2 diabetes diagnoses were determined by using ICD-9 codes that were retrieved from their clinical charts. The ICD-9 codes in the clinical charts indicated that patients at the Center had the diagnosis. However, we were unable to determine how well participants managed their type 2 diabetes, which would have been an interesting outcome to study. Second, we learned the importance of using multiple sources for data collection whenever possible. For example, in the ACES replication study, "licensed healthcare providers did not confirm participants' self-rated overall health with clinical evaluations" (Waite et al., 2013, p. 7). Future studies should include data that can be triangulated by combining self-report data with family member report or observations by clinical providers. MedFTs will continue to collaborate with the Center to include more systemic approaches to clinical research and to help them develop culturally sensitive family-centered approaches to care.

Important Skills

A variety of skills are needed to be an effective MedFT scientist-practitioner. Just as collaboration with the patient and other providers is essential to the practice of MedFT (Bischoff, Springer, Felix, & Hollist, 2011), collaboration is also important for conducting clinical research. It is important to effectively communicate with key stakeholders (e.g., clinical directors, providers, and patients) in order to manage any ongoing miscommunications or procedural issues that emerge. For example, both studies described in this segment (Bruner, Davey, et al. 2011; Bruner, Waite, et al., 2011; Lynch et al., 2013; Waite et al., 2013) were conducted in collaboration with clinical researchers in our Department of Couple and Family Therapy and in the Nursing Department within our college. We first contacted and met several times with a nursing colleague, and then, with her help, we met with the clinical director at the Center. If research is conducted in an academic setting, partnering with researchers from other departments and doing team science will bring additional skills and expertise to the research study. If the clinical research study is being conducted in a primary care medical setting, like the Center, meeting with the upper administration is essential for gaining access to and better understand the unique features of that site. We first partnered with the director of the Center who was then able to champion and be an advocate for our two studies. Additionally, we gave back to the Center by sharing our findings with the upper administration and with providers in order to transform and improve the current services being provided at the Center.

A MedFT scientist-practitioner needs to be flexible, sensitive to the needs of the community or clinic, adaptive, and have problem-solving skills because at any point during a clinical research study, obstacles will emerge that need to be overcome (e.g., buy-in from staff to participate in the study, logistics of scheduling, etc.). It is also important to note that when conducting research studies in clinical settings (effectiveness research), it is more difficult to control the research environment compared to conducting research in more controlled settings (e.g., efficacy trials). For example, in the collaboration study, providers had very busy schedules that affected their availability to participate in our focus group.

Finally, a scientist-practitioner needs to have excellent grant-writing skills in order to fund his or her clinical research. The first focus group study was supported by internal pilot funding from the Center's director and the second study was supported by a private foundation. Although the two projects are now completed, the Center's director, in collaboration with CFT faculty, has been applying for foundation funding to incorporate the lessons learned into the clinic. Future clinical research initiatives are actively being discussed by regularly meeting and seeking joint funding that support culturally sensitive and trauma-informed family-centered approaches to care. Research funding has become very competitive, and more universities expect their faculty to obtain external funding to support their programs of research. Grant writing requires the ability to propose one's idea in a convincing manner that effectively describes the significance and innovation of the project. There are many sources of grant funding, for example, internal university seed grants, private foundation grants, and the most competitive, federal grants (e.g., R03, R21, R01). Scientist-practitioners can take classes on grant writing to develop their grant-writing skills, but perhaps the best way to learn is by partnering with senior-funded clinical researchers and being mentored to do team science that can advance the MedFT field (e.g., cost-effectiveness and clinical outcome research).

Wayne Denton, MD, PhD, Marriage and Family Therapy Program, Florida State University

Scientist-Practitioner

To provide context, I was on the faculty of medical schools for 20 years in departments of psychiatry and am now on the faculty of the Marriage and Family Therapy (MFT) doctoral program at Florida State University. Most of my experience has been in the specialty mental health sector, although I am now doing research in a primary care medical clinic.

To do research in an academic medical center, it is useful to have some understanding of the differences between being on the faculty of a medical school and being on the faculty of a graduate school. The term "scientist-practitioner" is generally not used in medical schools. Rather, faculty are divided between "basic scientists" and "clinical scientists." To describe the difference simplistically, basic scientists study animals or cells in Petri dishes whereas clinical scientists study whole patients. While it is possible to be on the faculty of a graduate MFT program without being a scientist-practitioner, in medical schools, most faculty will consider themselves as clinical scientists. Thus, the scientist-practitioner discussion, as it exists in Psychology and MFT, is not one that I found to exist in medical schools. The discussion is more about boosting the research skills of clinical faculty. Whereas in a PhD program, the faculty may primarily be researchers who are being encouraged to apply their skills to clinical problems, in a medical school the faculty are primarily clinicians who are being encouraged to learn research skills that they can apply to the problems they are treating.

Overall, there is a tradition in academic medicine of combining research and clinical practice. I heard someone say once that "every patient should be enrolled in a protocol." That is, every patient should also be a research participant. While this goal is never completely reached even in the most academic of medical centers, it indicates that there is *generally* openness to research being conducted in academic medical centers. Traditionally, medical school faculty will build their careers by collecting data in their clinical work. A good example of how a successful career was built in this way can be found in Reifler (1992).

Currently, our MedFT research team is doing research in a community primary care medical clinic that is not part of an academic medical center and, thus, research is not part of their core mission. In fact, research participation could potentially be seen as a burden to their patients. We have addressed this in several ways. The first is that we became seen as valuable colleagues who "give" to the clinic and do not just "take." In meeting with the clinic leadership, I learned that they had a great need for behavioral health providers, and this became the avenue for joining them. I provided clinical service, and our doctoral students provided services as an internship in the clinic. The clinical services we provide have been appreciated and, I believe, facilitated an openness to research participation. The second approach was not so much intentional as it was a natural offshoot of doing clinical research. That is, our research projects themselves have been seen as somewhat valuable to the clinic. For example, MedFT students and I did a needs assessment study that addressed questions of interest to the clinic leadership. Subsequently, we have been doing research that provides treatment, and this was seen as making a positive contribution for the patients. Lastly, I am writing our community partner into the budget of research grant applications. Funds can be included to rent space for study staff, pay a portion of clinic staff salaries for the time they spend assisting us, etc. If we receive external research funding, our community partner clinic would receive a financial benefit from their collaboration with us.

Project Outcomes

In my first faculty position at the Wake Forest University School of Medicine, I was director of both an MFT clinic and an adult general Psychiatry clinic. Both clinics were training sites for psychiatry residents and other trainees, including MedFT graduate student interns. One of the challenges of doing research in a clinical setting is obtaining permission from the clinic leadership. Being the director of the clinics allowed me to bypass this step. We conducted a randomized trial of couple therapy in our MFT clinic by enrolling couples presenting for treatment without the need for any study advertising (Denton, Burleson, Clark, Rodriguez, & Hobbs, 2000). The therapists were residents in psychiatry receiving training in couple therapy. In the MFT clinic, we also did a study of supervision methods (Denton, Nakonezny, & Burwell, 2011) and included our MedFT trainees in evaluating a method of family assessment (Denton, Nakonezny, & Burwell, 2010). We did a "chart review" study in the general psychiatry clinic evaluating the role of marital status in the expenditures the patients accrued at the medical center (Denton, Reynolds, Burleson, & Anderson, 1999). Again, we did not advertise to recruit any of these research participants—they were patients who had self-referred for treatment.

In the medical clinic, where my MedFT students and I are presently working, we began by conducting a needs assessment. We surveyed clinic patients to assess their levels of depression, anxiety, substance use, couple and family discord, and other relevant clinical conditions. We found high levels of these problems among the patients and many patients were experiencing more than one of them. This led to the clinic administration instituting screening for depression and other behavioral health problems among all of their patients. There have also been other outcomes that have benefited our doctoral students including a national presentation (Woods, Priest, Fish, & Denton, 2012), a dissertation (Woods, 2012), and several publications in preparation or under review with student coauthors.

Lessons Learned

I believe the distinction between basic and clinical science can be applied to the study of families. Doctoral level MedFTs should be our "clinical scientists" deriving their research questions, at least in part, from their clinical (or supervisory) experiences. For example, if we add couple therapy, will people recover from depression more completely? Does it make a difference if the patients meet the people behind the mirror? Are communication avoiders experiencing more activation of their sympathetic nervous system? The clinician has access to data (i.e., from interaction with patients/clients) that the non-clinician does not. Developing a research question that will move the field forward is the most *important* part of study design. MedFT clinical scientists have the chance to use their creativity in their clinical experience to develop research questions that are interesting and important.

One of the most difficult parts of clinical research is recruiting the sample. Being a "director" of anything is going to take time away from your research. If it is a clinical assignment, can you get double duty by also using it for your research purposes? If you do not have your own patients to recruit from, you may have to use advertising which is less likely to attract people with significant clinical problems. Another alternative is to try and enlist the cooperation of clinical sites that are seeing the people you would like to include in your studies. This has to begin with enlisting the cooperation and support of key leaders in the organization. While they might be motivated by altruism to help you, do not count on it! Consider what you have to offer that could help them. If the key leaders are also in academia, they might be motivated by becoming a collaborator in your research and eventually participating in the writing of manuscripts for publication. Perhaps you can offer a service the clinic needs or can include them in the budget for a research grant. As addressed below, once you obtain the endorsement of the key leaders, you will then have to gain the support of clinicians and support staff actually working in the clinic on a day-to-day basis.

Important Skills

To be a successful MedFT clinical scientist, you must have mastery of the literature in your field combined with an ability to "read the tea leaves" about where the field is heading to develop research questions that will move the field forward. Then, you must have the networking skills to establish relationships with the key people whose support you will need to carry out the research. Strong social skills will be required to motivate clinic staff (and perhaps others) to cooperate with the needs of the study when there is no direct benefit to them from doing so. You will need to be able to assemble the team of your study staff and be able to keep the team intact until the study is completed while maintaining good relations with your community partner. The actual carrying out of the study may be where you are least needed! That is, with larger funded studies, you may hire someone to be a project manager and actually oversee implementation of the protocol. Of course, you may run the study yourself. In this case, you will need good organizational skills. With or without a project manager, you will need to ensure that the study is running smoothly, maintain the relationships necessary to see the project through to completion, and set the stage for your next study.

For funding research beyond the "pilot study" stage, grant-writing skills are both important and essential. The greatest expenses in MedFT research will be for people's time. If you are doing intervention research, it is most desirable to utilize therapists in your study who match the requirements that would be expected to deliver the intervention in the community. This usually means therapists who have completed their education and are licensed. This may also give your intervention a more fair evaluation than the use of volunteer student therapists. For the time required for a substantial study, you will need to be able to pay your therapists either a salary or by the hour. A larger study will also require more time for yourself and your co-investigators. Therefore, you may need funds to "buy out" time to release yourself and other key personnel from teaching and/or other duties. Additionally, payments to participants should be a fair compensation for participation time and greatly increase completion rates. Such payments are also expensive and can be included in grant budgets. Many resources are now available to help with grant-writing skills. University research offices are able to point investigators in the right direction if they need help in burnishing these skills.

Conclusion

These four models of MedFT scientist-practitioners demonstrate a variety of possible avenues for integrating research and practice. They offer valuable insights for conducting clinical research and articulate skills needed to be a successful scientist-practitioner. In doing so, they clarify how the field of MedFT can adopt its own way of producing clinical research and clinicians capable of utilizing this research to inform their practice. As discussed by our panelists, MedFT scientist-practitioners should be mindful of the following: developing a culture of research in clinical settings will require persistence, diligence, and collaboration; when conducting research, be attentive to the study population, setting-recruitment issues, and power dynamics; and identify potential collaborators and clearly articulate how the partnership can benefit them. Secondly, MedFT clinical researchers must adopt certain skills. The successful MedFT scientist-practitioner is flexible and adaptive; has strong research, methodology, and writing skills; understands how to evaluate and implement evidence-based practices; and can assemble and work in a multidisciplinary team.

Historically, MedFT practitioners and trainees have faced barriers in successfully implementing a scientist-practitioner model. Some of these include an unclear definition of what constitutes MedFT research and practice (Linville, Hertlein, & Prouty Lyness, 2007), lack of research support, inconsistent MedFT training curriculum (Tyndall, Hodgson, Lamson, White, & Knight, 2012), and a small number of leading MedFT researchers. The inconsistencies in defining MedFT research causes confusion over who conducts MedFT research and in identifying the leaders.

In order for MedFTs to adopt a scientist-practitioner model, they must actively address these concerns. Recently, the field has begun to do so. For example, Mendenhall, Pratt, Phelps, Baird, and Younkin (2014) outline a MedFT research agenda, provide a definition of MedFT research, and offer a lexicon to unite MedFT investigators in Chap. 13 of this book. They emphasize the need for MedFTs to address the clinical, operational, and financial worlds of health care. Earlier in 2003, Campbell outlined nine areas for MedFT intervention research, which also remains a relevant guide. Others have begun charting core competencies and training requirements to ensure a degree of standardization (Tyndall et al., 2012). They emphasize the need for strong clinical, research, and collaborative skills. Clinically, MedFTs are expected to have a strong working knowledge of social science and health-related literature (e.g., families and illness, physiology, pharmacology). Regarding research, MedFTs should be well versed in various methodologies (quantitative, qualitative, collaborative care) and advanced statistics. They are expected to both evaluate and design research and interventions from a biopsychosocial-spiritual perspective (Tyndall et al., 2012).

The establishment of MedFT as a unique and valuable part of our healthcare system relies on its ability to define itself, its research, and its interventions. Researchers and clinicians must not become complacent in their separate worlds. Instead, they must unite. Those who are primarily researchers need to understand the intricacies of clinical practice to produce meaningful translational work. Clinicians need to be active consumers and critics of research, implement evidence-based practices, and evaluate their own clinical skills. Our hope is that the examples put forth in this chapter make the path to establishing a MedFT scientist-practitioner model more clear and feasible.

Discussion Questions

1. What barriers or challenges do you encounter in creating or sustaining a scientist-practitioner model in your current workplace context? How can you overcome them?
2. What value would (or does) clinical research bring to your setting?
3. Take a moment to reflect on a research or quality improvement project that you are interested in doing (in your own clinic or with a community partner).
   (a) Explain the relevancy of this project to clinical care.
   (b) Identify all parties you would need buy-in from, and how you would approach them.
   (c) Does the study need funding? If so, what are potential funding sources?
4. What does it mean to be an active consumer and critic of research?
5. It is not uncommon for clinicians or researchers to become "silo-ed." That is, they may experience cutoff and isolation from other MedFTs, evidence-based research, and/or clinical practice. Identify scenarios and circumstances under which a MedFT may become silo-ed, the dangers this presents for a MedFT scientist-practitioner model, and ways this problem can be addressed.

References[1]

*Berge, J. M., Law, D. D., Johnson, J., & Wells, M. G. (2010). Effectiveness of a psycho-educational parenting group on child, parent, and family behavior: A pilot study in a family practice clinic with an underserved population. *Families, Systems & Health, 28*, 224–235. doi:10.1037/a0020907.

Berge, J. M., Neumark-Sztainer, D., & Prasad, S. (2013). *UMatter girls group: Healthy weight management in diverse youth using a health care home approach healthy foods*, Healthy Lives Institute [AM1]. Grant proposal to the National Institutes of Health.

Bischoff, R. J., Springer, P. R., Felix, D. S., & Hollist, C. S. (2011). Finding the heart of medical family therapy: A content analysis of medical family therapy casebook articles. *Families, Systems & Health, 29*, 184. doi:10.1037/a002463.

*Bruner, P., Davey, M., & Waite, R. (2011). Culturally sensitive collaborative care models: Exploration of a community based health center. *Families, Systems & Health, 29*, 155–170. doi:10.1037/a0025025.

Bruner, P., Waite, R., & Davey, M. (2011). Collaboration: Strategies for improving patient and population health outcomes. *International Journal of Integrated Care, 11*, 1–11. URN:NBN: NL:UI:10-1-101570/ijic2011-123

*Campbell, T. (2003). The effectiveness of family intervention for physical disorders. *Journal of Marital and Family Therapy, 29*, 263–281. doi:10.1111/j.1752-0606.2003.tb01204x.

Crane, D. R., & Hafen, M. (2002). Meeting the needs of evidence-based practice in family therapy: Developing the scientist-practitioner model. *Journal of Family Therapy, 24*, 113–124. doi:10.1111/1467-6427.00206.

Crane, D. R., Wampler, K. S., Sprenkle, D. H., Sandberg, J. G., & Hovestadt, A. J. (2002). The scientist-practitioner model in marriage and family therapy doctoral programs: Current status. *Journal of Marital and Family Therapy, 28*, 75–83. doi:10.1111/j.1752-0606.2002.tb01175.x.

Davey, M., Davey, A., Tubbs, C., Savla, T., & Anderson, S. (2012). Second order change and evidenced based practice. *Journal of Family Therapy, 34*, 72–90. doi:10.1111/j.1467-6427.2010.00499.x.

Denton, W. H., Burleson, B. R., Clark, T. E., Rodriguez, C. P., & Hobbs, B. V. (2000). A randomized trial of emotion-focused therapy for couples in a training clinic. *Journal of Marital and Family Therapy, 26*, 65–78. doi:10.1111/j.1752-0606.2000.tb00277.x.

Denton, W. H., Nakonezny, P. A., & Burwell, S. R. (2010). Reliability and validity of the global assessment of relational functioning (GARF) in a psychiatric family therapy clinic. *Journal of Marital and Family Therapy, 36*, 376–387. doi:10.1111/j.1752-0606.2009.00144.x.

Denton, W. H., Nakonezny, P. A., & Burwell, S. R. (2011). The effects of meeting a family therapy supervision team on client satisfaction in an initial session. *Journal of Family Therapy, 33*, 85–97. doi:10.1111/j.1467-6427.2010.00518.x.

Denton, W. H., Reynolds, D. L., Burleson, B. R., & Anderson, R. T. (1999). The role of marital status in health services expenditures for psychiatric outpatients. *Journal of Marital and Family Therapy, 25*, 383–392. doi:10.1111/j.1752-0606.1999.tb00255.x.

*Hodgson, J., Johnson, L. N., Ketring, S. A., Wampler, R. S., & Lamson, A. L. (2005). Integrating research and clinical training in marriage and family therapy training programs. *Journal of Marital and Family Therapy, 31*, 75–88. doi:10.1111/j.1752-0606.2005.tb01544.x.

*Linville, D., Hertlein, K. M., & Prouty Lyness, A. M. (2007). Medical family therapy: Reflecting on the necessity of collaborative healthcare research. *Families, Systems & Health, 25*, 85–97. doi:10.1037/1091-7527.25.1.85.

Lister, Z. D., Sieber, W. J., Ikeda, T., Lindeman, K., Morn, C., Johnson, J. L., … Fennessey, B. (2013, November). *Screening for depression in a patient centered medical home: PDSA*

[1] An asterisk has been use to note references that the chapter authors recommend for further reading.

cycles and beyond. Workshop presented at Society of Teachers of Family Medicine (STFM) Conference, San Diego, CA.

Lister, Z. D., Sieber, W. J., & Kallenberg, G. (2012, October). *Building the behaviorally enhanced PCMH: The development and implementation of an EHR-based system for the screening and management of depression in primary care*. Workshop presented at the annual meeting of the Collaborative Family Healthcare Association, Austin, TX.

Lynch, L., Waite, R., & Davey, M. (2013). Adverse childhood experiences and diabetes mellitus in adulthood: Support for a collaborative approach to care. *Contemporary Family Therapy, 35*, 639–655.

*Mendenhall, T. J., Pratt, K. J., Phelps, K. W., & Baird, M. A. (2012). Advancing medical family therapy through research: A consideration of qualitative, quantitative, and mixed-methods designs. *Contemporary Family Therapy, 34*, 187–203. doi:10.1007/s10591-012-9186-6.

Mendenhall, T. J., Pratt, K. J., Phelps, K. W., Baird, M. A., & Younkin, F. L. (2014). Advancing medical family therapy through qualitative, quantitative, and mixed-methods research. In J. Hodgson, A. Lamson, T. Mendenhall, & R. Crane (Eds.), *Medical family therapy: Advanced applications* (pp. 241–258). New York, NY: Springer.

Moon, J., Lounsberry, J., Berge, J., Wootten, M., Prasad, S., & Abbott, G. (2012). *Interprofessional care plan in primary care using an interdisciplinary team*. Academic Health Center. Minneapolis, MN: University of Minnesota.

National Committee for Quality Assurance (NCQA). (2011, March 28). Standards and guidelines for NCQA's patient-centered medical home (PCMH) 2011. Retrieved from www.ncqa.org/view-pcmh2011

Neumark-Sztainer, D., Story, M., Hannan, P. J., & Rex, J. (2003). New moves: A school-based obesity prevention program for adolescent girls. *Preventive Medicine, 37*, 41–51. doi:10.1016/S0091-7435(03)00057-4.

Neumark-Sztainer, D., Story, M., Tharp, T., Jaffee, L., Rex, J., Ackard, D., & Fedio, G. (2000). *New moves teacher's guide*. Minneapolis, MN: Division of Epidemiology, School of Public Health, University of Minnesota.

Panzer, P. G., & Bloom, S. L. (2003). Introduction to Sanctuary principles and practice in clinical settings [Special Section]. *Psychiatric Quarterly, 74*, 115–117.

Raimy, V. C. (1950). *Training in clinical psychology*. New York, NY: Prentice-Hall.

*Reifler, B. V. (1992). Reflections of a 16th year clinical scholar. *Journal of Clinical Epidemiology, 45*, 675–680.

Rosenthal, T. C. (2008). The medical home: Growing evidence to support a new approach to primary care. *Journal of the American Board of Family Medicine, 21*, 427–440.

Sieber, W. J., Newsome, A. M., Fiorella, M., & Mantilla, H. (2012). Translating patient self management research into primary care: Challenges and successes with group medical visits. *Translational Behavioral Medicine, 2*, 535.

*Sieber, W. J., Newsome, A., & Lillie, D. (2012). Promoting self-management in diabetes: Efficacy of a collaborative care approach. *Families, Systems & Health, 30*, 322–329. doi:10.1037/a0030714.

Tyndall, L. E., Hodgson, J. L., Lamson, A. L., White, M., & Knight, S. M. (2012). Medical family therapy: Charting a course in competencies. *Contemporary Family Therapy, 34*, 171–186. doi:10.1007/s10591-012-9191-9.

U.S. Preventive Services Task Force (USPSTF). (2009). Screening for depression in adults: U.S. Preventive Services Task Force recommendations. *Annals of Internal Medicine, 151*(11), 1–56.

Waite, R., Davey, M., & Lynch, L. (2013). Self-rated health and association with ACES. *Journal of Behavioral Health, 2*(3), 197–205.

Woods, S. B. (2012). *Examining the effects of family relationships on mental and physical health: Testing the biobehavioral model with an adult primary care sample* (Doctoral dissertation). Retrieved from http://diginole.lib.fsu.edu/etd/5277

Woods, S. B., Priest, J. B., Fish, J. N., & Denton, W. H. (2012, September). *Prevalence of relational discord in urban primary care*. Poster presented at the annual meeting of the American Association for Marriage and Family Therapy, Charlotte, NC.

Chapter 13
Advancing Medical Family Therapy Through Qualitative, Quantitative, and Mixed-Methods Research

Tai Mendenhall, Keeley Pratt, Kenneth Phelps, Macaran Baird, and Felisha Younkin

Over the past two decades, medical family therapy (MedFT) has emerged as a distinctive field within the larger behavioral health system. Since its foundation, it has adapted and evolved in response to the dynamic and ever-changing landscapes of health care, including the advent of healthcare maintenance organizations, the Patient Protection and Affordable Care Act, and development of patient-centered medical homes. To survive in this shifting climate, empirical evidence from core metrics is needed to track progress on healthcare quality, cost, patient and public engagement, and health outcomes (Institute of Medicine [IOM], 2013). In turn, these metrics may be used to earn favor by educators, clinicians, third-party payers, and policy makers for an integrated model of care. As we work to answer this call, scholars must cohesively define, characterize, and assess MedFT and identify research methods (qualitative, quantitative, and mixed methods) that bear promise to advance the approach and framework.

A Lexicon for Dissemination

Collaboratively oriented professionals (MedFTs included) have taken strides to build an empirical base supporting their work, raising important questions about how "collaboration" or "integrated care" is defined and measured (Peek, 2013; Peek & National Integration Academy Council, 2013; Reilly et al., 2012). We find ourselves in a similar position, as MedFT is often inconsistently defined from one article to the next (Linville, Hertlein, & Prouty-Lyness, 2007; Tyndall, Hodgson, Lamson, White, & Knight, 2012a, 2012b). This makes it difficult for scholars to assess which components or processes contribute to desired outcomes.

T. Mendenhall (✉)
University of Minnesota, ST Paul, MN, USA
e-mail: mend0009@umn.edu

J. Hodgson et al. (eds.), *Medical Family Therapy*, DOI 10.1007/978-3-319-03482-9_13,

Additionally, the comparison of MedFT to standard care alone and other collaborative models becomes increasingly problematic without a reliable definition.

Drawing from the foundational work of McDaniel, Hepworth, and Doherty (1992), alongside newer writings by McDaniel, Doherty, and Hepworth (2013), Linville et al. (2007), and Tyndall et al. (2012a, 2012b), key theoretical components of what MedFT looks like on the ground are now being synthesized. They include:

- Systems Theory: By recognizing that all parts of a system are forever interacting, adapting, and evolving (Goldenberg & Goldenberg, 2012; Whitchurch & Constantine, 1993), MedFTs understand that results of change in one part of a larger whole can—and oftentimes cannot—be predicted. By studying MedFT's complex and reciprocal impact(s) on patients' health, interpersonal relationships, family systems, team functionality, and healthcare systems, scholars honor their systemic heritage and unique contributions.
- Biopsychosocial–Spiritual (BPSS) Sensitivity: Scholars should be mindful of not perpetuating silo forms of assessment, where only psychological dimensions are researched. Instead, research (and indeed care) should include measures of biological, psychological, social, and spiritual elements (Engel, 1977, 1980; Rumbold, 2007; White, Williams, & Greenberg, 1996). MedFTs view these areas as mutually influential and maintain that they should be studied as such.
- Agency: Agency is defined as the active involvement and commitment to one's own care and a sense of making personal choices in dealing with illness and the healthcare system (McDaniel et al., 1992, 2013). This goal may be translatable to many psychosocial measures, including self-efficacy, autonomy, perceived competence, or locus of control.
- Communion: Communion centers on connectedness and being cared for, loved, and supported by a community of family members, friends, and professionals to prevent the fraying of emotional bonds by illness, disability, and contact with the healthcare system (McDaniel et al., 1992, 2013). As MedFTs approach research from a systemic viewpoint, it will be imperative to assess the ways that levels of community influence health, coping, and quality of life.
- Collaboration: MedFT practice involves active collaboration with providers representing multiple disciplines (e.g., Psychology, Social Work, Family Medicine, Pediatrics, Nursing, Psychiatry). We define this collaboration in accord to Peek's (2013) lexicon as a practice team "tailored to the needs of each patient and situation; with a shared population and mission; using a systematic clinical approach supported by office practice, leadership alignment, and a business model; and continuous quality improvement and measurement of effectiveness" (pp. 22–23).
- Three-World View of Health Care: Leaders in integrated health care have long called for sensitivity to how different stakeholders representing diverse "worlds" intersect (Peek, 2008). These include (a) the *clinical world* that endeavors to provide exceptional patient care; (b) the *operational world* that works to employ efficient, well-integrated, and patient-friendly systems; and (c) the *financial world* that acts to stay economically viable through cost-effective utilization of healthcare resources.

Implementing the Medical Family Therapy Research Agenda

As outlined above and elsewhere in this book, providers across disciplines have been increasing their efforts to collaborate with each other since the early 1990s (Campbell, 2003; Hodgson, Lamson, Mendenhall, & Crane, 2012; Linville et al., 2007; McDaniel et al., 1992, 2013). This movement is advancing in response to our burgeoning understanding and evidence that supports colocated and integrated services (Kessler & Miller, 2010; Peek, 2013; Singer, Friedberg, Kiang, Dunn, & Kuhn, 2012). More than 70 % of patients presenting for primary care visits have an underlying psychosocial comorbidity; it is thereby easy to understand how satisfaction with healthcare experiences correlates with the collaborative nature(s) of service sites (Alfuth & Barnard, 2000; Linderman, Koff, Freitag, Min, & Vandivier, 2011; Miller, Kessler, Peek, & Kallenberg, 2010). As efforts to extend "collaboration" broaden to actively include patients and families together with the professional members of multidisciplinary teams, MedFT is serving as both a commonsensical and natural bridge (Campbell, 2003; Harkness & Nofziger, 1998; Linville et al., 2007; Tyndall et al., 2012a).

MedFT's face validity for bringing together multiple disciplines and patients/families is not enough, however, to secure it a place at the integrated healthcare table. Health care is evolving fast, and it is thereby essential that all healthcare fields work hard to produce solid empirical evidence to survive (Miller, Mendenhall, & Malik, 2009). Scholars practicing MedFT must advance efforts to more systematically and thoroughly describe what it looks like vis-à-vis other practice types, assess which of its components and processes contribute to desired outcomes, and evaluate and compare MedFT to standard care alone and other collaborative models (Campbell, 2003; Crane, Hillin, & Jakubowski, 2005; Law & Crane, 2000; Law, Crane, & Berge, 2003; Mendenhall, Pratt, Phelps, & Baird, 2012; Miller et al., 2010; Peek, 2013; Proctor et al., 2010; Tyndall et al., 2012a). This work begins with establishing a shared lexicon (Peek, 2013; Peek & National Integration Academy Council, 2013), as outlined above, which will enable researchers and clinicians to consistently define and describe what they are doing (e.g., clinical techniques), the training of the clinicians who are doing it, the contexts in which the work is being carried out (e.g., primary, secondary, or tertiary sites), and the samples and health issues that are targeted (e.g., patients with a particular diagnosis vs. general clinic populations). Increased clarity across these and related foci will enable scholars to replicate the theory-driven studies that they conduct, which will ultimately serve to advance MedFT's credibility (Berger, Mamdani, Atkins, & Johnson, 2009; Campbell, 2003; Linville et al., 2007; Peek, 2013).

As we drive efforts to further our research agenda, we must draw upon both qualitative and quantitative methods (respectively and together). The following sections are organized as such. The authors begin with a discussion of qualitative research and how methods within this investigational frame can be advanced to inform knowledge across healthcare's three worlds (clinical, operational, and financial). We then highlight how quantitative methods can similarly target these worlds. We conclude with a consideration of how both qualitative and quantitative methods can be used together through mixed-methods approaches, specifically via community-based participatory research (CBPR) and practice-based research network (PBRN) platforms.

Advancing MedFT Through Qualitative Research

Qualitative methods should be purposively chosen according to each investigation's respective aims, scope, time frame, and resources. Examples of potential methodologies include content or thematic analysis of individual interviews, focus groups, case studies, and observational or ethnographic studies (Cohen & Crabtree, 2008; Denzin & Lincoln, 2011; Munhall, 2011; Peek, 2013).

Qualitative research in the clinical worlds of MedFT. Qualitative researchers within MedFT's clinical world must engage patients and families alongside all members of their healthcare team. It is important that researchers identify patients' and families' satisfaction levels and experiences with MedFT, from its initial introduction and integration into services to its conclusion (if applicable). For example, researchers could focus on the following questions: How was MedFT described to patients? Did it make sense as part of the treatment? Was it voluntary or did it feel forced? What types of interventions or methods did the MedFT employ? Which ones were most relevant or useful? Which components of the MedFT (or the larger collaborative efforts of the multidisciplinary team) most influenced agency, coping, skill development, disease management, or symptom improvement? Which components worked against beneficent outcomes?

Exploring providers' experiences with MedFT is also essential. How was MedFT introduced, conceptualized, or framed into the site's existing structure? Did therapists feel like valuable assets to a growing team or like an extra-wheel and nuisance to already-busy physicians and extenders (e.g., nurse practitioners, physician assistants)? Did medical providers see improved clinical care and decreased time burdens from the inclusion of MedFT? What types of interventions or collaborative sequences were the most useful in advancing care and achieving desired outcomes?

One way to explore these and related foci through qualitative methods would be to conduct key informant interviews with participants representing the respective voices of those involved in a MedFT intervention (i.e., patients, family members, providers). Following a semi-standardized format, interviewers could target key questions while simultaneously allowing for probes, elaboration, and rich discussions regarding elements of care that are most salient to those engaged. Using such a phenomenological approach, then, investigators could transcribe interviews verbatim and condense transcript texts into a gross database. Raw data could then be analyzed through an iterative data reduction method in which information is extracted and orchestrated into patterns, categories, and themes (Crabtree & Miller,

1999; Hsieh & Shannon, 2005; Kvale, 1997; Kvale & Brinkmann, 2009; Pope, Ziebland, & Mays, 2000). Knowledge gained through qualitative research about clinical processes will serve to inform efforts that position MedFT implementation as a justifiable disruption of standard care to patients, their families, and providers.

Qualitative research in the operational worlds of MedFT. Qualitative researchers within MedFT's operational worlds must extend to other members of the healthcare team (e.g., care coordinators, social workers, administers, medical assistants, dieticians, patient advocates), alongside aforementioned attention to patients, families, and providers. Integrated health care brings with it considerable complexity in referral sequences, follow-up and inter-staff/provider communication, and the coordination of care visits. With clinic staff, it is important to explore how MedFT was introduced or framed to them. Did it make sense in advancing the clinic's mission to improve health, or was it undemocratically announced as "one more thing" that they had to integrate into their work? What are the roadblocks to coordinating and scheduling visits that facilitate MedFT provision with biomedical care? What challenges have staff, MedFTs, and providers experienced in reaching or communicating with others about patients' and families' cases? What strategies have been the most useful in overcoming these challenges?

Qualitative researchers can help answer questions about the operational processes of connecting the dots of MedFT and integrated care. How easy is it to schedule joint meetings with different members of care teams? Are notes from a MedFT visit getting into the medical chart so that the medical provider knows what is going on when he/she sees the patient/family? Are patients and families seeing their providers collaborate with each other in a way that improves clinical processes because of this information sharing?

One way to explore these and related foci through qualitative methods would be to conduct ethnographic studies within care environments. Data collection methods employed through ethnography are designed to capture understandings about naturally occurring social sequences in select human settings, like an isolated tribal village, an inner-city gang, or a metropolitan primary care clinic (O'Reilly, 2005; Schensul, Schensul, & LeCompte, 1999; Van Maanen, 2011). Scholars could use key informant interviews with direct and indirect observations and field notes targeting a variety of clinical processes, from the appointment desk and hallway conversations about care coordination and multidisciplinary collaboration to team and clinical meetings. Data collected through these approaches tend to be extensive and complicated but offer a comprehensive and multi-sourced picture of social and group phenomena that cannot be well captured through straightforward questionnaires or related unimodal methodologies (Miller, Hengst, & Wang, 2003; Van Maanen, 2011).

Knowledge gained through qualitative research about operational processes will serve to inform efforts that position MedFT as a justifiable disruption of standard care to clinical staff and administration. Matching lessons learned to similar sites (e.g., by clinic size, staff size, logistics of space, scheduling sequences, and communication mediums) will enable clinic systems to modify the care they offer without having to reinvent the wheel. All involved will more readily accept and sustain MedFT within clinical practice because it is not experienced as inconvenient, laborious, complicated, or difficult to undertake.

Qualitative research in the financial worlds of MedFT. Empirically demonstrating the financial benefits of MedFT (and even "integrated care" more broadly) will be essential for it to survive within our contemporary large-scale markets of managed care and insurance companies (Campbell, 2003; Crane & Christenson, 2012; Law & Crane, 2000; Law et al., 2003). While quantitative methods are the principal means by which this will be accomplished, researchers and clinicians have much to gain in their implementation efforts from qualitative investigations that engage, especially, billing personnel and biomedical providers.

With billing personnel, qualitative inquiry can tap key barriers and challenges related to securing coverage for integrated services, advocating on behalf of patients/families to managed care organizations, negotiating blanket coverage for team care vs. behavioral health carve-outs, and/or advancing and securing outside receptivity to joint treatment plans. For biomedical team leaders, qualitative research can access key stakeholder views that maintain MedFT to be a valuable component of integrated teams, even if it is assessed as a singular service (for which fees are collected) that is not objectively "profitable." Other nonfinancial benefits, such as MedFT clinicians assisting primary care providers and/or other healthcare practitioners so that work is more time-efficient and/or satisfying in delivery, may serve as cost-offsets in the future (Proctor et al., 2010).

These foci, too, could be investigated qualitatively through a variety of methods. In addition to those already mentioned, focus group interviews with different and competing representatives of healthcare's different worlds could be useful. While analyzed with the same rigor as individual interviews, the interactive nature of group settings allows participants to talk with other group members (Hessy-Biber & Leavy, 2008; Oldenburg, Williams, McGonigal-Kenney, Maas, & Tripp-Reimer, 2011). As it relates to MedFT's operational worlds, this could uncover some of the gaps, respective and reciprocal perceptions or misperceptions that participants maintain about each other, and areas of agreement and/or conflict that they share. Ultimately, knowledge gained from research asking how billing personnel do their jobs will inform others who perform similar functions about how to introduce MedFT. Confidence in the utility of MedFT in improving healthcare providers' experiences with care and in advancing future cost-offsets will help buffer expense-related concerns about the tradeoffs of tangibly paying a MedFT team member and the less-tangible clinical and financial gains of doing so. As clinic administrators observe improved clinical processes, patient/family outcomes, and provider/care team satisfaction, they will likely be more receptive to implement or sustain MedFT.

Advancing MedFT Through Quantitative Research

Evaluative facets of implementation research call strongly for the application of quantitative methods (Miller et al., 2010). As we ask questions related to how

MedFT performs vis-à-vis other treatment approaches and/or what facets of care best predict desired clinical, operational, and/or financial outcomes, we must work to establish investigative designs that best fit with each project's unique aims, scope, time frame, and resources.

Quantitative research in the clinical worlds of MedFT. As Kessler and Miller (2010) point out, metrics are needed to provide standardized ways of assessing what MedFTs pragmatically do in clinical care and to be able to compare their role to the roles of others who operate within a healthcare setting. Furthermore, MedFT's emphasis on systems theory (Goldenberg & Goldenberg, 2012; Whitchurch & Constantine, 1993) should encourage researchers to gather as many data points as possible from each participant and worksite. For example, in examining a youth's well-child visit involving a MedFT as one of the care providers, we would want to consider the perspective of the child, caregiver(s), additional care providers, and important others who attended the visit. To conduct quantitative research involving such complex designs (experimental or nonexperimental), several types of methodologies could be applied. In a true experimental design, randomization, a control group, an experimental group, and pre- and posttests are all essential to determine whether the independent variables (IVs) have a significant effect on the dependent variables (DVs).

Randomized methods: In healthcare research, the most common conceptual methodology is between-groups designs, which tell us if groups' clinical outcomes are significantly different from each other and in what direction. We typically hypothesize that our experimental treatment is superior to a comparison group (or standard treatment) alone. To advance MedFT, we must determine how patients who receive MedFT (or experience it as part of their care team) differ from those who receive conventional care. For example, in a study designed to monitor diabetes management and depression levels for a group of adults receiving weekly outpatient treatment, the participating sample could be randomly assigned to a healthcare team with MedFT or a healthcare team without MedFT. Group results could then be compared across measures of metabolic control and mood.

Researchers employing randomized control trials (RCTs) are increasingly using non-inferiority and equivalence designs. Often the two are used interchangeably to refer to trials in which the primary objective is to show that a novel intervention is as effective as a standard intervention alone; e.g., MedFT is equally beneficial as standard practice (Green, Morland, Durkalski, & Frueh, 2008). Non-inferiority and equivalence designs further the between-groups design by determining if the effects of the two treatments are not clinically and statistically different. However, non-inferiority designs advance a one-sided test to determine if an intervention is no worse than standard intervention/treatment alone (as in the example above with diabetic control, inclusion is no worse than standard care), whereas equivalence designs employ a two-sided test that allows for the possibility that the novel intervention is not better than standard care. Non-inferiority designs can be of optimal value when a novel intervention, such as one that includes MedFT, has been developed that is more beneficial (e.g., easier to use, less costly, provides increased access, less side effects) when compared to standard care.

Nonrandomized methods: Pre-experimental designs, although the least able to determine causality and lacking random assignment, can still contribute to the advancement of MedFT. The one-shot case study, which contains an intervention and posttest, could be used when randomization and a control group are not possible. For example, a MedFT that is new to a healthcare team could measure family functioning and quality of life after being at a site for 1 year. A single-group pre-/posttest would be useful if randomization is not possible, and scholars have ample time to administer a pretest before the patient experiences MedFT as part of their team. In a static group comparison, participants can select if they would or would not like to see a MedFT as part of their visit (thereby assigning them into experimental and control groups), and pre-/posttests would be delivered regardless of group selection.

Quasi-experimental designs may be necessary to use when the researcher has little control over the IV (e.g., when there is no either control group or random assignment). Such studies may include conducting posttest-only analyses, such as the two-group posttest which contains random assignment but no pretest. Interrupted and equivalent time series designs can be used to measure the dependent variable over time through pretests and posttests when researchers are only looking at one group.

One particularly helpful nonrandomized method that could be used to determine how MedFT looks over several healthcare sites is the indirect comparisons method. This approach allows scholars to compare data from separate studies. This is particularly beneficial when there is a lack of sufficient evidence to compare trials. Well-conducted RCTs provide the most valid estimates if direct comparison interventions/treatment are feasible, but many interventions have not been directly compared in RCTs due to limitations in time, money, and resources. Their results could still be used to estimate the relative effects of different treatments; however, indirect methods may be the most promising, timely, and cost-beneficial way to determine how MedFT looks across different settings when compared to standard care.

Advanced methods: There has been a call for more complex statistical analyses that allow for the controlling of IVs and DVs while simultaneously analyzing dyads (e.g., couples, parent–child). Multilevel methods such as Hierarchical Linear Modeling (HLM) and Structural Equation Modeling (SEM) allow for nested structures (e.g., patients in therapies and patients in groups or repeated measures within one person). SEM is more of a confirmatory model (theory testing), whereas HLM is more of an exploratory model (theory development). HLM uses OLS regression and ANOVA, both of which are based on the general linear model (O'Connell & McCoach, 2004). HLM is useful for understanding relationships in hierarchical data structures, such as patients or physicians and extenders within healthcare settings (O'Connell & McCoach, 2004). For example, HLM would allow us to analyze whether there is a significant difference in mean patient outcome scores across different healthcare providers adjusted for appropriate covariates. Covariates may include patient characteristics (e.g., age, gender, diagnosis) and provider characteristics (e.g., disciplinary identification with MedFT, Psychology, Social

Work). SEM involves analyses with observed (manifest) variables, latent variables (variables which are not measured directly), or both (Schumacker & Lomax, 2004). Regression and ANOVA are included under SEM; often path diagrams are utilized to represent latent and observed variables (Schumacker & Lomax, 2004). An example using a SEM model in MedFT research could be to investigate patient–healthcare provider communication and its effects on patient satisfaction with different levels of integration in Family Medicine units. The variables of satisfaction with healthcare services, interpersonal treatment, contextual knowledge of the patient, and level of integration could be analyzed using multiple-group SEM.

Dyadic analysis assumes that dyads or dyad pairs are related or share something in common (Kenny, Kashy, & Cook, 2008). The fundamental concept around dyadic data analysis is nonindependence or that outcome scores or indexes are linked in some way. Examples of standard MedFT dyad designs could include student and supervisor pairs or provider and patient pairs. In dyadic analysis there are three major types of variables: between-dyad variables (all variation is between dyads), within-dyad variables (all variation is within dyads), and mixed variables (there is variation within and between dyads).

Quantitative research in the operational worlds of MedFT. Questions in the operational world should address how MedFTs function together with the team, the team's knowledge of and perceived value of MedFT, and support that is available from the office system for MedFT billing and coding. Similar to assessments that measure family cohesiveness or family functioning (e.g., the Family Assessment Device; Epstein, Bishop, & Levin, 1978), such metrics could be applied to the clinical team and their overall functioning with MedFT. The level of clarity and consistency for team members in the definition of MedFT and subsequent roles could be measured through their use of common space, language, level of training (individually and cohesively), and the degree to which they have achieved a shared practice culture. Quantitative assessments could be conducted for how individual team members believe that MedFT is part of their mission.

Electronic healthcare record (EHR) abstraction could be a useful tool in analyzing, at the population level, the degree to which care plans integrate MedFT components. For example, the EHR of patients from a specific clinic that employs one or more MedFTs could be analyzed to see if treatment plans include biological/physical, psychological, social, and spiritual components and how the multidisciplinary team plans on following up with the patient about their BPSS concerns and determining change has occurred. The reliability and efficiency of the office practice could be quantitatively assessed through the use of time stamping when patients walk in to their healthcare visit, when they are seen, who they are seen by, how long they are seen by each provider, their payment processing, and their exit. By providing descriptive time-stamped data, MedFT services can be quantified and compared to other services in that setting or with the clinical team cohesively.

Olson and Watson (2009) have adapted the Circumplex Model (conventionally applied to assess family functioning) to the study of work team dynamics. Leadership, for example, can have a significant impact on operational procedures and overall satisfaction with the clinical system. The Team Organizational Profile

(TOP) describes five leadership styles derived from assessments of cohesion (ranging from disengaged, somewhat connected, connected, very connected, and enmeshed) and flexibility (ranging from chaotic, very flexible, flexible, somewhat flexible, and rigid) scores. Leadership styles include uninvolved (high flexibility, low cohesion), controlling (low flexibility, low cohesion), permissive (high flexibility, high cohesion), micromanaging (low flexibility, high cohesion), and balanced. The balanced style is beheld as the most functional style, where group members have higher satisfaction scores and interpersonal working relationships. The TOP assessment can provide a quantitative way to compare clinical team operations across different clinical sites or to monitor improvement in team communication, satisfaction, and relationships.

Quantitative research in the financial worlds of MedFT. Crane and Christenson (2012) provided a summary of cost-effectiveness research for the profession and practice of MFT. They based their work on four sources of data, including a large health maintenance organization, the Kansas State Medicaid system, Cigna (a health insurance benefits management company), and a MFT training clinic. Three of these data sources represent healthcare systems which can provide valuable implications for future MedFT research in its financial world. Crane and Christenson reported that there is a potential for a medical cost-offset effect after couple or family therapy, with the largest reduction occurring for those patients who are recognized as high utilizers of care. They reported that higher treatment costs are not associated with covering MFT as a treatment option and highlighted several ways that cost savings from integrated care models could outweigh associated costs, including improved adherence to treatment recommendations, increased work productivity, and decreased malpractice suits. It will be important for integrated care with MedFT to show similar reductions and/or cost-offsets over time.

Advancing MedFT Through Mixed-Methods Research

Any of the qualitative or quantitative methods described above could be integrated together in a single study. Investigators must purposively assess the aims of their respective efforts and make decisions about which method(s) to employ in accord to said aims (Campbell, Gregory, Patterson, & Bybee, 2012; Leech, Dellinger, Brannagan, & Tanka, 2010). Platforms from which to do mixed-methods research that align well with the collaborative spirit of MedFT and the broader scientific community's call to produce new knowledge that advances implementation are myriad. We highlight two broad approaches here: community-based participatory research (CBPR) and practice-based research networks (PBRNs).

Community-Based Participatory Research (CBPR). The concept of CBPR evolved from *action research* in the 1940s and is characterized by investigations in which professionals partner with communities to generate knowledge and solve local problems (Agency for Healthcare Research and Quality [AHRQ], 2004;

Lewin, 1946). Several key assumptions permeate this work; the following are those most commonly recognized and advanced in professional literature: (1) democratic and equitable partnership between all project members (e.g., participants, community stakeholders, researchers) as collaborators through every stage of knowledge and intervention development; (2) promoting co-learning and capacity building between and among partners; and (3) cyclical processes in which problems are identified, solutions are developed within the context(s) of the community's existing resources, interventions are implemented, outcomes are evaluated according to what participants maintain is most important, and interventions are modified in accord with new information (Bradbury & Reason, 2003; LaVeaux & Christopher, 2009; Mendenhall & Doherty, 2005; Minkler & Wallerstein, 2011; Montoya & Kent, 2011; Scharff & Mathews, 2008; Strickland, 2006). See Chap. 14 (Mendenhall, Berge, & Doherty, 2014) for further description and discussion regarding this type of research.

Implementing MedFT through CBPR is defensible on the grounds that many are extending the call for research methods that are as collaborative as the care they seek to evaluate. By engaging all stakeholders in the research process, we are able to create knowledge that respective groups (e.g., healthcare providers, health economists, patients, and families) could not produce independently (Linville et al., 2007; Luzinski, 2012; Proctor et al., 2010; Restall & Strutt, 2008). Further, engaging the recipients of health care along with the usual players in service planning and evaluation is increasingly common because doing so enables them to have identifiable impacts. This leads to better advances in the acceptability, accessibility, and quality of what is ultimately offered (Jencius, 2004; Restall & Strutt, 2008; Stevenson et al., 2011).

A CBPR investigation of MedFT, for example, could advance clinical world understandings of patients'/families' health behaviors by qualitatively interviewing them about how MedFT/biomedical provider collaboration influenced decision-making and coping processes in diabetes management. Quantitative analysis could follow, incorporating foci identified by both patients/families (e.g., communication facility through couple/family inventories like the FACES-IV (Olson, 2011), depression through the Patient Health Questionnaire—Ninth Edition (PHQ-9; Kroenke, Spitzer, & Williams, 2001)) and providers (e.g., metabolic control/A1c) as important. Operational world understandings of administrative sequences could be assessed qualitatively through focus groups with front desk staff and care coordinators (e.g., challenges/strategies related to scheduling multiple providers) and quantitatively through time series evaluations of referral-to-next-visit waits and/or received communications between collaborating providers. Financial world understandings could be advanced by asking key stakeholders (e.g., insurance personnel, billing administrators) what is important as it relates to care finances and then followed up quantitatively by cost tracking, measuring cost-offset, or comparing different groups recognized as warranting further evaluative attention.

Practice-Based Research Networks (PBRNs). Practice-based research networks are defined as groups of ambulatory practices that are devoted to the primary care of patients and their families (AHRQ, 2011a, 2011b; Handley, Schillinger, &

Shiboski, 2011; Pace et al., 2009). By joining together, PBRNs are able to draw on the experience and insights of practicing clinicians to identify and frame research questions that can answer important questions about practice improvements. They work to link these questions with rigorous investigative methods, and they share (electronically and in manners approved by the Health Insurance Portability and Accountability Act [HIPAA]), track, and evaluate large medical record databases. PBRNs are designed in ways that enable researchers to produce findings quickly so that new knowledge is immediately relevant to contemporary clinical work and, at least in theory, more easily integrated and assimilated into everyday practice.

While several PBRNs exist in the United States, the Collaborative Care Research Network (CCRN) represents one that is especially well equipped to advance MedFT (American Association of Family Physicians [AAFP], 2009; Auxier et al., 2012; Miller et al., 2010). The CCRN was created so that clinicians could investigate integrated care through the examination of clinical, financial, and operational impacts of behavioral health on health outcomes of patients and families in primary care. An investigation of MedFT using this platform, for example, could endeavor to understand the processes and steps related to and between primary care providers' referrals for MedFT and patients'/families' initiation of services. Doing this across several clinics would facilitate a comparison of different sites' effectiveness in making referrals happen, as well as test (with a larger cumulative sample yielding more power) outcomes secondary to the care itself. Employing quantitative methods, researchers could collect data regarding referral (e.g., presenting problem), treatment initiation (i.e., was care initiated or not), and time lag between referral and treatment initiation through EMR review and simple descriptive and calculative methods. Qualitative key informant interviews could be employed to better understand providers' rationales for referring, clinic staff's experiences with making referrals work logistically and "stick" (i.e., sans no-shows), and patients'/families' understandings regarding the logic behind referrals made and experience with connecting from one provider to another. Standardized measures related to clinical outcomes (e.g., PHQ-9 scores) could be tracked and entered into electronic charts over the course of care. Focus group interviews could follow care termination to explore patients' and families' experiences with the collaborative efforts of their care team.

Summary and Discussion

As scholars strive to formalize a place for MedFT within the current healthcare landscape, it will be important to first standardize our professional identity. Drawing from the work of McDaniel et al. (1992, 2013), Linville et al. (2007), and Tyndall et al. (2012a, 2012b), researchers must include elements of systems theory, BPSS sensitivity to care, agency, communion, and interdisciplinary collaboration to remain true to the field's theoretical roots. Now that a standardized definition has been developed, future work can turn to the qualitative, quantitative, and mixed-methods approaches discussed above to advance our empirical base.

MedFT is situated with the challenge of being a relatively young presence within our US healthcare teams. In other fields, evidence-based practices (EBP) are expected and, indeed, the norm for clinical treatment and research design. In contrast, MedFT may benefit from practice-based evidence (PBE), known for utilizing a service-to-science model (opposite of EBP, which uses a science-to-service model) (Luzinski, 2012; Nicholson, Hinden, Biebel, Henry, & Katz-Leavy, 2007; Reupert & Maybery, 2009). According to Tyndall, Hodgson, Lamson, White, and Knight (2014) (see Chap. 2), there are currently 96 studies that document MedFT; none of which are RCTs or have a high-level experimental design (randomization, experimental/control group, pre-/posttests, and/or IVs/DVs). This further confirms the utility of practice-based evidence and research in moving us forward as we provide the foundation for solid empirical evidence to take place in the future.

We must evaluate MedFT across clinical, operational, and financial arenas. We can employ qualitative methods to tap patients', families', providers', and administrators' experiences with different care types and clinical procedures. We can advance quantitative methods to compare and track disease-related outcomes, cost-offset data, and intermember functioning and satisfaction in care teams. We can use mixed-methods approaches to simultaneously capture the richness of participants' experiences alongside objective measures of beneficent change. Wherever we choose to start and whatever we choose to do, we will be advancing MedFT because, at the present time, our field is so novel that there are more gaps in what we know than there are empirically supported areas of what we do.

Conclusion

To be clear, the authors are not advocating a campaign to "prove" MedFT's universal superiority over any other behavioral health field or framework, nor have we ever found interdisciplinary squabbling over who is "best" prepared to extend this level of clinical work helpful to advancing integration. We believe that graduate students within any discipline have a greater appreciation of clinical populations, treatment approaches, and interdisciplinary collaboration when they are exposed to each other's specialties and learn about how their own and other's respective efforts contribute to a larger mosaic of high-quality and effective care. It is through these rich training sequences that healthcare professionals across different disciplines can—provided they maintain the key elements of MedFT highlighted above—all practice MedFT. And just as there are some tasks in which a hammer is more appropriate than a screwdriver (and vice versa), there will be some scenarios in which MedFT is a better fit than a straightforward psychological assessment or social work intervention. In order for MedFTs to have a stable place at the healthcare table alongside all of their colleagues, we must catch up and establish our purpose (through the established definition of who we are and what we do) and utility (through efficacy and effectiveness research) to be there.

Discussion Questions

1. Consider the training facility, clinical practice, or agency in which you and/or others are working as a MedFT. What research question(s) is important to explore with key stakeholders (e.g., biomedical providers, behavioral health providers, administrators) there? Which of healthcare's three worlds are most pressing at this site at this time?
2. Consider the broader field(s) of integrated health care and MedFT's participation and evolution within this larger frame. What research question(s) is important to explore with key stakeholders across state, national, and/or international levels (e.g., managed care organizations, policy makers, educators/trainers)? Which of healthcare's three worlds are most pressing within these arenas at this time?
3. Brainstorm and design a study that could serve to answer the questions identified in #1 and/or #2, above. Are you exploring something—without attempting to change it—to create new knowledge? Are you advancing and evaluating an intervention? Who are your participants? What approach(es) will you use? Qualitative? Quantitative? Mixed methods?
4. Most graduate students pursuing MedFT intend to devote their careers primarily to clinical practice. How can training programs better engage new professionals to bridge their work with the research that is so important to securing MedFT's place within our healthcare system?
5. The authors maintain that they are not out to "prove" MedFT's effectiveness as superior to any other approach or framework. However, guild and organization leaders are often in direct competition with each other for healthcare dollars, and research data represent one of the means by which they do this. Are there circumstances in which, for example, comparing the respective clinical outcomes of a MedFT vs. a Psychologist or Social Worker would be indicated? Why or why not?

References[1]

Agency for Healthcare Research and Quality. (2004). *Community-based participatory research: Assessing the evidence*. Rockville, MD: AHRQ.

Agency for Healthcare Research and Quality. (2011a). *AHRQ support for primary care practice based research networks (PBRNs)*. AHRQ. Retrieved from http://www.ahrq.gov/research/pbrn/pbrnfact.htm

Agency for Healthcare Research and Quality. (2011b). *Primary care practice based research networks*. AHRQ. Retrieved March 19, 2012, from http://pbrn.ahrq.gov/portal/server.pt/community/practice_based_research_networks_%28pbrn%29__about/852

---

[1] An asterisk has been use to note references that the chapter authors recommend for further reading.

Alfuth, R., & Barnard, C. (2000). Family physicians and family therapists: Understanding the interdependent synergism. *Contemporary Family Therapy, 22*, 253–277. doi:10.1023/A:1007865506702.

American Academy of Family Physicians. (2009). *The collaborative care research network (CCRN)*. AAFP. Retrieved from http://www.aafp.org/online/en/home/clinical/research/natnet/get-involved/ccrn-info.html

Auxier, A., Runyan, C., Mullin, D., Mendenhall, T., Young, J., & Kessler, R. (2012). Behavioral health referrals and treatment initiation rates in integrated primary care: A Collaborative Care Research Network study. *Translational Behavioral Medicine, 2*, 337–344. doi:10.1007/s13142-012-0141-8.

Berger, M., Mamdani, M., Atkins, D., & Johnson, M. (2009). Good research practices for comparative effectiveness research: Defining, reporting and interpreting nonrandomized studies of treatment effects using secondary data sources. *Value in Health, 12*, 1044–1052. doi:10.1111/j.1524-4733.2009.00600.x.

Bradbury, H., & Reason, P. (2003). Action research: An opportunity for revitalizing research purpose and practices. *Qualitative Social Work, 2*, 155–175. doi:10.1177/1473325003002002003.

Campbell, T. (2003). The effectiveness of family interventions for physical disorders. *Journal of Marital and Family Therapy, 29*, 263–281. doi:10.1111/j.1752-0606.2003.tb01204.x.

Campbell, R., Gregory, K. A., Patterson, D., & Bybee, D. (2012). Integrating qualitative and quantitative approaches: An example of mixed methods research. In J. Leonard & D. Glenwick (Eds.), *Methodological approaches to community-based research* (pp. 51–68). Washington, DC: American Psychological Association.

Cohen, D., & Crabtree, B. (2008). Evaluative criteria for qualitative research in health care: Controversies and recommendations. *Annals of Family Medicine, 6*, 331–339. doi:10.1370/afm.818.

Crabtree, B., & Miller, W. (1999). *Doing qualitative research*. Thousand Oaks, CA: Sage Publications.

Crane, D., & Christenson, J. (2012). A summary report of the cost-effectiveness of the profession and practice of marriage and family therapy. *Contemporary Family Therapy, 34*, 204–216. doi:10.1007/s10591-012-9187-5.

Crane, D., Hillin, H., & Jakubowski, S. (2005). Costs of treating conduct disordered Medicaid youth with and without family therapy. *The American Journal of Family Therapy, 33*, 403–413. doi:10.1080/01926180500276810.

Denzin, N., & Lincoln, Y. (Eds.). (2011). *The SAGE handbook of qualitative research*. London: Sage.

Engel, G. (1977). The need for a new medical model: A challenge for biomedicine. *Science, 196*, 129–136.

Engel, G. (1980). The clinical application of the biopsychosocial model. *American Journal of Psychiatry, 137*, 535–544.

Epstein, N. B., Bishop, D. S., & Levin, S. (1978). The McMaster model of family functioning. *Journal of Marital and Family Therapy, 4*, 19–31.

Goldenberg, H., & Goldenberg, I. (2012). *Family therapy: An overview* (8th ed.). Belmont, CA: Brooks/Cole.

Green, C., Morland, L., Durkalski, V., & Frueh, B. (2008). Noninferiority and equivalence designs: Issues and implications for mental health research. *Journal of Traumatic Stress, 21*, 422–429. doi:10.1002/jts.20367.

Handley, M., Schillinger, D., & Shiboski, S. (2011). Quasi-experimental designs in practice-based research settings: Design and implementation considerations. *Journal of the American Board of Family Medicine: JABFM, 24*, 589–596.

Harkness, J., & Nofziger, A. (1998). Training in a collaborative context: What we did not know then...we know now. *Families, Systems & Health, 16*, 443–450. doi:10.1037/h0089868.

Hessy-Biber, S., & Leavy, P. (2008). *Handbook of emergent methods*. New York, NY: Guilford Press.
Hodgson, J., Lamson, A., Mendenhall, T., & Crane, R. (2012). Medical family therapy: Opportunity for workforce development in healthcare. *Contemporary Family Therapy, 34*, 143–146. doi:10.1007/s10591-012-9199-1.
Hsieh, H., & Shannon, S. (2005). Three approaches to qualitative content analysis. *Qualitative Health Research, 15*, 1277–1288. doi:10.1177/1049732305276687.
IOM (Institute of Medicine). (2013). *Core measurement needs for better care, better health, and lower costs: Counting what counts: Workshop summary*. Washington, DC: The National Academies Press.
Jencius, M. (2004). Citizen therapist: An interview with William Doherty. *The Family Journal, 12*, 82–88. doi:10.1177/1066480703258947.
*Kenny, D., Kashy, D., & Cook, W. (2008). *Dyadic data analysis*. New York, NY: Guildford Press.
*Kessler, R., & Miller, B. (2010). *A framework for collaborative care metrics*. Agency for Healthcare Research and Quality. Retrieved from http://www.ahrq.gov/research/collaborativecare/collab3.htm
Kroenke, K., Spitzer, R., & Williams, J. (2001). The PHQ-9: Validity of a brief depression severity measure. *Journal of General Internal Medicine, 16*, 606–613. doi:10.1046/j.1525-1497.2001.016009606.x.
Kvale, S. (1997). *Interviews: An introduction to qualitative research interviewing*. Thousand Oaks, CA: Sage Publications.
Kvale, S., & Brinkmann, S. (2009). *Interviews: Learning the craft of qualitative research interviewing* (2nd ed.). Los Angeles, CA: Sage.
LaVeaux, D., & Christopher, S. (2009). Contextualizing CBPR: Key principles of CBPR meet the indigenous research context. *Journal of Aboriginal and Indigenous Community Health 7*, 1–25. Retrieved from http://www.ncbi.nlm.nih.gov/pmc/articles/PMC2818123/
Law, D., & Crane, D. (2000). The influence of marital and family therapy on health care utilization in a health-maintenance organization. *Journal of Marital and Family Therapy, 26*, 281–291. doi:10.1111/j.1752-0606.2000.tb00298.x.
Law, D., Crane, D., & Berge, J. (2003). The influence of individual, marital, and family therapy on high utilizers of health care. *Journal of Marital and Family Therapy, 29*, 353–363. doi:10.1111/j.1752-0606.2003.tb01212.x.
Leech, N., Dellinger, A., Brannagan, K., & Tanka, H. (2010). Evaluating mixed methods research studies: A mixed methods approach. *Journal of Mixed Methods Research, 4*, 17–31. doi:10.1177/1558689809345262.
Lewin, K. (1946). Action research and minority problems. *Journal of Social Issues, 2*, 34–46. doi:10.1111/j.1540-4560.1946.tb02295.x.
Linderman, D. J., Koff, P. B., Freitag, T. J., Min, S. J., & Vandivier, R. W. (2011). Effect of integrated care on advanced chronic obstructive pulmonary disease in high-mortality rural areas. *Archives of Internal Medicine, 171*, 2059–2061. doi:10.1001/archinternmed.2011.576.
Linville, D., Hertlein, K., & Prouty-Lyness, A. (2007). Medical family therapy: Reflecting on the necessity of collaborative healthcare research. *Families, Systems & Health, 25*, 85–97. doi:10.1037/1091-7527.25.1.85.
Luzinski, C. (2012). Advancing the science of nursing, improving the quality of care. *Journal of Nursing Administration, 42*, 123–124. doi:10.1097/NNA.0b013e3182480754.
McDaniel, S., Doherty, W., & Hepworth, J. (2013). *Medical family therapy and integrated care* (2nd ed.). Washington, DC: American Psychological Association.
*McDaniel, S., Hepworth, J., & Doherty, W. (1992). *Medical family therapy: A biopsychosocial approach to families with health problems*. New York, NY: Basic Books.
Mendenhall, T., Berge, J., & Doherty, W. (2014). Engaging communities as partners in research: Advancing integrated care through purposeful partnerships. In J. Hodgson, A. Lamson, T. Mendenhall, & R. Crane (Eds.), *Medical family therapy: Advanced applications* (pp. 259–282). New York, NY: Springer.

Mendenhall, T., & Doherty, W. (2005). Action research methods in family therapy. In F. Piercy & D. Sprenkle (Eds.), *Research methods in family therapy* (2nd ed., pp. 100–117). New York, NY: Guilford Publications.

Mendenhall, T., Pratt, K., Phelps, K., & Baird, M. (2012). Advancing medical family therapy through research: A consideration of qualitative, quantitative, and mixed-methods designs. *Contemporary Family Therapy, 34*, 1–17. doi:10.1007/s10591-012-9186-6.

Miller, P., Hengst, J., & Wang, S. (2003). Ethnographic methods: Applications from developmental cultural psychology. In P. Camic & J. Rhodes (Eds.), *Qualitative research in psychology: Expanding perspectives in methodology and design* (pp. 219–242). Washington, DC: American Psychological Association.

*Miller, B., Kessler, R., Peek, C., & Kallenberg, G. (2010). *Establishing the research agenda for collaborative care*. Agency for Healthcare Research and Quality. Retrieved from http://www.ahrq.gov/research/collaborativecare/collab1.htm

Miller, B. F., Mendenhall, T. J., & Malik, A. D. (2009). Integrated primary care: An inclusive three-world view through process metrics and empirical discrimination. *Journal of Clinical Psychology in Medical Settings, 16*, 21–30. doi:10.1007/s10880-008-9137-4.

*Minkler, M., & Wallerstein, N. (Eds.). (2011). *Community-based participatory research for health: From process to outcomes*. San Francisco, CA: Jossey-Bass.

Montoya, M., & Kent, E. (2011). Dialogical action: Moving from community-based to community-driven participatory research. *Qualitative Health Research, 21*, 1000–1011. doi:10.1177/1049732311403500.

Munhall, P. (2011). *Nursing research*. Sudbury, MA: Jones & Bartlett Learning.

Nicholson, J., Hinden, B., Biebel, K., Henry, A., & Katz-Leavy, J. (2007). A qualitative study of programs for parents with serious mental illness and their children: Building practice-based evidence. *Journal of Behavioral Health Services & Research, 34*, 395–413. doi:10.1007/s11414-007-9063-5.

*O'Connell, A., & McCoach, D. (2004). Applications of hierarchical linear models for evaluations of health interventions: Demystifying the methods and interpretations of multilevel models. *Evaluation & the Health Professions, 27*, 119–151. doi:10.1177/0163278704264049.

Oldenburg, A., Williams, J., McGonigal-Kenney, M., Maas, M., & Tripp-Reimer, T. (2011). *Focus group process: Analysis of group interaction and participant insights*. Retrieved from http://hdl.handle.net/10755/160234

Olson, D. (2011). FACES IV and the circumplex model: Validation study. *Journal of Marital & Family Therapy, 37*, 64–80. doi:10.1111/j.1752-0606.2009.00175.x.

Olson, D., & Watson, R. (2009). *Team organization profile*. Roseville, MN: Life Innovations.

O'Reilly, K. (2005). *Ethnographic methods*. Abingdon, Oxford: Routledge.

Pace, W., Cifuentes, M., Valuck, R., Staton, E., Brandt, E., & West, D. (2009). An electronic practice-based network of observational comparative effectiveness research. *Annals of Internal Medicine, 151*, 338–340.

Peek, C. (2008). Planning care in the clinical, operational, and financial worlds. In R. Kessler (Ed.), *Collaborative medicine case studies* (pp. 25–38). New York, NY: Springer.

*Peek, C. (2013). Integrated behavioral health in primary care: A common language. In M. R. Talen & A. B. Valeras (Eds.), *Integrated behavioral health in primary care: Evaluating the evidence, identifying the essentials* (pp. 9–32). New York, NY: Springer.

*Peek, C., & National Integration Academy Council. (2013). *Lexicon for behavioral health and primary care integration: Concepts and definitions developed by expert consensus* (AHRQ Publication No. 13-IP001-EF). Retrieved from http://integrationacademy.ahrq.gov/sites/default/files/Lexicon.pdf

Pope, C., Ziebland, S., & Mays, N. (2000). Qualitative research in health care: Analyzing qualitative data. *British Medical Journal, 8*, 320–323. Retrieved from http://www.ncbi.nlm.nih.gov.ezp1.lib.umn.edu/pmc/articles/PMC1117368/

Proctor, E., Landsverk, J., Aarons, G., Chambers, D., Glisson, C., & Mittman, B. (2010). Implementation research in mental health services: An emerging science with conceptual, methodological, and training challenges. *Administration and Policy in Mental Health and Mental Health Services Research, 36*, 24–34. doi:10.1007/s10488-008-0197-4.

Reilly, S., Planner, C., Gask, L., Hann, M., Knowles, S., Druss, B., & Lester, H. (2012). Collaborative care approaches for people with severe mental illness. *The Cochrane Library*. doi:10.1002/14651858.CD009531

Restall, G., & Strutt, C. (2008). Participation in planning and evaluating mental health services: Building capacity. *Psychiatric Rehabilitation Journal, 31*, 234–238. doi:10.2975/31.3.2008.234.238.

Reupert, A., & Maybery, D. (2009). A "snapshot" of Australian programs to support children and adolescents whose parents have a mental illness. *Psychiatric Rehabilitation Journal, 33*, 125–132. doi:10.2975/33.2.2009.125.132.

Rumbold, B. D. (2007). A review of spiritual assessment in health care practice. *Medical Journal of Australia, 186*, S60–S62.

Scharff, D., & Mathews, K. (2008). Working with communities to translate research into practice. *Journal of Public Health Management and Practice, 14*, 94–98. doi:10.1097/01.PHH.0000311885.60509.61.

Schensul, S., Schensul, J., & LeCompte, M. (1999). *Essential ethnographic methods*. Walnut Creek, CA: AltaMira.

*Schumacker, R., & Lomax, R. (2004). *A beginner's guide to structural equation modeling*. Muhawah, NJ: Taylor & Francis.

Singer, S. J., Friedberg, M. W., Kiang, M. V., Dunn, T., & Kuhn, D. M. (2012). Development and preliminary validation of the patient perceptions of integrated care survey. *Medical Care Research and Review*. doi:10.1177/1077558712465654.

Stevenson, J. G., Beck, C., Heacock, P., Mercer, S. O., Hoskins, J. A., Doan, R., & Schnelle, J. F. (2011). A conceptual framework for achieving high-quality care in nursing homes. *Journal for Healthcare Quality, 22*, 31–36. doi:10.1111/j.1945-1474.2000.tb00137.x

Strickland, C. (2006). Challenges in community-based participatory research implementation: Experiences in cancer prevention with Pacific Northwest American Indian tribes. *Cancer Control, 13*, 230–236.

Tyndall, L., Hodgson, J., Lamson, A., White, M., & Knight, S. (2012a). Medical family therapy: A theoretical and empirical review. *Contemporary Family Therapy, 34*, 156–170. doi:10.1007/s10591012-9183-9.

Tyndall, L., Hodgson, J., Lamson, A., White, M., & Knight, S. (2012b). Medical family therapy: Charting a course in competencies. *Contemporary Family Therapy, 34*, 171–186. doi:10.1007/s10591-012-9191-9.

Tyndall, L., Hodgson, J., Lamson, A., White, M., & Knight, S. (2014). A review of medical family therapy: 30 Years of history, growth, and research. In J. Hodgson, A. Lamson, T. Mendenhall, & R. Crane (Eds.), *Medical family therapy: Advanced applications* (pp. 13–32). New York, NY: Springer.

Van Maanen, J. (2011). *Tales of the field: On writing ethnography*. Chicago, IL: University of Chicago Press.

Whitchurch, G., & Constantine, L. (1993). Systems theory. In P. Boss, W. Doherty, W. LaRossa, W. Schumm, & S. Steinmetz (Eds.), *Sourcebook of family theories and methods: A contextual approach* (pp. 325–352). New York, NY: Plenum Press.

White, K., Williams, T., & Greenberg, B. (1996). The ecology of medical care. *Bulletin of the New York Academy of Medicine, 73*, 187–212.

Chapter 14
Engaging Communities as Partners in Research: Advancing Integrated Care Through Purposeful Partnerships

Tai Mendenhall, Jerica Berge, and William Doherty

The call for interdisciplinary collaboration in health care is longstanding, and our collective efforts to engage in it are evolving across training programs and healthcare facilities today more than they ever have. Contemporary and cutting-edge advancements in the Patient-Centered Medical Home (PCMH) movement are arguably pushing team-based approaches in continuous and coordinated care toward the middle of the bell curve, wherein someday our integrated models of service delivery will represent the rule—instead of the exception—to how care is provided and carried out.

Our efforts, however, still often miss two things: (1) attention to the active roles that our patients and their families can play in cocreating health and well-being and (2) attention to the potential and collective power of larger patient communities to advance health. Instead, most care models continue to frame professionals as the expert carriers of knowledge and providers of services for patients and families who do not possess much knowledge and who function in ways that are relatively passive. Further, most of what we provide is delivered to patients one at a time, with no mechanism of connecting patients with each other along the way (Berge, Mendenhall, & Doherty, 2009; Doherty, Mendenhall, & Berge, 2010; Mendenhall & Doherty, 2005b).

This is a problem because arguably the greatest untapped resource for improving health is the knowledge, wisdom, and energy of individuals, families, and communities who face challenging health issues in their day-to-day lives (Doherty et al., 2010; Doherty, Mendenhall, & Berge, 2012). Consider, for example, the following questions: How does an adolescent recently diagnosed with diabetes really overhaul her lifestyle (and stick with it) across diet and physical activity arenas? Where is "the line" for this teen's parents between being supportive of her in disease management and being "nags"? How can a husband avoid burning out from supporting his mate whose pain is chronic and whose complaints are never ending?

T. Mendenhall (✉)
University of Minnesota Medical School, Minneapolis, MN, USA
e-mail: mend0009@umn.edu

J. Hodgson et al. (eds.), *Medical Family Therapy*, DOI 10.1007/978-3-319-03482-9_14,

How does he attend to his own health and needs while his partner continues to decline? How do families negotiate with and handle the often intrusive roles of insurance companies, health professionals, and/or social services?

As large national and international organizations focused on health (e.g., Agency for Healthcare, Research, and Quality [AHRQ]; National Institutes for Health [NIH]; World Health Organization [WHO]) have systematically called for—and advanced funding to support—collaborative and community-based efforts to address complex health and social problems ill-suited for conventional service delivery (Hodgson & Reitz, 2013), community-based participatory research (CBPR) has been put forth as a way to purposefully partner with our patients and their families (AHRQ, 2011; National Center on Minority Health and Health Disparities, 2011; NIH, 2013). This is an especially timely call within the arenas of MedFT (specifically) and integrated care (broadly), insofar as our strong emphases on collaborative and supportive relationships (between providers with each other and between providers with patients and families) are well underway. As we extend these emphases to communities of patients and families, we are able to create and implement new interventions—and with broader scope(s)—that neither professionals nor patients/families could create on their own.

Community-Based Participatory Research

As outlined in Chap. 13 of this book (Mendenhall, Pratt, Phelps, Baird & Younkin, 2014), "action research" was first coined in the 1940s, and many have since advanced investigative orientations in which professional investigators collaborate with communities to generate new knowledge and solve local problems (AHRQ, 2004; Berge et al., 2009; Lewin, 1946; Mendenhall & Doherty, 2005b). Approaches within this larger frame vary in the degrees to which researchers and community members facilitate group processes, make decisions and advance interventions, and undertake roles as co-learners (Bell et al., 2004; Cornwall & Jewkes, 1995; Wallerstein & Duran, 2006). These approaches have been recognized by unique and overlapping terminologies like "participatory research" (Classen et al., 2008; Torre & Fine, 2005), "participatory action research" (Baum, MacDougall, & Smith, 2006; Bell et al., 2004; Braithwaite, Coghlan, O'Neill, & Rebane, 2007; Cammarota & Fine, 2008; Kemmis & McTaggart, 2000; Pyrch, 2007; Pyrch & Castillo, 2001; Rahman & Fals-Borda, 1991), "critical action research" (DePoy, Hartman, & Haslett, 1999), "collaborative inquiry" (Kelly, Mock, & Tandon, 2001), "development leadership teams in action" (DELTA) (Haaland & Vlassoff, 2011), "cooperative inquiry" (Heron & Reason, 2001), and "appreciative inquiry" (Ludema, Cooperrider, & Barrett, 2001). Some have framed their efforts around healthcare practices (vs. specific diseases) in partnership with communities of patients, e.g., "practice-based participatory research (PBPR)" (Fauth & Tremblay, 2011), and still others have altogether excluded the word "research" so as to accentuate co-learning and change processes per se, e.g., "participatory action development" (Lammerink, Bury, & Bolt, 1999) and "participatory action learning" (Wilson, Ho, & Walsh, 2007). As national and international organizations focused on health have encouraged these types of efforts, the term "community-based participatory research" has been adopted as an inclusive umbrella (AHRQ, 2004; Edwards, Lund, Mitchell, & Anderson, 2008; Pan American Health Organization, 2004).

In CBPR, the "community" (however, it is defined) is recognized as a principal unit of identity, with lay members and professionals serving as collaborators across every stage of the process. This is remarkably different than the top-down, hierarchical methods of research and care that have conventionally been imposed upon our patient communities. Core assumptions guiding CBPR (see Fig. 14.1) advance these partnerships, from establishing project foci to implementing and evaluating interventions, to disseminating knowledge, and to refining practice in accord to said knowledge. Throughout this work, everyone works together in the context of flattened hierarchies, with each contributing expertise to a larger mosaic of understanding (Hacker, 2013; Minkler & Wallerstein, 2008; Mendenhall, Doherty, Berge, Fauth, & Tremblay, 2013).

Medical Family Therapists (MedFTs) are considerably well equipped to engage in this type of research, in large part, because the core principles that guide them are closely aligned with those that guide CBPR. MedFT's foundation in systems theory (Goldenberg & Goldenberg, 2012; Whitchurch & Constantine, 1993) and investment in advancing care with biopsychosocial-spiritual (BPSS) sensitivity (Engel, 1979, 1980; Rumbold, 2007; White, Williams, & Greenberg, 1996) embrace the complexities inherent to understanding any significant healthcare problem. Connecting individual patients' and families' experiences to larger contexts (e.g., healthcare systems, social systems) is an easy conceptual bridge for MedFTs, and this can push investigational queries and care interventions beyond any conventional one patient or family at-a-time approach. Extending care's focus in this manner also includes purposeful attention to the multiple providers involved in patients' and families' care, which is consistent with MedFT's investment in interdisciplinary collaboration and careful attention to healthcare's clinical, operational, and financial worlds (Peek, 2008). MedFT's value on agency (McDaniel, Doherty, & Hepworth, 2013; McDaniel, Hepworth, & Doherty, 1992) is a ready facilitator to patient and family engagement in CBPR as active participators and contributors to health, and its value on communion (McDaniel et al., 1992, 2013) advances doing so collectively.

Core Tenets Guiding Professional-Community Partnerships

Drawing from the core assumptions outlined above, the five tenets most relevant to the relationships maintained by CBPR collaborators are as follows:

Build upon existing strengths and resources. Whereas conventional approaches in health care begin with a "needs assessment" (i.e., deficit based) to

1. Recognition of the community as the principal unit of identity
2. Democratic and equitable partnership between all project members (e.g., community stakeholders, researchers) as collaborators through every stage of knowledge and intervention development
3. Building on the strengths and resources within the community
4. Promoting co-learning and capacity-building between and among partners
5. Deep investment in change that carries with it an element of challenging the status-quo and improving the lives of members in a community or practice
6. Cyclical process in which problems are identified, solutions to address problems are developed within the context(s) of the community's existing resources, interventions are implemented, outcomes are evaluated according to what is essential in the eyes of participants, and interventions are modified in accord with new information as necessary
7. Project members' humility and flexibility to accommodate changes as necessary across any part of a project
8. Disseminating findings and new knowledge to and by all partners and constituents in the investigative process
9. Recognition that CBPR can be a slow and messy process, especially during initial phases of development
10. Long-term engagement and commitment to the work

Fig. 14.1 Core assumptions of community-based participatory research (Hacker, 2013; Mendenhall et al., 2013; Minkler & Wallerstein, 2008)

inform professionals about what knowledge or resources to bring into a community, CBPR emphasizes the identification and advancement of local strengths, wisdom, and energies. This sets the stage for an equal valuing of professional and lay contributions to problem-solving (Mendenhall & Doherty, 2005a; Reason & Bradbury, 2001, 2006, 2008). For example, hosting a community forum wherein professionals ask patients and their families to share wisdom (e.g., "If a teen came into clinic today and was diagnosed with diabetes, what advice would you first offer to him or her? What would you tell the teen's parents?") sets a strength-based stage upon which a collective want to take action can naturally ensue. Indeed, considering the question "How can we all work together to improve health in our community?" feels very different than "How can professionals deliver more services to fix us?" (Berge, Mendenhall, & Doherty, 2009; Mendenhall et al., 2013).

Partner democratically and equitably. In contrast to conventional care, research, and public health initiatives (i.e., that are professionally led), CBPR projects are advanced with flattened professional hierarchies that honor the unique wisdom and expertise of everyone involved. While healthcare professionals and academic researchers bring with them an information and skill set regarding a disease or investigatory design, for example, patients bring with them an understanding of what it is like to live with the disease (Mendenhall et al., 2013). Patients' family members bring with them knowledge about how to best be supportive, tried-and-true strategies for accessing and affording indicated foods and medicines, and/or self-care so as to not experience compassion fatigue. Community leaders bring with them expertise and understanding about the local "pulse" and impact(s) that a health issue is having on their people. By recognizing and honoring all project members' respective contributions, patients, community stakeholders, healthcare providers, and academic researchers are able to collaborate through every stage of knowledge and intervention development—from early steps in building trust to later steps of evaluating a project and ensuring its long-term sustainability (Christopher, Watts, McCormick, & Young, 2008; Horowitz, Robinson, & Seifer, 2009; Israel, 2005; Wallerstein & Duran, 2010).

Learn and build capacity together. By focusing on each other's unique wisdoms and strengths and working together collaboratively, professionals and community members learn from each other. For example, as patients and families learn from providers about important information regarding a disease and its management (e.g., physical symptoms to watch for, good foods to eat, indicated amounts of exercise), they are also learning from other patients and families about where to find affordable foods or participate in physical activity safely. As providers learn from patients about local value systems regarding diet and health, they are able to advance more sensitive and culturally personalized care, suggestions, and dialogue (Bradbury & Reason, 2003; Doherty et al., 2010; Mendenhall et al., 2010; Minkler & Wallerstein, 2008).

Be (and stay) humble and flexible. Project members in CBPR maintain consistent humility regarding the extent of their knowledge and, along with this, receptivity to others' wisdom. They are responsive to new information that suggests indicated change across individual (e.g., a patient learning that she must alter a health-related routine) and/or project/community (e.g., modifying an intervention component in response to evaluation data that show it is not working) levels. This can be especially difficult for professional members of the team, as much of their medical or graduate training socializes them to function as unerring experts (Hayes, 1996; Mendenhall, 2002; Mendenhall & Doherty, 2003; Minkler, 2000; Minkler & Wallerstein, 2008). Rigidly staying the course, for example, with a project's original plan, may be consistent with professionals' training to abide by deliverables and research designs put forth to a funder, but in CBPR a project's course must flow with its cocreated processes and iterative cycles of data collection, analysis, and intervention development/refinement (Mendenhall et al., 2013).

Engage in and commit to the work for the long haul. CBPR projects can be very slow and messy to create and advance, especially during their early phases, as professionals and community members learn to work together and/or until a new initiative is firmly grounded in a professional or community organization. Our experience across several projects suggests that 1–2 years is a reasonable amount of time to expect between first meetings and the actual launching of action steps, implementation of new interventions, and collection of data relevant to program processes and/or outcomes and effectiveness. It is important that all participants understand this from the outset (i.e., so that they do not misinterpret a project's slow pace to represent failure) and that they are invested in working over the long haul (Doherty et al., 2010; Jones & Wells, 2007; Wallerstein & Duran, 2006, 2010).

Data Collection and Analyses in CBPR

An essential element in CBPR relates to the clarity of its "R," i.e., advancing a clear effort in the arenas that professional and lay communities would call "research." Because project participants are often dealing with novel problems within the unique contexts of local communities, they must be methodologically flexible and varied in order to best match data collection efforts with what is going on in the CBPR activity (McNicoll, 1999; Mendenhall & Doherty, 2005b). To be sensitive to the perspectives and needs of multiple participants, it is important to use methods and measures that have high face validity and practical (and immediate) utility. For this reason, CBPR researchers often gravitate toward qualitative methods of data collection during early phases of the work. Exploring, for example, participants' subjective experiences can serve to engage communities in identifying concerns that run deep and collectively within them. Monitoring intermember and intergroup processes as solutions are collaboratively and democratically developed and implemented can serve to inform others about how professionals and community members work best together. Exploring personal satisfaction with results of new interventions can further guide refinement of said interventions and inform later, more formal, evaluations. While objective (i.e., quantitative) measures of "success" can be created to assess a program's impact on a particular dependent variable (e.g., blood pressure or how many cigarettes somebody smokes per day), most CBPR researchers do not do this until after a project is comparatively underway.

To this end, a wide variety of qualitative data have been described in CBPR literature, including in-depth interviews (Lindsey & McGuinness, 1998; Mendenhall & Doherty, 2003; Mendenhall, Harper, Stephenson, & Haas, 2011), thematic and content analysis of group process notes and publicly available documents (Mendenhall & Doherty, 2003; Nichols, 1995), focus groups (Small, 1995), naturalistic case studies (Casswell, 2000), reflective journaling and meeting minutes (Hampshire, Blair, Crown, Avery, & Williams, 1999; Nichols, 1995), participant observation (Lindsey & McGuinness, 1998), oral histories (Small, 1995), and social network mapping (Bradbury & Reason, 2003). Access to many of these types of data is generally easy for investigators in CBPR, insofar as the very nature of the work requires that they be active participators in the projects that are being evaluated (Mendenhall & Doherty, 2005b; Mendenhall et al., 2013).

Whereas qualitative analyses are especially useful in helping investigators to understand participants' contexts, cultures, beliefs, attitudes, community practices, and subjective experiences related to CBPR processes, quantitative measures are usually and most usefully employed to evaluate the effectiveness of an intervention (Mendenhall & Doherty, 2005b; Reese, Ahern, Nair, O'Faire, & Warren, 1999). These efforts are also important on "political" grounds because formally testing for objective change in tangible measures helps to advance respect and regard by the broader scientific community that the effort being advanced is rigorous and credible (Minkler & Wallerstein, 2008; NIH, 2009).

In accord with basic tenets of CBPR, however, it is important to democratically involve participants in selecting what to evaluate or measure quantitatively. For example, in an initiative designed to reduce smoking on a local school campus, participants (researchers and community members) discussed how students' smoking prevalence was—and was not—an important measure of "success." Indeed, student participants saw the number of available after-school activities (which were advanced by the project to target the stress and boredom that students commonly attributed to smoking) was a more important quantitative measure of success (Mendenhall et al., 2011; Mendenhall, Whipple, Harper, & Haas, 2008). In another CBPR project, providers involved in a diabetes initiative for adolescents saw metabolic control as the most important evaluative dependent variable, whereas adolescent patients wanted to track school policies regarding whether students with diabetes were allowed to go on fieldtrips with their peers (Mendenhall & Doherty, 2007b). In these and other CBPR projects, what is quantitatively tested is up to the whole group to decide. It is important to note, too, that quantitative analyses in CBPR tend to remain "local"—i.e., for, by, and within the community in which a project is positioned (Mendenhall & Doherty, 2005b; Mendenhall et al., 2013). Efforts to test widespread generalizability (e.g., a randomized control trial) are less indicated than efforts to test local effectiveness (e.g., a single-group repeated-measures trial) because CBPR projects are designed purposefully to tap and reflect the unique challenges and resources of their resident communities (Hacker, 2013; Minkler & Wallerstein, 2008).

Ultimately, participants in CBPR tend to combine both qualitative and quantitative methods. This enables researchers to triangulate different sources of data, thereby increasing confidence in conclusions drawn (Hagey, 1997; Lindsey & McGuinness, 1998; McKibbin & Castle, 1996; Nichols, 1995). Throughout this and the cyclical processes of CBPR, all data that are collected and analyzed are presented back to the initiative's participants (Mendenhall & Doherty, 2005b; Meyer, 2000; Nichols, 1995). This facilitates an active and purposeful dialogue between providers, researchers, and community members about the meanings and usefulness of data, which then informs the creation and generation of ensuing action steps en route to collaboratively identified and mutually shared goals and to disseminating the work across varied and indicated arenas.

Disseminating CBPR

Disseminating research findings is another important aspect of community-based participatory research. By presenting results, researchers can communicate the success of a project, changes brought about by its labors, and the ongoing efforts that researchers/families/community members are doing to sustain the work. CBPR teams, then, collaborate fully in writing and disseminating study findings to professional/scientific communities, community-specific organizations, and the general public. To share knowledge with other professionals and the scientific community, they target refereed journals and local, national, and international conferences and forums. To share knowledge with community-specific organizations, the local community itself, and the general public, team members connect with community service providers and resources, e.g., targeting local and statewide public print and electronic media and community events/celebrations (Berge et al., 2009; Minkler & Wallerstein, 2008).

Action Strategies

In Fig. 14.2, the authors present a summary of action strategies for the initiation and conduct of CBPR in healthcare settings—or "Citizen Health Care"—based on their own and colleagues' collective experiences (Berge et al., 2009; Doherty & Mendenhall, 2006; Doherty et al., 2010; Mendenhall et al., 2010, 2013). In the early phases of a project's evolution, we have found that it is best to request little or no financial support from professional and/or administrative leaders because this helps to facilitate their buy-in while synchronously allowing the project to evolve without external pressures in terms of time or outcomes/deliverables. Proceeding in this manner is also important so as to convey to community members that the professionals' investment in the work is not wholly contingent upon being awarded a grant or some other kind of formal reward or accolade. This also enables professionals and community members to advance their attention to "go deep" in identifying health-related issues that are of great concern to all involved (Doherty et al., 2010, p. 392).

Before inviting a large group of community leaders to begin generating solutions and interventions, it is important for a small group of community members with personal experience (but without institutional constraints or priorities) to establish consensus in its focus and desire to proceed. As the project's membership is then strategically expanded and its momentum surges, community and citizen dimensions of the issue are examined, which then informs the development and implementation of action steps. Throughout this journey, democratic planning and decision-making are carried out through each step of the work. Professionals and community members continue to learn from each other, and project results continue

1. Get buy-in from key professional leaders and administrators.
   These are the gatekeepers who must support the initiation of a project based on its potential to meet one of the goals of the health care setting. However, we have found it best to request little or no budget, aside from a small amount of staff time, in order to allow the project enough incubation time before being expected to justify its outcomes.

2. Identify a health issue that is of great concern to both professionals and members of a specific community (clinic, neighborhood, cultural group in a geographical location).
   Stated differently, the issue must be one that a community of citizens actually cares about —not just something that we think they should care about. And the professionals initiating the project must have enough passion for the issue to sustain their efforts over time.

3. Identify potential community leaders who have personal experience with the health issue and who have relationships with the professional team.
   These leaders should generally be ordinary members of the community who in some way have mastered the health issue in their own lives and who have a desire to give back to their community. "Positional" leaders who head community agencies are generally not the best group to engage at this stage, because they bring institutional priorities and constraints.

4. Invite a small group of community leaders (3-4 people) to meet several times with the professional team to explore the issue and see if there is a consensus to proceed with a larger community project.
   These are preliminary discussions to see if a project is feasible and to begin creating a professional/citizen leadership group.

5. This group decides on how to invite a larger group of community leaders (10-15) to begin the process of generating the project.
   One invitational strategy we have used is for providers to nominate patients and family members who have lived expertise with a health issue and who appear to have leadership potential.

6. Over the next six months of biweekly meetings, implement the following steps of community organizing:

   i. Exploring the community and citizen dimensions of the issue in depth
   ii. Creating a name and mission
   iii. Doing one-to-one interviews with a range of stakeholders
   iv. Generating potential action initiatives, processing them in terms of the Citizen Health Care Model and their feasibility with existing community resources
   v. Deciding on a specific action initiative and implementing it

Fig. 14.2 (continued)

to inform intervention designs and revisions as indicated. Attention is paid consistently to identifying and developing new leaders, who then carry forward the project's efforts over time en route to its larger missions of effecting beneficent and widespread change.

7. Employ the following key processes:

    i. Democratic planning and decision making at every step. As mentioned before, this requires training of the professionals who bring a disciplined process model and a vision of collective action that does not lapse back into the conventional provider/consumer model, but who do not control the outcome or action steps the group decides to take.

    ii. Mutual teaching and learning among community members. Action initiatives consistent with the model first call upon the lived-experience of community members, with the support of professionals, rather than recruiting community members to support a professionally-created initiative.

    iii. Creating ways to fold new learnings back into the community. All learnings can become "community property" if there is a way for them to be passed on. Currently we have vehicles for professionals to become "learning communities," but few vehicles outside of Internet chat rooms for patients and families to become learning communities.

    iv. Identifying and developing leaders. The heart of community organizing is finding and nurturing people who have leadership ability but who are not necessarily heads of organizations with turfs to protect.

    v. Using professional expertise selectively—"on tap," not "on top." In this way of working, all knowledge is public knowledge, democratically held and shared when it can be useful. Professionals bring a unique font of knowledge and experience — and access to current research—to Citizen Health Care initiatives. But everyone else around the table also brings unique knowledge and expertise. Because of the powerful draw of the provider/consumer way of operating, professionals must learn to share their unique expertise when it fits the moment, and to be quiet when someone else can just as readily speak to the issue. A community organizing axiom applies here: Never say what someone in the community could say, and never do what someone else in the community could do.

    vi. Forging a sense of larger purpose beyond helping immediate participants. Keep the Big, Hairy, Audacious Goal (BHAG) in mind as you act in a local community. Citizen Health Care is not just about people helping people; it is about social change towards more activated citizens in the health care system and larger culture. This understanding inspires members of the Citizen Health Project about the larger significance of their work. It also attracts media and other prominent community members to seek to understand, publicize, and disseminate Citizen Health Care projects.

Fig. 14.2 Action strategies for CBPR and citizen health care (Doherty et al., 2010; Mendenhall et al., 2013)

Lessons Learned

Alongside attendance to the action strategies outlined above, there are a number of important lessons that the authors have learned in CBPR that could be helpful to know as one advances similar work; see Fig. 14.3 (Doherty & Mendenhall, 2006; Doherty et al., 2010; Mendenhall et al., 2010, 2013). First, doing this work does not

1. This work is about identity transformation as a citizen professional, not just about learning a new set of skills.
2. It is about identifying and developing leaders in the community more than about a specific issue or action.
3. It is about sustained initiatives, not one-time events.
4. Citizen initiatives are often slow and messy, especially during the gestation period.
5. You need a champion with influence in the institution.
6. Until grounded in an institution's culture and practices, these initiatives are quite vulnerable to shifts in the organizational context.
7. A professional who is putting too much time into a project is over-functioning and not using the model. We have found that the average time commitment to be on the order of 6-8 hours per month, but over a number of years.
8. External funding at the outset can be a trap because of timelines and deliverables, but funding can be useful for capacity building to learn the model, and for expanding the scope of citizen projects once they are developed.
9. The pull of the traditional provider/consumer model is very strong on all sides; democratic decision making requires eternal vigilance.

decision making requires eternal vigilance.

10. You cannot learn this approach without mentoring, and it takes two years to get good at it.

Fig. 14.3 Lessons learned in CBPR and citizen health care (Doherty et al., 2010; Mendenhall et al., 2013)

require a large amount of professionals' time (6–8 h per month, on average), but it does require a long-term commitment (several years or more). Second, learning how to do this kind of work requires mentorship. Simply reading about CBPR, listening to a presentation about it at a professional conference, or even checking in and consulting about it (in much the same way that therapy supervision looks when trainees conduct their work behind a one-way mirror), and then directly proceeding with a project can be likened to reading a book about how to ride a bicycle and then expecting to embark upon a trip without falling. There are no quick ways to teach professionals the public skills of engaging other citizens in CBPR or related community organizing projects with flattened hierarchies; direct observation and coaching (with frequent stops and starts, trials and errors, and discussion/processing) are necessary.

CBPR projects tend to be very vulnerable to falling apart without strong buy-in from an administrative leader and champion within the provider/researcher side of the professional-community partnership. This person does not have to be an active member of the CBPR per se, but he or she often plays a strong role in backing and supporting early efforts in getting something started, e.g., allowing professionals to devote time to the work, advocating for the project, and/or defending it against efforts by other administrative personnel who do not support it. Relatedly, CBPR projects can be vulnerable to shift in organizational contexts if they are not well grounded within an organization's culture before these shifts occur. For example, an early project called *Partners in Diabetes* (Mendenhall, 2002; Mendenhall & Doherty, 2003, 2007a) was disbanded when its partnering residency clinic transitioned to a private practice, whereas the *Family Education Diabetes Series* project (Doherty et al., 2010; Mendenhall et al., 2010) has survived several years of organizational, funding, and administrative changes since its establishment as a foundational part of its hosting organization's mission and services within its local American Indian community.

It is important to highlight how strong the pull of the traditional provider/consumer model is, too, and that maintaining democratic and collaborative efforts in CBPR requires interminable attention. This pull comes from both sides. For example, it can feel very natural for a provider to take over or offer solutions prematurely to a group, insofar as his socialization through graduate or medical school was such that this is what he is "supposed" to do in his "day job." It can feel equally natural for community members to defer to providers for leadership and guidance, because most of us have been socialized to be passive recipients of care when we see a physician (or physician assistant, nurse practitioner, etc.) and/or to follow authority figures' instructions (Doherty et al., 2010; Mendenhall et al., 2013).

Finally, CBPR must meet the needs of professionals for rewarding and satisfying work. We have found that if this public practice fits within one's values and vision, providers and researchers can experience an expanded sense of professional contribution, as well as a closer connection to and relationship with local communities. If health care is to be redesigned in the United States (and, indeed, most argue that it must be), doing so will require that we adopt new forms of partnership between professionals and the patient and family citizens that seek our care. The driving mission behind this work is to create a sustainable democratic model of health care that unleashes the capacity and energy of ordinary citizens as producers of health for themselves and their communities.

Sustainability of CBPR Projects

History is full of exceptional examples of "community projects" that ebbed or stopped altogether as soon as external funding ran out or their charismatic leader (s) left. A key tenet of CBPR is that projects do not follow this path, as extant community resources and energies are tapped and project ownership is collectively shared by a group of citizens that inhabit an initiative or are somehow connected to it (Doherty & Mendenhall, 2006; Mendenhall & Doherty, 2005b; Wallerstein & Duran, 2003). Through the collaborative processes outlined in this chapter, consecutive generations of lay and professional leaders work together to challenge the notion (frequently espoused by academic- and/or health-related fields and literature) that "care" or "research" can only be carried out if/when it is first funded by monies secured by professionals and/or that programs/interventions can only be sustained if funded by monies that are secured in such a manner. Consider specific projects, highlighted below, as examples of this sustainability:

The *Family Education Diabetes Series* (FEDS) is a CBPR project created through the collaborative efforts of providers at the University of Minnesota and local leaders in the Minneapolis/Saint Paul American Indian (AI) community (Mendenhall et al., 2010; Mendenhall, Seal, GreenCrow, LittleWalker, & BrownOwl, 2012). Initiated in 2001 without external funding, participants worked to engage low-income, urban-dwelling AIs and their families in an active forum of education, fellowship, and support through its mission to improve the health and well-being of AI people in manners that embrace their heritage, values, and culture (s). This work has functioned, and continues to function, with and without external funding. For example, intervention resources (e.g., food) have at times been provided through the collective contributions of participants, themselves, and at other times through local state and foundation grants. Professionals' involvement has sometimes been funded by grant monies; other times it has been advanced through voluntary means and/or viewed as part of "outreach" or "community-oriented" components within existing job descriptions.

The *Students Against Nicotine and Tobacco Addiction* (SANTA) initiative, begun in 2006, engages local providers in partnership with students, teachers, and administrators at the Hubert H. Humphrey Job Corps Center in St. Paul, MN, to address on-campus smoking. Its mission is to improve the health and well-being of students through smoking cessation, education, stress reduction, and support. As project members have worked together to answer the question "How do we keep SANTA going as an initiative that is owned and operated by the Job Corps community?" they have come to view its sustainability as both realistic and expected because (1) participating members are highly invested in SANTA surviving long after they have graduated, retired, or otherwise revised the foci of their current work and (2) no independent student-based group in the history of Job Corps has ever lasted as long as SANTA already has. The initiative continues to function with and without external funding, advancing a variety of lively on-campus activities, health and wellness education forums, and group and 1:1 supportive meetings (Mendenhall et al., 2008, 2011).

While most existing literature reflects the investigatory efforts of providers or professional researchers who conducted projects that they secured funding for to create, advance, and/or evaluate, CBPR does not function this way. This work supports the notion that both research and practice efforts can be advanced without depending on (or being delayed by) external funding. Indeed, waiting for external funding is conceptually inconsistent with CBPR tenets because to do so would require relying on professionals' efforts in grant writing while simultaneously prioritizing their needs for work-related status or laudation (which aligns with top-down, provider-driven sequences that are incompatible with authentic participatory approaches). To advance a project in such a way would be to place principal responsibility for an initiative's livelihood on professionals (Doherty et al., 2010; Mendenhall et al., 2010). In CBPR, professional expertise is best positioned as "on tap," not "on top."

CBPR and Integrated Care: Advancing the Research Agenda

As more healthcare providers and researchers—MedFTs included—engage in CBPR projects, what was once broadly viewed by academic and research institutions as flimsy or unscientific is now establishing a niche in the world(s) of valued healthcare research and service provision (Mendenhall & Doherty, 2005b; Minkler & Wallerstein, 2008; NIH, 2013). This evolution is advancing in synchrony with our increased emphases on patient-/family-centered medical homes, wherein comprehensive approaches are advanced within settings that facilitate partnerships between individuals/families and multidisciplinary care teams (Minkler & Wallerstein, 2008; Peek, 2013; Wallerstein & Duran, 2010). Through CBPR methods, patient/family community partnerships with providers are held up as an essential foundation to create care that is high quality, culturally competent, strength based, and effective (Chavez, Duran, Baker, Avila, & Wallerstein, 2003; Doherty et al., 2010; Tobin, 2000; Ward & Trigler, 2001). Over the last decade, projects driven by this approach have gained credibility through their ability to inform understanding of patients' experiences, improve or generate services, facilitate community outreach and engagement, enhance education, and augment cultural awareness (Chavez et al., 2003; Tobin, 2000; Ward & Trigler, 2001). Projects have advanced improvements in asthma (Brugge, Rivera-Carrasco, Zotter, & Leung, 2010), diabetes (Mendenhall & Doherty, 2003, 2007a), dental- and mouth-care practices (Watson, Horowitz, Garcia, & Canto, 2001), smoking cessation (Mendenhall et al., 2011), patient and practitioner satisfaction (e.g., through improved communication and problem-solving skills) (Hampshire et al., 1999; Lewis, Sallee, Trumbo, & Janousek, 2010; Lindsey & McGuinness, 1998; Meyer, 2000; Schulz et al., 2003), and a number of other significant healthcare foci (Doherty et al., 2012; Hacker, 2013; Mendenhall & Doherty, 2005b).

Efforts in CBPR are now proceeding to further advance the research agenda for integrated care by extending our attention beyond disease-specific arenas and narrowly defined clinical outcomes (AHRQ, 2011; Doherty et al., 2012; Fauth & Tremblay, 2011). Understanding(s) about the effects of specific strategies and care processes, levels of integration, and financial models of clinical outcomes is sorely needed, alongside regard for broader clinic- and health system(s)-level functioning (Miller, Kessler, Peek, & Kennenberg, 2010). In order to do this, we must first establish a common language and lexicon of terms and definitions to consistently guide researchers, systems (re)designers, experts in quality improvement and performance measurement, policymakers, and patients/citizens (Peek, 2013; Peek & National Integration Academy Council, 2013). This aligns well with CBPR's emphasis on involving all stakeholders collectively and throughout the aforementioned iterative process(es) of research and intervention development and improvement (Mendenhall & Doherty, 2005b; Minkler & Wallerstein, 2008). And it aligns well with MedFT's emphasis on involving all stakeholders collectively in care (McDaniel et al., 2013). Indeed, to do less would be to fall back on conventional provider-led, expert-driven methods of defining care parameters and to leave behind the voices of the very people that our efforts are supposed to help.

Following recommendations put forth by the AHRQ and Miller, Kessler, Peek, and Kennenberg (AHRQ, 2011; Miller et al., 2010), we must then begin asking descriptive questions to systematically create articulated pictures of how MedFT and related collaborative practices are carried out, followed by evaluative questions that assess outcomes across clinical, operational, and financial foci. CBPR is, again, well equipped to do this. By engaging all stakeholders in care processes, comprehensive descriptions of clinical practices can be gleaned (e.g., MedFTs can describe who they see in their practices and in what care settings; administrators can describe processes by which patients are identified and how care is coordinated and paid for; patients and family members can describe their experiences in working with care teams). To evaluate outcomes connected to a practice's care, engaged stakeholders' voices will similarly inform what is learned (e.g., providers and patients can describe clinical outcomes related to disease management; providers and administrators can describe health system processes related to clinic flow and interdisciplinary collaboration; administrators and patients can describe financial costs related to care initiation and maintenance). Efforts to engage in collaborative efforts such as these are now emerging, as leaders in the field are working to advance CBPR methods into larger health systems and as the pressure to produce high-quality evidence is felt more than ever before (Fauth & Tremblay, 2011; Mendenhall et al., 2013).

Quality of Evaluation and Strength of Research Evidence

While most agree that the guiding principles of CBPR are sensible in the design and implementation of interventions that target complex social and medical presentations (Berge et al., 2009; NIH, 2013), it is essential that the effectiveness of said interventions is demonstrated. Put simply: Does CBPR work? To answer this question, efforts to move past qualitative accounts (only) that capture this research process(es) and/or the understandings/resources it taps along the way are advancing quickly.

CBPR in health care has been advanced and evaluated across a broad range of foci, including (as noted earlier) obesity, diabetes, smoking cessation, asthma, dental- and mouth-care practices, preoperative fasting, accident reduction, safe sexual practices, midwifery, living with disabilities, and overall physical well-being (Barrett, 2011; Brugge et al., 2010; Davis & Reid, 1999; Doherty et al., 2010; Gallagher & Scott, 1997; Garwick & Auger, 2003; Hampshire et al., 1999; Lewis et al., 2010; Lindsey & McGuinness, 1998; Mendenhall & Doherty, 2005b; Meyer, 2000; Schulz et al., 2003; Stevens & Hall, 1998). The following is a brief, but more detailed, review of two of these topics.

CBPR Targeting Diabetes in the American Indian Community

Many providers and patient communities are beginning to engage in novel and collaborative partnerships that honor and tap resources across professional and lay groups where diabetes is of high concern, and CBPR is a leading methodology guiding this effort (Mendenhall & Doherty, 2003, 2005b; Mendenhall et al., 2010). Principal reasons justifying this approach in American Indian (AI) communities rest in its contrast to AIs' earlier experiences with conventional research (i.e., work conducted by outsiders through top-down, expert-driven methods) that has tended to benefit researchers more than Native people (e.g., advancing professionals' prestige and/or tenure), pathologized American Indians as dysfunctional, and not directly informed or enhanced the communities they were supposed to help (e.g., study results not shared or integrated/advanced into new services and outreach) (Burhansstipanov, Christopher, & Schumacher, 2005; Davis & Reid, 1999; Gone, 2009). Emerging projects support the utility of CBPR in cocreating medically sound programs that are sensitive to local customs and cultural traditions. For example, Castro, O'Toole, Brownson, Plessel, and Schauben (2009) found that integrating culturally relevant sequences like talking circles and community forums into standard education and exercise led to improvements in disease knowledge and management. Steckler and Linnan (2002) collaborated with AI and non-AI researchers and staff to incorporate cultural information into curricula for elementary school-aged children, alongside recognizing and emphasizing the importance of family and community involvement. Garwick and Auger (2003) partnered with AI teenagers to increase awareness of asthma and inform providers about how to offer more culturally sensitive, appropriate, and effective care. Potvin, Cargo, McComber, Delormier, and Macaulay (2003) partnered with AIs and local education systems to create sustainable school-based health programs that combine culturally relevant activities and health education. Mendenhall and colleagues (2010, 2012), in the *Family Education Diabetes Series* project presented above, have worked through university/clinic/community partnerships in CBPR to improve health in the American Indian community through significant reductions in weight and blood pressure, improvements in metabolic control (A1c), and increases in physical activity and healthy dietary practices.

CBPR Targeting Smoking Cessation in Adolescents and Young Adults

As the healthcare field(s) has begun to more aggressively address smoking cessation in teenagers and young adults, it has become increasingly clear that the unique challenges, resources, indicated interventions, and processes of implementing interventions for young people are not well understood by researchers positioned in academia who confront smoking from an adult-centric, top-down service-delivery approach. Consistent with the notion that the best person to talk with an adolescent is often another teenager, researchers are aligning with the CBPR principle that recognizes that the greatest untapped resource in our efforts is the lived experience and wisdom of the very individuals that we seek to influence. Through the employment of CPBR, Tsark (2001) addressed the need for culturally/ethnically appropriate and relevant approaches to reduce tobacco use among Native Hawaiians. The collaborative process was effective in the construction of a user-friendly survey tool to gather data from a broad range of community constituencies, community-specific findings with direct application to ongoing intervention design (s), and expanded local capacity for health promotion on a larger scale. Powers, Gillies, Madeley, and Abbot (1989) employed similar methods with a very different group. Engaging young mothers as active participators in CBPR to reduce smoking behaviors, the Nottingham Mother's Stop Smoking Project was designed and successfully implemented in a small New Zealand community. Burton et al. (2004) and Shelley et al. (2008) are currently working in partnership with the Chinese American community in New York City and have developed a multi-modal intervention to reduce smoking behaviors in young adults that encompasses awareness campaigns, telephone support and services, print materials, and neighborhood groups. In Pennsylvania and New Jersey, Ma and colleagues (2004) are similarly working to engage members of the local Asian community to address tobacco and cancer control. Mendenhall and colleagues (2008, 2011), in the *Students Against Nicotine and Tobacco Addiction* project (outlined above), have worked through university/clinic/community partnerships to improve adolescents' health through increased activities to reduce stress, increase readiness to change, and curb smoking.

CBPR Outcome Studies: What Do They Really Tell Us?

The common thread that runs through these and related projects is that CBPR methods serve to engage community members as active participators in research and care. Unlike conventional approaches (i.e., those that seek to design a single intervention that can be transported across different communities with positive quantitative results that are replicated time and again to prove its merit), CBPR researchers seek to develop interventions that are immediately relevant to the specific communities in which they are positioned. By addressing local and unique challenges in context, and tapping local wisdom and unique resources in context, participants in CBPR are increasingly (and repeatedly) showing the world that their efforts work. And while widespread generalizability of any single CBPR intervention is not realistic (or even sought), the immediate relevance and positive outcomes for local communities is seen as worth the trade-off (McGarvey, 1993; Mendenhall & Doherty, 2005b; Morrison & Lilford, 2001). CBPR outcome studies tell us, then, that engaging in such efforts where they have not heretofore been advanced is worth the risk. Others have done it; why not MedFTs?

Closing Thoughts

At the outset of this chapter, the authors maintained that the call for interdisciplinary collaboration in health care is something that most practicing providers have heard and that our early and collective efforts to answer this call are evolving across training programs and care facilities, alike. However, it is essential that we not forget to include the patients and families that we serve. Indeed, the greatest untapped resource for improving health is the knowledge, wisdom, and energy that they have acquired through facing and living with challenging issues in their everyday lives. MedFT's investments in agency and communion are readily facilitative of creating space to tap this resource and to advance research and new interventions that pair it collaboratively with providers' knowledge and expertise.

Through the use of CBPR methods, we all are able to contribute professional and personal pieces to a larger mosaic of care that nobody—clinicians, researchers, patients, family members, other community members—could, respectively, do by themselves. Ultimately, what we create can advance a broader scope than any (interdisciplinary, collaborative, or otherwise) top-down, provider-led one patient at-a-time model could reach. Projects are sustainable, too, because they are owned and operated by the communities that they are positioned in (vs. relying wholly on professional leadership or grant funding for support). Participants in CBPR believe in what they are doing and are energized by the collective energy they share to promote broad and meaningful change.

Discussion Questions

1. One of the tenets that guide community-based participatory research (CBPR) is that professionals and community members work together in the context(s) of flattened hierarchies so that each can contribute to a larger mosaic of knowledge. However, professionals are socialized through their training to be "experts" vis-à-vis patients who are socialized to be passive recipients of their care. In a CBPR project, how can professionals be vigilant about not rushing in to answer questions, problem-solving for the group, or take over meetings? How can community members feel safe and empowered to participate on par with professionals who they may have heretofore been intimidated by, hesitant to challenge, or overly reverent regarding?
2. The authors maintain that seeking out funding to begin a CBPR project can potentially sabotage the democratic process, timeframe, and tasks that its participants undertake. Additionally, CBPR efforts that are "owned and operated" by the communities in which they are positioned have demonstrated sustainability with and without external funding. If part of a professional's performance, however, is evaluated according to research dollars secured, how can she best engage in this type of work? Is CBPR only well matched for clinical

professionals who are not required to write grants or for university faculty who have already achieved tenure? Are there others ways that employers can think about CBPR in their evaluative efforts of employees?

3. Within your own community (defined by identification with a particular health challenge or patient population, clinic/hospital site, or geographic area), what is a "pressure point" for which conventional means of care or outreach have not worked? How could a CBPR project be explored and advanced to tackle this challenge? Who are your key stakeholders? What steps would you take to begin?

References[1]

Agency for Healthcare Research and Quality. (2004). *Community-based participatory research: Assessing the evidence*. Rockville, MD: AHRC. http://www.ncbi.nlm.nih.gov/books/NBK11852/.

Agency for Healthcare Research and Quality. (2011). A national agenda for research in collaborative care: Papers from the Collaborative Care Research Network research development conference. Agency for Healthcare Research and Quality. Retrieved from http://www.ahrq.gov/research/collaborativecare/.

Barrett, P. (2011). The Early Mothering Project: What happened when the words "action research" came to life for a group of midwives. In P. Reason & H. Bradbury (Eds.), *Handbook of action research: Participative inquiry and practice* (pp. 294–300). London: Sage.

Baum, F., MacDougall, C., & Smith, D. (2006). Participatory action research. *Journal of Epidemiology and Community Health, 60*, 854–857. doi:10.1136/jech.2004.028662.

Bell, J., Cheney, G., Hoots, C., Kohrman, E., Schubert, J., Stidham, L., ... Traynor, S. (2004). *Comparative similarities and differences between action research, participative research, and participatory action research*. Seattle, WA: Antioch University Seattle. Retrieved from http://arlecchino.org/ildottore/mwsd/group2final-comparison.html.

Berge, J., Mendenhall, T., & Doherty, W. (2009). Using Community-Based Participatory Research (CBPR) to target health disparities in families. *Family Relations, 58*, 475–488. doi:10.1111/j.1741-3729.2009.00567.x.

Bradbury, H., & Reason, P. (2003). Action research: An opportunity for revitalizing research purpose and practices. *Qualitative Social Work, 2*, 155–175. doi:10.1177/1473325003002002003.

Braithwaite, R., Coghlan, S., O'Neill, M., & Rebane, D. (2007). Insider participatory action research in disadvantaged post-industrial areas: The experiences of community members as they become community based action researchers. *Action Research, 5*, 61–74. doi:10.1177/1476750307072876.

Brugge, D., Rivera-Carrasco, E., Zotter, J., & Leung, A. (2010). Community-based participatory research in Boston's neighborhoods: A review of asthma case examples. *Archives of Environmental & Occupational Health, 12*, 70–76. doi:10.1080/19338240903390214.

Burhansstipanov, L., Christopher, S., & Schumacher, S. (2005). Lessons learned from community-based participatory research in Indian country. *Cancer, Cancer, Culture and Literacy Supplement*, 70–76. Retrieved from http://www.ncbi.nlm.nih.gov/pmc/articles/PMC3544402/.

[1] An asterisk has been use to note references that the chapter authors recommend for further reading.

Burton, D., Fahs, M., Chang, J., Qu, J., Chan, F., Yen, F., ... Shelley, D. (2004). Community-based participatory research on smoking cessation among Chinese Americans in Flushing, Queens, New York City. *Journal of Interprofessional Care, 18*, 443–445. doi: 10.1080/13561820400011412.

Cammarota, J., & Fine, M. (2008). *Revolutionizing education: Youth participation action research in motion*. New York: Routledge.

Casswell, S. (2000). A decade of community action research. *Substance Use and Abuse, 35*, 55–74. doi:10.3109/10826080009147686.

Castro, S., O'Toole, M., Brownson, C., Plessel, K., & Schauben, L. (2009). A diabetes self-management program designed for urban American Indians. *Public Health Research, Practice, and Policy, 6*, 1–8. http://198.246.124.29/pcd/issues/2009/oct/pdf/08_0147.pdf.

Chavez, V., Duran, B., Baker, Q. E., Avila, M. M., & Wallerstein, N. (2003). The dance of race and privilege in community-based participatory research. In M. Minkler & N. Wallerstein (Eds.), *Community Based Participatory Research for Health* (pp. 81–97). San Francisco: Jossey-Bass.

Christopher, S., Watts, V., McCormick, A., & Young, S. (2008). Building and maintaining trust in a community-based participatory research partnership. *American Journal of Public Health, 98*, 1398–1406. http://ajph.aphapublications.org/doi/pdf/10.2105/AJPH.2007.125757.

Classen, L., Humphries, S., Fitzsimons, J., Kaaria, S., Jimenez, J., Sierra, F., & Gallardo, O. (2008). Opening participatory spaces for the most marginal: Learning from collective action in Honduran hillsides. *World Development, 36*, 2402–2420. Retrieved from http://www.sciencedirect.com/science/article/pii/S0305750X08001708.

Cornwall, A., & Jewkes, R. (1995). What is participatory research? *Social Science Medicine, 41*, 1667–1676. doi:10.1016/0277-9536(95)00127-S.

Davis, S. M., & Reid, R. (1999). Practicing participatory research in American Indian communities. *American Journal of Clinical Nutrition, 69*, 755S–759S. http://ajcn.nutrition.org/content/69/4/755S.long.

DePoy, E., Hartman, A., & Haslett, D. (1999). Critical action research: A model for social work knowing. *Social Work, 44*, 560–569. doi:10.1093/sw/44.6.560.

Doherty, W., & Mendenhall, T. (2006). Citizen health care: A model for engaging patients, families, and communities as co-producers of health. *Families, Systems & Health, 24*, 357–362. doi:10.1037/1091-7527.24.3.251.

*Doherty, W., Mendenhall, T., & Berge, J. (2010). The Families & Democracy and Citizen Health Care Project. *Journal of Marital and Family Therapy, 36*, 389–402. doi:10.1111/j.1752-0606.2009.00142.x.

Doherty, W., Mendenhall, T., & Berge, J. (2012). Citizen Professional Center. University of Minnesota. Retrieved from http://www.cehd.umn.edu/cpc/projects.html.

Edwards, K., Lund, C., Mitchell, S., & Anderson, N. (2008). Trust the process: Community-based research partnerships. *Journal of Aboriginal and Indigenous Community Health, 6*, 187–199. http://www.ncbi.nlm.nih.gov/pmc/articles/PMC2942844/.

Engel, G. (1979). The need for a new medical model: A challenge for biomedicine. *Science, 196*, 129–136. doi:10.1126/science.847460.

Engel, G. (1980). The clinical application of the biopsychosocial model. *American Journal of Psychiatry, 137*, 535–544. doi:10.1093/jmp/6.2.101.

*Fauth, J., & Tremblay, G. (2011). Beyond dissemination and translation: Practice based participatory research. *Psychotherapy Bulletin*. Retrieved from http://www.divisionofpsychotherapy.org/wp-content/uploads/2011/03/Bulletin46-1.pdf.

Gallagher, E., & Scott, V. (1997). The STEPS project: Participatory action research to reduce falls in public places among seniors and persons with disabilities. *Canadian Journal of Public Health, 88*, 129–133. http://www.ncbi.nlm.nih.gov/pubmed/9170693.

Garwick, A. W., & Auger, S. (2003). Participatory action research: The Indian Family Stories Project. *Nursing Outlook, 51*, 261–266. doi:10.1016/j.outlook.2003.09.006.

Goldenberg, H., & Goldenberg, I. (2012). *Family therapy: An overview* (8th ed.). Belmont, CA: Brooks/Cole.

Gone, J. P. (2009). A community-based treatment for Native American historical trauma: Prospects for evidence-based practice. *Journal of Consulting and Clinical Psychology, 77*, 751–762. doi:10.1037/a0015390.

Haaland, A., & Vlassoff, C. (2011). Introducing health workers for change: From transformation theory to health systems in developing countries. *Health Policy and Planning, 16*(Suppl 1), 1–6. doi:10.1093/heapol/16.suppl_1.1.

*Hacker, K. (2013). *Community-based Participatory Research*. Thousand Oaks, CA: Sage.

Hagey, R. S. (1997). The use and abuse of participatory action research. *Chronic Disease & Cancer, 18*, 1–4. http://www.ncbi.nlm.nih.gov/pubmed/9188513.

Hampshire, A., Blair, M., Crown, N., Avery, A., & Williams, I. (1999). Action research: A useful method of promoting change in primary care? *Family Practice, 16*, 305–311. doi:10.1093/fampra/16.3.305.

Hayes, P. (1996). Is there a place for action research? *Clinical Nursing Research, 5*, 3–5. doi:10.1177/105477389600500101.

Heron, J., & Reason, P. (2001). The practice of co-operative inquiry: Research "with" rather than "on" people. In P. Reason & H. Bradbury (Eds.), *Handbook of action research: Participative inquiry and practice* (pp. 179–188). London: Sage.

Hodgson, J., & Reitz, R. (2013). The financial history and near future of collaborative care. In M. Talen & A. Valeras (Eds.), *Integrated behavioral health in primary care: Evaluating the evidence, identifying the essentials* (pp. 167–188). New York, NY: Springer.

Horowitz, C., Robinson, M., & Seifer, S. (2009). Community-based participatory research from margin to mainstream: A researchers prepared? *Circulation, 119*, 2633–2642. doi:10.1161/CIRCULATIONAHA.107.729863.

Israel, B. (2005). Introduction to methods in community-based participatory research for health. In B. Israel, E. Eng, A. Schulz, & E. Parker (Eds.), *Methods in Community Based Participatory Research for Health* (pp. 3–29). San Francisco, CA: Jossey-Bass.

Jones, L., & Wells, K. (2007). Strategies for academic and clinician engagement in community-participatory partnered research. *Journal of the American Medical Association, 296*, 407–410. doi:10.1001/jama.297.4.407.

Kelly, J., Mock, L., & Tandon, D. (2001). Collaborative inquiry with African American community leaders: Comments on a participatory action research process. In P. Reason & H. Bradbury (Eds.), *Handbook of action research: Participatory inquiry and practice* (pp. 348–355). London: Sage.

Kemmis, S., & McTaggart, R. (2000). Participatory action research. In N. Denzin & Y. Lincoln (Eds.), *Handbook of Qualitative Research* (pp. 567–605). Thousand Oaks, CA: Sage.

Lammerink, M., Bury, P., & Bolt, E. (1999). An introduction to participatory action development. *Participatory Learning and Action, 35*, 29–33. http://pubs.iied.org/pdfs/G01830.pdf.

Lewin, K. (1946). Action research and minority problems. *Journal of Social Issues, 2*, 34–46. doi:10.1111/j.1540-4560.1946.tb02295.x.

Lewis, K., Sallee, D., Trumbo, J., & Janousek, K. (2010). Use of community-based participatory research methods in adults' health assessment. *Journal of Applied Psychology, 40*, 195–211. doi:10.1111/j.1559-1816.2009.00570.x.

Lindsey, E., & McGuinness, L. (1998). Significant elements of community involvement in participatory action research: Evidence from a community project. *Journal of Advanced Nursing, 28*, 1106–1114. doi:10.1046/j.1365-2648.1998.00816.x.

Ludema, J., Cooperrider, D., & Barrett, F. (2001). Appreciative inquiry: The power of the unconditional positive question. In P. Reason & H. Bradbury (Eds.), *Handbook of action research: Participative inquiry and practice* (pp. 189–199). London: Sage.

Ma, G., Toubbeh, J., Su, X., & Edwards, R. (2004). ATECAR: An Asian American community-based participatory research model on tobacco and cancer control. *Health Promotion and Practice, 5*, 382–394. doi:10.1177/1524839903260146.

*McDaniel, S., Doherty, W., & Hepworth, J. (2013). *Medical family therapy and integrated care* (2nd ed.). Washington, DC: American Psychological Association.

McDaniel, S., Hepworth, J., & Doherty, W. (1992). *Medical family therapy: A biopsychosocial approach to families with health problems*. New York: BasicBooks/HarperCollins Publishers, Inc.
McGarvey, H. E. (1993). Participation in the research process. Action research in nursing. *Professional Nurse, 8*, 372–376. http://www.ncbi.nlm.nih.gov/pubmed/8446642.
McKibbin, E., & Castle, P. (1996). Nurses in action: An introduction to action research in training. *Curationis, 19*, 35–39. http://www.ncbi.nlm.nih.gov/pubmed/9283341.
McNicoll, P. (1999). Issues in teaching participatory action research. *Journal of Social Work Education, 35*, 51–62. http://www.jstor.org/discover/10.2307/23043442?uid=370764911&uid=3739736&uid=2134&uid=38193&uid=2&uid=70&uid=3&uid=67&uid=62&uid=3739256&sid=21101976949193.
Mendenhall, T. (2002). *Partners in diabetes: The process and evolution of a democratic citizenship initiative in a medical context* [dissertation]. University of Minnesota.
Mendenhall, T., Berge, J., Harper, P., GreenCrow, B., LittleWalker, N., WhiteEagle, S., & BrownOwl, S. (2010). The Family Education Diabetes Series (FEDS): Community-based participatory research with a Midwestern American Indian community. *Nursing Inquiry, 17*, 359–372. doi: 10.1111/j.1440-1800.2010.00508.x.
Mendenhall, T., & Doherty, W. J. (2003). Partners in diabetes: A collaborative, democratic initiative in primary care. *Families, Systems & Health, 21*, 329–335. doi:10.1037/1091-7527.21.3.329.
Mendenhall, T., & Doherty, W. (2005a). Partners in diabetes: A new initiative in primary care. In R. Kane, R. Priester, & A. Totten (Eds.), *Meeting the Challenge of Chronic Illness* (pp. 121–122). Baltimore, MD: John Hopkins University Press.
Mendenhall, T., & Doherty, W. J. (2005b). Action research methods in family therapy. In F. Piercy & D. Sprenkle (Eds.), *Research Methods in Family Therapy* (2nd ed., pp. 100–117). New York, NY: Guilford Publications.
Mendenhall, T., & Doherty, W. (2007a). Partners in diabetes: Action research in a primary care setting. *Action Research, 5*, 378–406. doi:10.1177/1476750307083722.
Mendenhall, T., & Doherty, W. (2007b). The ANGELS (A Neighbor Giving Encouragement, Love and Support): A collaborative project for teens with diabetes. In D. Linville & K. Hertlein (Eds.), *The Therapist's Notebook for Family Healthcare*. New York: Hayworth Press.
*Mendenhall, T., Doherty, W., Berge, J., Fauth, J., & Tremblay, G. (2013). Community-based participatory research: Advancing integrated health care through novel partnerships. In M. Talen & A. Valeras (Eds.), *Integrated behavioral health in primary care: Evaluating the evidence, identifying the essentials* (pp. 99–130). New York, NY: Springer.
Mendenhall, T., Harper, P., Stephenson, H., & Haas, S. (2011). The SANTA Project (Students Against Nicotine and Tobacco Addiction): Using community-based participatory research to improve health in a high-risk young adult population. *Action Research, 9*, 199–213. doi:10.1177/1476750310388051.
Mendenhall, T., Pratt, K., Phelps, K., Baird, M., & Younkin, F. (2014). Advancing medical family therapy through qualitative, quantitative, and mixed-methods research. In J. Hodgson, A. Lamson, T. Mendenhall, & R. Crane (Eds.), *Medical family therapy: Advanced applications* (pp. 241–258). New York: Springer.
Mendenhall, T., Seal, K., GreenCrow, B., LittleWalker, K., & BrownOwl, S. (2012). Family Education Diabetes Series (FEDS): Improving health in an urban-dwelling American Indian community. *Qualitative Health Research, 22*, 1524–1534. doi:10.1177/1049732312457469.
Mendenhall, T., Whipple, H., Harper, P., & Haas, S. (2008). Students Against Nicotine and Tobacco Addiction (S.A.N.T.A.): Community-based participatory research in a high-risk young adult population. *Families, Systems & Health, 26*, 225–231. doi:10.1037/1091-7527.26.2.225.
Meyer, J. (2000). Using qualitative methods in health related action research. *British Medical Journal, 320*, 178–181. http://www.ncbi.nlm.nih.gov/pmc/articles/PMC1128751/.

Miller, B., Kessler, R., Peek, C., & Kallenberg, G. (2010). *Establishing the research agenda for collaborative care*. Agency for Healthcare Research and Quality. Retrieved from http://www.ahrq.gov/research/collaborativecare/collab1.htm.

Minkler, M. (2000). Using participatory action research to build healthy communities. *Public Health Reports, 115*, 191–197. http://www.ncbi.nlm.nih.gov/pmc/articles/PMC1308710/pdf/pubhealthrep00022-0089.pdf.

Minkler, M., & Wallerstein, N. (2008). *Community based participatory research for health* (2nd ed.). San Francisco, CA: Jossey-Bass.

Morrison, B., & Lilford, R. (2001). How can action research apply to health services? *Qualitative Health Research, 11*, 436–449. doi:10.1177/104973201129119235.

National Center on Minority Health and Health Disparities. (2011). *NCMHD community based participatory research initiative*. National Institutes of Health. Retrieved from http://www.nimhd.nih.gov/our_programs/communityParticipationResearch.asp.

National Institutes of Health. (2009). *Summer institute: Community-based participatory research targeting the medically underserved*. National Institutes of Health. Retrieved from http://conferences.thehillgroup.com/si2009/about.html.

*National Institutes of Health (2013). *Community-based participatory research*. Retrieved from http://obssr.od.nih.gov/scientific_areas/methodology/community_based_participatory_research/.

Nichols, B. (1995). Action research: A method for practitioners. *Nursing Connections, 8*, 5–11. http://www.ncbi.nlm.nih.gov/pubmed/7777076.

Pan American Health Organization. (2004). *Participatory evaluation of healthy municipalities: A practical resource kit for action*. Washington, DC: Pan American Health Organization.

Peek, C. J. (2008). Planning care in the clinical, operational, and financial worlds. In R. Kessler & D. Stafford (Eds.), *Collaborative medicine case studies: Evidence in practice* (pp. 25–38). New York, NY: Springer.

*Peek, C. (2013). Integrated behavioral health in primary care: A common language. In M. R. Talen & A. B. Valeras (Eds.), *Integrated behavioral health in primary care: Evaluating the evidence, identifying the essentials* (pp. 9–32). New York, NY: Springer.

*Peek, C., & the National Integration Academy Council. (2013). *Lexicon for behavioral health and primary care integration: Concepts and definitions developed by expert consensus*. AHRQ Publication No.13-IP001-EF. Rockville, MD: Agency for Healthcare Research and Quality. Retrieved from http://integrationacademy.ahrq.gov/sites/default/files/Lexicon.pdf.

Potvin, L., Cargo, M., McComber, A. M., Delormier, T., & Macaulay, A. C. (2003). Implementing participatory intervention and research in communities: Lessons from the Kahnawake Schools Diabetes Prevention Project in Canada. *Social Science Medicine, 56*, 1295–1305. http://www.usask.ca/healthsci/che/chep/summer2007/day3/Implementing%20Participatory%20Intervention%20and%20Research%20in%20Communities.pdf.

Powers, F., Gillies, P., Madeley, R., & Abbot, M. (1989). Research in an antenatal clinic: The experience of the Nottingham Mothers' Stop Smoking Project. *Midwifery, 5*, 106–112. http://www.sciencedirect.com/science/article/pii/S0266613889800245#.

Pyrch, T. (2007). Participatory action research and the culture of fear: Resistance, community, hope and courage. *Action Research, 5*, 199–216. doi:10.1177/1476750307077324.

Pyrch, T., & Castillo, M. (2001). The sights and sounds of indigenous knowledge. In P. Reason & H. Bradbury (Eds.), *Handbook of action research: Participative inquiry and practice* (pp. 379–385). London: Sage.

Rahman, A., & Fals-Borda, O. (1991). *A self-review of PAR in action and knowledge: Breaking the monopoly with participatory action research*. London: Intermediate Technology Publications.

Reason, P., & Bradbury, H. (2001). *Handbook of action research: Participative inquiry and practice*. London: Sage.

Reason, P., & Bradbury, H. (2006). *Handbook of action research: Concise* (Paperbackth ed.). London: Sage.

Reason, P., & Bradbury, H. (2008). *The SAGE handbook of action research* (2nd ed.). Los Angeles: Sage.

Reese, D., Ahern, R., Nair, S., O'Faire, J., & Warren, C. (1999). Hospice access and use by African Americans: Addressing cultural and institutional barriers through participatory action research. *Social Work, 44*, 549–559. doi:10.1093/sw/44.6.549.

Rumbold, B. D. (2007). A review of spiritual assessment in health care practice. *Medical Journal of Australia, 186*, S60–S62.

Schulz, A., Israel, B., Parker, E., Lockett, M., Hill, Y., & Wills, R. (2003). Engaging women in community-based participatory research for health: The east side village health worker partnership. In M. Minkler & N. Wallerstein (Eds.), *Community-Based Participatory Research for Health* (pp. 293–315). San Francisco: Jossey-Bass.

Shelley, D., Fahs, M., Yerneni, R., Das, D., Nguyen, N., Hung, D., ... & Cummings, K. (2008). Effectiveness of tobacco control among Chinese Americans: a comparative analysis of policy approaches versus community-based programs. *Preventive Medicine, 47*, 530–536. doi: 10.1016/j.ypmed.2008.07.009.

Small, S. (1995). Action-oriented research: Models and methods. *Journal of Marriage and the Family, 57*, 941–955. http://www.jstor.org/stable/353414.

Steckler, A., & Linnan, L. (Eds.). (2002). *Process Evaluation for Public Health Interventions and Research*. San Francisco: Jossey-Bass.

Stevens, P., & Hall, J. (1998). Participatory action research for sustaining individual and community change: A model of HIV prevention education. *AIDS Education and Prevention, 10*, 387–402. http://psycnet.apa.org/psycinfo/1998-12882-001.

Tobin, M. (2000). Developing mental health rehabilitation services in a culturally appropriate context: An action research project involving Arabic-speaking clients. *Australian Health Review, 23*, 177–184. doi:10.1071/AH000177.

Torre, M., & Fine, M. (2005). Don't die with your work balled up in your fists: Contesting social injustice through participatory research. In B. Leadbeater & N. Way (Eds.), *Urban girls revisited: Building strengths* (pp. 221–240). New York: New York University Press.

Tsark, J. A. (2001). A participatory research approach to address data needs in tobacco use among Native Hawaiians. *Asian American and Pacific Islander Journal of Health, 9*, 40–48. http://www.ncbi.nlm.nih.gov/pubmed/11720413.

Wallerstein, N., & Duran, B. (2003). The conceptual, historical, and practice roots of community-based participatory research and related participatory traditions. In M. Minkler & N. Wallerstein (Eds.), *Community Based Participatory Research for Health* (pp. 27–52). San Francisco: Jossey-Bass.

Wallerstein, N., & Duran, B. (2006). Using community-based participatory research to address health disparities. *Health Promotion Practice, 7*, 312–323. doi:10.1177/1524839906289376.

*Wallerstein, N., & Duran, B. (2010). Community-based participatory research contributions to intervention research: The intersection of science and practice to improve health equity. *American Journal of Public Health, 100*, S40–S46. doi:10.2105/AJPH.2009.184036.

Ward, K., & Trigler, J. S. (2001). Reflections on participatory action research with people who have developmental disabilities. *Mental Retardation, 39*, 57–59. doi:10.1352/0047-6765.

Watson, M., Horowitz, A., Garcia, I., & Canto, M. (2001). A community participatory oral health promotion program in an inner-city Latino community. *Journal of Public Health Dentistry, 61*, 34–41. doi:10.1111/j.1752-7325.2001.tb03353.x.

Whitchurch, G., & Constantine, L. (1993). Systems theory. In P. Boss, W. Doherty, W. LaRossa, W. Schumm, & S. Steinmetz (Eds.), *Sourcebook of family theories and methods: A contextual approach* (pp. 325–352). New York: Plenum Press.

White, K., Williams, T., & Greenberg, B. (1996). The ecology of medical care. *Bulletin of the New York Academy of Medicine, 73*, 187–212. http://www.ncbi.nlm.nih.gov/pmc/articles/PMC2359390/?page=1.

Wilson, V., Ho, A., & Walsh, R. (2007). Participatory action research and action learning: Changing clinical practice in nursing handover and communication. *Journal of Children's and Young People's Nursing, 1*, 85–92. http://www.bipstar.co.uk/files/article.pdf.

Chapter 15
A Primer in Program Evaluation for MedFTs

Jackie Williams-Reade, Bobbi-Ann Gordon, and Wendy Wray

In health care today, most funding sources are looking for signs of evidence-based practices and measures of effectiveness. Utilizing the designs and methods of program evaluation has the potential to convey the relevance and value of including MedFTs to program beneficiaries and stakeholders. Program evaluation is the systematic assessment of social programs using social research procedures (Rossi, Lipsey, & Freeman, 2004) and is an imperative skill needed to promote the inclusion of behavioral health services. MedFTs provide unique contributions to program evaluation efforts because of their focus on contextual and relational issues that may impact program outcomes, especially as they pertain to patient care. Consider the following scenarios which illustrate when MedFTs may be called upon to conduct a program evaluation:

Scenario 1. A community health center is applying for state funding to enhance their efforts to address pediatric obesity in its local populace. The MedFT has been asked to assist in writing a proposal which requires a program evaluation plan that illustrates whether or not the project was successful and had the desired impact on the center's clientele.

Scenario 2. An integrated care setting serves patients with chronic pain. The number of patients to be seen individually is far beyond the capacity of the behavioral staff available. It has thereby been proposed by administration that group therapy services be implemented. While this will allow the MedFT to serve more patients, the medical team is concerned whether group therapy is as effective and beneficial as individual therapy.

Scenario 3. An integrated care setting has recently implemented the use of a PHQ-9 (Kroenke, Spitzer, & Williams, 2001) for all of its patients. While administrators originally considered this to be a relatively simple addition to the practice, it has significantly impeded staff workflow and it is not known how beneficial the

J. Williams-Reade (✉)
Loma Linda University, Loma Linda, CA, USA
e-mail: jreade@llu.edu

J. Hodgson et al. (eds.), *Medical Family Therapy*, DOI 10.1007/978-3-319-03482-9_15,

assessment is for patient care. Administration has asked the MedFT to help determine both staff and patient impact.

The above scenarios reflect today's culture of integrated care, including challenging patient populations, varied teams of providers and staff members, limited availability of resources, unique community contexts, and varied stakeholder influences. As a part of their job responsibilities, MedFTs will likely be called upon to help evaluate the effectiveness of their own interventions in a healthcare setting and implement appropriate processes, such as meaningful clinical quality procedures (HealthIT.gov, 2012). This chapter is designed to help MedFTs understand the process involved in planning, designing, and implementing a program evaluation with special emphasis on programs related to integrated care. The authors provide an overview of the frameworks, decision processes, methodology, and steps needed to carry out a program evaluation, alongside a bibliography of additional resources to assist in furthering relevant knowledge and skills.

Introduction to Program Evaluation

The term "program" refers to a collection of activities that are designed to reach certain objectives (Royse, Thyer, & Padgett, 2010). Program activities may include a variety of services which have been designed to impact participants or broader social change, such as interventions, research projects, policy development, promotion efforts, training or education initiatives, community building, administrative processes, etc. Program evaluation is the systematic assessment of these programs using social research procedures to ensure a program is providing appropriate social interventions that are producing intended outcomes (Rossi et al., 2004). While conventional research is used to prove significance, inform the broader scientific community, and provide for the possibility of replication, program evaluation is more often used to evaluate programmatic activities, inform internal decision makers, and incorporate findings into the improvement of an existing program. Program evaluation utilizes many of the same elements in conventional research activities, but it is conducted in real-life situations and often does not benefit from the controlled environments found in typical research protocols (Bamberger, Rugh, & Mabry, 2006).

Standards of Program Evaluation

Standards specific to program evaluation have been developed to ensure viable information is gathered (Yarbrough, Shulha, Hopson, & Caruthers, 2011). These standards are broken down into the following four areas: utility, feasibility, propriety, and accuracy. A program evaluation has utility when it provides information that will serve the necessary concerns of intended participants. The standard of

Table 15.1 Evaluation standard checklist

Utility	Feasibility	Propriety	Accuracy
• Evaluator credibility • Attention to stake-holders • Negotiated purposes • Explicit values • Relevant information • Meaningful processes and products • Timely and appropriate communication/reporting • Concern for consequences and influence	• Project management • Practical procedures • Contextual viability • Resource use	• Responsive to and inclusive orientation • Formal agreements • Human rights and respect (IRB approval) • Clarity and fairness • Transparency of disclosure • Conflicts of interest • Fiscal accountability	• Justified conclusions and decisions • Valid information • Reliable information • Explicit program and context descriptions • Information management • Sound designs and analyses • Explicit evaluation communication and reporting • Evaluation documentation • Internal meta-evaluation • External meta-evaluation

Adapted with permission from Yarbrough, D. B., Shulha, L. M., Hopson, R. K., & Caruthers, F. A. (2011). *The program evaluation standards: A guide for evaluators and evaluation users* (3rd ed.). Thousand Oaks, CA: Sage. Copyright 2010 Joint Committee on Standards for Educational Evaluation (JCSEE). http://www.eval.org/EvaluationDocumcents/progeval.html

feasibility ensures an evaluation will be realistic, prudent, diplomatic, and cost-effective so as not to overly burden those involved in the evaluation. Propriety standards promote ethical and legal components of program evaluation, especially as they relate to the well-being of participants and staff involved in the evaluation. Accuracy standards are designed to ensure that an evaluation will demonstrate scientific rigor and convey appropriate information regarding the program being evaluated. The above Table 15.1 provides more specific areas to consider when assessing compliance to these standards.

Phases of Program Evaluation

The first step to launching a program evaluation is creating a blueprint for how to proceed. In conjunction with the above standards, there are three main phases of program evaluation that are required to provide reliable results: planning, implementation, and utilization of findings (Kellogg, 2004a). In the following sections, the authors outline important details regarding how to proceed through each phase.

Planning

Primary tasks during the planning stage include determining the focus of program evaluation, assessment of resources, generate buy-in and input from key stakeholders, background review of the program, and formulation of evaluation questions (Center for Disease Control [CDC], 2011; Kellogg, 2004a).

Determining focus of program evaluation. The overall process of program evaluation can provide opportunities to identify values, strategies, strengths, and opportunities for change in a program. Proving effectiveness or improving programs are typical goals of evaluation; however, additional goals could include developing clear, common understanding of the program goals, establish and advance the program as an evidence-based practice, improve cost-effectiveness, provide evidence of need for additional resources, or prepare for external evaluations (Kellogg, 2004a). To achieve desired outcomes, an assessment of resources is required.

Assessment of resources. Common critiques regarding the feasibility of program evaluation include how expensive or time-consuming the activities will be and whether or not the team has the expertise needed to carry it out. In order to ensure the most appropriate and relevant programmatic activities will be carried out, it is important to consider the following questions in order to determine feasibility:

- **Time**. *Is this a short- or long-term project? Who is the sample population being evaluated? Are they easily accessible? How many individuals and what type of training will we need to implement the planned program evaluation activities?*
- **Money**. *What financial resources are available to you? Will you be funded to complete the evaluation or will you need to create a budget or acquire funding? Is the evaluation cost-effective?*
- **Expertise**. *Do you have access to a program evaluation expert on your team or will you need to hire a consultant? Who will provide overall leadership to the evaluation process? Do you have individuals who are available and prepared to speak with authority regarding the specifics of the programmatic activities you are evaluating?*

Stakeholder input and buy-in. Gaining stakeholder input and buy-in is an essential part of the program evaluation process. A stakeholder can be any number of individuals, groups, or organizations who have significant interest in how well a program functions (Rossi et al., 2004). While the primary goal of program evaluation is to improve the program's ongoing activities, each setting and/or stakeholder will have a variety of unique goals they consider most important. To help guide the purpose of the evaluation, it is important to identify the stakeholders related to the program and their unique perspectives, concerns, and planned use of the information that will be gathered. Finding out what the stakeholders want to know and how they will use the information will not only help ensure relevant and valuable information that is provided upon completion but aid in the uptake of any

Table 15.2 Stakeholders, goals, and application

Stakeholders: who will use the information?	Purpose and goals: what do they want to know?	Application: how will the results be used?
Administrators	Does MedFT meet expected outcomes?	To make decisions regarding funding, training, and expectations
Funding Agencies	How effective is the program?	To secure financial support
Professional review boards	Who does the program serve?	To justify the program
MedFTs	Are the behavioral health services meeting the needs of patients?	To make decisions about which services you offer to which patients
Patients and families	Am I receiving quality care?	To improve patient care

recommendations resulting from the evaluation. Stakeholders include those persons involved in or affected by the program and primary users of the evaluation (CDC, 2001). Examples of who may be stakeholders, their possible goals, and their intended application of program evaluation results are shown in Table 15.2.

Formulating the evaluation questions. Once a sense of stakeholder goals and purposes are outlined, formulation of the evaluation questions is the next step. These foundational questions will provide the overall purpose and focus of the program evaluation activities. For instance, will answers collected from the program evaluation help to improve patient satisfaction; answer questions posed by administrators, participants, or community members; assist stakeholders in better understanding the program and its results; improve the therapeutic interventions that are provided; assess patient satisfaction; and/or meet administrative requirements? Coming to agreement on which overarching questions are relevant to stakeholders is essential to ensure an agreed-upon purpose for the overall evaluation process and to help ensure programmatic activities promote utility and feasibility.

Background Review and Concept Mapping

A way to coordinate stakeholder input in the process of program evaluation is to include them in the background review. A background review includes gathering detailed background information about the program, including its mission, objectives, goals, and respective challenges and successes in order to determine which variables, processes, and outcomes are relevant to evaluate (Yarbrough et al., 2011). Background reviews help to ensure a common understanding of program goals and activities which provide the foundation on which subsequent decisions will be made. Providing a detailed description of the program helps facilitate the understanding of how program components relate to intended outcomes.

A common way to conceptualize the overall program involves concept mapping (Kane & Trochim, 2007). Concept mapping is a pictorial representation of the processes and steps involved in a program and used to help guide the planning and evaluation process. Concept mapping is an effective method for building consensus and group understanding among stakeholders regarding the key program components and how to measure for their utilization and effectiveness (Trochim, 1989). Typically, concept mapping includes the following six steps:

Preparation. To begin, the participants who will be involved in the concept mapping and the focus of the exercise must be selected. For instance, a variety of stakeholders may be selected to focus on mapping all of the outcomes they expect to see as a result of integrating behavioral health into current healthcare practice. Often, it is advantageous to include a facilitator for this process to maintain focus, progress, and understanding among individuals.

Generation of statements about the focus. At this time, stakeholders develop a set of statements that may describe the specific activities and outcomes related to the program. A wide variety of techniques can be used to generate ideas including brainstorming, interviews, focus groups, qualitative text analysis, etc. For instance, introducing the PHQ-9 (Kroenke et al., 2001) into the patient process flow could be the identified focus, and stakeholders could brainstorm as well as conduct interviews with staff and patients in order to elicit a broad range of statements regarding the specific needs and challenges related to this focus.

Structuring of statements. Once the statements are gathered, they must be organized. Borrowing analysis techniques from qualitative research, organization of the statements can be as simple as sorting similar statements into physical piles or in an electronic document, but can also be entered into a high-level computer program, such as CmapTools (Cañas et al., 2004), for more technical outputs. Using either method requires sorting and rating processes that must be agreed upon by the group in terms of importance to the overall goal. For instance, statements regarding implementation of the PHQ-9 (Kroenke et al., 2001) may be grouped into themes such as institutional resources required, mental health interventions to be used, impact on workflow, community resources for referral, training of staff, impact on community health, and many more. Participants then rate each statement according to their perceived sense of importance.

Representing the statements. Once rated, these statements are represented in a visual form or a concept map by using hand-drawn figures, statistical techniques, such as multidimension scaling and cluster analysis, or specialized software CmapTools (Cañas et al., 2004). Concept maps can take many shapes and forms. The following figure (Fig. 15.1) is one example of how a concept map helps visually portray the components of integrating a PHQ9 (Kroenke et al., 2001).

Interpretation of the maps. Once the concept map is created, the stakeholders create and agree upon their own meanings and interpretations of the findings. At this stage, it can be especially helpful to include a facilitator to help coordinate responses.

Utilization of findings. Finally, the maps are used to assist in addressing the original focus. This final step includes a discussion to determine action steps

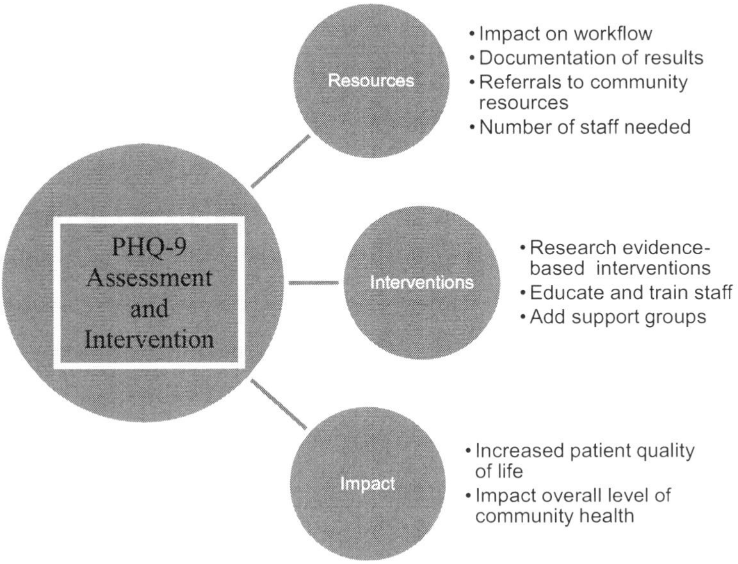

Fig. 15.1 Concept map for an integrated care setting contemplating the addition of adding a PhQ-9 (Kroenke et al., 2001) assessment and intervention protocol

regarding how the concept map may be used to enhance planning of the program or measuring the programmatic activities and outcomes.

The process of concept mapping provides the opportunity for stakeholders to define and organize concepts of their program into the identified issues, values, and strategies. Once the program is conceptualized this way, it becomes a frame of reference for the subsequent program evaluation activities. In addition, a concept map is often easily translated into the foundation of a logic model which will further focus the program evaluation.

Logic Model

The creation of a logic model is the final task in the background review stage. A logic model is used to provide a visual organization of the details of how a program is structured to meet its objectives (Taylor-Powell & Henert, 2008). Logic models depict the logic between the resources available to operate the program, the activities planned with those resources, and the expected results from the activities. Creating logic models further prepares the team for the evaluation as it facilitates outcome-oriented thinking, consensus, and accountability (Kellogg, 2004b). Logic models typically include the following components:

Inputs. Inputs are the resources available and utilized in order to deliver the program. Typically, inputs refer to physical resources such as staff (volunteers, type of staff), space (office space, buildings), time, funding (salaries, expenses), supplies, or equipment.

Activities. Activities are the actions or steps an organization takes to deliver a program or what the program does with the inputs. Activities include a variety of activities depending on what is being evaluated. In an integrated care setting, typical activities might include training providers, recruiting patients, delivering treatments, scheduling patients, providing interventions, creating collaborations among other staff or local/national agencies, implementing protocols, and charting in the medical record.

Participation. Participation reflects those who benefit from the activities. This can be both those who are direct beneficiaries of the services, such as patients or staff members, and indirect beneficiaries, including community agencies, policy makers, and others impacted by the provided service.

Outcomes. Outcomes reflect the impact or sought after changes of the program. These can vary in scope, including short-term, midterm, and long-term outcomes. Short-term outcomes relate to the immediate actions desired from the activity, while long-term outcomes are the overall impact and goals for the program. For example, by adding a MedFT to an integrated care setting, the short-term outcome might be an increased number of referrals to behavioral health, while the long-term outcome might be an increased percentage of patients who improve in overall health-related quality of life.

The logic model assists in understanding the link between these inputs, activities, participation, and outcomes by providing a concrete way to view a program's overall activities (Taylor-Powell & Henert, 2008). It should be detailed enough for the reader to grasp the major aspects of a program, but simplified to fit on only a few pages. It is important to remember that a logic model is a working document and can be adapted as the program develops. Below is an example of how a basic logic model is constructed, followed by a logic model specific to a project (Fig. 15.2).

Implementation

After completing the planning stage, the implementation of the program evaluation can begin. Using information collected in the planning phase, the type of evaluation needed is determined and a list of the potential evaluation questions is prepared along with a corresponding measure for each. There are many types of program evaluations, ranging from relatively simple designs to complex and labor-intensive ones. Some are used to form or enhance programs, while others are used to provide conclusive feedback. The common types of program evaluation can be placed into the following categories: formative, process, summative, and cost evaluations. The following table can be used as a guide to determine which type of evaluation is most

Outline of Logic Model

Inputs	Outputs		Outcomes		
	Activities	Participation	Short Term	Medium Term	Long Term
Available resources	What the program does	Who the program reaches	The overall changes and impact resulting from the program		
Staff Time Money Equipment Materials Partners	Deliver services Provide counseling Develop resources Train staff Build community relationships	Participants Patients Decision-makers Community agencies	Learning Awareness Knowledge Attitudes Skills Motivations	Action Behavior Practice Decision-making Policies Social Action	Greater Context Social Economic Civic Environmental

Logic Model for incorporating use of PHQ-9 (Kroenke, Spitzer, & Williams, 2001) in an integrated care setting

Inputs	Outputs		Outcomes		
	Activities	Participation	Short Term	Medium Term	Long Term
Staff (MedFT) Time (training, assessment, intervention, referral) Financial resources (staff, training, space) Materials (office space, assessment) Partners (local, state, national)	Provide assessments and interventions -PhQ-9 -Brief therapy -Support groups Develop educational pieces Conduct staff training Promote community resources	Patients Staff Local, state, national organizations Health care community	Increased knowledge and skills to address depression Increased staff skills in assessing patient quality of life	Increased coping skills Increased linkage to community resources Increased number of staff who screen and assess for depression	Reduction in depression symptoms, increased access to resources, improved quality of life Cost savings

Fig. 15.2 Example of logic model construction. Adapted with permission from Taylor-Powell, E., & Henert, E. (2008) *Developing a logic model: Teaching and training guide*. Madison, WI: University of Wisconsin-Extension, Cooperative Extension, Program Development and Evaluation. http://www.uwex.edu/ces/pdande

Table 15.3 Determining which type of evaluation is appropriate

Formative	Process	Summative	Cost evaluations
Is this program in early stages and needs feedback regarding implementation? Are services being used as originally intended?	How does the program work? Why do the patients seem much more at ease with this new intervention?	Is the program achieving the goals and objectives it was intended to accomplish? Are the patients getting better?	Does the benefit of achieving program goals exceed the cost of producing them? Does it cost less to use service A than service B?

appropriate to provide relevant information regarding previously identified evaluation questions and goals (Table 15.3).

Formative Evaluation

Formative evaluation is a method used during the inception and development of a program. It can be designed to monitor program delivery; to examine programmatic elements, such as procedures and interventions; or to measure the quality of program implementation. It is described as a form of evaluation that is change and improvement oriented. The data collected during a formative evaluation provide insight into program strengths and weaknesses and can be used to uncover barriers and discrepancies between the expected plan and program outcomes. Formative evaluation aids in developing an informed understanding of program dynamics and how program components work together (Newcomer, Hatry, & Wholey, 2010; Patton, 2012) (Table 15.4).

Formative evaluations can be integrated into the design of a program, ideally, as an ongoing activity; nonetheless, it can be conducted at different stages throughout the implementation process. A specific set of procedures is not required for conducting evaluations for program improvement. The information can be acquired through reviewing patient charts, progress notes, staff interviews, or patient observations (Royse et al., 2010). Common qualitative methods used in formative evaluations include focus groups, in-depth interviews, direct observation, and written documents. Focus groups and in-depth interviews can be designed to explore program developer, staff, and patient experiences. Factors that are identified during an initial analysis can help to construct the interview framework. These factors can also be used at a practical level to inform a shift or change needed in the development of a program. Focus group interviews provide insights into participants' experiences or beliefs regarding service issues. The group discussion stimulates respondents to talk freely, providing valuable clues to developing services that meet the particular needs of the intended recipients (Patton, 2002).

For example, the US Department of Veterans Affairs (VA) used formative evaluation during the implementation of two evidenced-based treatments (EBTs)

Table 15.4 Example questions to inform formative evaluation

Implementation focused	Patient centered	Program oriented	Staff oriented
What kinds of problems have emerged and how are these issues being addressed?	What are the characteristics of patients who are making progress and those who are not?	How has the program influenced the culture or climate within the organization?	How is staff adjusting to new program?
			How is staff adjusting to using a new intervention?
What is happening that is expected and/or not expected?	To what degree are patients improving and moving towards desired outcome?	What are the strengths and weaknesses of the program?	Are staff integrating new method or finding challenges to integrating new method?
How has the program affected internal operations?	What are patient perceptions of the program? What do they like, dislike, or want to change?	How well does the program fit with other programs within the organization?	
What new ideas or approaches have emerged that can be utilized and tested?			

in their VA Post-Traumatic Stress Disorder (PTSD) Residential Program (Cook et al., 2013). The VA's Northeast Program and Evaluation Center (NEPEC) facilitated the evaluation of 38 residential programs for veterans with PTSD. The VA was interested in how many providers were trained in one of the two EBTs, whether the training was being used, and providers' perceptions of the EBT's effectiveness. Information was collected through qualitative interviews, field notes, and participant observations. For each program, site visits were conducted over a 2-day period to interview program providers, directors, and staff. A semi-structured interview was developed using questions focused on training, use of EBTs, the quality of organizational leadership, and communication. Other qualitative measures included recording interviews, participant observations in treatment team meetings, and groups and field notes. The results revealed that implementation was not occurring at all sites, some providers were selective and did not use the EBT with all participants, and other findings indicated that one EBT seemed to be a better fit for residential treatment (Cook et al., 2013).

Process Evaluation

Evaluators analyzing program process are interested in how the purpose of the program's activities relate to desired results. Process evaluation attempts to explain why programs do or do not achieve their objectives (Rossi et al., 2004; Patton, 2012). This involves breaking down program services or patient activities into discrete components and documenting how each piece fits together. Process evaluators may pursue explanations for achievements, challenges, and changes by documenting day-to-day operations within the program setting, searching for distinct patterns and significant features that characterize the program. Process evaluations require attentiveness to quantitative and qualitative changes (Patton, 2012).

Process evaluations can include the purpose of describing a program, program monitoring, and quality assurance (Royse et al., 2010). While each purpose may have underlying objectives, a process evaluation may include a focus on one or a combination of the three. Process evaluations used to describe a program may capture data necessary to judge the intensity and reliability of service delivery. This can include data such as client sociodemographics, service usage, program activities, staff characteristics, client satisfaction data, and referral sources (Royse et al., 2010).

Process evaluation used for program monitoring seeks to understand what occurs in a program and the target population. Program evaluators often begin with examining the program's goals and objectives while making comparisons with routinely collected data, such as number of patients receiving services, types of services received, or the number of patients that complete a certain number of sessions. Program monitoring is viewed as the systematic and recurrent documentation of important components of program performance. It measures whether the program is functioning as intended or according to applicable standards (Rossi et al., 2004; Royse et al., 2010).

Quality assurance, as a form of process evaluation, aims to maintain standards of efficiency. This is often associated with subsequent reviews of clinical records and procedures for the adherence to treatment standards. Focus areas can include documentation of the presenting problem, diagnosis, treatment modality, and discharge planning. This information allows evaluators to determine if the level of treatment is consistent with overall established practice (Royse et al., 2010).

Process evaluations can be used to determine:

1. Are those persons receiving services the intended targets?
2. Are program functions being performed appropriately?
3. Does the program have qualified staff, necessary resources, and funding to support the program functions?
4. Does its governing board, funding agencies, and professional and legal standards enforce the program in compliance with requirement?
5. Are the participants satisfied with the services they receive?
6. Do the participants engage in the necessary follow-up protocols after the service is rendered?

As an evaluator's interest moves from understanding the various aspects of program process to determining program effects, a focus on summative evaluation is required (Patton, 2012).

Summative Evaluation

Summative evaluations measure the program's overall effectiveness and impact. This type of evaluation investigates to what extent the effects of the program are influencing the changes that occur for program participants. It is important for programs to have evidence that their services can effectively meet the needs of their patients. By determining the overall value of the program, stakeholders can make informed decisions regarding continuation or replication of the program (Patton, 2012). The following questions indicate the need for a summative evaluation:

1. Did our patients improve?
2. Are our interventions working?
3. Did the program achieve intended goals?
4. Should the program end or continue? Are we ready for expansion?
5. Can the measured outcomes be linked to the program?

Example from Scenario 3

A summative evaluation is conducted to determine the impact of adding a PHQ-9 (Kroenke et al., 2001) into patient care. The majority of the targeted patient groups reveal scores that indicate moderate to severe depression. Interventions associated with how to manage life stressors was implemented to reduce patients' levels of depression. To evaluate the effectiveness of the interventions, the next steps were to determine:

1. Outcome levels—the results of an outcome at a chosen point in time (level of depression among patients)
2. Outcome changes—the difference between outcome levels at different points in time
3. Program effects—the portion of an outcome change that can be attributed uniquely to the program as opposed to the influence of some other factors

It is important to note that when collecting quantitative data, that evaluators maximize reliability and validity. In conducting evaluations, using the right measurement tools (reliability) and measuring what you planned (validity) are key components in gaining effective results (Babbie, 2013; McKenzie, Neiger, & Thackeray, 2009). Sensitivity is utilized to detect changes or various outcomes that signify program effects. The sensitivity of an assessment is the magnitude to which the values on the assessment change when there is a change or difference in the entity being measured (Rossi et al., 2004).

Cost Evaluations

Costs continue to be a major concern to many stakeholders in today's healthcare climate, especially as budgetary constraints increase. As agencies seek to implement best practices or the most effective interventions, cost can be a key denominator (Fals-Stewart, Klostermann, & Yates, 2005). The ideal situation is to provide the most affordable services with the most favorable outcome, and cost evaluations can be quite helpful in making such a determination. Cost evaluations define "costs" as the monetary value placed on resources used. Further subdivision results in "direct" and "indirect" costs. Direct costs are those incurred to provide a treatment or service. Direct costs to deliver an intervention may include time, materials, equipment, supplies, and overhead costs for program operations. Indirect costs are resources lost due to the ailment or issue targeted by the program. This may include the cost of a decrease in productivity or loss of employment (Fals-Stewart et al., 2005; Riegg Cellini & Kee, 2010).

Cost evaluations can be applied at any point of time in a program's development or delivery. It can help to inform decisions when an agency is deciding between two or more treatments or programs. Cost evaluations require an accurate assessment of the cost-benefits and cost-effectiveness of delivering a service or carrying out program activities (Royse et al., 2010). It is important to note that cost evaluations can be complex and highly technical, requiring a specific framework or procedure and a thorough understanding of the steps (Fals-Stewart et al., 2005; Riegg Cellini & Kee, 2010; Rossi et al., 2004).

Cost-Effectiveness Analysis. Cost-effectiveness analysis relates the program costs program to its specific measures of effectiveness. Units of effectiveness refer to primary outcomes of the intervention or program. For example, reductions in patient symptoms, improvement in communication patterns, or academic performance can represent units of effectiveness. Cost-effectiveness can be calculated by dividing costs by the units of effectiveness, i.e., Cost-Effectiveness Ratio = Total Cost/Units of Effectiveness (Riegg Cellini & Kee, 2010).

Cost-Benefit Analysis. Cost-benefit analysis assigns a monetary value to the outcomes achieved. This is used to determine if the program's overall benefit to society exceeds the costs. It can be useful when comparing alternative programs. Cost-benefit analysis places a monetary value by weighing the costs of the programs against the monetary value of program benefits. The cost-benefits can be calculated by subtracting total benefits from the total cost of the program, i.e., Net Benefits = Total Benefits − Total Cost (Riegg Cellini & Kee, 2010).

Utilization of Findings

Evaluation efforts are only worthwhile if they are used appropriately. The findings of the program evaluation should be organized in such a way that they comply with the standards of propriety and utility to ensure the information gained will be accurate and used effectively (CDC, 2013; Yarbrough et al., 2011). How to best utilize the findings will depend upon the specific purpose. Evaluation findings can be utilized for several purposes, including direct or instrumental, conceptual, or persuasive (Leviton & Hughes, 1981; Rossi et al., 2004). Direct or instrumental utilization refers to the specific use of evaluation findings that are translated into a concrete, usable form such as a protocol or guideline that informs practice (e.g., decision-making regarding specific interventions related to patient care decisions). Conceptual utilization refers to the use of evaluation findings to influence thinking about an issue, but many not result in changed actions or behavior (e.g., providing evidence to help shape an institution's policy). Persuasive utilization is the use of evaluation findings to inform and influence others regarding their stance on an issue (e.g., utilizing information to advocate for appropriate reimbursement for behavioral health integration). Utilization also includes considering how to best convey findings to stakeholders which can include media releases, community meetings, videos, website content, white papers or briefs, presentations, etc.

Conclusion

Program evaluation is an important bridge between the work of MedFTs and evidence-based practice. In this era of rapid changes in health care and emphases on effective and efficient care models, program evaluation is an increasingly important and valuable tool for MedFTs. We know that in order to function optimally, any organization or group of individuals needs to continually assess and adapt its functioning in order to meet agreed-upon objectives and goals in the face of a myriad of changes. Each question asked in program evaluation offers the opportunity to gather and integrate new information to assist in the adjustment to the changes in health care. Program evaluation is a way for MedFTs to serve as vital and responsive members of the healthcare team by taking an active role in the shared mission of providing high-quality and effective health care to patients. Through program evaluation, MedFTs can evaluate their practice beyond subjective appraisals, measures of billable hours, or patient visits and provide systematic evidence of their effectiveness to other healthcare professionals, insurance companies, policy makers, the public, or patients and family members.

Discussion Questions

1. After reviewing this chapter, what are some programmatic activities that could be evaluated at your integrated care setting? Are the programmatic goals and activities clearly articulated and understood by staff? Are you achieving your outcomes?
2. Based on what you have learned in this chapter, what initial steps would you take to investigate the feasibility of a program evaluation? Who are the stakeholders that need to be involved? What are the programmatic activities that need to be evaluated? What designs and methods make sense for your evaluation purposes? What would you choose as your evaluation questions?
3. If you were to suggest a program evaluation at your integrated care setting, what are some possible challenges you might encounter? How might you address these challenges?
4. Revisit the three scenarios shared at the opening of the chapter. Think through how you might address these various scenarios using the program evaluation basics covered in this chapter.

References[1]

Babbie, E. (2013). *The practice of social research* (13th ed.). Belmont, CA: Cengage Learning.

Bamberger, M., Rugh, J., & Mabry, L. (2006). *Real World evaluation: Working under budget, time, data, and political constraints*. Thousand Oaks, CA: Sage.

Cañas, A. J., Hill, G., Carff, R., Suri, N., Lott, J., Eskridge, T., …, Carvajal, R. (2004). CmapTools: A knowledge modeling and sharing environment. Concept Maps: Theory, methodology, technology. In A. J. Cañas, J. D. Novak, & F. M. González (Eds.), *Proceedings of the 1st International Conference on Concept Mapping* (Vol. 1, pp. 125–133). Pamplona, Spain: Universidad Pública de Navarra.

Centers for Disease Control and Prevention (CDC). (2001). *A framework for program evaluation*. Retrieved http://www.cdc.gov/eval/framework/index.htm.

Centers for Disease Control and Prevention (CDC). (2011). *Developing an effective evaluation plan*. Retrieved http://www.cdc.gov/obesity/downloads/CDC-Evaluation-Workbook-508.pdf.

Centers for Disease Control and Prevention (CDC). (2013). *Developing an effective evaluation report*. Retrieved http://www.cdc.gov/eval/materials/Developing-An-Effective-Evaluation-Report_TAG508.pdf.

Cook, J. M., O'Donnell, C., Dinne, S., Bernardy, N., Rosenheck, R., & Hoff, R. (2013). A formative evaluation of two evidence-based psychotherapies for PTSD in VA residential treatment programs. *Journal of Traumatic Stress, 26*, 56–63. doi:10.1002/jts.21769.

Fals-Stewart, W., Klostermann, K., & Yates, B. T. (2005). Assessing the costs, benefits, cost-benefit ratio, and cost-effectiveness of marital and family treatments: Why we should and how we can. *Journal of Family Psychology, 19*, 28–39. doi:10.1037/0893-3200.19.1.28.

HealthIT.gov. (2012). *Meaningful use. Policy making, regulation and strategy*. Retrieved http://www.healthit.gov/policy-researchers-implementers/meaningful-use.

[1] An asterisk has been use to note references that the chapter authors recommend for further reading.

*Holden, D. J., & Zimmerman, M. A. (2009). *A practical guide to program evaluation*. Thousand Oaks, CA: Sage.

Kane, M., & Trochim, W. M. K. (2007). *Concept mapping for planning and evaluation*. Thousand Oaks, CA: Sage.

*Kapp, S. A., & Anderson, G. R. (2010). *Agency-based program evaluation: Lessons from practice*. Thousand Oaks, CA: Sage.

Kroenke, K., Spitzer, R. L., & Williams, J. B. (2001). The PHQ-9: Validity of a brief depression severity measure. *Journal of General Internal Medicine, 16*, 606–613. doi:10.1046/j.1525-1497.2001.016009606.x.

Leviton, L. C., & Hughes, E. F. X. (1981). Research on the utilization of evaluations: A review and synthesis. *Evaluation Review, 5*, 525–548. doi:10.1177/0193841X8100500405.

*Maxwell, J. A. (2009). Designing a qualitative study. In L. Bickman & D. J. Rog (Eds.), *Applied social research methods* (pp. 214–253). Thousand Oaks, CA: Sage.

McKenzie, J. F., Neiger, B. L., & Thackeray, R. (2009). *Planning, implementation, & evaluating health promotion programs: A primer* (5th ed.). San Francisco, CA: Pearson Education.

Newcomer, K. E., Hatry, H. P., & Wholey, J. S. (2010). Planning and designing useful evaluations. In J. S. Wholey, H. P. Hatry, & K. E. Newcomer (Eds.), *Handbook of program evaluation* (3rd ed., pp. 5–29). San Francisco, CA: Jossey-Bass.

Patton, M. (2002). *Qualitative research and evaluation methods* (3rd ed.). Thousand Oaks, CA: Sage.

Patton, M. (2012). *Essentials of utilization-focused evaluation*. Thousand Oaks, CA: Sage.

*Posavac, E. J. (2011). *Program evaluation—Methods and case studies* (8th ed.). Upper Saddle River, NJ: Prentice Hall.

Riegg Cellini, S., & Kee, J. E. (2010). Cost-effectiveness and cost-benefit analysis. In J. S. Wholey, H. P. Hatry, & K. E. Newcomer (Eds.), *Handbook of program evaluation* (3rd ed., pp. 493–530). San Francisco, CA: Jossey-Bass.

Rossi, P., Lipsey, M., & Freeman, H. (2004). *Evaluation: A systematic approach* (7th ed.). Thousand Oaks, CA: Sage.

Royse, D., Thyer, B. A., & Padgett, D. K. (2010). *Program evaluation: An introduction* (5th ed.). Belmont, CA: Wadsworth.

*Sutherland, S., & Katz, S. (2005). Concept mapping methodology: A catalyst for organizational learning. *Evaluation and Program Planning, 28*, 257–269. doi:10.1016/j.evalprogplan.2005.04.017.

Taylor-Powell, E., & Henert, E. (2008). *Developing a logic model: Teaching and training guide*. Madison, WI: University of Wisconsin-Extension, Cooperative Extension, Program Development and Evaluation. Retrieved http://www.uwex.edu/ces/pdande.

Trochim, W. (1989). An introduction to concept mapping for planning and evaluation. *A Special Issue of Evaluation and Program Planning, 12*, 1–16. doi:10.1016/0149-7189(89)90016-5.

*United Way of America. (1996). *Measuring program outcomes: A practical approach*. Arlington, VA: United Way of America.

W. K. Kellogg Foundation. (2004a). *Evaluation handbook*. Battle Creek, MI: Kellogg Foundation.

W. K. Kellogg Foundation. (2004b). *Logic model development guide: Using logic models to bring together planning, evaluation, and action*. Battle Creek, MI: W.K. Kellogg Foundation.

Yarbrough, D. B., Shulha, L. M., Hopson, R. K., & Caruthers, F. A. (2011). *The program evaluation standards: A guide for evaluators and evaluation users* (3rd ed.). Thousand Oaks, CA: Sage.

Chapter 16
Dissemination and Implementation Science: Research for the Real-World Medical Family Therapist

Jodi Polaha and Beth Nolan

For many, the inspiration to work in Medical Family Therapy (MedFT) is based upon a desire to serve patients and families in settings where they are most likely to seek help, such as primary care clinics, specialty healthcare practices, or hospitals. Using the models and methods of Dissemination and Implementation Science (D&I Science), MedFTs, whose primary focus is clinical care or clinical research, have the opportunity to directly improve the quality of patient care while advancing science. In fact, it is the MedFT's contact with patients and the systems in which they seek help that makes this kind of research possible. This chapter describes an emerging scientific discipline closely aligned with the discipline of clinical care and how MedFTs are well positioned to make an important impact.

Evidence-Based Treatments

Evidence-based treatments (EBTs) have been a critical theme across many health professions' training programs since the 1990s (Claridge & Fabian, 2005). Today, the field of behavioral health boasts an armamentarium of psychosocial interventions with demonstrated efficacy across wide-ranging presenting problems and populations. Indeed, for behavioral health researchers, it is a point of pride to discuss the empirically supported merits of various psychosocial interventions such as cognitive behavior therapy (CBT) for anxiety in adults (Otte, 2011) or parent behavior management training for treating behavior problems in young children (Shriver & Allen, 2008). Each of these examples has accumulated dozens of studies, has shown moderate to strong effect sizes in meta-analytic reviews (Fabiano et al. 2009; Hofmann & Smits, 2008; Norton & Price, 2007), and has

J. Polaha (✉)
Department of Psychology, East Tennessee State University, Johnson City, TN, USA
e-mail: polaha@mail.etsu.edu

J. Hodgson et al. (eds.), *Medical Family Therapy*, DOI 10.1007/978-3-319-03482-9_16,

outperformed medication therapy in some cases (Charach et al., 2013; Roshanaei-Moghaddam et al., 2011).

Unfortunately, within the field of behavioral health research, the sense of triumph with this accomplishment is tempered by increasing evidence that many clinicians outside of academic settings do not use EBTs. For example, in spite of the evidence for CBT for anxiety disorders, most psychologists reported they did not use exposure or response prevention for obsessive-compulsive disorder (Freiheit, Vye, Swan, & Cady, 2004). This "scientist-practitioner gap" has been demonstrated in a number of studies and across a wide range of presenting concerns and community-based settings (e.g., Babione, 2010; Meehl, 1987; Ruscio & Holohan, 2006; Stewart & Chambless, 2007).

In addition to low uptake by clinicians, evidence is increasing that many patients are not necessarily attracted to the EBTs that have been developed (Kreuter & Hovmand, 2012). In the case of behavioral parent training, high attrition rates in community-based deployment of this intervention are well documented (Jensen & Grimes, 2010). While there are many potential explanations for why parents might discontinue this type of treatment (see Werba, Eyberg, Boggs, & Algina, 2006 for a review), one possibility is that these treatments, often formatted as 8–12, 1-h individual or group sessions, are not well matched with the desires and interests of the parents who need them.

Another troubling concern is the realization that both the methods and administrative process of science have significant shortcomings. Kreuter and Hovmand (2012) used a system dynamics modeling approach to show that while using "business as usual" in our current science, in the best case scenario only one in 33 funded studies actually gain traction as a treatment in community-based settings. Moreover, these authors showed that in the optimistic case, it takes 21 years for the results of a large, well-designed study to make an impact on clinical practice. These findings have grave fiscal implications; in 2012, research grants from the National Institutes of Health (NIH) totaled nearly $16 billion (Office of Statistical Analysis and Reporting, Office of Research Information Systems, & Office of Extramural Research, 2012). A telling example of this problem comes from academic settings, in which many of these studies are conducted, where researchers are evaluated based on the "impact factor" of the journals they publish in (and that are read by other academics) rather than the impact of their work on practitioners, patients, families, and others in the community (Brumback, 2009; Brishoux & Cook, 2009).

To date, the net result is that the field of behavioral health, including both clinical and research enterprises, has had little demonstrated public health impact. Broad studies of the young adult population, for example, show a one standard deviation increase in most problem scores across the past 70 years (Twenge et al., 2010). Looking at the literature on behavior problems in children, Collishaw, Maughan, Goodman, and Pickles (2004) found increases in parents' ratings of adolescent conduct problems over the past 20 years. Blunt comments regarding Psychology can be applied to the entire field of behavioral health:

> Ultimately, the public will judge Psychology on its contribution—or lack thereof—to societal improvement. Societal upheaval and individual dysfunction seem to be steadily worsening, and Psychology cannot proffer any comprehensive, understandable solutions that can be readily implemented. Psychology's lasting contributions are pitifully small compared to the advances in medicine that have resulted in an astounding increase in longevity and the quality of life (pp. 103–104).

Translating Science to the Real World

As the behavioral health field has recognized the relative impotency of its research, there has been a direct challenge to engage research that is a better match for use in the "real world" (e.g., Dodge, 2011). In fact, researchers are beginning to view the deployment of science for the explicit purpose of improving practice as an ethical obligation (Hoagwood & Olin, 2002; Hyman, 1999). More recently, the field is garnering momentum around this turn and D&I Science is showing some promise to better bridge the "bench to bedside" transition. The development of this relatively new field has significant implications for bringing the real-world experiences and knowledge of MedFTs to bear on the mental/behavioral health of people everywhere.

Consider this: impact = effectiveness × reach (Miller, Munoz, & Christensen, 2010). As discussed, the behavioral health field has made a significant dent in the *effectiveness* element in this equation, but with little *impact* because it has lacked *reach*. Considering reach helps program planners describe and evaluate the extent to which their program attracts its intended audience (Klesges, Estabrooks, Glasgow, & Dzewaltowski, 2005). In this equation, "reach" refers to both implementation and dissemination. While D&I Science often appears as one endeavor, the distinct areas of implementation and dissemination research stand alone in the literature as well.

Implementation Science

Evidence about the effectiveness of an intervention does not explicitly drive clinicians or consumers to implement it. Rather, scientific evidence garnered under controlled settings only describes an intervention that would work to achieve the desired outcomes in a restricted experimental context (Brownson, Colditz, & Proctor, 2012). A simple example is that while most people know that speeding is one of the greatest contributors to traffic accidents, many people continue to speed (US Department of Transportation, National Highway Traffic Safety Administration, & National Center for Statistics and Analysis, 2012). The issue is not one of lack of knowledge; most drivers can see the posted speed limits signs, know how to monitor their speed, and what the consequences for speeding are (e.g., accidents, speeding tickets). That is to say, the evidence is well disseminated, but this alone is not sufficient to produce successful implementation.

Implementation research addresses "reach" by employing approaches to introduce or change evidence-based health interventions within human service settings in a way that helps them gain better traction and follow-through. Defined implementation research as a discipline with the purpose of developing a field of knowledge to describe *how* interventions are translated to the practice setting. The National Institutes of Health has called for implementation research looking at how service systems and setting characteristics influence prevention and treatment program implementation, as well as strategies to improve the adoption and implementation of evidence-based treatment innovations. Many MedFTs have a wealth of knowledge about real-world factors affecting implementation, and this kind of savvy is essential to developing a sophisticated study of implementation.

Dissemination Science

Reach is also about dissemination or spreading EBTs to a broad audience. Dissemination has been described as "how information about mental healthcare interventions is created, packaged, transmitted, and interpreted among various stakeholder groups" (Chambers, Ringeisen, & Hickman, 2005, p. 313). Presently, there are many efforts to disseminate EBTs, such as websites that describe EBTs for clinicians or consumers (e.g., Association for Behavioral and Cognitive Therapies (ABCT)) or smartphone applications that put an EBT for managing a panic attack or quitting smoking in a place that is inexpensive and accessible to many people (Enota et al., 2011; Gallo, Comer, & Barlow, 2013; Smith et al., 2011).

Importantly, as described in the speeding example above, the act of dissemination alone does not ensure widespread reach. Dissemination Science is focused on evaluating the complex factors that influence the speed at which, and the likelihood that, such interventions are taken up by a broad audience (Greenhalgh, Robert, MacFarlane, Bate, & Kyriakidou, 2004). Dissemination Science is focused on innovation in getting treatments to places where they are needed, including tailoring interventions to aid in dissemination (instead of expecting a one-size-fits-all treatment to be deployed across wide-ranging settings) and using comprehensive, multilevel approaches rather than single-source messages (Brownson et al., 2012).

Characteristics of Dissemination and Implementation Science

Presently, the field of D&I Science encompasses the gamut of studies engaged in questions around implementation and dissemination. It is emerging models and methods designed to improve our scientific methods, allowing us to study ways to gain better reach and results with EBTs. It is a new and evolving field, with much strength but also with the kind of disorganization that comes with rapid growth and innovation (Brownson et al., 2012; Glasgow et al., 2012). Several core features characterize it as a focus on stakeholders/consumers, engagement of transdisciplinary teams, incorporation of novel partners and methods, and an emphasis on scaling-up and sustainability.

Focus on Stakeholders/Consumers

One of the hallmarks of D&I Science is the direct study and integration of findings for those individuals—administrators, community members, providers, or patients—who might support, engage, or consume EBTs. Methods for optimizing stakeholder input are wide-ranging, but one of the most well-known methods is community-based participatory research (CBPR). CBPR is a method for uniting clinical scientists with the people in communities to give the community a voice in the development of research questions, design, choice of methods, and results interpretation, as well as critical input regarding implementation (Minkler & Wallerstein, 2008) . At the fifth Annual NIH D&I Science conference in 2012, CBPR was named one of the most important innovations to the field. CBPR involves a collaborative approach to planning, conducting, and interpreting findings. It can be an incredibly effective method for translating EBTs to the real world such that many barriers will be addressed or avoided altogether. Results from studies using CBPR provide numerous examples of the utility of stakeholder involvement on the improved outcomes (Minkler & Wallerstein, 2008). There are many CBPR resources available for researchers seeking information and training in this area; the reader is referred to Chapter 14 (Mendenhall, Berge, & Doherty, 2014) in this book for more information.

Another method of engaging stakeholder and customer input is to build stakeholder or consumer feedback into the design of the study itself. Building stakeholder involvement from the beginning of the decision-making process can better inform all aspects of the effort. Many D&I projects engage "implementation teams" who meet regularly to provide iterative feedback to the needs assessment, adaptation, implementation, and maintenance phases. This can be accomplished using focus groups, community meetings, patient panels, or other types of qualitative methods. Alternately, quantitative methods in which consumers or stakeholders rate the utility, accessibility, effectiveness, or acceptability of a treatment may be used. There are a number of online resources for finding such measures. As an example, the National Cancer Institute (NCI) is compiling a Grid-Enabled Measures system, cataloging hundreds of measures and including information about their validity and reliability (NCI, 2012).

MedFTs in clinical settings may already be gathering some consumer feedback in the form of satisfaction surveys with patients and families or may understand how to gain this information in a way that fits in with practice flow without adding a complex set of procedures. Likewise, MedFTs who are already engaged to regular meetings with providers, administrators, or even patient advocacy groups have access to a "captive" implementation team for strategically assessing the uptake of interventions. These are simple ways a MedFT can begin to focus on stakeholders and customers.

Engagement of Transdisciplinary Teams

Another focus in D&I Science is the engagement of multiple disciplines. In seeking an explanation for our lack of potency on a large scale, it has become clear that the science of behavioral health, like many other fields, is "siloed," meaning that research is published in field-specific journals which are read by a narrow audience (Young, Ionnidis, & Al-Ubaydli, 2008). Moreover, research in behavioral health is not informed by research in other fields, including basic psychological research (Guerra, Graham, & Tolan, 2011; Sussman, Valente, Rohrbach, Skara, & Pentz, 2006; Zerhouni, 2003). The larger field of translational research and D&I Science pushes cross-pollination of methods, findings, and analyses across basic to applied science and across a wide range of health disciplines.

MedFTs working in healthcare settings may have many colleagues from various disciplines such as family or specialized medicine, nursing, public or allied health, and pharmacy with whom they already collaborate to provide patient care. This group could form a regular research team, reading each other's literature around a particular problem and collecting data together. An excellent starting point, consistent with D&I Science and relevant to administrators and practitioners alike, is answering straightforward questions about the utility (e.g., time saved, greater patient/provider satisfaction), cost-benefit (e.g., fewer procedures or emergency room visits needed), or feasibility (e.g., how quickly it was adopted, time to engage procedure, cost of procedure) of team-based care or another best-practice procedure that has been implemented in the clinic.

Incorporation of Novel Partners and Methods

D&I Science is characterized by a strong sense of creativity and innovation in determining how to better implement or disseminate treatments. Often this involves engaging partners who are not commonly engaged in behavioral health research (Brownson, Drisinger, Colditz, & Proctor, 2012; Porges, 2006). For example, the first author of this chapter is engaged with a team of researchers that includes a digital media and marketing expert. This individual has never conducted health sciences research before but has expertise in using online/digital formats to sell products. In this group, he is providing expertise on how to market behavioral health treatment. Moreover, this expert has connected the team with a private for-profit media group who manages websites, which has the potential to track online traffic and user habits (i.e., data that could prove useful in disseminating EBTs).

Likewise, a strong theme within D&I Science is innovation in methodology (Brownson et al., 2012). In particular, this field gravitates away from time-intensive, inflexible designs, such as randomized controlled trials. Instead, the field is finding ways to keep research more pragmatic and gain rapid results that can potentially have an immediate impact on the way services are delivered in the real world. As an example of this trend, the NIMH (2013) recently noted in a funding announcement that "the R34 provides the opportunity for 'high risk, high reward studies' and these will be of high priority" (para. 8) and that the federal funder encourages applications that place a premium on two key features: innovation and impact. Innovation, in this context, refers to technological solutions that have not been applied to the mental health service continuum (screening, assessment, intervention, referral, monitoring).

For a MedFT, D&I Science pushes the envelope of creativity and encourages innovative thinking about how to get a treatment implemented or disseminated and how to study it. Novel partnerships will bring new resources to bear on clinical practice and research. Moreover, novel approaches to research that encompass a more flexible, rapid pace mean that MedFTs can fit D&I-consistent research designs into regular clinical practice and use research outcomes to promote changes, new service, or policy directions within their organization in a timely manner. This may sound like the familiar quality improvement (QI) initiatives often engaged in these settings. In fact, QI is a way to "sell" D&I Science to healthcare administration. Data from good D&I studies should have clear and relevant implications for improving the quality of care within the setting(s) where the research was conducted.

Emphasis on Scaling-Up and Sustainability

D&I Science is characterized by studies which, at the outset, have an eye toward long-term and big picture impact (Brownson et al., 2012). "Sustainability" refers to how well an intervention continues to deliver its identified benefits over time, including after grant funding for research is concluded (Shediac-Rizkallah & Bone, 1998). Another important concept, "scale-up," is defined as strategic efforts to address the impact of new, evidence-based treatments so as to benefit more people and to foster policy and program development (Mittman et al., 2009; Simmons, Fajans, & Ghiron, 2007).

As investigators in D&I Science focus on capturing the meaning of these two concepts, they ask questions such as: What contextual factors affect sustainability and scale? How can we best plan for sustainability and scale-up? And how do we maintain or grow programs in settings with limited resources (Mittman et al., 2009)? As with many concepts in D&I Science, these ideas are viewed flexibly and dynamically. There is recognition that service systems change, stakeholders vary, and implementation is a process. Thus, maintaining the effects of an EBT, or bringing them to a larger audience, is not likely to happen via a static program. Instead, it is important to build in evaluative mechanisms that allow adaptation of that program to natural change(s). Again, MedFTs in real-world settings have their finger on the pulse of critical variables that can affect sustainability and scale-up, and they can make important contributions to this literature.

Exemplary Models

The field of D&I Science is a still relatively new, evolving discipline concerned with how to best deploy and utilize EBTs to improve health (Eccles & Mittman, 2006; Glasgow et al., 2012). Like all science, it is guided by theoretical models which provide a systematic way to design, conduct, and evaluate interventions (Green & Kreuter, 2005). In a recent review, Tabak, Khoong, Chambers, and Brownson (2012) identified 109 theoretical models consistent with D&I Science, across a wide range of disciplinary endeavors. Below, we provide an overview of two strong models, RE-AIM (Glasgow, Vogt, & Boles, 1999) and Fixsen, Naoom, Blase, Friedman, and Wallace's (2005) implementation framework, with examples of their application to integrated care (an area where MedFTs are increasingly engaged).

Reach, Effectiveness, Adoption, Implementation, and Maintenance (RE-AIM)

For large-scale D&I research, the RE-AIM framework can inform program decision making, planning, and measurement of program impact (Glasgow, Vogt, & Boles, 1999). **Reach** is the extent to which a program attracts the targeted population. In particular, RE-AIM focuses on establishing the population denominator so that program outcomes can include the proportion of the population reached. **Effectiveness** refers to program outcomes. RE-AIM provides planning tools to guide design and data collection to best document the effectiveness of the program. **Adoption** is similar to Reach, but the denominator is collected at the setting level, rather than the population level. In other words, Adoption calls for planning to establish a means for capturing the number of individuals most likely to be served in the targeted setting (e.g., collecting participation rates, screening rates, etc.). While Effectiveness is a collection of the outcomes measure, Adoption is a collection of process measures. **Implementation** refers to intervention fidelity or the extent to which different components of an intervention are delivered as intended. Implementation calls for planning to establish a means of tracking the way the intervention is delivered, likely employing process measures. Finally, **Maintenance** extends Implementation, as it calls for planning at both the individual participant level and the setting level. At the *individual level* in Maintenance, the team would plan for the long-term effects of the intervention on both outcomes and the quality of life of the target group. For example, how will participants maintain their new low weight after they are no longer participants? At the *setting level* in Maintenance (the practice, department, or institution), the team would plan for the sustainability of the program. In other words, was the program written into the service system's procedures manual? Is the process being taught at orientation? What resources are available to offset the new costs?

Example of RE-AIM. RE-AIM can provide researchers and their organizational and community partners a broad planning process for success in the near and long term. As an example, the second author worked with an organization that used RE-AIM to help in planning to expand their integrated physical health/behavioral healthcare program beyond the single practice into a multi-practice group.

With regard to *Reach*, the group defined the target population as all of their practice patients 14 years of age and older and created a monthly denominator to include all scheduled and walk-in appointments with a primary care provider (PCP) visit. For *Effectiveness*, the practice adopted the reliable measures they used in their pilot program with empirically derived benchmarks for achieving goals based on the visit number for each measure. For example, one measure for depression symptom screening, the Patient Health Questionnaire-9 questions (PHQ9) was administered with the expectation that there would be a 50 % reduction in score by week 8 (Kroenke, Spitzer, & Williams, 2001).

For *Adoption*, the practices chose to include all practices in their group but paid special attention to one of the practices with a low patient volume. The practice was small enough not to have been able to support a full-time behavioral health provider alone; however, by sharing a full-time equivalent clinician, they could provide for the behavioral health needs of their patients across all three practices.

For *Implementation*, the practices included the percent of PCP-visit patients screened, based on the denominator established under Reach. They also included a variety of other process measures such as the proportion of those patients who received a personal introduction to the behavioral health provider and the proportion of patients who returned for a second visit, if clinically recommended. Each of these process measures under Adoption provided weekly feedback to the practice as to how well they were adopting the package of EBTs associated with their goal of being a fully integrated practice.

For *Maintenance*, the practices choose to examine grant opportunities so as to support the program while they worked to acquire provider credentialing and establish large enough caseloads to cover a portion of their costs. From a consumer perspective, all patients were screened at each visit, regardless of their current or former use of behavioral health services at the practice. Thus, the team could tell if they were improving the overall behavioral health of their practices or at least maintaining the gains they had achieved through integrated care.

Overall, the use of RE-AIM at the planning stage helped the team to understand all components of their program, and it helped them reach full strength faster than the previous pilot program. Also, they had a clear understanding of their process goals and clinical and practice benchmarks and were able to predict when they could reach sustainability. In fact, by being able to calculate when they felt they would be able to reach their financial stability goal, the team was able to report to their funding organization that they beat that goal *and* were thus invited to apply for a second grant to support a new initiative.

Fixsen's Implementation Framework

Implementing an EBT across multiple sites or within a large organization while ensuring sustainability is a significant challenge. Implementation Science aims to provide guidance with such a challenge, with methods to promote systematic uptake, establishment, and maintenance of the treatment into routine mental health practice (Eccles & Mittman, 2006). This process is outlined in the comprehensive synthesis of the literature on successful intervention research involving implementation by the work of Fixsen and colleagues (2005).

The advantage of the Fixsen's Implementation framework lies in its specificity; it provides detail on how to implement EBTs. Fixsen et al. (2005) determined that there were seven critical elements of a successful implementation: (1) **selection** to determine the appropriate implementation team, identify the appropriate EBT, and recruit staff to attend the in service; (2) **preservice training** on the specific EBTs; (3) expert **consultation and coaching** of staff and administration to carry out their newly acquired skill; (4) **staff evaluation** to assess the use and behavior change desired regarding the trained skill; (5) **program evaluation** to assess and provide feedback on key aspects of the performance of the organization around the new skill; (6) **facilitative administrative supports** to insure data collected are fed back to administration to focus and inform decision making; and (7) **systems intervention** to identify financial, organizational, and human resources required to support the work of the practitioners. Only with the use of all seven core components in planning and implementation can the likelihood for success be ensured.

MedFTs can use the seven core implementation components to create a comprehensive and specific list of tasks to be completed as the work toward full implementation. For example, under the implementation component "selection," researchers identify any staff, supervisors, new hires, etc., and who should participate in the training. Work on this component should also include preplanning such as selecting the implementation team who will be helping start the new program. For every task identified, a responsible party is assigned along with a due date and any relevant details regarding the ongoing progress of the task. Updating this list at each team meeting can provide a clear, up-to-date picture of how to go about implementing the program step by step.

Example of Fixsen's Framework. The utility of this model can be seen using an example of a primary care office who implemented an integrated care program. Using the Fixsen et al. (2005) implementation framework, the team first established a core implementation team consisting of the medical director, practice manager, and an RN or staff member in the practice for whom multiple individuals identified as a natural leader. This enabled the core implementation team to have at least one person with authority in the organization (such as hire/fire authorization or someone with access to budget decisions). This team was necessary to conduct the next step: contract an external consultant to help them understand all aspects of the EBTs associated with creating an integrated care practice. They then met and, using the seven Fixsen et al. (2005) implementation components as a guide, brainstormed all tasks necessary under each of the seven categories. To illustrate this, below is a partial table of some of the tasks they identified under each of the seven core implementation components. The dark gray bars are the interpretation of the seven core implementation components.

Task Toward Implementation	Due	Leader	Progress to date
Select & dedicate staff			
Establish the Core Implementation Team			
Hire BHP			
Identify consulting Pharmacist and Psychiatrist			
All staff trained on model			
Train BHP on health education coaching			
Train MDs in substance use harm reduction model			
Train BHP on Problem Solving Therapy			
Train RNs on screening tools			
Supporting implementation (Consult/Coaching)			
Create a process flow for universal patient screening			
Train billing manager on reimbursement codes			
Create EMR access for BHP			
Start universal screening			
Establish MH insurance processes			
Establish referral process to specialty TMT			
Establish Feedback to Support Team (Staff Eval)			
Establish protocol for weekly call with psychiatrist			
Establish BHP coaching sessions for PST			
Establish Feedback to Program (Program Eval)			
Track weekly appointments made/missed/kept			
Measurept progress on harm reduction goals			
Measure pt progress on PHQ9			
Establish Administrative Supports			
Create data sharing policies			
Create crisis response policies			
Plan for Sustainability via Systems Interventions			
Meet with Managed Care Organizations			
Track revenue captured vs expenditures			

All of the above tasks were expanded on as the team grew in their understanding of the program. Throughout the process, the "due dates," parties responsible for tasks ("leaders"), and open dialogues about successes and barriers ("progress to date") helped to facilitate a highly functional core implementation team.

Further Training in Dissemination and Implementation Science

Beyond this chapter, there are a variety of ways to gain knowledge and skills for MedFTs to launch their own research on implementation. Below is a list of D&I resources for academic, clinical, and student/trainee MedFTs.

Recommendations for Academic MedFTs

MedFTs in an academic setting may find the following resources and ideas helpful to expand their current areas of research into D&I Science:

- Subscribe to and read the journal *Implementation Science* to get a sense of studies encompassed within and advanced by this field.
- The *Dissemination and Implementation in Health* e-Newsletter is distributed monthly and contains up-to-date information regarding webinars, calls for manuscripts, and grant deadlines. In addition, this newsletter highlights important recent publications in the field.
- The NIH Conference on the Science of Dissemination and Implementation is held nearly annually with wide-ranging presentations across all health disciplines and engaging all aspects to D&I work (NIH, 2013). It provides an excellent "first sampling" experience for a research-savvy professionals interested in learning more about the field.
- Two different week-long training experiences are available for those who have accomplished research track records and some experience doing D&I research. Funded by the NIH, these include the following: (1) Training Institute for the Dissemination and Implementation Research in Health (TIDIRH) and (2) the Implementation Research Institute.

Recommendations for Clinical MedFTs

MedFTs with daily access to clinical settings may find the following resources and ideas helpful to include D&I research into their practices:

- Reach out to an academic partner. By looking outside one's own discipline—to medicine, public health, nursing, or other disciplines—one can find an academic researcher who is trained in D&I Science (or has research interests consistent with it). Academics need partners in the community, because while academics can provide some technical expertise around models, measures, analyses, or manuscript development, community-based professionals can provide end-point perspectives, facilitate staff buy-in, and elicit administrative support to make the project doable and the results meaningful.
- Strengthen basic program evaluation skills or quality improvement research. An online search can identify publications and ongoing webinars which are periodically offered by federal agencies (e.g., the NICHQ recently offered a QI webinar series).
- Do not be intimidated by research methodology. Ultimately, the permanent product or archival data (such as medical records or therapy notes) you already have in your practice may have significant information contained. Kreuter and Hovmand (2012) point out that building the sophisticated models and methods is

important but, in the end, the field needs active research projects. To illustrate this point, in the first author's first position in a clinical/training site, she collected medical record data (with the help of undergraduate research assistants) during the year before and after she trained primary care staff to conduct an evidence-based assessment protocol. The results were published in *Pediatrics*, which is a leading clinical journal in the field. One does not have to be a trained methodologist to make a significant contribution to science.

Recommendations for Graduate Students Training in MedFT

MedFTs in training may find the following resources and ideas helpful to explore areas of research into D&I Science:

- Choose thesis/dissertation topics around end-point use. Rather than asking "Does this treatment work?" ask "Does this treatment work in this particular setting with these practitioners using this user-friendly format?"
- Consider conducting your thesis/dissertation or other project in a real-world setting where you are already familiar with stakeholders, teams, and clinical flow, such as a practicum placement or externship. Undergraduate students considering health professions (e.g., Medicine, Nursing, Psychology, or allied disciplines like Physical Therapy) are often motivated to earn credit hours or resume-building opportunities by helping a MedFT collect data in a healthcare setting. For the student, this experiential learning opportunity would be invaluable. The first author cites the example of her own student, Natasha Gouge, whose dissertation focused on cost-effectiveness in a rural pediatric practice where she had completed her externship. The results of this investigation showed that the practice made over $1,000 each day they had a behavioral health student on site. These data are currently unpublished, but it is noteworthy that she used the findings in her job talks and was able to retain a competitive offer.
- Using the suggestions above, especially the annual conference held by the NIH, the newsletter, and journals, start a journal club and get immersed in D&I literature.
- Seek out a graduate program that offers focused training in D&I Science.

Conclusion

D&I Science is an evolving field designed to close the research-practice gap. MedFTs are perfectly poised to advance this science due to the positions that they hold within health service settings and through their daily contact with patients and families. RE-AIM (Glasgow, Vogt, & Boles, 1999) and the Fixsen and colleagues' (2005) implementation framework are two well-designed frameworks around which one can build and execute a sound study using D&I Science principles.

Discussion Questions

1. Consider one study or body of research with which you are familiar. Are its aims consistent with D&I Science? If so, how? If not, how could a study be designed to bring the characteristics of D&I Science to bear on this area?
2. Looking at research teams in your science community, what entrepreneurial relationships exist? What relationships could exist to further a research question or interest you have had? What would an ideal transdisciplinary team look like in your area of interest?
3. Community engagement is a critical element in D&I Science. How have you engaged communities and/or stakeholders in research that you have conducted in the past? How might you improve these practices so that communities/ stakeholders provide iterative feedback throughout your current (or a new) research study?

References[1]

Babione, J. M. (2010). Evidence-based practice in psychology: An ethical framework for graduate education, clinical training, and maintaining professional competence. *Ethics and Behavior, 20* (60), 443–453. doi:10.1080/10508422.2010.521446.

Brischoux, F., & Cook, T. (2009). Juniors seek an end to the impact factor race. *Bioscience, 59*, 238–239. doi:10.1525/bio.2009.59.8.2.

*Brownson, R. C., Colditz, G. A., & Proctor, E. K. (2012). *Dissemination and implementation in research and health: Translating science into practice*. New York, NY: Oxford Press.

Brownson, R. C., Dreisinger, M., Colditz, G. A., & Proctor, E. K. (2012). The path forward in dissemination and implementation research. In R. C. Brownson, G. A. Colditz, & E. K. Proctor (Eds.), *Dissemination and implementation in research and health: Translating science into practice*. New York, NY: Oxford Press.

Brumback, R. A. (2009). Impact factor wars: Episode V—The empire strikes back. *Journal of Child Neurology, 24*, 260–262. doi:10.1177/0883073808331366.

Charach, A., Carson, P., Fox, S., Ali, M. U., Beckett, J., & Lim, C. G. (2013). Interventions for preschool children at high risk for ADHD: A comparative effectiveness review. *Pediatrics, 131*, e1584. doi:10.1542/peds.2012-0974. originally published online 1 April 2013.

Chambers, D. A., Ringeisen, H., & Hickman, E. E. (2005). Federal, state, and foundation initiatives around evidence-based practices in child and adolescent mental health. *Child and Adolescent Psychiatric Clinics of North America, 14*, 307–327. doi:10.1016/j.chc.2004.04.006.

[1] An asterisk has been use to note references that the chapter authors recommend for further reading.

Claridge, J. A., & Fabian, T. C. (2005). History and development of evidence-based medicine. *World Journal of Surgery, 29*, 547–553. doi:10.1007/s00268-005-7910-1. DOI:%2010.1007/s00268-005-7910-1.

Collishaw, S., Maughan, B., Goodman, R., & Pickles, A. (2004). Time trends in adolescent mental health. *Journal of Child Psychology and Psychiatry, 45*, 1350–1362. doi:10.1111/j.1469-7610.2004.00335.x.

Dodge, K. A. (2011). Context matters in child and family policy. *Child Development, 82*, 433–442. doi:10.1111/j.1467-8624.2010.01565.x.

Eccles, M. P., & Mittman, B. S. (2006). Welcome to implementation science. *Implementation Science, 1*, 1. doi:10.1186/1748-5908-1-1. Published online. DOI:10.1186%2F1748-5908-1-1#pmc_ext.

Eonta, A. M., Christon, L. M., Hourigan, S. E., Ravindran, N., Vrana, S. R., & Southam-Gerow, M. (2011). Using everyday technology to enhance evidence-based treatments. *Professional Psychology: Research and Practice, 42*(6), 513–520. doi:10.1037/a0025825.

Fabiano, G. A., Pelham, W. E., Jr., Coles, E. K., Gnagy, E. M., Chronis-Tuscano, A., & O'Connor, B. C. (2009). A meta-analysis of behavioral treatments for attention-deficit/hyperactivity disorder. *Clinical Psychology Review, 29*, 129–140. doi:10.1016/j.cpr.2008.11.001. DOI:10.1016/j.cpr.2008.11.001#doilink.

*Fixsen, D. L., Naoom, S. F., Blase, K. A., Friedman, R. M., & Wallace, F. (2005). Implementation research: A synthesis of the literature. Tampa, FL: University of South Florida, Louis de la Parte Florida Mental Health Institute, The National Implementation Research Network (FMHI Publication #231). Retrieved from http://nirn.fpg.unc.edu/sites/nirn.fpg.unc.edu/files/resources/NIRN-MonographFull-01-2005.pdf.

Freiheit, S. R., Vye, C., Swan, R., & Cady, M. (2004). Cognitive-behavioral therapy for anxiety: Is dissemination working? *The Behavior Therapist, 27*, 25–32.

Gallo, K. P., Comer, J. S., & Barlow, D. H. (2013). Direct-to-consumer marketing of psychological treatments for anxiety disorders. *Journal of Anxiety Disorders, 27*, 793–801. doi:10.1016/j.janxdis.2013.03.005.

Glasgow, R. E., Vogt, T. M., & Boles, S. M. (1999). Evaluating the public health impact of health promotion interventions: the RE-AIM framework. *American Journal of Public Health, 89*, 1322–1327. doi:10.2105/ajph.89.9.1322.

*Glasgow, R. E., Vinson, C., Chambers, D., Khoury, M. J., Kaplan, R. M., & Hunter, C. (2012). National Institutes of Health Approaches to Dissemination and Implementation Science: Current and future directions. *American Journal of Public Health, 102*, 1274–1281. doi:10.2105/AJPH.2012.300755.

Green, L. W., & Kreuter, M. W. (2005). *Health program planning: An educational and ecological approach* (4th ed.). New York: McGraw-Hill.

Greenhalgh, R., Robert, G., MacFarlane, R., Bate, P., & Kriakidou, O. (2004). Diffusion of innovations in service organizations: Systematic review and recommendations. *Milbank Quarterly, 82*, 581–629. doi:10.1111/j.0887-378X.2004.00325.x.

Guerra, N. G., Graham, S., & Tolan, P. H. (2011). Raising healthy children: Translating child development research into practice. *Child Development, 82*(1), 7–16. doi:10.1111/j.1467-8624.2010.01537.x.

Hoagwood, K., & Olin, S. S. (2002). The NIMH blueprint for change report: Research priorities in child and adolescent mental health. *Journal of the American Academy of Child and Adolescent Psychiatry, 41*, 760–767. doi:10.1097/00004583-200207000-00006.

Hofmann, S. G., & Smits, J. A. (2008). Cognitive-behavioral therapy for adult anxiety disorders: A meta-analysis of randomized placebo-controlled trials. *Journal of Clinical Psychiatry, 69*, 621–632.

Hyman, S. E. (1999). Protecting patients, preserving progress: Ethics in mental health research. *Academic Medicine, 74*, 258–259.

Jensen, S. A., & Grimes, L. K. (2010). Increases in parent attendance to behavioral parent training due to concurrent child treatment groups. *Child & Youth Care Forum, 39*, 239–251. doi:10.1007/s10566-010-9101-y.

Klesges, L. M., Estabrooks, P. A., Glasgow, R. E., & Dzewaltowski, D. (2005). Beginning with the application in mind: Designing and planning health behavior change interventions to enhance dissemination. *Annals of Behavioral Medicine, 29*, 66S–75S. doi:10.1207/s15324796abm2902s_10.

Kreuter, M. W. & Hovmand, P. S. (2012). Does marketing enhance dissemination? Results from a system dynamics simulation study. *Paper presented at the 5th Annual NIH conference on the Science of Dissemination and Implementation*. Bethesda, MD.

Kroenke, K., Spitzer, R. L., & Williams, J. B. (2001). The PHQ-9: Validity of a brief depression severity measure. *Journal of General Internal Medicine, 16*, 606–613. doi:10.1046/j.1525-1497.2001.016009606.x.

Meehl, P. E. (1987). Theory and practice: Reflections of an academic clinician. In E. F. Bourg, R. J. Bent, J. E. Callan, N. F. Jones, J. McHolland, & G. Stricker (Eds.), *Standards and evaluation in the education and training of professional psychologists: Knowledge, attitudes, and skills* (pp. 7–23). Norman, OK: Transcript Press.

Mendenhall, T., Berge, J., & Doherty, W. (2014). Engaging communities as partners in research: Advancing integrated care through purposeful partnerships. In J. Hodgson, A. Lamson, T. Mendenhall, & R. Crane (Eds.), *Medical family therapy: Advanced applications* (pp. 259–282). New York: Springer.

Miller, W., Munoz, R., & Christensen, C. (2010). Expanding evidence based psychological services: From traditional therapy to self-help books to internet interventions. *Clinical round table presented at the annual meeting of the Association for Behavioral and Cognitive Therapies*. San Francisco, CA.

Minkler, M., & Wallerstein, N. (Eds.). (2008). *Community-based participatory research for health: From process to outcomes* (2nd ed.). San Francisco, CA: Jossey Bass.

Mittman, et al. (2009). *Practical guidance for scaling up health service innovations*. Geneva: World Health Organization. Retrieved from http://www.expandnet.net/PDFs/WHO_ExpandNet_Practical_Guide_published.pdf.

National Cancer Institute (NCI). (2012). *Grid enabled measures database: A community site for researchers*. Retrieved from http://cancercontrol.cancer.gov/brp/gem.html.

National Institutes of Health (NIH). (2013). *Offices of Behavioral and Social Science Research/NIH conference on the Science of Dissemination and Implementation*. Retrieved from http://obssr.od.nih.gov/index.aspx, and http://obssr.od.nih.gov/scientific_areas/translation/dissemination_and_implementation/index.aspx.

Norton, P. J., & Price, E. C. (2007). A meta-analytic review of adult cognitive-behavioral treatment outcomes across the anxiety disorders. *Journal of Nervous Mental Disease, 195*, 521–531. doi:10.1097/01.nmd.0000253843.70149.9a.

Office of Statistical Analysis and Reporting, Office of Research Information Systems, & Office of Extramural Research. (2012). *Research grants: Funding by mechanism*. Retrieved from http://report.nih.gov/NIHDatabook/Charts/Default.aspx?showm=Y&chartId=43&catId=2.

Otte, C. (2011). Cognitive behavioral therapy in anxiety disorders: Current state of the evidence. *Dialogues in Clinical Neuroscience, 13*(4), 413–421.

Porges, S. W. (2006). Asserting the role of biobehavioral sciences in translational research: The behavioral neurobiology revolution. *Development and Psychopathology, 18*, 923–933. doi:10.1017/S0954579406060457.

Roshanaei-Moghaddam, B., Pauly, M. C., Atkins, D. C., Baldwin, S. A., Stein, M. B., & Roy-Byrne, P. (2011). Relative effects of CBT and pharmacotherapy in depression versus anxiety: Is medication somewhat better for depression and CBT somewhat better for anxiety? *Depression and Anxiety, 28*, 560–567. doi:10.1002/da.20829.

Ruscio, A. M., & Holohan, D. R. (2006). Applying empirically supported treatments to complex cases: Ethical, empirical, and practical considerations. *Clinical Psychology: Science and Practice, 13*(2), 146–162. doi:10.1111/j.1468-2850.2006.00017.x.

Shriver, M. D., & Allen, K. D. (2008). *Working with parents of noncompliant children*. Washington, DC: APA. doi:10.1037/11791-009.

Shediac-Rizkallah, M. C., & Bone, L. R. (1998). Planning for the sustainability of community-based health programs: Conceptual frameworks and future directions for research practice and policy. *Health Education Research, 13*, 87–108.

Simmons, R., Fajans, P., & Ghiron, L. (2007). Introduction. In R. Simmons, P. Fajans, & L. Ghiron (Eds.) *Scaling up health service delivery: From pilot innovations to policies and programmes* (pp. vii–xvii). Geneva: World Health Organization. Retrieved from http://whqlibdoc.who.int/publications/2007/9789241563512_eng.pdf.

Smith, R. E., Fagan, C., Wilson, N. L., Chen, J., Corona, M., Nguyen, H., . . . Shoda, Y. (2011). Internet-based approaches to collaborative therapeutic assessment: New opportunities for professional psychologists. *Professional Psychology: Research and Practice, 42*(6), 494–504. doi:10.1037/a0025392.

Stewart, R. W., & Chambless, D. L. (2007). Does psychotherapy research inform treatment decisions in private practice? *Journal of Clinical Psychology, 63*(3), 267–281. doi:10.1002/jclp.20347.

Sussman, S., Valente, T. W., Rohrbach, L. A., Skara, S., & Pentz, M. A. (2006). Translation in the health professions: Converting science into action. *Evaluation in the Health Professions, 29*, 7–31. doi:10.1177/0163278705284441.

*Tabak, R. G., Khoong, E. C., Chambers, D. A., & Brownson, R. (2012). Bridging research and practice: Models for dissemination and implementation research. *American Journal of Preventative Medicine, 43*, 337–350. doi:10.1016/j.amepre.2012.05.024. DOI:10.1016/j.amepre.2012.05.024#doilink.

Twenge, J. M., Gentile, B., DeWall, C. N., Ma, D., Lacefield, K., & Schurtz, D. R. (2010). Birth cohort increases in psychopathology among young Americans, 1938–2007: A cross-temporal meta-analysis of the MMPI. *Clinical Psychology Review, 30*, 145–154. doi:10.1016/j.cpr.2009.10.005.

US Department of Transportation, National Highway Traffic Safety Administration, & National Center for Statistics and Analysis. (2012). *Traffic safety facts: 2010 data*. Washington, DC: DOT HS 811 636. Retrieved from http://www-nrd.nhtsa.dot.gov/Pubs/811636.pdf.

Werba, B. E., Eyberg, S. M., Boggs, S. R., & Algina, J. (2006). *Behavior Modification, 30*, 618–646. doi:10.1177/0145445504272977.

Young, N. S., Ioannidis, J. P. A., & Al-Ubaydli, O. (2008). Why current publication practices may distort science. *PLoS Medicine, 5*(10), e201. doi:10.1371/journal.pmed.0050201.

Zerhouni, E. (2003). The NIH roadmap. *Science, 302*, 63–72. doi:10.1126/science.1091867.

Chapter 17
Advancing Health Equity in Medical Family Therapy Research

Melissa Lewis, Laurelle Myhra, and Monique Walker

> *As doctors, it is our job to overcome these natural (biased) tendencies and make patients from all backgrounds comfortable. As members of the public, however, we must continue to be dissatisfied with the disparity in medical outcomes among different racial groups.*
>
> Shaw and Armin (2011, p. 254)

Introduction

In both the medical and behavioral health fields, US minorities experience worse health outcomes when compared to nonminority members (Department of Health and Human Services [HHS] [HHS], 2011). Specifically, "characteristics such as race or ethnicity, religion, socioeconomic status (SES), gender, age, behavioral health status, disability, sexual orientation or gender identity, geographic location, or other characteristics historically linked to exclusion or discrimination are known to influence health status" (HHS, 2011, p. 2). Possible causes of these health disparities include lack of insurance, poor access to care, poor quality of care, less preventative care, low patient centeredness (e.g., not providing appropriate language services, cultural incompetence, devaluing patient and family belief systems or opinions), low income, and poor health behaviors (e.g., dietary risks, sedentary lifestyle, substance abuse) (Agency for Healthcare Research & Quality [AHRQ] [AHRQ], 2011; Hasnain-Wynia et al., 2010, Healthy 2020, 2012; HHS, 2011). In addition, social inequities and higher rates of stress related to prolonged

M. Lewis (✉)
University of Minnesota Medical School, Duluth, MN, USA
e-mail: melewis@d.umn.edu

J. Hodgson et al. (eds.), *Medical Family Therapy*, DOI 10.1007/978-3-319-03482-9_17,

and systematic oppression are powerful and often ignored contributors to health disparities (Healthy 2020, 2012).

While Engel's seminal work (1977) stressed the importance of including the biological, psychological, and social aspects of health in care, it was less specific about how social inequities affect health outcomes. Unfortunately, overt and covert racism and heterosexism contribute to unequal and poorer health experiences for minorities living in the United States. Among minorities, stress, discrimination, and unfair treatment have been linked to negative health outcomes (Al-Khatib et al., 2012; Troxel, Matthews, Bromberger, & Sutton-Tyrrell, 2003). For example, low socioeconomic status (SES) and discrimination are linked to increases in body mass index (BMI), tobacco use, hypertension, and reduced physical activity (Rutledge et al., 2003; Subramanyam et al., 2012; Williams & Leavell, 2012). Further, among racial minorities, SES and neighborhood safety have been linked to increased blood pressure as early as adolescence (McGrath, Matthews, & Brady, 2006). Among the lesbian, gay, bisexual, transgender, and queer (LGBTQ) population, health disparities include higher risk for certain types of cancer—especially breast cancer in women (Buchmueller & Carpenter, 2010) and prostate cancer in men (Hart, Coon, Kowalkowski, & Latini, 2011)—and mental illness, particularly depression, anxiety, and suicidal ideation (Healthy 2020, 2012; Krehely, 2009). In addition, LGBTQ individuals are more likely to smoke (Lee, Griffin, & Melvin, 2009), drink alcohol (Hughes, 2005), use drugs (Hunt, 2012), and engage in other risky behaviors when compared to heterosexual individuals (Healthy 2020, 2012; Krehely, 2009).

The primary purpose of this chapter is to guide MedFTs toward culturally humble and reflexive healthcare delivery and research production to reduce health disparities (Shaw & Armin, 2011). To this end, the authors will provide recommendations for every step in the research process, but not before this content is nested in its appropriate context: self of the researcher reflections from each author and information about the history of research with minority populations. The authors use the term Medical Family Therapists (MedFTs) to imply *both* a clinician and researcher, because the role of clinician-researcher is a collaborative and circular process whereby research informs care and vice versa. There is a need to better bridge gaps between both (a) research and practice and (b) researchers working within their respective fields (e.g., behavioral health and medical health) through collaboration. Just as operating in the silos of biological, psychological, social, and spiritual health has resulted in fractioned and less effective care, research and clinical practice typically occur in isolation from one another.

Guidelines set forth in this chapter are informed by critical race theory (Curtis, 2006) or, more specifically, a decolonizing framework (Smith, 1999; Duran, Firehammer, & Gonzalez, 2008). The decolonizing framework addresses power dynamics and reveals untold or subjugated truths that inform healing methods through increasingly egalitarian research strategies. Through this framework, research is more likely to reflect the health experiences of underserved communities.

Locating Our Multiple Selves

We contend that an important aspect of being a MedFT is reflexivity and humility, which involves identifying similarities and differences within salient social locations, such as race, ethnicity, age, gender, class, sexual orientation, and religion, and acknowledging how these factors can influence clinical care with patients and the way(s) in which research is conducted (Jorgensen, 2011; Walker, Read, & Priest, 2013; Watts-Jones, 2010). Below we first "locate" ourselves in order to increase transparency regarding our social locations, values, and research interests.

The first author is bicultural (Caucasian and Cherokee) and a dual citizen of the Cherokee Nation and the United States (i.e., political citizenship to both sovereign nations). She earned her PhD in MedFT, is a Licensed Marriage and Family Therapist, and is an AAMFT-Approved Supervisor. She has taught didactic and clinical courses to Marriage and Family Therapy (MFT) and medical students and has conducted mixed-methods research on the integration of behavioral health services in medical settings with indigenous communities (e.g., those residing in the United States and Canada) and military couples. She specialized in MedFT because of her belief that health is holistic, systemic, family focused, community based, and informed by intergenerational knowledge. Her dual identities (political and cultural) inform the work that she does and the lens that she utilizes.

The second author is of mixed heritage including Ojibwe and Scandinavian. She is a health researcher and a Licensed Marriage and Family Therapist whose work has focused on health disparities among American Indians, including communities' strengths and vulnerabilities, culturally tailored care, and conducting responsible and intentional research. Her passion stems from her early life experiences growing up on the Red Lake reservation. Although mostly positive, she witnessed the intergenerational effects of cultural loss and trauma in her community. Because of her modest upbringing, it has been important for her to be cognizant of power differentials when providing therapy and engaging communities in research.

The third author identifies as a Black (and African-American), queer, feminist family therapist and mixed-methods researcher. She is a passionate social justice advocate and activist and is dedicated to raising awareness about how issues of race, ethnicity, religion, gender, gender identity, sexuality, and sexual orientation influence clinical and research processes. Her passion for working with patients of color and LGBTQ individuals, couples, and families comes from her understanding of how her own multiple and intersecting identities have shaped her life experiences and views of the world. She is especially committed to creating safe spaces for Black youth and understanding experiences of Black families during the coming out process. She is uniquely aware of the positions of privilege and subjugation that she occupies and tries to remain intentional about addressing issues of power, privilege, hierarchy, and injustice in her research and clinical work.

History of Minorities in Medicine and Research

Minority groups have disproportionately been victims of unethical medical and research practices that include painful, deceitful, life-threatening, and culturally inappropriate interventions throughout the history of the United States, usually for the benefit of the majority members. It is important to remember that discrimination in medical settings is merely a microcosm of discrimination that occurs at the larger societal level. Racism notably commenced in the United States less than 300 years ago through the implementation of laws (e.g., slave codes prohibited carrying of firearms and having servants, for instance) and popular scientific inquiry (e.g., classification of nature attempted to prove that races were scientifically different) (Goodman, Moses, & Jones, 2012). These acts followed, most clearly, with the forcible removal of Africans from their homeland to be used brutally as unpaid workers in the United States, as well as the attempted colonization of indigenous peoples. Before this time, discrimination occurred not on the basis of skin tone, but by religion, SES (i.e., stratification by income and other economic factors), or class (i.e., stratification by occupation and other economic factors). Further, government and scientific bodies did not follow the social belief system that the scientific notion of race was a dividing line for legal rights. Shortly after this time, genocide and eugenics based on skin color occurred around the world (e.g., in Germany, Australia, and the United States). Hierarchical grouping preferences, and therefore hierarchical qualities of life, are still at the root of discrimination today.

Racism that occurs at a societal level is inevitably reflected in the medical research of the time period. To illustrate this point, we will review a few historical periods and corresponding medical interventions and research during those times. The field of Gynecology was created by Dr. Marion Sims in 1845, who conducted excruciating and invasive vaginal experiments on African slaves in the United States with no anesthesia (Washington, 2006). From these experiments, he invented a fistula repair and then offered this procedure to White patients with the benefit of anesthesia. During the period of segregation in the United States, the Tuskegee Syphilis Study was initiated in 1932 to learn about disease progression. Participants were African-American men who were not given antibiotics until 1972, despite penicillin being the standard treatment since 1947 (Washington, 2006). In a study from 1940 to 1953, the US government funded research that infected Guatemalan citizens with sexually transmitted infections, but the ethical violations related to this research were not investigated until 2010 (Presidential Commission for the Study of Bioethical Issues, 2011).

In the same vein as eugenics and genocide, population control measures (e.g., sterilization programs) were funded by the US government under the Nixon and Bush Sr. administrations. These programs targeted poor minorities, especially within indigenous communities, as well as citizens from Columbia, Bolivia, and Puerto Rico, with the intent of sterilizing 25 % of the world's population (Park, 2012). Latin American victims of this practice were offered $5.00 for the procedure. In the mid-1970s, Indian Health Services (IHS) facilities advanced nontherapeutic sterilizations on up to 75 % of its patients. Women were told that their social services benefits would be taken from them if they did not get sterilized (Lawrence, 2000). The last documented forced sterilization in the United States occurred in 1981 (Park, 2012).

Ethical violations continue even under today's strict Institutional Review Board (IRB) and Health Insurance Portability and Accountability Act (HIPAA) regulations. In 2002, the Havasupai tribe of Arizona sued Arizona State University for using biomarkers without their permission (Hendricks, 2004; Trimble, Scharron-del Rio, & Bernal, 2010). Researchers had initially gained informed consent to gather DNA materials to study diabetes but also collected handprints from participants all the while knowing that they would do a study on inbreeding. In addition, without obtaining an updated informed consent, researchers later used the DNA material to study schizophrenia and historical migration patterns that were not requested by the community. Further, the "creation story" of the Havasupai tribe relates to the tribe being born out of the Grand Canyon, yet researchers were attempting to invalidate this belief and show that they migrated to the Grand Canyon instead. In total, fifteen of the twenty-three published articles covered content that was not given consent for. Studying another culture's religion or worldview in an attempt to disprove or devalue their belief systems is indicative of both investigative misconduct and researcher ethnocentrism.

Microaggressions and colorblind racism represent the most prevalent forms of racism today. Microaggressions include insulting comments that are commonplace and brief and usually go unnoticed by the sender of the message (Sue et al., 2007). The seemingly subtle undertones make the racist components difficult to identify and even more difficult to address but are harmful nonetheless (Sue, 2010). Similarly, colorblind racism is a type of racism that is covert but specifically denies the history and experiences of minorities living in the United States by attempting to ignore social inequities. Messages that are categorized as microaggressions or colorblind racism increase feelings of comfort around privilege for majorities (Fryberg, 2010) and cause stress in minority groups (Holoien & Shelton, 2011). Examples of these racial tribulations include grabbing one's purse or locking car doors when a minority member walks by, saying "you don't look Black" or "I couldn't even tell that you are disabled" and using terms like "that is so ghetto," "that's retarded," or "that's gay."

These inherent but masked belief systems may unintentionally guide the focus of research or the way in which research studies are conducted. Looking back at the previous example of sterilization, the research was founded on the underlying belief that minority women have too many children. This racist belief continues today, with the commonplace notion that single, minority women disproportionately and undeservedly draw on the welfare system. This belief may then influence how a researcher quantifies intervention success. Using an outcome variable like number of pregnancies as a predictor of health for minority women (and not for majority women and families) is an example of a research-placed microaggression. These research decisions go unchecked and have an enormous influence on the participants and the communities in which they live. A research participant disclosed, "At times, there is subtle racism in researchers who come into tribal communities, and [they] think they are helping us, but there is a latent attitude of the 'ignorant Indians' on the reservation" (NCAI Policy Research Center and MSU Center for Native Health Partnerships, 2012, p.17).

To avoid subtle and overt discrimination in research, it is critical that MedFTs spend time learning about and engaging in dialogue around (a) the history of the people that they are treating and researching, (b) the current and historical relationship between this population and that of the dominant culture, and (c) the history of the land in which they are living on. Further, addressing the self of the researcher through location of self, addressing biases, and learning how to engage the community around these issues, although challenging, will allow the MedFT researcher to engage in a more culturally humble manner, create more collaborative relationships, and produce more effective and relevant research outcomes.

Self of the Medical Family Therapy Researcher

Historically, researchers who have worked with minority groups have focused on problem-saturated stories that describe why these communities experience so much illness and disease, often from the perspective that the minorities' intrinsic "problems" are the cause of their poor health (e.g., "bad" genes, "bad" health habits, and "bad" relationships) (Duran, 2006; McGrath et al., 2006; Rutledge et al., 2003). This type of causal explanation originates from larger societal views of minorities, and perpetuates the practice of blaming minorities for their negative health outcomes (Duran, 2006). In the larger behavioral and medical health fields, there has recently been a focus on more cultural understanding and sensitivity (Anderson, Scrimshaw, Fullilove, Fielding, & Normand, 2003; Dana & Allen, 2008; Hunt, 2001; Kirmayer, 2012; NAHO, 2008; Rincón, 2009; Wendt & Gone, 2012; Whitbeck, 2006). For example, there has been an increase in the last two decades of literature pertaining to providers' cultural understandings and awareness, and how these interventions influence patient outcomes (Betancourt, Green, Carrillo, & Ananeh-Firempong, 2003; Papps & Ramsden, 1996; Renganathan, 2009; Shaw & Armin, 2011).

Self-Evaluation in Research

Understanding and using one's "self" is being increasingly recognized as an integral part of the behavioral science research process because it is clear that "what we see and what we hear in fieldwork settings is affected by our backgrounds, proclivities, and social locations" (Jorgensen, 2011, p. 115). Instead of ignoring or denying how we influence the research process, we suggest that acknowledging and understanding these influences is vital to the research process in both quantitative and qualitative MedFT research.

Self-evaluation techniques have been traditionally applied to qualitative research (Goldstein, 2003); however, we suggest that locating oneself and being self-reflexive is necessary for quantitative and mixed-method MedFT researchers as well because our understandings are shaped by our prior experiences and social locations (Jorgensen, 2011). The authors suggest the following techniques to locate oneself in one's research project: (a) researcher reflexivity (described in more detail, below), (b) enhancing trustworthiness (through methods such as prolonged engagement), which both contribute to (c) enhancing trustworthiness (the qualitative equivalent to reliability and validity) Berg & Smith, 1988; Goldstein, 2003; Kvale, 1996; Nicholls, 2009; Pezalla, Pettigrew & Miller-Day, 2012; Simon, 2006). Credibility requires assessing the congruency between the observations and findings of reality. Guba and Lincoln (1981) have suggested that credibility is one of the most important factors in establishing trustworthiness, which deals with the aspects of truth value, applicability, consistency, and neutrality.

Bracketing is an important method for practicing reflexivity. This technique requires stepping back and challenging one's previously held notions and biases in order to allow for more engagement with the current research. For example, the third author, is a queer-identified researcher who investigates LGBTQ populations, practices bracketing by journaling about her biases, assumptions, and hypotheses at the outset of a research project as a way of putting distance between her personal experiences and beliefs and what she may expect to discover. This process continues throughout data collection and analysis and is important because she may be more prone to looking *for* specific outcomes or themes in research based on her connections and experience with the research. Instead, the third author wants to be sure that she remains open and able to see and hear what emerges from the data.

The MedFT researcher is not simply an objective observer of human behavior and health outcomes without personal biases and beliefs, but is inherently embedded within the research process and, therefore, influences the outcomes. The *researcher-as-instrument* perspective thereby defines investigators as active contributors to the research who must first address their belief systems and identify their biases. This includes interpreting prior studies, choosing theoretical frameworks to guide the design of the study, developing a primary aim to examine, choosing the instruments or measures, and collecting and analyzing data (Guba & Lincoln, 1981; Pezalla et al., 2012). The authors also recommend that the MedFT researcher has a clear understanding of why he/she is conducting the research; what beliefs are already held about the variables and behaviors being examined, the value of using varying sampling approaches, data collection strategies, data analysis methods (i.e., triangulation), and theoretical lenses; and what outcomes are expected.

Cultural Humility and Cultural Safety

Cultural humility and cultural safety are critical components for the development of a MedFT researcher. Personal awareness of beliefs and biases must continue to be navigated over time, which is an idea that opposes previously held notions of cultural competence as an outcome or destination. Tervalon and Murray-Garcia (1998) differentiate between cultural humility and cultural competence and describe the former as a process that requires:

> Humility as individuals continually engage in self-reflection and self-critique as lifelong learners and reflective practitioners, humility in how physicians bring into check the power imbalances that exist in the dynamics of physician–patient communication by using patient focused interviewing and care, and humility to develop and maintain mutually respectful and dynamic partnerships with communities on behalf of individual patients and communities in the context of community-based clinical and advocacy training models. (p. 118).

In MedFT research, cultural humility has great value because it recognizes the importance of attending to the multiple social locations of patients and providers using community engagement to lessen the hierarchical and power imbalances inherent in the research process (Doherty & Mendenhall, 2006). The authors suggest that MedFT researchers who are engaging vulnerable populations adopt a culturally humble perspective. This perspective promotes (a) the reflexive process that the authors believe is integral in research and (b) attention to the community's voice is valued. The focus of cultural humility is on the growth and increased awareness of the researcher, which marks a distinct shift from historical practice in healthcare research settings (Anderson et al., 2003). Additionally, a stance of cultural humility acknowledges the expertise and importance of participants and their communities as agents of change in the research process and in having agency within the change process.

Cultural safety describes the importance of attending to the social, historical, political, and economic circumstances that help to create power differences and inequalities in health during clinical or research encounters (Anderson et al., 2003; Kirmayer, 2012; Polaschek, 1998). The goals of cultural safety, according to Polaschek (1998), are to (a) highlight researchers' beliefs and attitudes; (b) learn from participants, especially those who are different from the researcher; (c) disengage from the process of victim blaming; (d) attend to sociohistorical, political, linguistic, economic, and spiritual processes; and (e) provide culturally appropriate interventions as defined by the people they serve.

The ability of providers, researchers, and institutions to become more self-reflexive is a critical component for delivering ethically and culturally sensitive services. A self-reflexive approach promotes a leveling of the hierarchy between researchers and participants, shared decision-making about healthcare goals and treatment, and ownership of clinical research within minority communities to create a new paradigm regarding power and privilege. MedFTs should work to understand their own cultural identities and empower their participants to understand theirs in order to provide culturally appropriate research that promotes the well-being of diverse individuals, families, and communities (Kirmayer, 2012; Polaschek, 1998).

The Minority Researcher

"In-group" researchers are equally vulnerable to incorporating bias into their work as are "outsiders." Both must resist the urge to become experts in a community, whether they are members of the community or have worked with members of the community for 20 years. For instance, the process of learning the experimental method may require minority researchers to learn a new way of evaluating the world which may or may not fit with their home communities' current beliefs.

If a minority researcher finds a way to balance old and new belief systems and is able to complete graduate school, another particularly challenging time period follows. Postgraduation is a time filled with much enthusiasm to take learned knowledge and apply it to communities in need. However, a researcher may use research techniques (i.e., techniques learned from a Western education) that are offensive and possibly damaging to community members (NCAI Policy Research Center and MSU Center for Native Health Partnerships, 2012). For example, a minority researcher may return to her home community and ask questions about sensitive topics such as family relationships, sex, or health without first following the proper protocol in that community because she has not tracked her own changing belief systems over time. Minority members, similar to nonminority members, must use critical and evaluative self-of-researcher techniques to monitor their overt and hidden biases. One researcher commented:

> I'm a Native person but I never presume, even when I am home that I really know. And, the other thing, I guess, kind of a rule, is to listen... I listen and look and learn. Because if you presume that you know what is going on, you have made your first mistake. (NCAI Policy Research Center and MSU Center for Native Health Partnerships, 2012, p. 20).

Very rarely are minority students or faculty members educated or mentored to utilize their local and cultural knowledge to address health issues. Instead, the underlying message is that they must use Western principles of science, medicine, and research only. Further, popular theories of health that have been developed by or with minority communities rarely are credited to the minority community; instead, credit is given to the researcher (e.g., Maslow's hierarchy of needs and the Blackfoot community, Virginia Satir and the Tiyospaye community) (Bodin, 1988; Coon, 2006). It is suggested here that educators learn how to address self-of-researcher in methodology courses and encourage students to utilize their own cultures as a tool alongside other research tools.

Identifying One's Personal Research Value and Role

MedFTs hold tremendous power and privilege in that they can influence healthcare delivery, policy, and outcomes. This privilege must be taken seriously, with every research project developed and completed with care and thoughtful critique. Even further, MedFT researchers should identify their personal *research value* and, therefore, their *role* to ground and center themselves in the research community (Villegas, 2013). For example, the first author's research *value* is that strengthening indigenous family and community relationships (e.g., via acknowledging tribal sovereignty and privileging indigenous ways of being) protects against medical and behavioral health risks. Therefore, her *role* is to empower indigenous families and communities. Examples of research projects that she can engage in may be quantitative or qualitative, address diabetes or early childhood interventions, aim to change healthcare delivery or policy, etc., as long as her values and roles remain consistent and transparent.

Identifying researcher role and value will (a) organize and direct the researcher's projects and portfolio, (b) identify the researcher's identity (including strengths and biases), and (c) identify one's central responsibility to the field and research participants. Further, research role and value identification will situate the researcher in the larger research community. A role implies that a team of others with differing specific skills is needed to work on a project collaboratively. For example, when the researcher is brainstorming a research project, she will talk with local healthcare providers, patients, community members, other researchers involved in similar research, and local or national advocacy groups, instead of searching for gaps in literature through academic reviews alone.

Engaging Communities in Health Research

As outlined above, minority groups in the United States have long been victims of unethical research practices. Due to this disconcerting history, ethnic and sexual minorities often distrust researchers (Spears et al., 2011). Therefore, investigators should not attempt to remove themselves from this history, but rather locate themselves within it and prepare to humbly address power differentials as they carry forward their work.

Community-Based Participatory Research

For many critical and feminist researchers, community-based participatory research (CBPR) represents a valuable approach that is sensitive to over-researched and undervalued ethnic and minority groups (Wallerstein & Duran, 2003). CBPR has gained increased recognition over the last decade as a viable and culturally tailored research methodology in which researchers and community members form long-term partnerships to ultimately reduce health disparities in a manner that is empowering to minority groups (Israel et al., 2003; Minkler, 2005; Rhodes, Malow, & Jolly, 2010). Successful CBPR partnerships have led to community action and improved health outcomes that are defined as priorities by both the community members and the research team (Dulmus & Cristalii, 2012; Israel, Eng,

Schulz, & Parker, 2005; Loh & Sugerman-Brozan, 2002; Minkler, 2005; Rhodes et al., 2010).

A central tenet of CBPR, as described in detailed in Chap. 14 of this text (Mendenhall, Berge, & Doherty, 2014), is the formation of a multidisciplinary research team which includes outsiders and insiders from the community, both professionals and lay members (Eng et al., 2005). It is important to remember that the representatives or key stakeholders in the community may not represent the majority of the community, so it is imperative to engage the community and establish relationships to fully understand the community's needs and strengths. This requires attending community events, meeting community members, and becoming a noticeable ally. Engaging community members in the research process helps to ensure the quality and integrity of the research as well as increase the likelihood of observing change in health outcomes (Minkler, 2005).

The way in which communities are engaged in health research should be uniquely tailored to culture and context (LaVeaux & Christopher, 2009; Wallerstein & Duran, 2003) and with the needs and priorities of the community at the forefront (Rhodes et al., 2010). For example, in a review of CBPR tenets as applied to indigenous communities, LaVeaux and Christopher (2009) highlighted important and unique sociohistorical factors including considering historical experience with research (e.g., top-down, abusive), health issues (e.g., diabetes, cardiovascular disease), considering tribal sovereignty, differentiating between tribal and community membership, and recognizing tribal diversity. Successful CBPR partnerships should lead to sustainable prevention services, interventions, and changes in policy and procedures, through ethical research designs that fully incorporate cultural context and knowledge (Rhodes et al., 2010).

Culturally Tailored Assessments

A debate continues in translational health research about the appropriateness of adapting and applying evidence-based practices to groups whose worldviews and experiences may not have been considered when first developing a particular intervention (Novins et al., 2011). Further, because of the disproportionate lack of funding to conduct evaluation research, many culturally specific treatment approaches have not been developed or validated with, or disseminated to, minority communities (Beauvais, 1998; Duran & Duran, 1995; Legaspi & Orr, 2007; Novins et al., 2011). Researchers and providers often agree that culturally tailored prevention and treatment, when possible, can enhance outcomes by building upon cultural strengths (Gone, 2003; Walters, Simoni, & Evans-Campbell, 2002; Weaver & Brave Heart, 1999; Whitbeck, 2006). The process of developing culturally tailored programs requires reflective researchers who prioritize the wisdom and belief systems of the individual community. Therefore, a dynamic and long-term partnership with the community is key to the successful development and evaluation of culturally tailored programs (Eng et al., 2005; Israel et al., 2003).

Before developing a research study, the authors recommend that researchers first develop a relationship with the community to consider together how they can frame a study to best benefit the community. Determining the needs and assets of the community requires multidirectional knowledge sharing and shared decision-making to ensure authentic research designs, culturally tailored implementation, and development of realistic interventions and prevention programs (Israel, Schulz, Parker, & Becker, 2001; Rhodes et al., 2010; Schulz et al., 2002). The assessment should draw upon a wide range of resources, including extant epidemiology data and literature (published and unpublished), and these findings should be triangulated with cultural knowledge from community members and key stakeholders (Eng et al., 2005; Harris, Jerome, & Fawcett, 1997; Rhodes et al., 2010; Wallerstein & Duran, 2010).

The goal of assessment in research and practice is to enhance knowledge and inform care; however, the utility and validity of assessments with minority groups continue to be in question for a number of reasons, including lack of normative data for minority groups (Malgady & Colon-Malgady, 2008), lack of quality cultural training (Dana, 2005; Lie, Lee-Rey, Gomez, Bereknyei, & Braddock, 2010), lack of evaluation of cultural trainings (Dana & Allen, 2008), and little or no supervision regarding how to use multicultural assessments (Allen, 2007). Researchers and providers need to increase access to culturally tailored assessments and interventions in order to decrease health disparities. Assessments should be developed with a community voice and cultural knowledge. With a CBPR approach, this may be achieved with or without funding (Rhodes et al., 2010).

Data Ownership

Ownership of data or knowledge inherently involves issues of power and privilege, which is a delicate issue when engaging communities of minority status. Historically, researchers and their respective universities have been the perceived data owners secondary to their roles of storing, compiling, identifying findings, and deciding how to share or disseminate the knowledge (Rhodes et al., 2010). Data ownership is a historically unacknowledged privilege that goes unexamined until ethical, institutional, legal, or professional issues emerge from the research participants and their communities (Cashman et al., 2008; Lazarus, Duran, Caldwell, & Bulbulia, 2012; Wallerstein & Duran, 2006). Communities should feel empowered to act in their best interests, negotiating risks and benefits as equitable partners in the research process (Minkler, 2005; Rhodes et al., 2010; Wallerstein & Duran, 2006). In order to ensure community members' full consent of the proposed use of the data and that the use of data will directly benefit them, communication about data ownership must take place at the beginning of the partnership (Lazarus et al., 2012; Wallerstein & Duran, 2006).

The role of the IRB has traditionally been to protect human subjects from harm; however, IRBs do not assess whether or not a community has benefitted from research. The authors support the recommendation that IRBs protect human subjects but also assert that IRBs should encourage projects that provide more direct benefit to the community that is studied (Community-Campus Partnerships for Health, 2009; Wallerstein & Duran, 2006). Until this paradigmatic change occurs, the responsibility falls on the research team to ensure that a democratic partnership has been built and that the research products or post-research actions benefit the community in ways that the community deems appropriate. The direct benefits or post-research actions that may be most significant in reducing health disparities are effective interventions and prevention programs, policy changes, and community capacity building (Lazarus et al., 2012).

Democratic participation on the part of the community is necessary for the feasibility and sustainability of post-research community programs (Lazarus et al., 2012; Wallerstein & Duran, 2010). The authors recommend the use of community boards over individual community representatives to increase representation and diversity of views and experiences. Community boards should be active in the research process, engaged in decision-making around interpretation of the research findings, and translating findings into action (Lazarus et al., 2012; Wallerstein & Duran, 2010).

Capacity Building in Research

A major strength of CBPR is the goal of strengthening communities through sustainable partnerships that focus on capacity building (Dulmus & Cristalii, 2012; Harris et al., 1997; Lazarus et al., 2012; Minkler & Wallerstein, 2008; Wallerstein & Duran, 2006). As a part of the research design, capacity building includes engaging community members in a wide variety of roles, including researchers, research assistants, cultural informants, and community liaisons that help to keep the community's needs at the forefront of the research. In the case of CBPR, professional and lay community members also engage in research by providing interventions and supervision of interventions and by monitoring and evaluating programs to increase the potential for success (Cashman et al., 2008; Jones, Koegel & Wells, 2008).

Done well, capacity building can empower and enhance pride in cultural knowledge and practices and can also provide benefits equitably to community members (e.g., health workers) engaged in the research process in the same manners as it does for paid researchers or academics. Historically, outcomes or products of research for professionals have included grant funding, publications, tenure, and/or other benefits, while research participants and community members have not experienced parallel or analogous gains. For instance, community health workers or project managers may watch as a master's level student becomes a doctoral student and as doctoral student becomes the principal investigator for a project that the community member has been working on longer, has put more hours into, and has more familiarity with. This scenario, of course, is ripe for contentious relationships. Further, unemployed community members may participate on research teams in hopes of securing financial compensation or a future position, and these may never come to fruition (Minkler, 2004, 2005). Regardless of whether community members value or want to advance their education or careers through Western ways of knowing, researchers must acknowledge the inherent systemic biases toward advancing those within the system and should attempt to move away from these discriminatory practices.

Translation and Dissemination Plans

The translation of research to practice is a vitally important step in reducing health disparities and requires a great deal of time, energy, and community input (Lazarus et al., 2012; Wallerstein & Duran, 2010). To ensure the feasibility and sustainability of effective programs, community members should have tangible post-research outcomes (Wallerstein & Duran, 2010). This might include the training of a specific number of community members to provide an intervention and/or the development of manuals for sustainable programming within communities after funding ends. Ideally MedFT researchers, regardless of funding, will stay connected to the community.

Dissemination of health research and best practices are an important part of ethical MedFT research and practice to reduce health disparities in underprivileged communities. An important but challenging aspect of dissemination is closing the gap between researchers, communities, participants, decision-makers, and practitioners to facilitate relevant research, effective practice, and prevention efforts (Elliott et al., 2003; MacLean, 1996; Rhodes et al., 2010). Researchers and communities have differing interests in knowledge production; communities desire to address specific problems and researchers may lose sight of the action that should follow research (Lazarus et al., 2012). Further, the length of time from theory creation to intervention is approximately 17 years (Green, Ottoson, García, & Hiatt, 2009). The populations that suffer most from this delay are minorities because they are more likely to die from disease than are nonminorities (Rutledge et al., 2003).

Higher standards and expectations in research are needed in order to shift the culture of academia from being tenure focused to promoting community engagement (Community-Campus Partnerships for Health, 2009; Wallerstein & Duran, 2006). Increased attention is needed specifically within the arenas of researchers' dissemination plans and their accountability to the communities that they study (Lazarus et al., 2012; Williams et al., 2010). Community members and stakeholders should be actively engaged in the interpretation of research findings as well as deciding how to communicate and act upon the said findings (Lazarus et al., 2012; Minkler, 2005; Wallerstein & Duran, 2010).

In line with community engagement principles, dissemination strategies should be tailored to the individual community. Dissemination practices must go beyond the standard publication in peer-reviewed journals and pamphlets and include bringing the findings back to the community in meaningful ways (Wallerstein & Duran, 2010). This is not to say that community members would not be interested in journal articles or pamphlets, but rather that dissemination efforts need to be expanded to more directly engage communities around wellness. A review of grantees' efforts to communicate research findings back to community members and lay persons found that 88 % of grantees developed at least one website, 60 % held oral presentations, 15 % created public service recordings, and 9 % participated in television or radio talks (Willis, Salazar, Jefferies, Foster-Bey, & Disney, 2010). Findings may be best disseminated through community-specific events and talks and local media outlets (e.g., newspapers, radio, television, art) in a way that celebrates movement toward decreasing health disparities.

The increased use of technology for dissemination of research findings suggests a need for collaboration with technology experts to develop tools specific to community needs (Willis et al., 2010). Technology can also help to improve participants and stakeholders' participation with regular access to updates and opportunities to contribute more to the research process. This increased involvement may foster increased trust in the research process. For example, technology could be used to obtain culturally tailored dissemination strategies from the community. Tablets have been used to obtain informed consent and participant information, and a personal log-in allows for participants to make changes including withdrawing at any point in the research process (Kaye & Kanellopoulou, 2011). Tablets may also be used with participants to triangulate research findings for external validity and/or for verification/clarification of interpretation. The effectiveness of the use of diverse technologies needs further exploration.

Conclusion

While health disparities in this country are substantial products of historical and present-day discrimination, MedFTs with appropriate training and a desire to learn about health equity may take active roles in closing this gap. HHS (2011) has proposed four possible ways to reduce health disparities in the United States: (a) gathering more data on minority populations, (b) making data transparent and useful to the public, (c) incentivizing improvements in healthcare delivery for minorities, and (d) properly evaluating interventions via an awareness and sensitivity for diverse populations. On the ground, these changes would increase the number and quality of community-based healthcare teams, patient-centered medical homes, care coordination, improvement strategies such as wellness promotion, language services and cultural competency, electronic health records (EHR), insurance recipients, access to dental care for children, and research that examines the risk factors of cardiovascular disease (HHS, 2011). While these suggestions are important in reducing health disparities, they are top-down proposals that would be best coupled with research that is community driven and that addresses the root causes of the disparities (e.g., sociopolitical-historical factors).

More specific examples of targeted improvements for research include utilizing community health workers, increasing diversity of the healthcare workforce, closing language gaps, empowering community capacity, increasing culturally appropriate outreach and preventative services such as in-home programs to support early childhood development, promoting community-based participatory research (CBPR) (Sandoval et al., 2012), and reducing dissemination time of research from publication to utilization in practice (HHS, 2011). Not only have these changes been proposed, but there is already an increase in the number of research projects that utilize local knowledge, empower communities, and cocreate research agendas and clinical interventions (Chilisa, 2011).

Health inequities in the United States include differences in quality of life, access to treatment, rates and severity of disease, morbidity, and mortality based on race, class, gender, and sexual and gender identity. Multidisciplinary, integrated teams that include MedFTs have the potential to become effective agents in reducing health disparities by acknowledging patient and community history, by utilizing self-of-researcher methods, and by implementing participant-centered research techniques and methodologies. When healthcare systems are free from discrimination and inequality in service access and when care delivery is advanced in a manner wherein every person has the opportunity to achieve optimal health irrespective of social location, health equity will be achieved (Centers for Disease Control and Prevention [CDC], 2009).

Reflection Questions

1. Describe a research project that could result in the reduction of health disparities.
2. How do beliefs, biases, and assumptions held by the researcher about the participant population shape the research process?
3. What steps would need to be taken to ensure that a community is in agreement with a proposed research agenda?
   (a) What might motivate participants and their families to take part in this research project?
   (b) What are the outcomes that the community might like to see? Why?
4. What questions would need to be asked of potential research collaborators in order to assess their beliefs and biases about the researcher's sample of interest?
5. What steps should a researcher take to better understand a community's current and historical experiences?

Acknowledgments The authors would like to thank Melissa Walls and Maureen Davey for their assistance in reviewing this chapter

References[1]

Agency for Healthcare Research & Quality [AHRQ]. (2011). *National healthcare disparities report, 2011. Detailed methods appendix*. Rockville, MD. Retrieved from http://www.ahrq.gov/qual/nhdr11/methods/index.html

Allen, J. (2007). A multicultural assessment supervision model to guide research and practice. *Professional Psychology: Research and Practice, 38*(3), 248.

Al-Khatib, S. M., Hellkamp, A. S., Hernandez, A. F., Fonarow, G. C., Thomas, K. L., Al-Khalidi, H. R., ..., Peterson, E. D. (2012). Trends in use of implantable cardioverter defibrillator therapy among patients hospitalized for heart failure: Have the previously observed sex and racial disparities changed over time? *Circulation*, 25, 1094–1101. doi:10.1161/CIRCULATIONAHA.111.066605

Anderson, L. M., Scrimshaw, S. C., Fullilove, M. T., Fielding, J. E., & Normand, J. (2003). Culturally competent healthcare systems. A systematic review. *American Journal of Preventive Medicine, 24*(3), 68–79. doi:10.1016/S0749-3797(02)00657-8.

Beauvais, F. (1998). American Indians and alcohol. *Alcohol Health & Research World, 22*, 253–259. Retrieved from http://pubs.niaaa.nih.gov/publications/arh22-4/toc22-4.htm

Berg, D. N., & Smith, K. K. (1988). *The self in social inquiry: Researching methods*. London, NY: Sage.

Betancourt, J. R., Green, A. R., Carrillo, J. E., & Ananeh-Firempong, O. (2003). Defining cultural competence: A practical framework for addressing racial/ethnic disparities in health and health care. *Public Health Reports, 118*, 293–302. doi:10.1007/s11606-007-0481-0.

Bodin, A. M. (1988). Virginia Satir: A memorium. *Journal of Family Psychology, 2*, 117. doi:10.1037/h0084987.

Buchmueller, T., & Carpenter, C. S. (2010). Disparities in health insurance coverage, access, and outcomes for individuals in same-sex versus different-sex relationships, 2000–2007. *American Journal of Public Health, 100*, 489–495. doi:10.2105/AJPH.2009.160804

Cashman, S. B., Adeky, S., Allen, A. J., III, Corburn, J., Israel, B. A., Montaño, J., ..., Eng, E. (2008). The power and the promise: Working with communities to analyze data, interpret findings, and get to outcomes. *American Journal of Public Health, 98*, 1407–1417. doi:10.2105/AJPH.2007.113571

Centers for Disease Control and Prevention [CDC]. (2009). National Center for Health Statistics. Chronic disease prevention and health promotion. Retrieved from http://www.cdc.gov/chronicdisease/healthequity/index.htm

*Chilisa, B. (2011). *Indigenous research methodologies*. Thousand Oaks, CA: Sage.

Community-Campus Partnerships for Health. (2009). Community-based participatory research and research ethics. Retrieved from http://depts.washington.edu/ccph/irbhome.html

Coon, D. (2006). Abraham H. Maslow: Reconnaissance for eupsycia. In D. A. Dewsbury, L. T. Benjamin Jr., & M. Wertheimer (Eds.), *Portraits of Pioneers in Psychology* (Vol. 6, pp. 255–273). Washington, DC: American Psychological Association and Lawrence Erlbaum Associates.

Curtis, A. (2006). A brief introduction to critical race theory, narrative inquiry, and educational research. In A. Curtis & M. Romney (Eds.), *Colour, race and English language teaching: Shades of meaning* (pp. 1–10). Mahwah, NJ: Lawrence Erlbaum Associates Publishers.

Dana, R. H. (2005). *Multicultural principles, applications, and examples*. Mahwah, NJ: Lawrence Erlbaum Associates.

Dana, R. H., & Allen, J. (Eds.). (2008). *Cultural competence training in a global society*. New York, NY: Springer.

[1] An asterisk has been use to note references that the chapter authors recommend for further reading.

Department of Health and Human Services [HHS]. (2011). HHS action plan to reduce racial and ethnic health disparities. Washington, DC, Retrieved from http://minorityhealth.hhs.gov/npa/templates/content.aspx?lvl=1&lvlid=33&ID=285

Doherty, W. J., & Mendenhall, T. J. (2006). Citizen health care: A model for engaging patients, families, and communities as co-producers of health care. *Families, Systems and Health, 24*, 251–263. doi:10.1037/1091-7527.24.3.251.

Dulmus, C. N., & Cristalii, M. E. (2012). A university-community partnership to advance research in practice settings: The HUB research model. *Research on Social Work Practice, 22*, 195–202. doi:10.1177/1049731511423026.

Duran, E. (2006). *Healing the soul wound: Counseling with American Indians and other native peoples*. New York, NY: Teachers College Press.

Duran, E., & Duran, B. (1995). *Native American postcolonial psychology*. New York, NY: State University of New York Press.

Duran, E., Firehammer, J., & Gonzalez, J. (2008). Liberation psychology as the path toward healing cultural soul wounds. *Journal of Counseling & Development, 86*, 288–295. doi:10.1002/j.1556-6678.2008.tb00511.x.

Elliott, S. J., O'Loughlin, J., Robinson, K., Eyles, J., Cameron, R., Harvey, D., . . ., Gelskey, D. (2003). Conceptualizing dissemination research and activity: The case of the Canadian heart health initiative. *Health Education & Behavior, 30*(3), 267–282. doi:10.1177/1090198103030003003

Eng, E., Moore, K. S., Rhodes, S. D., Griffith, D., Allison, L., Shirah, K., & Mebane, E. (2005). Insiders and outsiders assess who is "the community": Participant observation, key informant interview, focus group interview, and community forum. In B. A. Israel, E. Eng, A. J. Schulz, E. Parker (Eds.). *Methods for conducting community-based participatory research for health* (pp. 77–100). San Francisco, CA: Jossey-Bass.

Engel, G. L. (1977). The need for a new medical model: A challenge for biomedicine. *Science, 196*, 129–136. doi:10.1126/science.847460.

Fryberg, S. M. (2010). When the world is colorblind, American Indians are invisible: A diversity science approach. *Psychological Inquiry, 21*, 115–119. doi:10.1080/1047840X.2010.483847.

Goldstein, A. (2003). Researcher on the couch: Is "understanding the self" critical for qualitative research? Center for Kvalitativ Metodeudvikling v/Psykologisk Institut, Århus Universitet. Retrieved from http://bs2.auinstallation28.cs.au.dk/fileadmin/site_files/filer_psykologi/dokumenter/CKM/NB35/goldstein.pdf

Gone, J. P. (2003). American Indian mental health service delivery persistent challenges and future prospects. In J. S. Mio & G. Y. Iwamasa (Eds.), *Culturally diverse mental health: The challenges of research and resistance* (pp. 211–229). New York: Brunner-Routledge.

Goodman, A. H., Moses, Y. T., & Jones, J. L. (2012). *Race: Are we so different?* Oxford, UK: American Anthropological Association.

Green, L. W., Ottoson, J. M., García, C., & Hiatt, R. A. (2009). Diffusion theory and knowledge dissemination, utilization, and integration in public health. *Annual Review of Public Health, 30*, 151–174. doi:10.1146/annurev.publhealth.031308.100049.

Guba, E. G., & Lincoln, Y. S. (1981). The evaluator as instrument. In E. G. Guba & Y. S. Lincoln (Eds.), *Effective evaluation* (pp. 128–152). San Francisco, CA: Jossey-Bass.

Harris, K. J., Jerome, N. W., & Fawcett, S. B. (1997). Rapid assessment procedures: A review and critique. *Human Organization, 56*, 375–378.

Hart, S., Coon, D., Kowalkowski, M., & Latini, D. (2011). 163 gay men with prostate cancer report significantly worse HRQOL than heterosexual men. *The Journal of Urology, 185*, e68–e69. doi:10.1016/j.juro.2011.02.231.

Hasnain-Wynia, R., Kang, R., Landrum, M. B., Vogeli, C., Baker, D. W., & Weissman, J. S. (2010). Racial and ethnic disparities within and between hospitals for inpatient quality of care: An examination of patient-level hospital quality alliance measures. *Journal of Health Care for the Poor and Underserved, 21*, 629–648. doi:10.1353/hpu.0.0281.

Healthy People 2020. (2012). Lesbian, gay, bisexual, and transgender health. Retrieved from http://www.healthypeople.gov/2020/topicsobjectives2020/overview.aspx?topicid=25

Hendricks, L. (2004). *Havasupai file $25 M suit vs ASV* (p. A1). Flagstaff, AZ: Arizona Daily Sun.

HHS. (2011). *HHS action plan to reduce racial and ethnic disparities: A nation free of disparities in health and health care*. Washington, DC: U.S. Department of Health and Human Services.

Holoien, D. S., & Shelton, J. N. (2011). You deplete me: The cognitive costs of colorblindness on ethnic minorities. *Journal of Experimental Social Psychology, 48*, 562–565. doi:10.1016/j.jesp.2011.09.010.

Hughes T. L. (2005). Alcohol use and alcohol-related problems among lesbians and gay men. *Annual Review of Nursing Research, 23*, 283–325. Retrieved from http://www.ncbi.nlm.nih.gov/pubmed/16353369

Hunt, L.M. (2001). Beyond cultural competence: Applying humility to clinical settings. *The Park Ridge Center Bulletin, 24*, 3–4. Retrieved from http://www.med.unc.edu/pedclerk/files/hunthumility.pdf

Hunt, J. (2012). Why the gay and transgender population experiences higher rates of substance use. Retrieved from http://www.americanprogress.org/issues/lgbt/report/2012/03/09/11228/why-the-gay-and-transgender-population-experiences-higher-rates-of-substance-use/

Israel, B. A., Eng, E., Schulz, A. J., & Parker, E. A. (2005). Introduction to methods in community-based participatory research for health. In B. A. Israel, E. Eng, A. J. Schulz, & E. Parker (Eds.), *Methods for conducting community-based participatory research for health* (pp. 3–26). San Francisco, CA: Jossey-Bass.

Israel, B. A., Schulz, A. J., Parker, E. A., & Becker, A. B. (2001). Community-based participatory research: Policy recommendations for promoting a partnership approach in health research. *Education for Health (Abingdon), 14*, 182–197. doi:10.1080/13576280110051055.

Israel, B. A., Schulz, A. J., Parker, E. A., Becker, A. B., Allen, A. J., & Guzman, R. (2003). Critical issues in developing and following community based participatory research principles. In M. Minkler & N. Wallerstein (Eds.), *Community based participatory research for health* (pp. 53–76). San Francisco, CA: Jossey-Bass.

Jones, L., Koegel, P., & Wells, K. B. (2008). Bringing experimental design to community-partnered participatory research. In M. Minkler & N. Wallerstein (Eds.), *Community based participatory research for health: Process to outcomes* (pp. 67–85). San Francisco, CA: Jossey-Bass.

Jorgensen, J. (2011). Reflexivity in feminist research practice: Hearing the unsaid. *Women & Language, 34*(2), 115–119. Retrieved from http://web.ebscohost.com.libproxy.temple.edu/ehost/pdfviewer/pdfviewer?sid=f587289-a29a-4b34-83e9-e21c4ed32bc3%40sessionmgr15&vid=2&hid=1

Kaye, J., & Kanellopoulou, N. (2011). *Dynamic informed consent. EnCoRe Project. HeLEX Oxford Centre for Health, Law, and Emerging Technologies.* UK: Oxford University.

Kirmayer, L. J. (2012). Rethinking cultural competence. *Transcultural Psychiatry, 49*, 149–164. doi:10.1177/1363461512444673.

Krehely, J. (2009, December 21). How to close the LGBT health disparities gap: Disparities by race and ethnicity. Retrieved from http://www.americanprogress.org/wp-ontent/uploads/issues/2009/12/pdf/lgbt_health_disparities_race.pdf

Kvale, S. (1996). *InterViews: An introduction to qualitative research interviewing*. London, UK: Sage.

LaVeaux, D., & Christopher, S. (2009). Contextualizing CBPR: Key principles of CBPR meet the Indigenous research context. *Pimatisiwin, 7*, 1–16. Retrieved from http://www.pimatisiwin.com/online/wp-content/uploads/2009/07/01Contents.pdf

Lawrence, J. (2000). The Indian Health Service and the sterilization of Native American women. *The American Indian Quarterly, 24*, 400–419. doi:10.2307/1185911.

Lazarus, S., Duran, B., Caldwell, L., & Bulbulia, S. (2012). Public health research and action: Reflections on challenges and possibilities of community-based participatory research. In J. Maddock (Ed.), *Public health – Social and behavioral health*. InTech: Manhattan, NY. doi:10.5772/38411.

Lee, G. L., Griffin, G. K., & Melvin, C. L. (2009). Tobacco use among sexual minorities in the USA: 1987 to May 2007: A systematic review. *Tobacco Control, 18*, 275–282. doi:10.1136/tc.2008.028241.

Legaspi, A., & Orr, E. (2007). Dissemination research on community health and well-being: A collaboration between Alaska Native villages and the Academe. *American Indian and Alaska Native Mental Health Research, 14*(1), 24–43. doi:10.5820/aian.1401.2007.28.

Lie, D. A., Lee-Rey, E., Gomez, A., Bereknyei, S., & Braddock, C. H., III. (2010). Does cultural competency training of health professionals improve patient outcomes? A systematic review and proposed algorithm for future research. *Journal of General Internal Medicine, 26*, 317–325. doi:10.1007/s11606-010-1529-0.

Loh, P., & Sugerman-Brozan, J. (2002). Environmental justice organizing for environmental health: case study on asthma and diesel exhaust in Roxbury, Massachusetts. *Environmental Health Perspectives, 584*, 110–124. doi:10.1177/000271620258400108.

MacLean, D. R. (1996). Positioning dissemination in public health policy. *Canadian Journal of Public Health, 87*(supp 2), S40-S43. Retrieved from http://www.ncbi.nlm.nih.gov/pubmed/9002342

Malgady, R. G., & Colon-Malgady, G. (2008). Building community test norms: Considerations for the ethnic minority populations. In L. A. Suzuki & J. G. Ponterotto (Eds.), *Handbook of multicultural assessment: Clinical, psychological, and educational application* (3rd ed., pp. 34–51). New York, NY: Wiley.

McGrath, J. J., Matthews, K. A., & Brady, S. S. (2006). Individual versus neighborhood socioeconomic status and race as predictors of adolescent ambulatory blood pressure and heart rate. *Social Science & Medicine, 63*, 1442–1453. doi:10.1016/j.socscimed.2006.03.019.

Mendenhall, T., Berge, J., & Doherty, W. (2014). Engaging communities as partners in research: Advancing integrated care through purposeful partnerships. In J. Hodgson, A. Lamson, T. Mendenhall, & R. Crane (Eds.), *Medical family therapy: Advanced applications* (pp. 259–282). New York: Springer.

Minkler, M. (2004). Ethical challenges for the "outside" researcher in community-based participatory research. *Health Education & Behavior, 31*, 684–701. doi:10.1177/1090198104269566.

Minkler, M. (2005). Community-based research partnerships: Challenges and opportunities. *Journal of Urban Health, 82*, ii3–ii12. doi:10.1093/jurban/jti034.

Minkler, M., & Wallerstein, N. (2008). *Community-based participatory research for health: From process to outcomes*. San Francisco, CA: Jossey-Bass.

National Aboriginal Health Organization [NAHO]. (2008). *Cultural competency and safety: A guide for health care administrators, providers and educators*. Ottawa, Canada: NAHO.

NCAI Policy Research Center and MSU Center for Native Health Partnerships. (2012). *"Walk softly and listen carefully": Building research relationships with tribal communities*. Washington, DC: NCAI Policy Research Center and MSU Center for Native Health Partnerships.

Nicholls, R. (2009). Research and indigenous participation: Critical reflexive methods. *International Journal of Social Research Methodology, 12*, 117–126. doi:10.1080/13645570902727698.

Novins, D. K., Aarons, G. A., Conti, S. G., Dahlke, D., Daw, R., Fickenscher, A., . . ., Spicer, P. (2011). Use of the evidence base in substance abuse treatment programs for American Indians and Alaska Natives: Pursuing quality in the crucible of practice and policy. *Implementation Science, 6*(63), 1–12. doi:10.1186/1748-5908-6-63

Papps, E., & Ramsden, I. (1996). Cultural safety in nursing: The New Zealand experience. *International Journal of Quality in Health Care, 8*, 491–497. doi:10.1093/intqhc/8.5.491.

Park, Y. (2012). *The dark side: Immigrants, racism and the American way*. Bloomington, IN: iUniverse.

Pezalla, A. E., Pettigrew, J., & Miller-Day, M. (2012). Researching the researcher-as-instrument: An exercise in interviewer self-reflexivity. *Qualitative Research, 12*, 165–185. doi:10.1177/1468794111422107.

Polaschek, N. R. (1998). Cultural safety: A new concept in nursing people of different ethnicities. *Journal of Advanced Nursing, 27*, 452–457. doi:10.1046/j.1365-2648.1998.00547.x.

Presidential Commission for the Study of Bioethical Issues. (2011). *"Ethically impossible" STD research in Guatemala from 1946–1948*. Washington, DC: Bioethics Commission. Retrieved from http://bioethics.gov/sites/default/files/Ethically-Impossible_PCSBI.pdf

Renganathan, S. (2009). Exploring the researcher-participant relationship in a multiethnic, multicultural and multilingual context through reflexivity. *Qualitative Research Journal, 9*(2), 3–17. doi:10.3316/QRJ0902003.

Rhodes, S. D., Malow, R. M., & Jolly, C. (2010). Community-based participatory research (CBPR): A new and not-so-new approach to HIV/AIDS prevention, care, and treatment. *AIDS Education and Prevention, 22*, 173–183. doi:10.1521/aeap.2010.22.3.173.

Rincón, A. M. (2009). Practicing cultural humility. In T. Berthold, J. Miller, & A. Avila-Esparza (Eds.), *Foundations for community health workers* (pp. 135–154). San Francisco, CA: Jossey-Bass.

Rutledge, T., Reis, S. E., Olson, M., Owens, J., Kelsey, S. F., Pepine, C. J., . . ., Matthews, K. A. (2003). Socioeconomic status variables predict cardiovascular disease risk factors and prospective mortality risk among women with chest pain. *Behavior Modification, 27*, 54–67. doi:10.1177/0145445502238693

Sandoval, J. A., Lucero, J., Oetzel, J., Avila, M., Belone, L., Mau, M., . . ., Wallerstein, N. (2012). Process and outcome constructs for evaluating community based participatory research projects: A matrix of existing measures. *Health Education Research, 27*, 680–690. doi:10.1093/her/cyr087

Schulz, A. J., Parker, E. A., Israel, B. A., Allen, A., Decarlo, M., & Lockett, M. (2002). Addressing social determinants of health through community-based participatory research: The East Side Village Health Worker Partnership. *Health Education & Behavior, 29*, 326–341. doi:10.1177/109019810202900305.

Shaw, S., & Armin, J. (2011). The ethical self-fashioning of physicians and health care systems in culturally appropriate health care. *Culture, Medicine & Psychiatry, 35*, 236–261. doi:10.1007/s11013-011-9215-1.

Simon, G. M. (2006). The heart of the matter: A proposal for placing the self of the therapist at the center of family therapy research and training. *Family Process, 45*, 331–344. doi:10.1111/j.1545-5300.2006.00174.x.

Smith, L. T. (1999). *Issues in indigenous research: Decolonizing methodologies research and indigenous people*. London: Zed Books.

Spears, C. R., Nolan, B. V., O'Neill, J. L., Arcury, T. A., Grzywacz, J. G., & Feldman, S. R. (2011). Recruiting underserved populations to dermatologic research: A systematic review. *International Journal of Dermatology, 50*, 385–395. doi:10.1111/j.1365-4632.2010.04813.x.

Subramanyam, M. A., Diez-Roux, A., Hickson, D. A., Sarpong, D. F., Sims, M., Taylor, H. A., . . ., Wyatt, S. B. (2012). Subjective social status and psychosocial and metabolic risk factors for cardiovascular disease among African Americans in the Jackson heart study. *Social Science & Medicine, 74*, 1146–1154. doi:10.1016/j.socscimed.2011.12.042

*Sue, D. W. (2010). Microaggressions, marginality, and oppression: An introduction. In D. W. Sue (Ed.), *Microaggressions and marginality: Manifestation, dynamics, and impact* (pp. 3–22). Hoboken, NJ: Wiley.

*Sue, D. W., Capodilupo, C. M., Torino, G. C., Bucceri, J. M., Holder, A. M. B., Nadal, K. L., & Esquilin, M. (2007). Racial microaggressions in everyday life. *American Psychologist, 62*, 271–286. doi:10.103770003-066X.624.271

Tervalon, M., & Murray-García, J. (1998). Cultural humility versus cultural competence: A critical distinction in defining physician training outcomes in multicultural education. *Journal of Health Care for the Poor and Underserved, 9*, 117–125. doi:10.1353/hpu.2010.0233.

Trimble, J. E., Scharron-del Rio, M., & Bernal, G. (2010). In D. C. Sack & A. Ali (Eds.), *Cultural perspectives on women's depression: Self-silencing, psychological distress and recovery* (pp. 73–95). New York: Oxford.

Troxel, W. M., Matthews, K. A., Bromberger, J. T., & Sutton-Tyrrell, K. (2003). Chronic stress burden, discrimination, and subclinical carotid artery disease in African American and Caucasian women. *Health Psychology, 22*, 300–309. doi:10.1037/0278-6133.22.3.300.

Villegas, M. (2013). Charting a course for Native health research. *Presentation presented at RICH Indigenous Health Symposium: Global Approaches to Health Promotion*. Duluth, MN

Walker, S., Read, S., & Priest, H. (2013). Use of reflexivity in a mixed-methods study. *Nurse Researcher, 20*(3), 38–43. doi:10.1038/ejhg.2012.286.

*Wallerstein, N. B., & Duran, B. (2003). The conceptual, historical and practical roots of community based participatory research and related participatory traditions. In M. Minkler & N. Wallerstein (Eds.), *Community-based participatory research for health: From process to outcomes* (pp. 27–52). San Francisco, CA: Jossey-Bass.

Wallerstein, N. B., & Duran, B. (2006). Using community-based participatory research to address health disparities. *Health Promotion Practice, 7*, 312–323. doi:10.1177/1524839906289376.

Wallerstein, N. B., & Duran, B. (2010). Community-based participatory research contributions to intervention research: The intersection of science and practice to improve health equity. *American Journal of Public Health, 100*, S40–S46. doi:10.2105/AJPH.2009. 184036.

Walters, K. L., Simoni, J. M., & Evans-Campbell, T. (2002). Substance use among American Indians and Alaska Natives: Incorporating culture in an "Indigenist" stress-coping paradigm. *Public Health Reports, 117*, S104–S117. Retrieved from http://publichealthreports.org/

*Washington, H. A. (2006). *Medical apartheid: The dark history of the medical experimentation on Black Americans from colonial times to the present*. New York: Random House Digital.

Watts-Jones, T. D. (2010). Location of self: Opening the door to dialogue on intersectionality in the therapy process. *Family Process, 49*, 405–420. doi:10.1111/j.1545-5300.2010.01330.x.

Weaver, H. N., & Brave Heart, M. Y. (1999). Examining two facets of American Indian identity: Exposure to other culture and the influence of historical trauma. *Journal of Human Behavior and the Social Environment, 2*, 19–33. doi:10.1300/J137v02n01_03.

Wendt, D. C., & Gone, J. P. (2012). Rethinking cultural competence: Insights from indigenous community treatment settings. *Transcultural Psychiatry, 49*, 206–222. doi:10.1177/1363461511425622.

Whitbeck, L. B. (2006). Some guiding assumptions and a theoretical model for developing culturally specific preventions with Native American people. *Journal of Community Psychology, 34*, 183–192. doi:10.1002/jcop.20094.

Williams, D. R., & Leavell, J. (2012). The social context of cardiovascular disease: Challenges and opportunities for the Jackson heart study. *Ethnicity & Disease, 22*(S1), 15–21. doi:10.1016/j.pcad.2013.03.007.

Williams, R. L., Willging, C. E., Quintero, G., Kalishman, S., Sussman, A. L., & Freeman, W. L. (2010). Ethics of health research in communities: Perspectives from the southwestern United States. *Annuals of Family Medicine, 8*, 433–439. doi:10.1370/afm.1138.

Willis, T. J., Salazar, R. M., Jefferies, T., Foster-Bey, J., & Disney, L. D. (2010). *Communicating community-based participatory research findings to non-scientific communities: Lessons learned from the Community Networks Program (CNP)*. Retrieved from http://www.iiis.org/CDs2010/CD2010SCI/BMIC_2010/PapersPdf/BA302FJ.pdf

Part III
Policy

Chapter 18
Policy and Practice: A Primer on the Past, Present, and Future of Healthcare Reform in the United States

Todd Edwards, Jo Ellen Patterson, Joseph Scherger, and Susanna Vakili

Traditionally, training in family therapy master's programs has focused on preparing future therapists to serve individuals, couples, and families. Students that graduate from clinical programs commonly go to work in community behavioral health or private practice settings that function in a fee-for-service manner. Unfortunately, most training programs seldom include business or public policy perspectives of clinical work. Students frequently enter the professional world unaware of macro-level influences of health care systems, such as the broader political and economic context of behavioral health care. As more relational therapists identify as medical family therapists (MedFTs) and go to work in healthcare settings that are being radically changed by new healthcare policies, they can no longer focus exclusively on microlevel, face-to-face interventions with their patients. Instead, MedFTs must be aware of the broader influences that both expand and limit opportunities for individual therapists and their patients. The purpose of this chapter is to provide a primer on healthcare policy for MedFTs and to describe current and proposed changes that will revolutionize the delivery of healthcare services to families in the United States.

Health Care in the United States

The method of healthcare delivery in the United States has evolved into being one of the most ineffective healthcare systems in the world (Davis, Schoen, & Stremikis, 2010). In 2011, the United States spent more on health care per capita than any other nation. While expenditures far exceed those of other developed countries, the resulting healthcare quality is much lower (Berwick, Nolan, & Whittington, 2008). The following rankings illustrate the disparity between the

T. Edwards (✉)
University of San Diego, San Diego, CA, USA
e-mail: tedwards@sandiego.edu

J. Hodgson et al. (eds.), *Medical Family Therapy*, DOI 10.1007/978-3-319-03482-9_18,

cost and quality of health care in the United States (Murray & Frenk, 2010): 39th among nations on infant mortality, 37th among nations on life expectancy, 39th on male life expectancy, and 39th on female life expectancy.

In addition to these changes in life expectancy, multimorbidity is becoming a rule rather than an exception (Edwards et al., 2012). For example, more than 25 % of patients in the United States have two or more chronic conditions, which frequently include behavioral health problems, such as substance-use disorders, disorders of cognitive impairment, and developmental disabilities (Anderson, 2010; Vogeli et al., 2007). Unfortunately, multiple health conditions can result in receiving care from different providers who may not communicate or coordinate treatment plans within or across contexts. In fact, lack of care coordination results in one in seven hospitalized Medicare patients experiencing a healthcare error and one in five Medicare patients being released from a hospital only to be readmitted within 30 days (Berenson & Burton, 2011). The sharing of information between providers or healthcare contexts is cumbersome and often incomplete, resulting in care that takes too long to deliver and is sometimes inaccurate, unsafe, and costly. As a result of miscommunication or lack of collaboration, primary care providers are left to work with patients on treatment and health goals without having the patient's complete biopsychosocial healthcare history.

Healthcare Reform

One groundbreaking report that has shaken health care over the past decade is *Crossing the Quality Chasm*, written by the Institute of Medicine (IOM) in 2001. The IOM experts described the gulf between the type of health care that Americans should receive and the care that is typically provided (i.e., great disparities were described based on patient accessibility, sociodemographics, and receipt of quality and equitable treatment in health care). In response to these disparities and the chasm in health care, the IOM created six aims (i.e., care that is safe, patient centered, equitable, timely, efficient, and effective) and ten rules for improvement (e.g., care should be continuous, tailored to patient needs, transparent, based on scientific evidence) (IOM, 2001).

A fundamental overhaul in health care was described as the only way to bridge the chasm, something that has started but is only beginning to deliver improved quality to populations of patients. According to Dentzer (2011), 10 years subsequent to the IOM report, some progress had been made in patient safety and quality improvement, but much work still needs to be done. Robust information systems, redesign of care to improve the health of populations, and practice via interdisciplinary teams are hallmarks of this overhaul and are currently described as the Triple Aim, Accountable Care Organizations (ACOs) and Patient-Centered Medical Homes (PCMHs) (Berwick et al., 2008). These movements are described in this chapter and form a strategy for the successful integration of MedFTs in the emerging healthcare systems that are positioned to succeed under the Affordable Care Act (ACA) in the United States.

The ACA passed during the Obama Administration sets the course for a more organized and universal healthcare system in the United States (Abrams, Nuzum, Mika, & Lawlor, 2011). The ACA mostly focuses on access to care, but ensuring quality care at affordable costs will lead efforts forward. President Barack Obama appointed CEO Donald Berwick on July 7, 2010, to head the Centers for Medicare and Medicaid Services to stimulate changes in health care and quality improvement. He served until December 2, 2011, when a nurse by training, Marilyn Tavenner, replaced him in that position. Healthcare reform has resulted in chaos and political turbulence as politicians work to advocate for their solutions. Leaders agree that healthcare needs to change, but in what order and to whose benefit remain uncertain. Next are three examples of quality initiatives included in the considerations for healthcare reform.

Key Initiatives to Change Health Care

Health care is changing from a service delivered by one professional to one person to a system of care covering a population of people (including their families) by multidisciplinary teams. While the individual is not diminished in these systems, better value is delivered to a community and the costs of care are sustainable. This section addresses three unifying constructions that reflect a new system of care: Triple Aim, ACOs, and PCMHs.

Triple Aim Initiative

The Triple Aim began as an initiative by the Institute for Healthcare Improvement (IHI) in 2008 as part of a shift of this organization toward improving population health (Berwick et al., 2008). Donald Berwick's transition from founder and CEO of IHI to the director of the Centers for Medicare and Medicaid Services in Washington led to the integration of the Triple Aim into policies for ACOs (described below), fundamental to value-based care under the Affordable Care Act (Berwick et al., 2008). The three parts of the Triple Aim are as follows: (a) improving the individual experience of care, (b) improving the health of populations, and (c) reducing the per capita costs of care for populations.

The goals of the Triple Aim are to improve the individual experience of care and health of populations and reduce the per capita costs of care for populations. These goals are interdependent and must be balanced with each other in implementing a business model for a healthcare organization. There are many barriers to implementing the Triple Aim, including physician-centric care, little foreign competition to spur domestic change, and a system that motivates hospitals to maximize profits by admitting patients and providing a high volume of services (Berwick et al., 2008).

In order for the Triple Aim to be accomplished, three key elements must be incorporated into the design of the healthcare system (Berwick et al., 2008): (a) identifying and tracking a defined group of people over time that would be treated by a healthcare system, (b) accepting that the healthcare system will be constrained by the decisions made by those who manage the system (e.g., how much money will be spent on health care for the population) and those who receive the care, and (c) establishing an integrator (a single organization) who accepts responsibility for the three components of the Triple Aim and who will coordinate the services of all healthcare providers. With its focus on population health, the experience of getting care, and better management of healthcare costs, the Triple Aim provides an important framework for health care in the twenty-first century.

Accountable Care Organizations

The ACO is a response to the goals of the Triple Aim and grew out of several issues (Berwick et al., 2008) for example (a) complaints by healthcare providers, policymakers, and analysts about incentives in the current fee-for-service system that motivates providers to prescribe as many services as possible, thereby driving up healthcare costs for patients; (b) patient objections to the Health Maintenance Organization's (HMO) perceived intrusion into patient care decisions; and (c) a recognition that HMOs had failed to become the integrators of quality, cost-effective care, and instead have become entities that were defined more by their organizational structure rather than their aims and performance, and were viewed as managing money, not care.

The ACO refers to a group of providers and suppliers of services (e.g., hospitals, healthcare providers who voluntarily work together to coordinate all services for a group of Medicare beneficiaries). In addition to the coordination of care, Berenson and Burton (2011) stated that responsibilities for members of an ACO include "investment in infrastructure and redesigned care processes for high quality and efficient service delivery" (p. 3). The goal of an ACO is to avoid unnecessary duplication of services, prevent medical errors, and provide the right care to patients, especially the chronically ill, at the right time. Three central characteristics differentiate ACOs from HMOs and other existing health plan providers (Berenson & Burton, 2011): (a) shared savings (e.g., providers are eligible for bonuses from Medicare if patient care costs fall below a projected amount); (b) accountability for quality (e.g., shared savings are determined in part by a variety of quality metrics); and (c) free choice (e.g., patients who are part of an ACO can seek care from another provider). Accountable health care delivered to a population of patients has become the goal of health systems and thus the embodiment of the principles of the Triple Aim in action, which can only be punctuated when situated in PCMHs.

Patient-Centered Medical Home

The PCMH is defined as a group of people in a community who share the goal of improving the health of their community (American Academy of Family Physicians (AAFP), American Academy of Pediatrics (AAP), American College of Physicians (ACP), & American Osteopathic Association (AOA), 2007). The PCMH movement is the microsystem response to providing coordinated care in every setting. The medical home concept originated in the 1960s as a way to improve the delivery of care to children with special healthcare needs (Sia, Tonniges, Osterhus, & Taba, 2004). It is being applied to primary health care as a means for lowering costs, improving quality through the use of disease registries and health information technology, and increasing access to care. The PCMH concept has been piloted in demonstration projects and practices throughout the country (see www.pcpcc.org for examples). The results of these efforts are being assessed on an ongoing basis and are being incorporated into a feedback loop that results in changes to the PCMH model to improve its ability to achieve its intended outcomes (Stange et al., 2009).

In 2007, the major US primary care organizations agreed on a set of guiding principles for the PCMH (AAFP et al., 2007). These principles included a personal physician to provide first-contact, continuous, and comprehensive care; physician-directed medical practice that takes responsibility for the ongoing care of patients; whole-person orientation for all stages of life; coordinated or integrated care team; quality and safe context; a plan that enhances access to care; and a payment system that recognizes value to the patient.

Is the PCMH, with its commitment to physician-directed care, really patient centered? It depends on what is meant by patient-centered care. To some, being patient centered means that the focus is on the patient, not just the disease (deGruy & Etz, 2010). Another view is to add the patient to the care team or even place him or her at the center of the team (Berenson et al., 2008). Shared decision making has emerged as a desired care model, especially when the evidence is not completely clear on what tests and treatments are preferred, such as with screening and treatment for breast or prostate cancer. In such situations, patient preference becomes paramount and often drives the medical decision making. These concepts allow for patient centeredness through a more active and engaged participation from everyone involved while converting the traditional role of physician as the one in control of healthcare practices into provider as a collaborator or a coach.

The PCMH and behavioral health needs. The PCMH concept has much to offer patients, but it will not reach its full potential without addressing behavioral health needs (Croghan & Brown, 2010; deGruy & Etz, 2010). According to Scherger (2012), psychosocial problems are frequent in health care and usually are masked by physical complaints. More than just patient centeredness, the integration of behavioral health services will enable the PCMH to meet its goals of enhanced access and coordinated and high-quality care (Hunter & Goodie, 2010). While more studies are needed to deepen the support for collaborative services across the full range of behavioral health needs and available professions, there is strong evidence that integrated care improves outcomes for patients with depression (Katon et al., 2010). Below, we offer a case example that illustrates the benefits of an integrated care model:

A 72-year-old male patient sought help from his family physician for low back pain, fatigue, and a general lack of motivation. During the interview, his physician learned that his symptoms began a few months after the patient retired from a successful career in the military and the death of his wife. After ruling out serious medical conditions and concluding that the patient's repeated somatic symptoms were likely related to sadness, fear, and anxiety associated with major life changes, the physician decided to recommend a treatment plan that combined medical and behavioral health services. The physician had a close, collaborative relationship with a MedFT and was able to confidently refer the patient for therapy and work with the therapist in monitoring the patient's progress. After a 4-month course of an SSRI and 6 months of family-oriented therapy via traditional and integrated care, the patient was able to regain and sustain a euthymic mood and reconnect with friends and neighbors, an outcome that he had not been able to achieve in the past.

The integrated care described in this case addresses all of the principles (labeled above) in relation to a successful PCMH model. The patient's experience of care was seamless rather than fragmented (principle a). Costs were reduced through unnecessary medical testing beyond the initial medical evaluation (principle g). Principles b and d were achieved through an integrated care model that allowed the patient to receive both traditional and integrated care services while maintaining physical health care. Seamlessness resulted from a patient introduction between the primary care provider and the therapist (principle d). The patient was not left to negotiate a new appointment or continuously describe the problem to new providers (principles e and f). Costs are reduced by having the patient seen by a MedFT that was already on site (principle f). Furthermore, there is no barrier to professional collaboration, a serious and frustrating problem with independent private practice. The additional potential benefits of integrated care could include (a) improved sensitivity and accuracy of behavioral health problem identification among partnering primary care providers (principle e); (b) contributions to increased screening, detection, and intervention (principles b and c); (c) attention to context and relationships, such as key life transitions, and the strengthening of social connections (principles b and c); and (d) possibly earlier prevention of health and substance-use issues (principles a and b) (Edwards et al., 2012).

As currently defined, PCMHs can adequately treat patients with mild-to-moderate behavioral health problems. However, most of the PCMH pilot projects have not addressed behavioral health despite evidence that behavioral problems are common and are increasingly being treated in the primary care setting (Croghan & Brown, 2010). In addition, they have not addressed the family as the unit of care. Several policy actions will be required to facilitate the integration of high-quality behavioral health services into the PCMH model, such as equipping primary care practices with the necessary tools to effectively screen for, diagnose, and coordinate treatment for behavioral health issues (Croghan & Brown, 2010). The development of such new policies and their advocacy for acceptance in health system design would come from participation in organizations such as the Patient-Centered Primary Care Collaborative, the Center for Studying Health System Change, and the IHI.

Behavioral Health and Healthcare Policy in the Future

The Affordable Care Act supports the implementation of health homes by including sections that require reform in the way that Medicare/Medicaid services are reimbursed. The Act also enables states to care for Medicaid patients with chronic illnesses, including behavioral health and substance-use disorders, through the establishment of health homes. The term "health home" is used in the ACA to convey that a comprehensive care model ensures quality and efficiency. Health homes could expand upon the concept of medical homes by being explicit about the incorporation of behavioral health and substance use and community support into the model. Health homes are a core element of the ACOs, and adoption of the ACA may accelerate their growth and implementation (National Council for Community Behavioral Healthcare, 2011).

In 2009, Thomas Smith, director for the New York City Mental Healthcare Monitoring Initiative, and Lloyd Sederer, director of the New York State Office of Mental Health, proposed a mental health home that would integrate primary and preventative care, focus and apply practices based on scientific evidence, and establish networks of support and outreach for patients within their families and communities. In a mental health home, the roles and responsibilities of those who are primary caretakers for people with serious and persistent mental illnesses would need to be designed. Psychiatrists would be performing many activities that are currently being performed by primary care providers and would need to be willing and able to adopt this new type of role (Moran, 2010).

PCMHs are similar to health homes; models have been piloted across the country to test ways of implementing higher quality and lower cost comprehensive care. To be successful, PCMHs will need to have relationships with specialists and hospitals that can provide services in areas such as behavioral health and substance use. The ACP (2010) advocates for a set of core principles that would apply to a provider (a PCMH neighbor) who partners with a health home to deliver specialty services. Clinical relationships that a PCMH could have with a partner include pre-consultation exchange (a brief exchange of information regarding a patient), formal consultations (involving more detailed assessment procedures and treatment recommendations), co-management (the PCMH and specialist work together in treating the patient), and transfer to specialty care.

A PCMH would likely work with several specialists, and the ACP recommends that incentives be developed to encourage the development of sustaining relationships between behavioral health and substance abuse specialists and PCMHs. MedFTs wanting to participate as a PCMH neighbor would need to be able to fulfill the quality requirements that guide PCMHs. MedFTs with a proven ability to partner with federally qualified health centers or other primary care providers will likely have an advantage in partnering with PCMHs.

An ACO could comprise multiple PCMHs/health homes. While the ACO will be responsible for clinical and administrative functions, behavioral health and substance abuse providers will be able to participate in both areas and to share in the savings plans like the type that is being developed by Medicare. Given the high prevalence of behavioral health and substance-abuse issues, practitioners in these areas that can deliver high-quality, efficient services will be sought after by ACOs. MedFTs will need to team with ACOs in achieving the Triple Aim of improving patient health, improving the patient experience of care, and reducing cost. Accordingly, MedFTs will need to be able to perform a variety of functions, including (a) participating in team-based care; (b) using standardized assessment tools to track patient progress; (c) working with patients in participating in the management of their own care; (d) using a systemic approach to managing referrals; (e) being available after hours to address urgent situations and make clinical data available for such care; (f) using health information systems to track care coordination and transitions; (g) being able to work effectively with diverse populations; (h) being trained and skilled in providing evidence-based behavioral interventions, assessments, and treatments; (i) incorporating the use of electronic means for tracking and sharing patient information; and (j) participating in data gathering and reporting activities to support the ACO's requirement to manage its performance.

Sometimes the most difficult step for MedFTs is knowing how to initiate the conversations with key personnel to join a health home. To participate in health homes and ACOs, a MedFT may want to begin by identifying potential healthcare partners and developing relationships with these individuals. MedFTs may want to prepare a list of assessments that they are qualified to use and comfortable in using so that these can be discussed with partners. MedFTs may appear more competent if they are able to describe their understanding of population health management, the Triple Aim, and ways to measure health outcomes. All in all, MedFTs should be prepared to discuss their understanding of integrated care models, including the use of technology systems (e.g., electronic health records) and ways to transition into team-based health homes.

These recommendations suggest that MedFTs should learn more about business practices, team-based care, evidence-based treatments, and screening tools for assessment. Thus, MedFT training programs or postgraduate MedFT supervisors should incorporate these practices into courses or meetings in order to maximize the MedFT competence and confidence in health homes. In addition, programs can include an introduction to policy issues that affect the work of MedFTs. As US healthcare policy continues to rapidly evolve, training programs must stay abreast of the changes.

Families and Healthcare Policy

An obvious question for MedFTs with regard to healthcare policy is the following: Where do families and relational therapy fit in this context? MedFTs who are trying to stay up to date with the ever-changing evidence for new clinical treatments may feel that healthcare policy is beyond their work scope. However, the inclusion of family concerns in health policy should be a concern for all MedFTs because policy and financing support the clinical context where MedFTs deliver care.

As the healthcare delivery context evolves, MedFTs advocating for family-based care face some specific challenges. While clinically they recognize the critical roles that families play in healthcare delivery, operational and payment systems might make it challenging to provide family-based care (Patterson, Peek, Heinrich, Bischoff, & Scherger, 2002). However, policy work is being done to advocate for the family in health care, in particular there are foci on children and youth, elderly, and caregivers, along with patients with disabilities.

Children and Youth

The Committee on Psychosocial Aspects of Child and Family Health; the Committee on Early Childhood, Adoption, and Dependent Care; and the Section on Developmental and Behavioral Pediatrics (2012) make several recommendations for changes in policies and services related to youth and pediatric care, including a family-centered pediatric medical home. A pediatric medical home would (a) support children's emerging social-emotional-linguistic skills and encourage the adoption of positive parenting techniques; (b) screen for toxic stress (e.g., maternal depression, parental substance abuse, domestic violence, hunger, social isolation); (c) expand the ability of the medical home to serve children at risk; and (d) identify local resources that address the risks for toxic stress. This chapter is based on the converging, multidisciplinary science of human development that suggests that early experiences can have a lasting effect on children's brains, genetic predispositions, and overall health. Thus, adult mental and physical diseases should be viewed as developmental disorders that begin early in life but may not manifest for many years (Schonkoff, Garner, the Committee on Psychosocial Aspects of Child and Family Health, Committee on Early Childhood, Adoption, and Dependent Care, and Section on Developmental and Behavioral Pediatrics, 2012). Given MedFTs' systemic training and developmental knowledge, they are well prepared to develop and implement policies and practices that can benefit children.

The Elderly and Their Family Caregivers

In addition to children, seriously ill and aged family members are other groups that need family-based care. As the US population ages and elderly family members grow increasingly dependent on family members for care, healthcare delivery systems must grapple with ways to include family-based care. Family members play a significant role in caregiving and often struggle with fears about how to be a caregiver, have guilt about not being able to do more for their loved one as they balance multiple responsibilities in their lives, and are confused about their caregiving role (Patterson, 2012). Current legal and operational barriers exacerbate these emotions for families because they limit family members' access to information that would help them better understand their loved one's condition and more effectively function as a caregiver (Patterson, 2012).

Wolff (2012) describes many barriers to supporting families, such as legal challenges that exclude family members from both knowledge and decision-making capacity about their loved ones. Family members often struggle with fear about how to be caregivers and feel guilty about not being able to do more for their loved one as they balance multiple responsibilities (Wolff, 2012). Current legal and operational barriers exacerbate these emotions for families because they limit family members' access to information that would help them better understand their loved one's condition and more effectively function as a caregiver. When a patient leaves the physician's office or the hospital, his or her care often becomes the primary responsibility of family members.

Wolff suggests that the role of family in patient health care is complicated, but that families serve "as the backbone of medical and long-term care delivery" (Wolff, 2012, p. 1530). She believes that families' contributions must be measured and documented before they can be valued by policymakers. She offers specific policy recommendations that could be easily implemented into any healthcare setting in order to assist families, including the following: (a) ensure that health information is made available to family members according to patients' expressed wishes, (b) routinely document important aspects of family function that influence caregiving into the medical record, (c) screen family caregivers who are at risk for burnout and make sure that they receive routine care, and (d) document family members' presence and identity at a patient's healthcare visit, including any differing perspectives on the problem.

In an effort to further address these issues, the United Hospital Fund has implemented a program called Transitions in Care-Quality Improvement Collaborative (TIC-QuIC), which just completed its first-round intervention in 2011 (Levine, 2011). The goal was to improve transitions for chronically or seriously ill patients between settings (e.g., from hospital to home) by providing training for family caregivers. The results showed that caregivers reported better preparation and staffs reported a decrease in their post-discharge workload. The TIC-QuIC project is one example of the powerful benefits of including family members as part of the healthcare team.

Patients with Disabilities

Other groups that particularly benefit from family-based healthcare services and policies include families with members who have physical or mental disabilities. For example, returning veterans with post-traumatic stress disorder or traumatic brain injury and their families need family-based care (Patterson, 2012). An editorial in the *Journal of the American Medical Association* calls for integrated care, treatments that include narrative processes that strengthen social connections, and inclusion of family members "who have their own unique perspectives, are essential participants in the veteran healing process and also need their own support" (Hoge, 2011, p. 551). The following case illustrates the important role of families in the care of family members with comorbid physical and mental illness:

A hospitalized male patient had both leukemia and bipolar disorder. During his hospital stay he became violent but was restrained. His family had little understanding of his recent diagnosis of bipolar disorder and felt panicked as they watched their loved one decline. Citing legal reasons and hospital policy, the floor nurses said that they could not provide the family any information about his erratic behavior. Eventually his 60-year-old wife and 82-year-old mother awoke at 4:00 a.m. so that they could be at the hospital by 5:00 a.m. in case the oncologist rounded early. When that effort failed, they "camped out" in the physician's office waiting room for five hours only to be told that the oncologist did not have consent (from a manic patient) to release medical information to them. While this difficult situation unfolded, the wife's unspoken fear was that her violent husband would be sent home and she would be fully responsible for his care. She simultaneously felt terrified of his violent behavior and fearful of watching his painful death. She felt overwhelmed.

While all patients could benefit from family-centered medical homes, patients who depend on family members for daily care, such as children, the elderly, disabled veterans, and others, must have care that includes consideration of the family. MedFTs who are competent in working within health delivery systems can serve as strong advocates for the inclusion of family-based care in both micro (clinical work) and macro (service delivery, policy, payment) systems.

Conclusions

Team-based care is seen as vital to healthcare reform (Alpert, 2013). Currently, the core team usually includes physicians, nurses, physician assistants, pharmacists, and possibly social workers (Weinstein, Brandt, Gilbert, & Schmitt, 2013). Unfortunately, MedFTs are frequently excluded from these teams. For example, in a recent Center for Studying Health System Change newsletter describing Portland, Oregon's efforts for national health reform, a discussion about collaborative culture and care made no mention of MedFT (Tu, Mechanic, Boukus, & Draper, 2013). As a wider audience becomes aware of this fact, their integration into and involvement within health care will inevitably increase.

As MedFTs increasingly participate in contemporary healthcare teams, such as PCMH practices, they must also become an integral part of the healthcare policy and advocacy discussion. One important group for the MedFT community to join is the Patient-Centered Primary Care Collaborative (www.pcpcc.org). This Washington DC-based organization is the central location for advocacy and development of multidisciplinary medical homes. MedFTs must become aware of this organization and closely follow their conferences and publications. Another important group for MedFTs to follow is the Center for Studying Health System Change, also in Washington DC (www.hschange.com). Finally, MedFTs should become involved in the conferences of the IHI in Boston (www.ihi.org). This organization has been leading healthcare reform since the 1990s.

In addition to these groups, behavioral health (e.g., American Association for Marriage and Family Therapy) and collaborative healthcare (Collaborative Family Healthcare Association) organizations need to ensure that its members are seated at the tables where these important and opportune conversations are taking place. As new models of healthcare delivery are being invented for the twenty-first century that replace independent physician practice, there is a great need and opportunity for MedFTs to play a leadership role in the future of healthcare delivery.

Questions for Reflection

1. Healthcare policy and reform can appear quite distant and removed from the daily work of MedFTs. How might healthcare policy inform your work with patients?
2. What aspects of healthcare reform give you hope and optimism in your role as a MedFT? What aspects worry you?
3. This chapter references the work of Jennifer Wolff (2012), who makes specific recommendations to better care for families. Which of the recommendations do you value the most?
4. Given your experiences, what potential policy initiatives would you like to see implemented to optimize care for families?
5. How could your voice as a MedFT inform the development of healthcare policy in the United States? What obstacles might you face in this effort?

References[1]

*Abrams, M., Nuzum, R., Mika, S., & Lawlor, G. (2011). *Realizing health reform's potential: How the Affordable Care Act will strengthen primary care and benefit patients, providers, and payers*. The Commonwealth Fund. Retrieved from http://www.commonwealthfund.org/~/media/Files/Publications/Issue%20Brief/2011/Jan/1466_Abrams_how_ACA_will_strengthen_primary_care_reform_brief_v3.pdf

Alpert, J. S. (2013). The team approach—Go team!! *The American Journal of Medicine, 126*, 275. doi:10.1016/j.amjmed.2012.09.013.

*American Academy of Family Physicians (AAFP), American Academy of Pediatrics (AAP), American College of Physicians (ACP), & American Osteopathic Association (AOA). (2007). *Joint principles of the patient-centered medical home*. Retrieved from http://www.medicalhomeinfo.org/Joint%20Statement.pdf

American College of Physicians. (2010). *The patient-centered medical home neighbor: The interface of the patient-centered medical home with specialty/subspecialty practices*. Retrieved from http://www.acponline.org

Anderson, G. (2010). *Chronic care: Making the case for ongoing care*. Princeton, NJ: Robert Woods Johnson Foundation. Retrieved from http://www.rwjf.org/content/dam/farm/reports/reports/2010/rwjf54583

*Berenson, R. A., & Burton, R. A. (2011). Accountable care organizations in Medicare and the private sector: A status update. *Timely Analysis of Immediate Health Policy Issues*, 1–12. Washington, DC: The Urban Institute. Retrieved from http://www.urban.org/uploadedpdf/412438-Accountable-Care-Organizations-in-Medicare-and-the-Private-Sector.pdf

Berenson, R. A., Gans, D. N., Zuckerman, S., Merrell, K., Underwood, W. S., & Williams, A. F. (2008). A house is not a home: Keeping patients at the center of practice redesign. *Health Affairs, 27*, 1219–1230. doi:10.1377/hlthaff.27.5.1219.

*Berwick, D. M., Nolan, T. W., & Whittington, J. (2008). The triple aim: Care, health, and cost. *Health Affairs, 27*, 759–769. doi:10.1377/hlthaff.27.3.759.

Committee on Psychosocial Aspects of Child and Family Health, Committee on Early Childhood, Adoption, and Dependent Care, and Section on Developmental and Behavioral Pediatrics. (2012). Early childhood adversity, toxic stress, and the role of the pediatrician: Translating developmental science into lifelong health. *Pediatrics, 129*, e224–e231. doi:10.1542/peds.2011-2662.

*Croghan, T. W., & Brown, J. D. (2010). *Integrating behavioral health treatment into the patient centered medical home* (AHRQ Publication No. 10-0084-EF). Rockville, MD: Agency for Healthcare Research and Quality. Retrieved from http://brittenassociates.com/documents_pcmh/AHRQ/Mental%20Health%20in%20the%20PCMH-July1.pdf

Davis, K., Schoen, C., & Stremikis, K. (2010). *Mirror, mirror on the wall: How the performance of the U.S. Health Care System compares internationally*. The Commonwealth Fund. Retrieved from http://www.commonwealthfund.org/~/media/Files/Publications/Fund%20Report/2010/Jun/1400_Davis_Mirror_Mirror_on_the_wall_2010.pdf

deGruy, F. V., & Etz, R. S. (2010). Attending to the whole person in the patient-centered medical home: The case for incorporating behavioral healthcare, substance abuse care, and health behavior change. *Families, Systems & Health, 28*, 298–307. doi:10.1037/a0022049.

Dentzer, S. (2011). Still crossing the quality chasm—Or suspended over it? *Health Affairs, 30*, 554–555. doi:10.1377/hlthaff.2011.0287.

Edwards, T. M., Svab, I., Ivbijaro, G., Scherger, J., Clarke, D., & Kallenberg, G. A. (2012). Multimorbidity in primary care behavioral health. In G. Ivbijaro (Ed.), *Companion to primary care mental health* (pp. 672–686). Geneva, Switzerland: World Health Organization.

[1] An asterisk has been use to note references that the chapter authors recommend for further reading.

Hoge, C. (2011). Interventions for war-related posttraumatic stress disorder: Meeting veterans where they are. *Journal of the American Medical Association, 306*, 549–551. doi:10.1001/jama.2011.1096.

Hunter, C. L., & Goodie, J. L. (2010). Operational and clinical components for integrated-collaborative behavioral healthcare in the patient-centered medical home. *Families, Systems & Health, 28*, 308–321. doi:10.1037/a0021761.

Institute of Medicine. (2001). *Crossing the quality chasm: New health system for the 21st century*. Retrieved from http://www.iom.edu/Reports/2001/Crossing-the-Quality-Chasm-A-New-Health-System-for-the-21st-Century.aspx

Katon, W. J., Lin, E. H. B., Von Korkff, M. V., Ciechanowski, P., Ludman, E. J., Young, B., ... McCulloch, D. (2010). Integrated care for patients with depression and chronic illnesses. *New England Journal of Family Medicine, 363*, 2611–2620. doi:10.1056/NEJMoa1003955

Levine, C. (2011). Improving transitional care for involving family caregivers. *National Health Policy Forum*, October 28, 2011. Retrieved from http://www.uhfnyc.org/assets/968

Moran, M. (2010). Medical home needs remodeling to provide optimal MH care. *Psychiatric News*. Retrieved from http://psychnews.psychiatryonline.org/newsarticle.aspx?articleid=113684&RelatedNewsArticles=true

Murray, C. J. L., & Frenk, J. (2010). Ranking 37th—Measuring the performance of the U.S. Health Care System. *The New England Journal of Medicine, 362*, 98–99.

National Council for Community Behavioral Healthcare. (2011, January). *Partnering with health homes and accountable care organizations*. Retrieved from http://www.thenationalcouncil.org

Patterson, J. (2012, November 6). *JAMA advocates for families in healthcare* [web log comment]. Retrieved from http://www.cfha.net/blogpost/753286/153313/JAMA-Advocates-for-Families-in-Healthcare

*Patterson, J. E., Peek, C. J., Heinrich, R. L., Bischoff, R. J., & Scherger, J. (2002). *Mental health professionals in medical settings: A primer*. New York, NY: Norton.

*Scherger, J. (2012, October 10). *Do medical family therapists bring value to healthcare*? [web log comment]. Retrieved from http://www.cfha.net/blogpost/753286/151901/Do-Medical-Family-Therapists-Bring-Value-to-Health-Care

Schonkoff, J. P., Garner, A. S., & the Committee on Psychosocial Aspects of Child and Family Health, Committee on Early Childhood, Adoption, and Dependent Care, and Section on Developmental and Behavioral Pediatrics. (2012). The lifelong effects of early childhood adversity and toxic stress. *Pediatrics, 129*, e232–e246. doi:10.1542/peds.2011-2663.

Sia, C., Tonniges, T. F., Osterhus, E., & Taba, S. (2004). History of the medical home concept. *Pediatrics, 113*, 1473–1478.

Stange, K., Nutting, P. A., Miller, W. L., Jaen, C. R., Crabtree, B. F., Flocke, S. A., & Gill, J. M. (2009). Defining and measuring the patient-centered medical home. *Journal of General Internal Medicine, 25*, 601–612. doi:10.1007/s11606-010-1291-3

Tu, H. T., Mechanic, R., Boukus, E. R., Draper, K. (2013, July). *Portland, Oregon: Health insurance market geared up for national health reform*. Center for Studying Health System Change. Retrieved from http://www.hschange.org/CONTENT/1368/

Vogeli, C., Shields, A. E., Lee, T. A., Gibson, T. B., Marder, W. D., Weiss, K. B., & Blumenthal, D. (2007). Multiple chronic conditions: Prevalence, health consequences, and implications for quality, care management, and costs. *Journal of General Internal Medicine, 22*, 391–395. doi:10.1007/s11606-007-0322-1

*Weinstein, R. S., Brandt, B. F., Gilbert, J. H., & Schmitt, M. H. (2013). Bridging the quality chasm: Interdisciplinary teams to the rescue? *The American Journal of Medicine, 126*, 276–277. doi:10.1016/j.amjmed.2012.10.014.

Wolff, J. (2012). Family matters in health care delivery. *Journal of the American Medical Association, 308*, 1529–1530. doi:10.1001/jama.2012.13366.

Chapter 19
Family Therapists in Primary Care Opportunities for Integration Throug… Advocacy

Jennifer Hodgson, Melissa Fox, and Angela Lamson

The infrastructure of the American healthcare system has created a distinct crevasse between the behavioral health and physical healthcare systems. However, American adults have repeatedly indicated that primary care is where they prefer to have their mental health needs addressed (Kessler & Stafford, 2008; Reiss-Brennan, 2010; Strosahl, 1994). For over three decades, this desire has made primary care the nation's de facto mental healthcare system (deGruy, 1996; Regier, Goldberg, & Taube, 1978; Regier et al., 1993; Strosahl, 2005). Strikingly, up to 70 % of primary care visits have a psychosocial component (Fries, Koop, & Beadle, 1993; Gatchel & Oordt, 2003).

Primary care providers, or PCPs (e.g., physicians, nurse practitioners, physician assistants), are the main source of identifying and treating mental health disorders. However, they often lack both time and the advanced psychosocial diagnostic training needed to make clinical assessments and identify subclinical concerns before they become problematic. As a result, many disorders go undiagnosed and/or untreated (Bitar, Springer, Gee, Graff, & Schydlower, 2009; Kessler, Chiu, Demler, & Walters, 2005; Kessler & Stafford, 2008; McCann & LeRoux, 2006; Reiss-Brennan, 2010). In a recent national survey, 63 % of urban and suburban and 71 % of rural physicians working in primary care claimed that in addition to the aforementioned issues, inadequate access to mental health services affects their patients' health negatively (Robert Wood Johnson Foundation, 2011). A third issue for PCPs is patients' inability to pay for necessary treatments. For example, 71 % (suburban), 73 % (rural), and 77 % (urban) of PCPs would like to write prescriptions for behavioral health services and have the cost covered by the healthcare system. However, while not all mental health disorders require psychotropic intervention (Kessler et al., 2005), impairments have been shown to impact one's overall

J. Hodgson (✉)
East Carolina University, Greenville, NC, USA
e-mail: hodgsonj@ecu.edu

J. Hodgson et al. (eds.), *Medical Family Therapy*, DOI 10.1007/978-3-319-03482-9_19,

g (especially at home and in social relationships), and even more so than on physical disorders (Druss et al., 2009). Given that up to 84 % of the most ommon primary care symptoms are not found to have an organic cause and typically include expensive and sometimes unnecessary testing (Kroenke & Mangelsdorff, 1989), it seems logical that MedFTs could make a contribution by focusing on the systemic picture and interventions that target biopsychosocial-spiritual (BPSS) outcomes.

Numerous pioneering authors and organizations have argued that an integrated system that offers medical and mental health treatment simultaneously is sorely needed (e.g., Alfuth & Barnard, 2000; Cummings, 2001; deGruy, 1996; Druss & Bornemann, 2010; Future of Family Medicine Project Leadership Committee, 2004; Hepworth & Cushman, 2005; Institute of Medicine [IOM], 2002; Levant, House, May, & Smith, 2006; President's New Freedom Commission on Mental Health, 2003; Strosahl, 1994), especially given that approximately 25 % of American adults (Druss et al., 2009; Kessler et al., 2005) and 11 % of children (US Department of Health and Human Services, 2010) have diagnosable mental health disorders (American Psychiatric Association, 2013). Although many medical and behavioral health clinicians want to unify their efforts, those working in primary care often lack the time, in-depth training, and billing structures to do so (Blount, DeGirolamo, & Mariani, 2006; Butler et al., 2008; Dickinson & Miller, 2010; Peek & Heinrich, 1998; Robinson & Reiter, 2007). Furthermore, not all behavioral health providers (BHPs) have been trained to address issues that extend past the individual patient (McDaniel, Hepworth, & Doherty, 1992), and/or to work in a primary care setting (Blount, 1998; Dickinson & Miller, 2010; Patterson, Peek, Heinrich, Bischoff, & Scherger, 2002; Robinson & Strosahl, 2009; Strosahl, 2005). Recently, subsets of primary care and behavioral health providers have developed various integrated applications within the fragmented system to address these barriers and strengthen the possibilities for integrated care models to succeed (e.g., Blount et al., 2006; Butler et al., 2008; Collins, Hewson, Munger, & Wade, 2010; Funk & Ivbijaro, 2008; Lopez, Coleman-Beattie, Jahnke, & Sanchez, 2008; Mauer, 2006, 2009; Mauer & Jarvis, 2010; Miller, Kessler, & Peek, 2011; Robinson & Reiter, 2007; Russell, 2010; Tyndall, Hodgson, Lamson, White, & Knight, 2012a).

Recent systematic reviews have found support for the utility of integrated care in improving depression (Archer et al., 2012; Thota et al., 2012), anxiety (Archer et al., 2012), chronic care for both physical and behavioral health of patients (Woltmann et al., 2012), as well as for couples and families (Tyndall et al., 2012a). Integrated care has also been demonstrated to improve global mental health functioning in primary care patients (Bryan et al., 2012; Ray-Sannerud et al., 2012). Bryan and colleagues (2012) found that the degree of improvement was associated with the number of behavioral health consultant appointments that patients attended and that a behavioral health intervention was also effective for patients with severe baseline impairment.

This chapter illustrates an opportunity for MedFTs to punctuate how their relational, systemic, and collaborative skills are prime for providing integrated care. The paradigm shift from traditional behavior health settings to integrated primary care is discussed, highlighting: (a) how MedFTs can contribute at various levels of integration, (b) the clinical, operational, and financial barriers that MedFTs need to be aware of as they enter healthcare settings to provide co-located and integrated care services, and (c) possible solutions to barriers and recommendations for how MedFTs can become more of a presence in the integrated care movement.

The Role of Family in Health Care

The Institute of Medicine (IOM) recognizes the roles that families play in individual health and has been recommending their inclusion in primary care since 1994. McDaniel and colleagues (2005) asserted, "The family represents what may be the most important challenge and opportunity for today's primary care provider" (p. viii). Involving family members in individual patient care can be influential to the success and efficiency of treatment plans. Family inclusion can range from acknowledging family influence on individual health to specifically incorporating family, friends, and caregivers into routine care (IOM, 1994, 2001; McDaniel et al., 2005). Family intervention involves skills that few behavioral health professionals have, making systemically trained providers a unique contributor to healthcare settings (Tyndall et al., 2012a; Tyndall, Hodgson, Lamson, White, & Knight, 2012b).

Some of the pioneers of the family therapy field were first trained as physicians (e.g., Lyman Wynne, Murray Bowen, Nathan Ackerman, Milton Erickson, Salvador Minuchin) and focused their research and progress on the functioning of the family. Therefore, there is a legacy of relational therapists who have worked in healthcare settings. Family therapists have been practicing in pediatric settings since the 1970s and in research and teaching settings with family medicine providers since the 1980s (Doherty, McDaniel, & Hepworth, 1994). The history of interdisciplinary work is punctuated by Dym and Berman who in 1985 issued a call for "collaboration between family therapist and family physician" (p. 66). In 1986, they described in detail a fully integrated model in which family therapists and family physicians saw all patients together, forming conjoint treatment plans. By 1992, family therapist–physician collaboration had been formally named as "Medical Family Therapy" (McDaniel et al., 1992).

McDaniel et al. (1992) defined MedFT as the, "biopsychosocial treatment of individuals and families who are dealing with medical problems. As we conceptualize it, MedFT works from a biopsychosocial systems model and actively encourages collaboration between therapists and other health professionals" (p. 2). Since nearly 20 years had passed, Tyndall, Hodgson, White, Lamson, and Knight (2010) wanted to study if the definition of MedFT had evolved after advancements have been documented in the science and practice of it. After completing a yearlong

Dephi study, an expert MedFT panel lengthened its description to include what follows below.

> [Medical Family Therapy is...] an approach to healthcare sourced from a BPS-S [biopsychosocial-spiritual] perspective and marriage and family therapy, but also informed by systems theory. The practice of MedFT spans a variety of clinical settings with a strong focus on the relationships of the patient and the collaboration between and among the healthcare providers and the patient. MedFTs are endorsers of patient and family agency and facilitators of healthy workplace dynamics. (pp. 68–69).

Systems theorists hold that the most logical way to work with and study individuals is to consider their biological, relational, and sociocultural influences (Bowen, 1978; Von Bertalanffy, 1968). Engel's biopsychosocial (BPS) approach (1977, 1980) helped to extend systems thinking to a healthcare setting by developing a conceptualization of medical problems as best understood in the contexts of biological, psychological, and social factors. MedFTs are also trained to recognize the roles that spirituality (i.e., belief systems and meaning) may play in treatment (Hodgson, Lamson, Mendenhall, & Crane, 2012; Hodgson, Lamson, & Reese, 2007; Linville, Hertlein, & Prouty Lyness, 2007; Seattle Pacific University, 2010; Tyndall et al., 2012a; 2012b). The addition of spiritual awareness to systems theory and Engel's BPS model (1977, 1980) forms the BPSS approach (Hodgson et al., 2012; Katerndahl, 2008; Onarecker & Sterling, 1995; Prest & Robinson, 2006; Wright, Watson, & Bell, 1996). MedFTs apply this model routinely in their research and clinical work with patients, families, and members of the healthcare system (Tyndall et al., 2012a, 2012b).

Some debate exists as to whether MedFT is a separate field, subdiscipline of family therapy, framework, or an orientation. Tyndall and colleagues (2010) examined this debate in depth. For purposes of this chapter, the term "MedFT" will be used to refer to behavioral health providers who are trained in family intervention and/or family therapy and who work in healthcare settings, bridging physical and BPSS health. Gaining competency in MedFT requires specific training in family therapy models and interventions, behavioral health interventions, brief evidence-based models, the BPSS approach, and healthcare clinical, operational, and financial domains before they begin integration into a healthcare practice (see Chap. 3 in this text for more information; Tyndall, Hodgson, Lamson, White, & Knight, 2014). This training is critical because MedFTs often work side-by-side with PCPs who are aware of interactions between relational and health challenges, but lack the time, training, and compensation necessary to fully address these challenges (American Academy of Family Physicians, 2011; Hepworth & Cushman, 2005; Peyrot et al., 2005; Robinson & Reiter, 2007; Strosahl, 1994). In these cases, MedFTs can use their specialized relational, systemic, and diagnostic training to develop integrated treatment plans and deliver interventions that improve outcomes, especially through the venue of integrated primary care.

Integrated Primary Care

Integrated primary care is the general "service that unifies medical and mental health care in a primary care setting, and the practice of avoiding the dichotomy of 'physical' or 'mental' in defining the problems brought by a patient" (Blount, 1998, p. xi). The basic format of this model consists of PCPs and BHPs collaborating side-by-side with patients to develop, implement, monitor, and evaluate treatment (e.g., Blount et al., 2006; Butler et al., 2008; Collins et al., 2010; Funk & Ivbijaro, 2008; Lopez et al., 2008; Mauer, 2006, 2009; Mauer & Jarvis, 2010; Miller et al., 2011; Robinson & Reiter, 2007; Russell, 2010). However, because the term "integration" has many interpretations and descriptors, it may look different at various healthcare sites, making it difficult to replicate and evaluate (Miller et al., 2011; Peek, 2013).

A variety of taxonomies have been written to describe the levels of integration that a healthcare system can adopt. The most notable taxonomy was written by Doherty, McDaniel, and Baird in 1996. They identified five levels of integrated care ranging from minimal collaboration (BHPs and PCPs work in separate locations and rarely connect) to full integration (BHPs and PCPs working side by side). In 2003, Blount collapsed Doherty et al.'s (1996) five levels of integration into three broader categories: coordination, co-location, and integration. Then in 2010, Collins et al. merged the work of Doherty et al. (1996) and Blount (2003) into one taxonomy. The evolution of integration then inspired Heath, Romero, and Reynolds in 2013 to expand the five levels of integration to six. Retaining the work of Doherty et al. (1996) and Blount (2003), they broke out the three categories into two levels each in order to accommodate more descriptive characteristics so organizations can capture patient and staff experiences, as well as better evaluate their efforts toward integration.

Then in 2013, two separate teams of experts on behavioral health integration identified needed improvements in how integration is assessed and categorized. Heath et al. (2013) expanded Doherty et al.'s (1996) five levels to six levels, taking more of a developmental approach to achieving full behavioral health integration. At the same time, Peek in collaboration with the National Integration Academy Council (2013), published a lexicon model permitting integration sites to track their evolution across seven specific areas: (a) type of spatial arrangement, (b) type of collaboration, (c) level of shared workflows, (d) degree of shared care plans, and (e) degree of use of shared record, and (f) level of shared culture and training, and (g) level of organizational alignment. They believe that the lexicon method allows for a rich meaningful dialogue to take place between the supervisors, supervisee, and the site's "clinicians, care systems, health plans, payers, researchers, policymakers, business modelers and patients working for effective, widespread implementation on a meaningful scale" (p. 1), promoting a common language.

When providers strictly adhere to a coordinated care approach, it invites BHPs and PCPs to discuss patient referrals, but these contacts are rare; therefore, co-location of care is the first step to having medical and behavioral health providers coexist in the same healthcare setting. Co-located providers might work in a manner described as collaborative or even integrated but contact between them is typically through inter-office referrals or when crisis consults are needed. They might also never communicate with each other about shared patients. While co-location most commonly takes place in healthcare settings, The National Council for Community Behavior Healthcare ([NCCBH], 2009) advocated for a bidirectional model of integration where medical services are brought into behavioral health settings as well. This means that in addition to having behavioral health providers integrated into healthcare settings, medical providers should also be integrated into behavioral health settings.

There is some debate on whether or not integration is best assessed on a continuous or dichotomous basis. Unlike Heath et al.'s (2013) six levels of integration where organizations can be assigned a specific level number, in the "Primary Care Behavioral Health" model (PCBH; Robinson & Reiter, 2007; Robinson & Strosahl, 2009), integration is seen as continuous and may be implemented in three different ways: (a) behavioral health consulting, (b) specialty consulting, and (c) integrated care services. This is similar to the beliefs shared by the Lexicon model developers (Peek & NIAC, 2013).

In behavioral health consulting, on-site BHPs are contacted by a PCP for help with mild to moderate patient behavioral health issues. The BHP will speak with the PCP outside the exam room, provide a brief assessment in the exam room, or talk with the patient about scheduling a brief return appointment, if time is limited. The BHP then provides the PCP with feedback. In specialty consulting, BHPs join other members of the healthcare team in the exam room for patients with more serious issues, but the PCP still initiates the consult. Finally, in an integrated program, patients with the most serious issues and commonly high utilizers of healthcare services are always seen by the PCP and BHP simultaneously as part of the standard of care for that particular issue (e.g., chronic pain).

In most instances, the PCBH model takes the place of a traditional 50-min psychotherapy appointment (Robinson & Strosahl, 2009). The consult model allows for the BHP to immediately be available to the PCP and patient, with a shared treatment plan made collaboratively before the visit ends, ideally, or within a few days. The treatment plan may consist of psychoeducation and patient self-management with PCP/BHP follow up. In addition, the patient will likely have several consult sessions to see the BHP for more intensive skill building, or a referral to specialty mental health services for issues too complex to treat in primary care (Strosahl, 1997).

Because MedFT was developed in family medicine training programs (McDaniel et al., 1992), a logical fit exists between integration and the principles of MedFT (i.e., systemic orientation with a focus on agency, communion, and the influence of families/relationships on overall health and well-being). However, despite the reciprocal influences of behavioral, physical, and relational health, clinical models that sufficiently address all three are not easily achieved in today's fragmented, time- and cost-driven private sector (Doherty, 2007; Patterson et al., 2002; Robinson & Strosahl, 2009). The following section presents a brief overview of the possible barriers that MedFTs may experience as they assume employment in primary care settings.

Barriers and Strategies to Integration

Although MedFTs have an important role in the integrated care system, policy changes are needed to remove the barriers to integration impacting most BHPs (Blount, 2003; Dickinson & Miller, 2010; Kathol, Butler, McAlpine, & Kane, 2010; Levant et al., 2006). The Three-World view framework (Peek, 2008) offers a structure for reviewing each barrier and identifying where changes are needed. Using this framework, each healthcare system is seen as having three branches (or "worlds"): clinical, operational, and financial. The clinical branch is concerned with quality of clinical care and good provider–patient relationships. The operational branch is concerned with realistic, accessible care, and smooth flow between triage and treatment. The financial branch is concerned with cost-effective care as well as billing and receiving.

To have an effective, affordable, and efficient system, each branch must work together, as a change in one will invariably impact the others (IOM, 2001; Peek, 2008; Waldman, Smith, & Hood, 2003). The individual functions of the branches and the dynamic interactions between them can be conceptualized in terms of family dynamics, particularly first and second order change (Watzlawick, Weakland, & Fisch, 1974). Sometimes only one family member changing his or her thoughts and behavior can allow the family as a whole to reach some sort of stabilization (first order change). The problem itself may remain, but the system is functioning at least a little better. Over time, the new patterns and rules can lead to resolution of the problem (second order change). These patterns are easier to change when all family members are present, and if all branches are attended to, but change in just one person or branch can initiate change in the family or healthcare system. Similar to how family therapy training programs often structure their didactics around working with each person and also within the family system, the "Three-World view" (Peek, 2008) will be used here to help relational providers who are interested in working in primary care settings understand the hurdles they, and the healthcare system, must clear before achieving a fully functioning integrated partnership.

Clinical World

Barrier

Training differences often present an obstacle as medical and BHPs are generally not given instructions on how to work together (Blount, 1998, 2003; Blount & Bayona, 1994; O'Donohue, Cummings, & Cummings, 2009; Patterson et al., 2002; Robinson & Reiter, 2007). The process of integrating care is not always smooth, nor is it innate (Oser & O'Donohue, 2009; Robinson & Reiter, 2007; Tyndall et al., 2012b). Psychosocial health training is becoming more prevalent in medical education, but barriers to including the full range of necessary training have persisted (Association of American Medical Colleges [AAMC], 2011). Training for many PCPs still tends to emphasize the biological aspects of health (AAMC, 2011; Astin, Soeken, Sierpina, & Clarridge, 2006; McDaniel et al., 2005; Patterson et al., 2002), while most BHP training tends to focus on the psychosocial and/or relational aspects of health (Edwards & Patterson, 2006; McDaniel et al., 2005; Patterson et al., 2002). To prepare both sets of providers to function effectively in an integrated care setting, cross training should occur helping to advance integration through early exposure to one another's content and shared learning opportunities. While BHPs generally do not want to see a bleeding patient any more than PCPs want to walk into the exam room and see a crying patient, both are frequent occurrences in primary care settings and BHPs and PCPs need to know what to do when faced with these situations. In healthcare contexts, BHPs are aware that many patients have biomedical health issues, but often feel these issues are outside the scope of their training and thus PCPs should address them (Edwards & Patterson, 2006). Likewise, PCPs often feel overwhelmed by patients' psychosocial concerns and might appreciate someone who is trained, both in educating patients (e.g., how to make healthy choices or how to implement changes) and in addressing general psychosocial issues (Blount et al., 2006; deGruy, 2000; Robert Wood Johnson Foundation, 2011).

Alfuth and Barnard (2000) contended that to advance integration both BHPs and PCPs need to have a shared interest and respect for one another's unique language and culture. In practice, however, any multidisciplinary team of professionals "may not readily appreciate each other's strengths or recognize weaknesses except in crisis situations" (IOM, 2001, p. 131). Lack of insight into each other's traditionally separate worlds can result in differences of opinion that stem from deep-seated values combined with conflicting professional ethics about what is considered to be good clinical care (see special issue on ethics and integrated care in *Families, Systems, & Health*, volume 31, 2013). Conflicts can sometimes be resolved, but have also been identified as a common reason for the failure of integrated care projects.

Part of the conflict stems from the fact that the competencies needed for integrated care are different from those needed for traditional therapy (O'Donohue, Cummings, & Ferguson, 2003). Although many therapists working in integrated settings feel comfortable in their surroundings (Doherty, 2007), others feel out of place, isolated, and underappreciated (Edwards & Patterson, 2006). Thus, competencies often set a baseline for what therapists should know to function as well as possible in their environment. There are several practice-based lists or texts that address behavioral health competencies in varying degrees, but most are not comprehensive across a variety of integrated care models or settings (e.g., O'Donohue et al., 2009; Patterson et al., 2002; Robinson & Reiter, 2007; Strosahl, 2005) and others are discipline specific (Interorganizational Work Group on Competencies for Primary Care Psychology Practice, 2013; National Association of Social Workers, 2005). However, only one known list has been put forward for MedFTs (see Chap. 3; Tyndall et al., 2014). Tyndall et al. (2012b) constructed a list of competencies specifically for MedFTs, as most resources do not mention specific competencies needed for BHPs providing integrated primary care (IPC) services beyond psychoeducational support for families about the patient's illness and understanding how the illness impacts the family and vice versa. While training differences may or may not significantly affect the basic competencies needed for integrated care, Strosahl (2005) asserted that a clarification of differences in scope of practice between BHP disciplines would benefit not only BHPs but also integrated teams and, ultimately, patients by including important and complementary skill sets. For example, not all BHPs are trained to provide family therapy, understand and advocate for community resources, or conduct psychometric testing.

The idea behind competency is that while each specific integrated care site requires flexibility in methods and models used by BHPs (deGruy & Etz, 2010), consistency in the core competencies of integration would allow for good patient care and open the door for the evaluation of factors contributing to this care (Strosahl & Robinson, 2008). At present, integrated care practitioners and hiring professionals have little a priori evidence of the exact skills or disciplines needed for providing integrated care. To date, no research could be located that formally examines how closely integrated care experts from a wide range of settings agree upon core competencies, or how consistent training opportunities prepare BHPs for this work. Nor does research exist that determines whether one discipline is more prepared or capable of running the behavioral health services in a primary care setting; therefore, the most prepared provider versus a specific discipline-type is a more logical choice.

Strategy

Master's level MedFTs are poised to apply their systemic training to clinical work in a healthcare setting. Doctoral level MedFTs have additional skills and training in administration and research, which are critical to designing, implementing, maintaining, and expanding integrated care programs based on measureable outcomes. However, without training in MedFT, therapists may struggle to apply a systems orientation to working collaboratively within primary healthcare systems.

Web sites and continuing education workshops along with local, regional, and national conferences focused on integrated care (e.g., Agency for Healthcare Research and Quality's Academy for Integrating Behavioral Health and Primary Care (www.integrationacademy.ahrq.gov/), Collaborative Family Healthcare Association (www.CFHA.net), Integrated Behavioral Health Project (www.ibhp.org), National Council for Behavioral Health (www.thenaitonalcouncil.org/), and SAMSHA-HRSA Center for Integrated Health Solutions (www.integration.samhsa.gov)) offer opportunities for BHPs to learn how to adapt their traditional psychotherapy training to a healthcare setting. The opportunities for specific training in MedFT range from weeklong intensives to postgraduate certificates, master's, or doctoral training tracks/programs (see Chap. 3; Tyndall et al., 2014) with varying expectations of learning outcomes and degrees of exposure to MedFT knowledge and skills.

Based on one's level of MedFT training, BHPs can approach primary care practices and highlight how their training, which includes attending to family dynamics and intervening appropriately based on level of training, makes them well suited for contributing to interdisciplinary team efforts of promoting, operationalizing, evaluating, disseminating, and refining integrated care for individuals, families, and healthcare teams. These efforts can also include identifying which competencies and systemic components are most crucial to successful outcomes. As a final clinical strategy, MedFTs should implement competency-based protocols at their clinics and evaluate and conduct new research on these competencies (See Chap. 3 for more information on MedFT competencies; Tyndall et al., 2014. See Chaps. 11–16 on research and design; Lewis, Myhra, & Walker, 2014; Mendenhall, Berge, & Doherty, 2014; Mendenhall, Pratt, Phelps, Baird, & Younkin, 2014; Polaha & Nolan, 2014; Williams-Reade, Gordon, & Wray, 2014; Zak-Hunter et al., 2014).

Operational World

Barrier

The fragmented healthcare system and competing goals of each "world" present major obstacles to harmonious balance between primary and behavioral health care (Hodgson et al., 2012; Peek, 2008; President's New Freedom Commission on Mental Health, 2003). Medical and behavioral health systems are typically trained and reimbursed to operate and attend to issues differently (Thielke, Vannoy, & Unutzer, 2007), with PCPs seen as "care managers" responsible for a patient's overall health and depending on level of integration, BHPs serving as specialists for patients who meet a provider or system's referral criteria (Blount, 2003; Collins et al., 2010; Doherty et al., 1996; Heath et al., 2013). When these two systems are combined, the providers can have a pragmatic culture clash (Kathol et al., 2010).

Therefore, having buy-in from senior clinical and administrative leaders for operational overhaul (Dickinson & Miller, 2010; Kathol et al., 2010; Strosahl, Baker, Braddick, Stuart, & Handley, 1997) is an integral component to smoothing out this clash. Even when all stakeholders prefer an integrated system, merging BHPs of any kind into daily operations of a busy clinic can present a formidable challenge (Kessler, 2008a).

Operational challenges generally center on the logistics of triaging and treating patients. This may include not having enough time or space for patients to be seen or not having a seamless referral and consultation process, for example "the physicians had to call an '800' number to arrange for a therapist colleague to walk down the hall and join a consultation with a patient" (Blount, 1998, p. xii). For PCPs, it may take time to learn to offer a referral in a way the patient is likely to accept (McDaniel et al., 2005). For MedFTs, learning to integrate with PCPs may also take artful logistics, especially in a fast-paced setting where patients spend less than 15 min in an exam room on average. Lastly, not all electronic medical record (EMR) systems have templates for psychosocial information, much less stored, in a manner accessible to physicians (Crane, 2011). Also, EMR systems organized by individual patients make it difficult to link family members together to capture shared medical history (Crane, 2011; McDaniel et al., 2005). Simply co-locating a BHP within the primary care clinic will generally not be successful; the BHP must be immersed and integrated in practice operations (Alfuth & Barnard, 2000; Kessler, 2008a; O'Donohue et al., 2003).

Strategy

Medical family therapists would benefit from workforce development on how to practice collaboratively within the time and space issues common to healthcare settings (see Chap. 4 for more information on merging culture and context; Trudeau-Hern, Mendenhall, & Wong, 2014); the first lesson is that there is often very little of each available. Consequently, families are not usually included in direct patient care (McDaniel et al., 2005), and MedFTs must find ways to adapt their evidence-based systemic approaches to brief therapy opportunities. Working more with individuals than families does not mean that MedFTs must abandon their relational focus and training. Rather, they can emphasize to prospective employers how they are positioned to provide relationally oriented care while acknowledging the realities of the healthcare system. Systems theorists highlight that "a family orientation has more to do with how one thinks about the patient than it does with how many people are in the exam room" (McDaniel et al., 2005, p. 43). When marketing their skills, therapists can point to research demonstrating improved clinical outcomes when relational therapy is added to routine medical care (e.g., Crane & Christenson, 2008; Law & Crane, 2000; Law, Crane, & Berge, 2003; see Chap. 22 for a summary report on family therapy cost-effectiveness research; Crane & Christenson, 2014).

Medical family therapists will want to remember that the operational world calls for realistic, accessible care, and smooth flow between triage and treatment. Realistic care means refraining from using one modality in structured 50-min sessions to using flexible treatment methods in unstructured 5–30 min consults with 50–90 different patients weekly in a fast-paced, unpredictable climate filled with interruptions (Alfuth & Barnard, 2000; Patterson et al., 2002; Strosahl, 2005). Accessible care requires therapists to work in crowded exam rooms instead of quiet offices with comfortable couches (Seaburn, Lorenz, Gunn, Gawinski, & Mauksch, 1996). Smooth flow between triage and treatment means learning how to integrate services without interrupting the workflow while adding value to the patient encounter and healthcare team.

Financial World

Barrier

The cost of adding BHPs in a reimbursement system, where their services are "carved-out" from medical care, is perhaps the most frequently cited barrier to integration (Hodgkin, Horgan, Garnick, Merrick, & Goldin, 2000; Kathol et al., 2010; Levant et al., 2006; Robinson & Strosahl, 2009). Sometimes administrators bypass this issue by starting grant-funded or student-volunteered pilot projects that achieve clinical and operational success. But often, once the grant funding or the student interns used for the pilot project are gone, so is the project (Barry & Frank, 2006; Kathol et al., 2010; Robinson & Strosahl, 2009).

Lack of uniform insurance coverage for BHPs under the Center for Medicare and Medicaid Services (CMS) is part of why pilot projects are not sustainable. "Together, Medicare, Medicaid, and CHIP [Children's Health Insurance Program] financed $823.8 billion in health care services in 2008—slightly more than one-third of the country's total health care expenditures and almost three-fourths of all public spending on health care" (Klees, Wolfe, & Curtis, 2012, p. 4). So while there is a great deal of money available in the system, it is a tangled mess of outdated policies and misinformation about the benefits of IPC and those trained to provide it.

Medicaid alone provides more behavioral health care than any other insurer (American Association of Marriage and Family Therapy [AAMFT], 2012a). Reimbursement by CMS is especially important for Federally Qualified Community Health Centers, as over 70 % are providing integrated care (Lardiere, Jones, & Perez, 2011). However, some BHPs struggle with getting reimbursed due to archaic policies and a lack of general understanding about their knowledgebase and training. For example, approximately 38 states at least partially recognize family therapists as Medicaid eligible providers, but they are completely shut out of nationally run Medicare (AAMFT, 2012a, 2012b). Furthermore, Medicaid billing for integrated care is more complicated than billing for traditional mental health visits. Therapists may be able to bill "incident-to" a physician or psychologist, but must be diligent in working with their local offices to code this correctly (Kessler, 2008b). Full CMS recognition will allow therapists to independently use Health and Behavior Codes (H&B). These codes are a fairly recent strategy that improves sustainability by allowing same-day billing by PCPs for medical components of care and BHPs for psychosocial components of care related to the physical diagnosis (Kessler, 2008b; Levant et al., 2006; Miyamoto, 2006). These codes allow BHPs to bill for treatment of issues that affect patients' health (e.g., coping with a new diabetes diagnosis) but do not meet criteria for a DSM 5 (American Psychiatric Association, 2013) diagnosis.

All BHPs still use traditional psychiatric/psychotherapy codes for DSM 5 diagnoses; however, same day billing of DSM 5 and H&B codes is not generally permitted (Chaffee, 2009; Miyamoto, 2006; North Carolina Center of Excellence for Integrated Care, 2011), thus limiting the range of integrated care services and foci. While some private insurers limit the use of H&B codes to BHPs in carve-out networks, misinterpret and/or do not recognize the codes (Kessler, 2008b), others either continue to require a DSM 5 diagnosis for reimbursement or will not reimburse for H&B codes if the patient has a co-occurring DSM 5 diagnosis. H&B codes are a big step forward, but confusion surrounding their purpose and CMS rules can prevent payment for services to patients with co-occurring diagnoses or subclinical symptoms, maintain the perception of behavioral health as a disease (Robinson & Strosahl, 2009), marginalize family-based treatment, and present a philosophical challenge for strength-based MedFTs (Yapko, 2008).

Another key financial barrier is that integrating services has required significant up-front expenditures, including added salaries, resources to design new systems, and training costs (Chaffee, 2009). Since the 1960s, these expenses have been shown to slowly give way to cost savings of about 25 %, as clinical outcomes improve, making care more efficient by decreasing the need for services (e.g., Chiles, Lambert, & Hatch, 1999, 2002; Crane & Christenson, 2008; Cummings, 2001; Cummings, Cummings, & Johnson, 1997; Cummings & Follette, 1968, as cited in Cummings, 2001; see Chap. 22 for a review of family therapy cost-effectiveness research; Crane & Christenson, 2014). Eventually, organizational startup costs are fully offset by savings in medical costs (Levant et al., 2006). This phenomenon has been found in nearly 100 published studies (Levant et al., 2006).

Researchers studying family therapy services in primary care settings have demonstrated 21 % cost savings in general populations (Law & Crane, 2000). Importantly, 50 % lower costs and 38–78 % fewer services have been reported for high-utilizing patients (Crane & Christenson, 2008; Law et al., 2003). High-utilizers are the 10 % of patients who account for nearly 70 % of primary care visits (Berk & Monheit, 2001), yet typically have no organic etiology for their symptoms (Kroenke & Mangelsdorff, 1989). Interestingly, costs were also reduced by up to 57 % for these patients' family members (Law et al., 2003). A recent systematic review has also demonstrated the economic value of integrated care specifically for the treatment of depression (Jacob et al., 2012).

With so much research showing cost-offset, one must wonder why cost continues to be a barrier to integration. The answer is deceptively simple: (a) specific clinical and operational processes must be in place for the offset effect to be seen (Cummings, 2002); and (b) in a healthcare system dominated by third-party payers, most are not willing to spend the up-front money needed for system change knowing it will take 18–36 months for the cost to be offset (Chaffee, 2009; Levant et al., 2006). Thus, integration efforts will continue to be curtailed unless all insurance carriers support a financial overhaul (Barry & Frank, 2006; Butler et al., 2008; Robinson & Strosahl, 2009).

Strategy

Clinically, reimbursement policies are the main obstacle for employers in hiring MedFTs to provide direct patient care. Knowing the value of MedFTs within integrated care, both financially and intangibly, can be important to jumping reimbursement hurdles. MedFTs are particularly affected by the currently fragmented system, especially in the financial world. For now, some organizations are so convinced of the power of integrated care that they hire MedFTs or other BHPs despite the fact that their salaries cannot be offset by insurance reimbursement (Robinson & Strosahl, 2009). Also, grant funding is increasingly available for this work, allowing therapists to offset their salaries for the first few years to help build integrated models (Collins, 2009; Hodgson & Reitz, 2013). According to Korda and Eldridge (2011), there are ways in which integrated care payment-incentives introduced with the Patient Protection and Affordable Care Act can be used to promote positive systemic change. Strategies may include bundled or episode-based payment approaches, gain-sharing, and performance-based payment that incentivizes providers' care team collaboration and/or patients' treatment adherence and self-management (Korda & Eldridge, 2011). Founded by providers with a systemic perspective, the CFHA (www.CFHA.net) is working hard to advocate for integrated care reimbursement models that are sustainable and promote integrated care where behavioral health providers and medically trained providers can work in tandem.

It is important that MedFTs become familiar with successful models of integrated care. For example, models within military healthcare systems and HMOs have a closed financial system wherein the funder and providers are the same organization. Thus, the "insurer" pays for medical services and the providers' salary or contracts (Cummings, O'Donohue, & Cummings, 2009). In this type of staff model, cost risks are offset by gains and the financial system and thus able to absorb the cost of integration (Robinson & Strosahl, 2009). Other systems are leading the way in integrated care and provide a template for financial reform (see Chap. 23 for more information on financial models for MedFT; Marlowe, Capoblanco, & Greenberg, 2014).

Although closed systems like military and staff models make financial barriers easier, reimbursement is necessary for integrated care to succeed in open systems, as well (Miyamoto, 2006; Robinson & Strosahl, 2009). Although state requirements vary, MedFTs are qualified to assess, diagnose, and treat individuals experiencing behavioral health issues (US Government Printing Office via GPO Access, 2009), and are uniquely trained to also address relational concerns. As noted earlier, CMS recognition continues to be a concern. However, some MedFTs (based on training discipline) are not actually prohibited from CMS reimbursement, but rather are simply not included in the list of providers who must be reimbursed, despite being recognized as a core behavioral health profession (AAMFT, 2012b). CMS recognition will help expand what MedFTs can contribute to a healthcare visit and also improve patient access to behavioral health services.

Lastly, family therapists trained in MedFT are currently under-represented compared with other BHPs in regard to state and federal advocacy efforts as a whole. Initial steps to correct this include increasing involvement in and contributions to Political Action Committees (Yapko, 2008), meeting with local and state CMS and private insurance personnel, and getting involved with grassroots organizations invested in changing healthcare laws, specifically reimbursement policies.

Conclusion

Widespread system change is needed in order to support the type of care that patients are demanding today (Druss & Bornemann, 2010). If we as a society of professionals and consumers do not act soon, the opportunity to integrate behavioral and biomedical health care could be lost. Although there are barriers to such integration, it is hoped that this chapter will spark interest for therapists, who are already familiar with first and second order change, and lend structure to the vision of how small changes at the local level can lead to larger ones at the national level.

Current efforts at integration offer MedFTs an entryway into the changing healthcare system (Hodgson et al., 2012; Ruddy & McDaniel, 2003). Demonstrating our natural fit with primary care and advocating for policy changes are critical to securing our place. Understanding and being able to speak to the priorities of stakeholders in each branch of the "Three-World view" is paramount; MedFTs must capitalize on their systemic skills to master this key component of collaboration. To that end, "there is an emerging consensus in the policy community about the central importance of 'aligning incentives' so that providers, payers, the research community, and consumers are all focused on identifying and learning to use the most effective health care" (Robert Wood Johnson Foundation, 2009 p. 1). In striving to find their place within the idealized new system, MedFT clinicians, trainers, program developers, researchers, and policy advocates are well poised to help each of these voices be heard and understood by others, demonstrating how their systemic orientation and family focus can become part of the solution to our nation's broken healthcare system.

Discussion Questions

1. Based on the Primary Care Behavioral Health model (Robinson & Reiter, 2007; Robinson & Strosahl, 2009), what model of integrated care would you be most comfortable with and why? Please explain your response from a clinical, operational, and financial perspective.
2. Who are the various stakeholders represented in each domain of the Three-World view (Peek, 2008; Peek & Heinrich, 1998)?
3. In your current context, identify one clinical, operational, and financial barrier that may be impeding advancement of integrated care? Identify a strategy for overcoming each barrier.
4. When confronting the barriers noted above, which one do you think would be most important to address first, and why?
5. What are the current family therapy advocacy efforts in your state? Specifically, what is being done to advance opportunities for family therapists in healthcare settings? If unsure, contact your state's AAMFT division president to find out. Reflect on which of the advocacy efforts are paving the way for family therapists in healthcare settings and which are needed to further promote family therapists in primary care contexts.

References[1]

*Alfuth, R., & Barnard, C. P. (2000). Family physicians and family therapists: Understanding the interdependent synergism. *Contemporary Family Therapy, 22*, 253–277. doi:10.1023/A:1007865506702.

American Academy of Family Physicians. (2011). *Mental health care services by family physicians* [position paper]. Retrieved from http://www.aafp.org/online/en/home/policy/policies/m/mentalhealth careservices.html

*American Association of Marriage and Family Therapy. (2012a). *State advocacy: Medicaid fact sheet*. Retrieved from http://www.aamft.org/imis15/Content/Advocacy/State_Advocacy.aspx

American Association of Marriage and Family Therapy. (2012b). *Federal advocacy: Medicare fact sheet*. Retrieved from http://www.aamft.org/imis15/Content/Advocacy/Federal_Issues.aspx

American Psychiatric Association. (2013). *Diagnostic and statistical manual of mental disorders* (5th ed.). Arlington, VA: Author.

[1] An asterisk has been use to note references that the chapter authors recommend for further reading.

Archer, J., Bower, P., Gilbody, S., Lovell, K., Richards, D., Gask, L., & Coventry, P. (2012). Integrated care for depression and anxiety problems [Systematic Review]. *Cochrane Database of Systematic Reviews 2012*. Retrieved from http://ovidsp.ovid.com/ovidweb.cgi?T=JS&CSC=Y&NEWS=N&PAGE=fulltext&D=coch&AN=00075320-100000000-05157

Association of American Medical Colleges. (2011). *Behavioral and social science foundations for future physicians: Report of the behavioral and social science expert panel*. Washington, DC: Author. Retrieved from https://www.aamc.org/download/271020/data/behavioralandsocialsciencefoundations forfuturephysicians.pdf

Astin, J. A., Soeken, K., Sierpina, V. S., & Clarridge, B. R. (2006). Barriers to the integration of psychosocial factors in medicine: Results of a national survey of physicians. *Journal of the American Board of Family Medicine, 19*, 557–565.

Barry, C. L., & Frank, R. G. (2006). Commentary: An economic perspective on implementing evidence-based depression care. *Administration and Policy in Mental Health and Mental Health Services Research, 33*, 21–25. doi:10.1007/s10488-005-4234-2.

Berk, M. L., & Monheit, A. C. (2001). The concentration of health care expenditures, revisited. *Health Affairs, 20*(2), 9–18.

Bitar, G. W., Springer, P., Gee, R., Graff, C., & Schydlower, M. (2009). Barriers and facilitators of adolescent behavioral health in primary care: Perceptions of primary care providers. *Families, Systems & Health, 27*, 346–361. doi:10.1037/a0018076.

Blount, A. (Ed.). (1998). *Integrated primary care: The future of medical & mental health collaboration*. New York, NY: Norton.

*Blount, A. (2003). Integrated primary care: Organizing the evidence. *Families, Systems & Health, 21*, 121–133. doi:10.1037/1091-7527.21.2.121.

Blount, A., & Bayona, J. (1994). Toward a system of integrated primary care. *Family Systems Medicine, 12*, 171–182.

Blount, A., DeGirolamo, S., & Mariani, K. (2006). Training the integrated care practitioners of the future. *Families, Systems & Health, 24*, 111–119. doi:10.1037/1091-7527.24.1.111.

Bowen, M. (1978). *Family therapy in clinical practice*. Northvale, NJ: Jason Aronson.

Bryan, C. J., Corso, M. L., Corso, K. A., Morrow, C. E., Kanzler, K. E., & Ray-Sannerud, B. (2012). Severity of mental health impairment and trajectories of improvement in an integrated primary care clinic. *Journal of Consulting and Clinical Psychology, 80*, 396–403. doi:10.1037/a0027726.

*Butler, M., Kane, R. L., McAlpine, D., Kathol, R. G., Fu, S. S., Hagedorn, H., & Wilt, T. J. (2008). *Integration of mental health/substance abuse and primary care No. 173* (AHRQ Publication No. 09-E003). Rockville, MD: Agency for Healthcare Research and Quality. Retrieved from http://www.ahrq.gov/clinic/tp/mhsapctp.htm#Report

Chaffee, B. (2009). Financial models for integrated behavioral health care. In L. C. James & W. T. O'Donohue (Eds.), *The primary care toolkit: Practical resources for the integrated behavioral care provider* (pp. 19–30). New York, NY: Springer. doi:10.1007/978-0-387-78971-2_3.

Chiles, J. A., Lambert, M. J., & Hatch, A. L. (1999). The impact of psychological interventions on medical cost-offset: A meta-analytic review. *Clinical Psychology: Science and Practice, 6*, 204–219. doi:10.1093/clipsy/6.2.204.

Chiles, J. A., Lambert, M. J., & Hatch, A. L. (2002). Medical cost-offset: A review of psychological interventions on medical utilization over the past three decades. In N. A. Cummings, W. T. O'Donohue, & K. E. Ferguson (Eds.), *The impact of medical cost-offset on practice and research: Making it work for you*. Reno, NV: Context Press.

Collins, C. (2009). Integrating behavioral and mental health services into the primary care setting. *North Carolina Medical Journal, 70*, 248–252. Retrieved from http://www.ncmedicaljournal.com/

Collins, C., Hewson, D. L., Munger, R., & Wade, T. (2010). *Evolving models of behavioral health integration in primary care*. Report commissioned by the Milbank Memorial Fund.

*Crane, D. R. (2011). Does family therapy reduce health care costs for more than the identified patient? *Clinical Child Psychology and Psychiatry, 16*, 3–4. doi:10.1177/1359104510397607.

*Crane, D. R., & Christenson, J. D. (2008). The medical offset effect: Patterns in outpatient services reduction for high utilizers of health care. *Contemporary Family Therapy, 30*, 127–138. doi:10.1007/s10591-008-9058-2.

Crane, D., & Christenson, J. (2014). A summary report of cost-effectiveness: Recognizing the value of family therapy in healthcare. In J. Hodgson, A. Lamson, T. Mendenhall, & R. Crane (Eds.), *Medical family therapy: Advanced applications* (pp. 419–436). New York, NY: Springer.

Cummings, N. A. (2001). A new vision of healthcare for America. In N. A. Cummings, W. O'Donohue, S. C. Hayes, & V. Follette (Eds.), *Integrated behavioral healthcare: Positioning mental health practice with medical/surgical practice* (pp. 19–37). San Diego, CA: Academic Press.

Cummings, N. A. (2002). Are healthcare practitioners economic illiterates? *Families, Systems & Health, 20*, 383–394. doi:10.1037/h0089593.

Cummings, N. A., Cummings, J. L., & Johnson, J. N. (Eds.). (1997). *Behavioral health in primary care: A guide for clinical integration* (pp. 37–58). Madison, CT: Psychosocial Press.

Cummings, N. A., O'Donohue, W. T., & Cummings, J. L. (2009). The financial dimension of integrated behavioral/primary care. *Journal of Clinical Psychology in Medical Settings, 16*, 31–39. doi:10.1007/s10880-008-9139-2.

deGruy, F. (1996). Mental health care in the primary care setting. In M. S. Donaldson, K. D. Yordy, K. N. Lohr, & N. A. Vanselow (Eds.), *Primary care: America's health in a new era*. Washington, DC: Institute of Medicine.

deGruy, F. V. (2000). Mental health diagnoses and the cost of primary care. *The Journal of Family Practice, 49*, 311–313.

*deGruy, F. V., & Etz, R. E. (2010). Attending to the whole person in the patient-centered medical home: The case for incorporating mental healthcare, substance abuse care, and health behavior change. *Families, Systems & Health, 28*, 298–307. doi:10.1037/a0022049.

Dickinson, W. P., & Miller, B. F. (2010). Comprehensiveness and continuity of care and the inseparability of mental and behavioral health form the patient-centered medical home. *Families, Systems & Health, 28*, 348–355. doi:10.1037/a0021866.

Doherty, W. J. (2007). Fixing health care: What role will therapists play? *Psychotherapy Networker, 31*, 24–60.

*Doherty, W. J., McDaniel, S. H., & Baird, M. A. (1996). Five levels of primary care/behavioral healthcare collaboration. *Behavioral Healthcare Tomorrow, 5*, 25–27.

Doherty, W. J., McDaniel, S. H., & Hepworth, J. (1994). Medical family therapy: An emerging arena for family therapy. *The Association for Family Therapy, 16*, 31–46. doi:10.1111/j.1467-6427.1994.00775.x.

*Druss, B. G., & Bornemann, T. (2010). Improving health and healthcare for persons with serious mental illness: The window for US federal policy change. *Journal of American Medical Association, 303*, 1972–1973. doi:10.1001/jama.2010.615.

Druss, B. G., Hwang, I., Petukhova, M., Sampson, N. A., Wang, P. S., & Kessler, R. C. (2009). Impairment in role functioning in mental and chronic medical disorders in the United States: Results from the national comorbidity survey replication. *Molecular Psychiatry, 14*, 728–737. Retrieved from http://www.nature.com/mp/index.html

Dym, B., & Berman, S. (1985). Family systems medicine: Family therapy's next frontier? *The Family Therapy Networker, 9*, 20–66.

Dym, B., & Berman, S. (1986). The primary health care team: Family physician and family therapist in joint practice? *Family Systems Medicine, 4*, 9–21.

*Edwards, T. M., & Patterson, J. E. (2006). Supervising family therapy trainees in primary care medical settings: Context matters. *Journal of Marital and Family Therapy, 32*, 33–43. doi:10.1111/j.1752-0606.2006.tb01586.x.

*Engel, G. L. (1977). The need for a new medical model: A challenge for biomedicine. *Science, 196*, 129–136. doi:10.1126/science.847460.

*Engel, G. L. (1980). The clinical application of the biopsychosocial model. *American Journal of Psychiatry, 137*, 535–544. Retrieved from http://ajp.psychiatryonline.org/
Fries, J., Koop, C., & Beadle, C. (1993). Reducing health care costs by reducing the need and demand for medical services. *New England Journal of Medicine, 329*, 321–325. doi:10.1056/NEJM199307293290506.
Funk, M., & Ivbijaro, G. (2008). *Integrating mental health into primary care—A global perspective.* Geneva, Switzerland: World Health Organization. Retrieved from www.who.int/mental_health/policy/Mental%20health%20+%20primary%20care %20final%20low-res%20140908.pdf
Future of Family Medicine Project Leadership Committee. (2004). The future of family medicine: A collaborative project of the family medicine community. *Annals of Family Medicine, 2* (Supp. 1), S3–S32. Retrieved from http://www.annfammed.org/
Gatchel, R. J., & Oordt, M. S. (2003). *Clinical health psychology and primary care: Practical advice and clinical guidance for successful collaboration.* Washington, DC: American Psychological Association.
Heath, B., Wise Romero, P., & Reynolds, K. (2013). A standard framework for levels of integrated care. Washington, DC: SAMSHA-HRSA Center for Integrated Health Solutions. Retrieved from http://www.integration.samhsa.gov/resource/standard-framework-for-levels-of-integrated-healthcare
Hepworth, J., & Cushman, R. A. (2005). "Biopsychosocial"—Essential but not sufficient. *Families, Systems & Health, 23*, 406–409. doi:10.1037/1091-7527.23.4.406.
Hodgkin, D., Horgan, C. M., Garnick, D. W., Merrick, E. L., & Goldin, D. G. (2000). Why carve out? Determinants of behavioral health contracting choice among large US employers. *The Journal of Behavioral Health Services & Research, 27*, 178–193. doi:10.1007/BF02287312.
*Hodgson, J., Lamson, A. L., Mendenhall, T., & Crane, R. (2012). Medical family therapy: Opportunity for workforce development in healthcare. *Contemporary Family Therapy, 34*, 143–146. doi:10.1007/s10591-012-9199.
*Hodgson, J. L., Lamson, A., & Reese, L. (2007). The biopsychosocial-spiritual interview method. In D. Linville & K. M. Hertlein (Eds.), *The therapist's notebook for family health care: Homework, handouts, and activities for individuals, couples, and families coping with illness, loss, and disability* (pp. 3–12). New York, NY: Haworth Press.
Hodgson, J. L., & Reitz, R. (2013). The financial history and near future of collaborative care. In M. Talen & A. Valeras (Eds.), *Integrated behavioral health in primary care: Evaluating the evidence, identifying the essentials.* New York, NY: Springer.
Institute of Medicine. (1994). *Defining primary care: An interim report.* Washington, DC: National Academies Press. Retrieved from http://www.nap.edu/
*Institute of Medicine. (2001). *Crossing the quality chasm: A new health system for the 21st century.* Washington, DC: National Academies Press.
Institute of Medicine. (2002). *Fostering rapid advances in healthcare: Learning from systems demonstrations.* Washington, DC: National Academies Press. Retrieved from http://www.nap.edu/
Interorganizational Work Group on Competencies for Primary Care Psychology Practice. (2013). *Competencies for psychology practice in primary care.* Retrieved from http://www.apa.org/ed/resources/competencies-practice.pdf
Jacob, V., Chattopadhyay, S. K., Sipe, T. A., Thota, A. B., Byard, G. J., & Chapman, D. P. (2012). Economics of integrated care for management of depressive disorders: A community guide systematic review. *American Journal of Preventive Medicine, 42*, 539–549. doi:10.1016/j.amepre.2012.01.011.
Katerndahl, D. A. (2008). Impact of spiritual symptoms and their interactions on health services and life satisfaction. *Annals of Family Medicine, 6*, 412–420. doi:10.1370/afm.886.
*Kathol, R. G., Butler, M., McAlpine, D. D., & Kane, R. L. (2010). Barriers to physical and mental condition integrated service delivery. *Psychosomatic Medicine, 72*, 511–518. doi:10.1097/PSY.0b013e3181e2c4a0.

Kessler, R. (2008a). How I learned about integrated care by failing miserably: The deadly sins of integration. In R. Kessler & D. Stafford (Eds.), *Collaborative medicine case studies: Evidence in practice* (pp. 39–50). New York, NY: Springer. doi:10.1007/978-0-387-76894-6_4.
Kessler, R. (2008b). Integration of care is about money too: The health and behavior codes as an element of a new financial paradigm. *Families, Systems & Health, 26*, 207–216. doi:10.1037/a0011918.
Kessler, R. C., Chiu, W. T., Demler, O., & Walters, E. E. (2005). Prevalence, severity, and comorbidity of twelve-month DSM-IV disorders in the National Comorbidity Survey Replication (NCS-R). *Archives of General Psychiatry, 62*, 617–627. doi:10.1001/archpsyc.62.6.617.
Kessler, R., & Stafford, D. (2008). Primary care is the de facto mental health system. In R. Kessler & D. Stafford (Eds.), *Collaborative medicine case studies* (Evidence in practice, pp. 9–24). New York, NY: Springer. doi:10.1007/978-0-387-76894-6_2.
Klees, B. S., Wolfe, C. J., & Curtis, C. A. (2012). *Brief summaries of Medicare and Medicaid: Title XVIII and Title XIX of The Social Security Act as of December 31, 2012*. Baltimore, MD: Centers for Medicare & Medicaid Services, Department of Health and Human Services. Retrieved from http://www.cms.gov/Research-Statistics-Data-and-Systems/Statistics-Trends-and-Reports/MedicareProgramRatesStats/Downloads/MedicareMedicaidSummaries2012.pdf
Korda, H., & Eldridge, G. N. (2011). Payment incentives and integrated care delivery: Levers for health system reform and cost containment. *Inquiry, 48*, 277–287.
Kroenke, K., & Mangelsdorff, D. (1989). Common symptoms in ambulatory care: Incidence, evaluation, therapy and outcome. *American Journal of Medicine, 86*, 262–266. doi:10.1016/0002-9343(89)90293-3.
Lardiere, M. R., Jones, E., & Perez, M. (2011). *2010 assessment of behavioral health services provided in federally qualified health centers*. Retrieved from http://www.nachc.com/client/NACHC%202010%20Assessment%20of%20Behavioral%20Health%20Services%20in%20FQHCs_1_14_11_FINAL.pdf
*Law, D. D., & Crane, D. R. (2000). The influence of marital therapy on health care utilization in a health-maintenance organization. *Journal of Marital and Family Therapy, 26*, 281–291. doi:10.1111/j.1752-0606.2000.tb00298.x.
*Law, D. D., Crane, D. R., & Berge, J. M. (2003). The influence of individual, marital, and family therapy on high utilizers of health care. *Journal of Marital and Family Therapy, 29*, 353–363. doi:10.1111/j.1752-0606.2003.tb01212.x.
Levant, R. F., House, A. T., May, S., & Smith, R. (2006). Cost offset: Past, present, and future. *Psychological Services, 3*, 195–207. doi:10.1037/1541-1559.3.3.195.
Lewis, M., Myhra, L., & Walker, M. (2014). Advancing health equity in medical family therapy research. In J. Hodgson, A. Lamson, T. Mendenhall, & R. Crane (Eds.), *Medical family therapy: Advanced applications* (pp. 319–340). New York, NY: Springer.
*Linville, D., Hertlein, K. M., & Prouty Lyness, A. M. (2007). Medical family therapy: Reflecting on the necessity of collaborative healthcare research. *Families, Systems & Health, 25*, 85–97. doi:10.1037/1091-7527.25.1.85.
Lopez, M., Coleman-Beattie, B., Jahnke, L., & Sanchez, K. (2008). *Connecting body and mind: A resource guide to integrated health care in Texas and the United States*. Austin, TX: Hogg Foundation for Mental Health.
Marlowe, D., Capobianco, J., & Greenberg, C. (2014). Getting reimbursed for MedFT: Financial models toward sustainability. In J. Hodgson, A. Lamson, & T. Mendenhall (Eds.), *Medical family therapy: Advanced applications*. New York, NY: Springer.
Mauer, B. (2006). *Behavioral health/primary care integration: The four quadrant model and evidence-based practices*. Rockville, MD: National Council for Community Behavioral Healthcare.
Mauer, B. (2009). *Behavioral health/primary care integration and the person-centered healthcare home*. Washington, DC: National Council for Community Behavioral Healthcare.

Mauer, B., & Jarvis, D. (2010). *The business case for bidirectional integrated care: Mental health and substance use services in primary care settings and primary care services in specialty mental health and substance use settings*. Integration Policy Initiative.

McCann, C. M., & LeRoux, P. (2006). Individual, family, and group therapy for adolescents. *Adolescent Medicine Clinics, 17*, 217–231. doi:10.1016/j.admecli.2005.09.003.

McDaniel, S. H., Campbell, T. L., Hepworth, J., & Lorenz, A. (2005). *Family-oriented primary care* (2nd ed.). New York, NY: Springer.

McDaniel, S. H., Hepworth, J., & Doherty, W. J. (Eds.). (1992). *Medical family therapy: A biopsychosocial approach to families with health problems*. New York, NY: Basic Books. doi:10.1080/01926189208250882.

Mendenhall, T., Berge, J., & Doherty, W. (2014). Engaging communities as partners in research: Advancing integrated care through purposeful partnerships. In J. Hodgson, A. Lamson, T. Mendenhall, & R. Crane (Eds.), *Medical family therapy: Advanced applications* (pp. 259–282). New York, NY: Springer.

Mendenhall, T., Pratt, K., Phelps, K., Baird, M., & Younkin, F. (2014). Advancing medical family therapy through qualitative, quantitative, and mixed-method research. In J. Hodgson, A. Lamson, T. Mendenhall, & R. Crane (Eds.), *Medical family therapy: Advanced applications* (pp. 241–258). New York, NY: Springer.

Miller, B. F., Kessler, R., & Peek, C. J. (2011). *A national agenda for research in collaborative care: Papers from the Collaborative Care Research Network Research Development Conference (AHRQ Publication No. 11-0067)*. Rockville, MD: Agency for Healthcare Research and Quality.

Miyamoto, R. E. S. (2006). Billing effectively with the new health and behavior current procedural terminology codes in primary care and specialty clinics. *Journal of Clinical Psychology, 62*, 1221–1229. doi:10.1002/jclp.20299.

National Association of Social Workers. (2005). *NASW standards for social work practice in health care settings*. Retrieved from http://www.socialworkers.org/practice/standards/NASWHealthCareStandards.pdf

National Council for Community Behavioral Healthcare. (2009). *Behavioral health/primary care integration and the person-centered healthcare home*. Retrieved from http://www.cbhc.org/2009/04/09/behavioral-health-primary-care-integration-and-the-person-centered-healthcare-home/

North Carolina Center of Excellence for Integrated Care. (2011). *Behavioral health provider billing and coding: ICARE 102—billing/coding/documentation*. Retrieved from http://www.icarenc.org/index. php?option=com_frontpage&Itemid=1

O'Donohue, W. T., Cummings, N. A., & Cummings, J. L. (2009). The unmet educational agenda in integrated care. *Journal of Clinical Psychology in Medical Settings, 16*, 94–100. doi:10.1007/s10880-008-9138-3.

O'Donohue, W. T., Cummings, N. A., & Ferguson, K. E. (2003). Clinical integration: The promise and the path. In N. A. Cummings, W. T. O'Donohue, & K. E. Ferguson (Eds.), *Behavioral health as primary care: Beyond efficacy to effectiveness* (pp. 15–30). Reno, NV: Context Press.

Onarecker, C. D., & Sterling, B. C. (1995). Addressing your patient's spiritual needs. *Family Practice Management, 2*, 44–49. Retrieved from http://www.aafp.org/online/en/home/publications/journals/fpm.html

Oser, M., & O'Donohue, W. T. (2009). How to determine the need: A readiness assessment system. In L. C. James & W. T. O'Donohue (Eds.), *The primary care toolkit: Practical resources for the integrated behavioral care provider* (pp. 3–12). New York, NY: Springer. doi:10.1007/978-0-387-78971-2_1.

Patterson, J., Peek, C. J., Heinrich, R. L., Bischoff, R. J., & Scherger, J. (2002). *Mental health professionals in medical settings: A primer*. New York, NY: Norton.

*Peek, C. J. (2008). Planning care in the clinical, operational, and financial worlds. In R. Kessler & D. Stafford (Eds.), *Collaborative medicine case studies: Evidence in practice* (pp. 25–38). New York, NY: Springer. doi:10.1007/978-0-387-76894-6_3.

*Peek, C. J. (2013). Integrated behavioral health in primary care: A common language. In M. R. Talen & A. B. Valeras (Eds.), *Integrated behavioral health in primary care: Evaluating the evidence, identifying the essentials* (pp. 9–32). New York, NY: Springer.

Peek, C. J., & Heinrich, R. L. (1998). Integrating primary care and behavioral health in a health care organization: From pilot to mainstream. In A. Blount (Ed.), *Integrated primary care: The future of medical and mental health collaboration* (pp. 167–202). New York, NY: Norton.

*Peek, C. J. & National Integration Academy Council. (2013). *Lexicon for behavioral health and primary care integration: Concepts and definitions developed by expert consensus* (AHRQ Publication No.13-IP001-EF). Rockville, MD: Agency for Healthcare Research and Quality. Retrieved from http://integrationacademy.ahrq.gov/sites/default/files/Lexicon.pdf

Peyrot, M., Rubin, R. R., Lauritzen, T., Snoek, F. J., Matthews, D. R., & Skovlund, S. E. (2005). Psychosocial problems and barriers to improved diabetes management: Results of the cross-national diabetes attitudes, wishes and needs (DAWN) Study. *Diabetic Medicine, 22*, 1379–1385.

Polaha, J., & Nolan, B. (2014). Dissemination and implementation science: Research for the real world medical family therapist. In J. Hodgson, A. Lamson, & T. Mendenhall (Eds.), *Medical family therapy: Advanced applications*. New York, NY: Springer.

President's New Freedom Commission on Mental Health. (2003). *Achieving the promise: Transforming mental health care in America*. Rockville, MD. Retrieved from http://store.samhsa.gov/product/SMA03-3831

*Prest, L. A., & Robinson, W. D. (2006). Systemic assessment and treatment of depression and anxiety in families: The BPSS model in practice. *Journal of Systemic Therapies, 25*, 4–24. doi:10.1521/jsyt.2006.25.3.4.

Ray-Sannerud, B. N., Dolan, D. C., Morrow, C. E., Corso, K. A., Kanzler, K. E., Corso, M. L., & Bryan, C. J. (2012). Longitudinal outcomes after brief behavioral health intervention in an integrated primary care clinic. *Families, Systems, & Health, 30*, 60–71. doi:10.1037/a0027029

Regier, D. A., Goldberg, I. D., & Taube, C. A. (1978). The de facto US mental health services system: A public health perspective. *Archives of General Psychiatry, 35*, 685–693. Retrieved from http://archpsyc.ama-assn.org/

Regier, D. A., Narrow, W. E., Rae, D. S., Manderscheid, R. W., Locke, B. Z., & Goodwin, F. K. (1993). The de facto US mental and addictive disorders service system: Epidemiologic catchment area prospective 1-year prevalence rates of disorders and services. *Archives of General Psychiatry, 50*, 85–94. Retrieved from http://archpsyc.ama-assn.org/

*Reiss-Brennan, B. (2010). Cost and quality impact of Intermountain's mental health integration program. *Journal of Healthcare Management, 55*, 97–113. Retrieved from http://www.ache.org/pubs/jhmtoc.cfm

Robert Wood Johnson Foundation. (2009). Academy health policy brief. *Public perspectives on health delivery system reforms: Changes in health care financing & organization*. Retrieved from http://www.academyhealth.org/files/HCFO/HCFOPolicyBrief0609.pdf

*Robert Wood Johnson Foundation. (2011). *Healthcare's blindside: The overlooked connection between social needs and good health*. Retrieved from www.rwjf.org/vulnerablepopulations/product. jsp?id=73646

Robinson, P. J., & Reiter, J. T. (2007). *Behavioral consultation and primary care: A guide to integrating services*. New York, NY: Springer.

Robinson, P. J., & Strosahl, K. D. (2009). Behavioral health consultation and primary care: Lessons learned. *Journal of Clinical Psychology in Medical Settings, 16*, 58–71. doi:10.1007/s10880-009-9145-z.

*Ruddy, N. B., & McDaniel, S. H. (2003). Medical family therapy. In T. L. Sexton, G. R. Weeks, & M. S. Robbins (Eds.), *Handbook of family therapy: The science and practice of working with families and couples* (pp. 365–379). New York, NY: Brunner-Routledge.

Russell, L. (2010). *Mental health care services in primary care: Tackling the issues in the context of health care reform*. Washington, DC: Center for American Progress.

Seaburn, D. B., Lorenz, A. D., Gunn, W. B., Jr., Gawinski, B. A., & Mauksch, L. B. (1996). *Models of collaboration: A guide for mental health professionals working with health care practitioners*. New York, NY. Basic Books.

Seattle Pacific University. (2010). *Medical family therapy (MDFT) program overview: Program philosophy*. Retrieved from http://www.spu.edu/depts/spfc/medical/Overview/philosophy.asp

Strosahl, K. (1994). New dimensions in behavioral health/primary care integration. *HMO Practice, 8*, 176–179. doi:10.1016/S1077 7229(05)80084-7.

Strosahl, K. (1997). Building primary care behavioral health systems that work: A compass and a horizon. In N. A. Cummings, J. L. Cummings, & J. N. Johnson (Eds.), *Behavioral health in primary care: A guide for clinical integration* (pp. 37–58). Madison, CT: Psychosocial Press.

Strosahl, K. (2005). Training behavioral health and primary care providers for integrated care: A core competencies approach. In W. T. O'Donohue, M. R. Byrd, N. A. Cummings, & D. A. Henderson (Eds.), *Behavioral integrative care: Treatments that work in the primary care setting* (pp. 15–52). New York, NY: Brunner-Routledge.

Strosahl, K., Baker, N. J., Braddick, M., Stuart, M. E., & Handley, M. R. (1997). Integration of behavioral health and primary care services: The group health cooperative model. In N. A. Cummings, J. L. Cummings, & J. N. Johnson (Eds.), *Behavioral health in primary care: A guide for clinical integration* (pp. 61–86). Madison, CT: Psychosocial Press.

Strosahl, K., & Robinson, P. (2008). The primary care behavioral health model: Applications to prevention, acute care and chronic condition management. In R. Kessler & D. Stafford (Eds.), *Collaborative medicine case studies: Evidence in practice* (pp. 85–96). New York, NY: Springer. doi:10.1007/978-0-387-76894-6_8.

Thielke, S., Vannoy, S., & Unutzer, J. (2007). Integrating mental health and primary care. *Primary Care: Clinics in Office Practice, 34*, 571–592. doi:10.1016/j.pop.2007.05.007.

Thota, A. B., Sipe, T. A., Byard, G. J., Zometa, C. S., Hahn, R. A., McKnight-Eily, L. R., ... Williams, S. P. (2012). Integrated care to improve the management of depressive disorders: A community guide systematic review and meta-analysis. *American Journal of Preventive Medicine, 42*, 525–538. doi:10.1016/j.amepre.2012.01.019

Trudeau-Hern, S., Mendenhall, T., & Wong, A. (2014). Preparing to be a medical family therapist: Bridging the multiple worlds of healthcare. In J. Hodgson, A. Lamson, T. Mendenhall, & R. Crane (Eds.), *Medical family therapy: Advanced applications* (pp. 55–76). New York, NY: Springer.

*Tyndall, L., Hodgson, J., Lamson, A., White, M., & Knight, S. (2012a). Medical family therapy: A theoretical and empirical review. *Contemporary Family Therapy, 34*, 156–170. doi:10.1007/s10591-012-9183-9.

*Tyndall, L. E., Hodgson, J. L., Lamson, A. L., White, M., & Knight, S. M. (2012b). Medical family therapy: Charting a course in competencies. *Contemporary Family Therapy, 34*, 171–186. doi:10.1007/s10591-012-9191-9.

Tyndall, L., Hodgson, J., Lamson, A., White, M., & Knight, S. (2014). Medical family therapy: Charting a course in competencies. In J. Hodgson, A. Lamson, T. Mendenhall, & R. Crane (Eds.), *Medical family therapy: Advanced applications* (pp. 33–54). New York, NY: Springer.

*Tyndall, L., Hodgson, J., White, M., Lamson, A., & Knight, S. (2010). *Medical family therapy: Conceptual clarification and consensus for an emerging profession* (Unpublished doctoral dissertation). East Carolina University, Greenville, NC.

U.S. Department of Health and Human Services, Health Resources and Services Administration, Maternal and Child Health Bureau. (2010). *The National Survey of Children's Health 2007*. Rockville, MD: Author. Retrieved from http://mchb.hrsa.gov/nsch/07emohealth/national/mhs/pages/2mhs.html

US Government Printing Office via GPO Access. (2009). *Code of federal regulations–Title 42–Public Health–Chapter 1–Public health service, Department of health and human services–Part 5, Appendix C–Designation of health professional(s) shortage areas* (10-01-2009 version, pp. 74–78). Retrieved from http://edocket.access.gpo.gov/cfr_2009/octqtr/pdf/42cfr5AppC.pdf

Von Bertalanffy, L. (1968). *System theory: Foundations, development, applications*. New York, NY: George Braziller.
Waldman, J. D., Smith, H. L., & Hood, J. N. (2003). Corporate culture: The missing piece of the healthcare puzzle. *Hospital Topics, 81*, 5–14. doi:10.1080/00185860309598010.
Watzlawick, P., Weakland, J., & Fisch, R. (1974). *Change: Principles of problem formation and problem resolution*. New York, NY: Norton.
Williams-Reade, J., Gordon, B.-A., & Wray, W. (2014). A primer in program evaluation for MedFTs. In J. Hodgson, A. Lamson, T. Mendenhall, & R. Crane (Eds.), *Medical family therapy: Advanced applications* (pp. 283–300). New York, NY: Springer.
Woltmann, E., Grogan-Kaylor, A., Perron, B., Georges, H., Kilbourne, A. M., & Bauer, M. S. (2012). Comparative effectiveness of collaborative chronic care models for mental health conditions across primary, specialty, and behavioral health care settings: Systematic review and meta-analysis. *The American Journal of Psychiatry, 169*, 790–804. doi:10.1176/appi.ajp.2012.11111616.
Wright, L. M., Watson, W. L., & Bell, J. M. (1996). *Beliefs: The heart of healing in families and illness*. New York, NY: Basic Books.
Yapko, M. D. (2008). Skills or pills? What MFTs can do better than antidepressant medications. *Family Therapy Magazine, 7*, 18–23.
Zak-Hunter, L., Berge, J., Lister, Z., Davey, M., Lynch, L., & Denton, W. (2014). Medical family therapy scientist-practitioners. In J. Hodgson, A. Lamson, & T. Mendenhall (Eds.), *Medical family therapy: Advanced applications*. New York, NY: Springer.

Chapter 20
The Ethics of Integration: Where Policy and Practice Collide

Cathy Hudgins, Sandra Rose, Peter Fifield, and Steve Arnault

For anyone working in an Integrated Primary Care (IPC) setting, ethical challenges routinely arise due to a variety of contextual and procedural factors. Situations can become more complicated when diverse professionals interface, each holding to their own discipline's code of ethics. Medical family therapists (MedFTs), along with healthcare providers, are asked to adhere to both the ethical standards of their specific disciplines and the legal standards set forth by state and federal guidelines, all of which can differ by specialty. If this issue was not complicated enough, there are additional and often differing sets of guidelines embedded in IPC contexts, including the specific policies established by the setting. Efforts to comply with multiple regulations can serve as a challenge when laws and ethics do not cleanly interface with contextual policies that are intended to protect the patient. This tug of war can actually impede optimum care when they conflict.

This chapter addresses some of the common ethical issues that arise in IPC settings and offers practices that MedFTs and other IPC providers can use while keeping patients at the center of care and protecting their rights. Wherein practitioners of MedFT are the focus for this chapter, the information provided here is applicable across the system of IPC providers, including differing types of behavioral health providers (BHPs). Greatest attention is given to policy and practice implications for MedFTs who function in IPC settings, including guidance via federal and state statutes when applicable on how to maximize patient care in the context of an integrated system.

C. Hudgins (✉)
Center of Excellence for Integrated Care, North Carolina Foundation for Advanced Health Programs, Cary, NC, USA
e-mail: cmhudgins@radford.edu

J. Hodgson et al. (eds.), *Medical Family Therapy*, DOI 10.1007/978-3-319-03482-9_20,

MedFT Ethics

Whether practicing in an IPC or a traditional specialty behavioral healthcare setting MedFTs are bound by their discipline-specific ethical standards. We have chosen to focus on the challenges identified as most prominent in IPC practice and research, including (a) client confidentiality; (b) informed consent; and (c) exploitive, dual, and multiple relationships. Before discussing these challenges specifically, it is important to review the role that ethical guidelines play in IPC settings.

Throughout this chapter, case studies will be presented to illustrate concepts. The following decision-making model will provide a framework for each case study discussed in this chapter, assuring that most aspects of a situation have been explored in a standardized manner. Providers are encouraged to process ethical dilemmas as they are encountered by moving through the steps outlined in the following decision-making model (developed by the authors of this chapter):

1. Clarify the facts and their context.
2. Explore the applicability of federal and state statutes.
3. Explore the applicability of professional codes of ethics.
4. Consult agency policy and procedure manual.
5. Seek supervision or consult with a colleague of equal or greater experience.
6. Define options with consideration of the clinical ramifications.
7. Implement and document.
8. Critique the process.

By navigating through these steps, the result as noted by Runyan, Robinson, and Gould (2013), will be "care [that] will come closer to the bar of compassion when the patient (rather than our disciplines) is the focus of care (p. 7)." All of these ingredients are steps that providers should navigate when faced with ethical challenges, but in IPC, providers do not and should not feel as though they are managing these eight steps in isolation.

Despite the assumption of uniformity in IPC systems, contexts all have at least some subtle differences. For example, statutes governing IPC may differ from state to state. Thus, providers would be wise to research and understand the healthcare statutes and rules impacting the care of patients who cross state lines or who reside in a different state from the provider [i.e., couples whereby one partner is deployed elsewhere]. This would also apply to providers who practice in multiple states (e.g., trauma responders, multiple state licensees). Legal and ethical standards also differ between BHPs and primary care providers (PCP) of all types, including nurse Practitioners, physician assistants, and physicians. Therefore, policies and protocols for information sharing, informed consent, and confidentiality require careful review under federal and state law, as well as per professional code of ethics and context specific guidelines. Discrepancies are most apparent in the laws and ethics that involve patient confidentiality and informed consent and those which determine the relationships between providers and patients.

Currently, there is a resounding call in health care for laws, rules, and ethical guidelines to be revised and align more with an IPC model (Hudgins, Rose, Fifield, & Arnault, 2013; Runyan et al., 2013). The following section will address common ethical challenges in IPC, including aspects of case law that set a precedent and act as guidance (Hudgins et al., 2013) on how to manage ethical violations, Health Insurance Portability and Accountability Act laws (HIPAA, 1996), and Federal Alcohol and Drug Confidentiality Laws (42CFR-Part 2; Substance Abuse Services, 2011), as well as policy implications and practice considerations.

Confidentiality

Confidentiality is the ongoing process of protecting the information shared between provider and patient as part of care. Grounded in federal and state law, and codified by professional guilds, this process forms the foundation of the therapeutic relationship and establishes trust and confidence in a provider's ability to understand and treat patients. In IPC settings, confidentiality is one of the most difficult responsibilities to navigate. Expectations for privacy by those who have been trained in relatively closed environments (e.g., traditional or specialty behavioral health practices) may seem unrealistic to those operating in IPC settings, where there are relatively open physical spaces, easy flow of information, and an immense volume and velocity of patient and provider interactions (Reiter & Runyan, 2013; Runyan et al., 2013). To further complicate these matters, requesting and receiving receipt and release of information from a patient, and then sharing patient information between providers, can be a complex process: One that providers must quickly and seamlessly navigate or face ethical challenges.

Federal Statutes

Providers may sometimes feel as though they are in the cross fire between federal statutes and flexibility in offering best patient care. These experiences may be amplified in IPC settings where providers strive to strengthen the collaboration between patients and their diverse care team. Unfortunately, some are left feeling conflicted about their interpretation of the law and their belief in practice toward efficient patient care. The bottom line is that federal laws must be followed for patient protection in all settings, with HIPAA being the most prominent guideline.

HIPAA

HIPAA includes provisions for patient safety and dictates rules for communication of protected health information (PHI), irrespective of provider type (HIPAA, 1996). Thus, conduct pertaining to confidentiality should be clear to both provider and patient. However, under this relatively liberal law, PHI may be communicated to a PCP for treatment purposes without a patient's authorization, provided a patient is notified of the provider's privacy policies. Most healthcare settings require a written signature by the patient acknowledging that healthcare information is communicated for health purposes in this way. It is then the dual accountability of providers to follow the PHI provisions and for patients to understand the implications for documents signed.

No distinction is made in relation to confidentiality between medical and behavioral health (in relation to these contexts) according to HIPAA, except in the case of "psychotherapy notes." HIPAA defines these notes as that which is created by a "mental health professional documenting or analyzing the contents of a conversation during a private counseling session or a group, joint, or family counseling session, and are separated from the rest of the individual's medical record (Section 45CFR 164.501; HIPAA, 2007)." The definition excludes "medication prescription and monitoring, counseling session start and stop times, the modalities and frequencies of treatment furnished, results of clinical tests, and any summary of the following items: diagnosis, functional status, the treatment plan, symptoms, prognosis, and progress to date" even when conducted by a BHP.

There is minimal guidance regarding how to differentiate "psychotherapy notes" from "progress notes" in the electronic medical record (EMR). However, the consensus appears to be that typical BHP encounter notes would not fall under the definition of psychotherapy notes, as they are not documenting "process-oriented" notes of traditional psychotherapy. Moreover, psychotherapy notes are, by definition, separate from the rest of the healthcare record. However, separation of records alone does not render a behavioral progress note to then become a psychotherapy note. Some examples of psychotherapy note content include: clinician interpretations, transference and countertransference content, relational problems, and specific sensitive detail of past sexual abuse. Psychotherapy notes differ from regular clinical records and receive special confidentiality protection under HIPAA (2007; Section CFR 45, Part 164.524) from other clinical records, which may be exchanged without *specific* permission from the patient. Furthermore, physically integrating the psychotherapy information into one document does not make the excluded information protected. By adhering to standard progress note structure (such as a SOAP note format), one might minimize unnecessary or overly inclusive information in an encounter note that does not benefit patient care or provider treatment options.

According to Reitz, Common, Fifield, and Stiasny (2012), there is very little consensus on best practices for securing and maintaining confidentiality within IPC documentation processes to ensure HIPAA compliance. One approach is to construct confidentiality protocol such that providers limit the sensitive content in BHP encounter notes and permit widespread access across healthcare providers and to those managing payment, all of whom are well trained on respectful, accountable, and effective confidentiality practices. Alternatively, some EMR systems enable security settings to be associated with specific charts and the BHP or other providers can set the appropriate security level (e.g., labeled as "behavioral" health or "substance use") at time of entry, with access on a need-to-know basis among staff. EMR security audit trails can be undertaken as well, to ensure compliance with healthcare context security protocols.

42CFR Part 2

MedFTs practicing in IPC settings that provide specialized substance abuse services must maintain an additional layer of confidentiality to protect patient information. The Federal Drug and Alcohol Confidentiality Law (42CFR Part 2) imposes restrictive rules upon providers who are designated within "programs," by dictating the protection of alcohol and drug information. A covered "program" is one that receives federal funds (such as a Federally Qualified Health Clinic or programs reimbursed by Medicare) and meets the following criteria:

1. If a provider is *not* a general medical care facility, then the provider meets Part 2's definition of a "program" if it is an individual or entity that holds itself out as providing, *and* provides alcohol or drug abuse diagnosis, treatment, or referral for treatment.
2. If the provider is an identified unit within a general medical care facility, it is a "program" if it holds itself out as providing, *and* provides, alcohol or drug abuse diagnosis, treatment or referral for treatment.
3. If the provider consists of medical personnel or other staff in a general medical care facility, it is a program if its primary function is the provision of alcohol or drug abuse diagnosis, treatment or referral for treatment *and* is identified as such specialized medical personnel or other staff within the general medical care facility (SAMSHA, 2011, p. 6).

Many MedFTs in IPC settings offer some substance abuse services, including screening, assessment, and perhaps some elements of treatment or management. Both behavioral health and healthcare providers are covered by this regulation if they "primarily" assess or treat substance abuse disorders, as in criteria three listed above. Consistent with this interpretation, is guidance from the Legal Action Center, which states . . .

> Generalist mental health providers who work in general health centers are NOT 'programs' covered by 42 C.F.R. unless they meet the definition of a 'program' because they are part of (1) a specialized unit or, are (2) specialized staff (whose primary function is to provide drug or alcohol diagnosis, treatment or referral), as defined in Part 2's definition of a program (K. O'Neil, Personal communication, May, 26, 2011).

Generalist BHPs and PCPs who do not meet the three requirements do not require special authorization from the rest of the treatment team for alcohol and drug information, thus confidential information is more freely exchanged to maximize collaborative treatment efforts. Specialists, such as Licensed Alcohol and Drug Counselors or PCPs who predominantly prescribe Suboxone or who practice in specialized substance abuse units within a health center may be examples of "programs." These providers require the specific patient Part 2 authorizations to release alcohol and drug information to other providers even within the same treatment team or healthcare system. These providers must also obtain Part 2 authorization to provide an alcohol or drug diagnosis or other substance abuse information to third-party payers for reimbursement. Given the sensitivity of this information, even if not required, it is prudent that patients be specifically notified via informed consent materials that confidential content related to alcohol and drug information is exchanged with PCPs within the IPC system. They should also be made aware that this information will be transmitted to third parties for billing and, if the system's policies permit, to outside healthcare professionals who may be referred for their care.

The Legal Action Center's Web site (Legal Action Center, n.d.) provides model forms, including that which combines HIPAA and Part 2 elements as well as sample Qualified Service Organization Agreements (QSO). All of these can facilitate communication between professional organizations and Part 2 covered entities. These recommendations can then be cross-checked against other mandatory guidelines, such as state laws and discipline specific professional code of ethics.

State Statutes

Requirements for procedures related to the exchange of confidential communication is not limited to federal law, but must also be followed via state statutes. In many states, for example, confidential discussions between patients and physicians, as well as between patients and BHPs, are defined similar to communication between lawyers and their clients. However, the licensing statute for the four behavioral health disciplines regulated by the omnibus New Hampshire Board of Mental Health Practice (e.g., Clinical Mental Health Counselors, Clinical Social Workers, Pastoral Psychotherapists, and Marriage and Family Therapists), not only prescribes specific language which must be included in informed consent materials provided to patients, but also includes the specific means for delivery of materials to patients in order to assure confidentiality. The cumbersome provisions of this law were obviously not borne in the context of IPC, where MedFTs meet patients in exam rooms to discuss behavioral health modifications. MedFTs and other providers who practice in IPC settings should check their state licensing statutes to determine what specific laws apply to practice in their specialty and how this might differ from that of their healthcare colleagues.

Case Law

Case law illustrates how some courts may elevate communication between a licensed BHP and a patient, beyond that of a PCP and patient. Although the privacy protections for patients of PCPs and MedFTs are similarly viewed by statute, a court ruling in New Hampshire singled out the importance of privilege between a Psychologist and patient beyond even that of a doctor–patient and a lawyer–client. In the case of Berg v. Berg (2005), the opinion of the New Hampshire Supreme court asserted that the therapist–patient privilege may be even more compelling than that behind the usual physician–patient privilege because of the greater demand for confidence and trust that the patient needs to enter treatment and the need to make disclosures important for psychotherapy versus that which may be required in the treatment of physical ailments. The court cited an opinion by the New Jersey Supreme Court, which noted that communication "will frequently be even more personal, potentially embarrassing, and more often readily misconstrued than those between attorney and client. Made public and taken out of context, the disclosure of notes from therapy sessions could have devastating personal consequences for the patient and his or her family (Section II)."

What may be implied from this case, as well as that from HIPAA's unique treatment of psychotherapy notes and Part 2 regulation, is that the greater the sensitivity of the information generated and documented, and the greater harm that could result from disclosure, the more confidentiality safeguards must be built into practices by the MedFT. This is usually not a problem when the focus of treatment is on lifestyle management or health behaviors. However, patients may view the role of the MedFT differently than they do their PCP's, offer information that may exceed the minimal sensitivity seen in a typical 15-min medical encounter, and expect more privacy in communications with MedFTs. This may result, for example, in more willingness to admit alcohol and drug abuse, marital concerns, or disclosures related to sexuality. Thus, MedFTs must navigate complex circumstances with their healthcare peers who share confidentiality as collaborators, while also honoring MedFT–patient relationships when sensitive information is shared (e.g., having an affair, gambling addictions). In these cases, informed consent procedures pertaining to access of charts or exchange of information must be adequately addressed with patients. In particular, both collaborating colleagues and patients must understand the MedFTs' role, how it differs from therapists who function in traditional therapy contexts, and how information is shared among the team.

Professional Code of Ethics

All behavior health and medical disciplines have a code of ethics that offer clarity in regard to the expectation for confidentiality within the provider–patient relationship. All codes of ethics describe the limits of confidentiality, release of information, and use and protection of patient information. The challenge within IPC settings is not a lack of awareness for confidentiality, but in the lack of understanding among providers in how these codes overlap or diverge from one another. MedFTs, because of their relational training, are uniquely attuned to the system's needs, so finding balance between their ethical codes and those of their colleagues should be a skill in which they can contribute to the collaborative team. Flexibility, communication, and cross-training are key strategies found to increase the IPC team's ability to navigate these ethical quandaries in a fast-paced, complex healthcare environment (Hodgson, Mendenhall, & Lamson, 2013; Reiter & Runyan, 2013).

To help understand how team members from diverse professions perceive confidentiality, Curtis and Christian (2012) provided a comprehensive discussion of ethical guidelines across disciplines, including an interpretation of ethical codes for both PCPs and BHPs. These authors use excerpts from five professional codes of ethics to suggest how to resolve the quandary of whose ethics trumps whose when collaborating. Ethical issues related to sharing information and mandated reporting (key elements related to confidentiality) are the focus of this resource. They prefaced these recommendations with the note that even seasoned IPC team members may experience conflict when attempting to develop policies and protocols related to confidentiality. Hodgson et al. (2013) also provided a review of nine leading professional organizations' ethical guidelines, including those written for MedFTs, and use clinical case studies to illustrate issues related to confidentiality and informed in IPC settings.

What follows is a case study pertaining to confidentiality, followed up with the decision-making model (described earlier in the chapter) that MedFTs can use to navigate federal, state, and professional codes of ethics.

Case Study: Confidentiality Decision-Making Model

> Mr. Johnson, a 53-year-old male is seen with his wife for a follow-up appointment. He has been diagnosed with renal failure, and the focus of the session is on the lifestyle adjustments the couple will need to make to promote health, intimacy, and overall quality of life. During the session, Mrs. Johnson brings up the fact that her husband typically drinks several beers every evening. Upon this disclosure, Mr. Johnson becomes angry with his wife and initially denies the alcohol use. After some discussion, he relents but asks that the MedFT not disclose his drinking to his PCP primarily because his physician is the son of his boss.
>
> **Discussion**: This case represents a common dilemma faced in an IPC setting. When considering the eight elements of the decision-making model, the MedFT should first review the facts that were shared by both husband and wife and then consider relevant statutes. Applying the decision model we come to understand Mr. Johnson's situation more clearly. Mr. Johnson appeared to feel betrayed by

his wife and seemed concerned about the information about his alcohol use getting back to his boss and thus feared losing his job. A review of the applicable statutes reveals that 42 CFR Part 2 may come into play providing protection to the substance use information. However, after a careful review of the statute and consultation with her supervisor, the MedFT thinks that she, and the practice in which she works, do not meet the criteria as a "program" under this statute. Therefore, they believe 42 CFR part 2 does not apply to this context. The code of ethics and the practice's policy and procedure manual both speak to upholding the patient's rights and the primacy of the patient's right to decision-making. Further, Mr. Johnson signed the practice's participation agreement indicating that he understands and agrees that mental health and substance abuse information is shared among providers. The MedFT is aware that the patient has the right to rescind this at any time and has effectively done so.

The situation now rests on the clinical ramifications of the MedFT's choice of action. She needs to weigh the risks of telling or not telling the PCP about the use of alcohol which may impact the prognosis of Mr. Johnson's renal failure. Additionally, she is concerned about her ongoing therapeutic relationship with her patient, understanding that Mr. Johnson will see her revealing this information as a breach of trust. Ethically, it is paramount to engage in conversation with Mr. Johnson regarding the importance of this information and how his alcohol use directly relates to his overall medical care. This conversation may help him to see that his wife is acting out of concern. It is often beneficial in these situations to point out the dilemma that the MedFT is in and partner with the patients to find a solution. In this case, reassurance from the PCP that the information will be held in confidence may be the key. Mr. Johnson may either realize that the trust with this PCP is genuine, thereby strengthening his relationship with his healthcare team or he may need to get a referral to new providers so that he can better address all aspects related to his health. This situation would then be documented accordingly, and then processed by the MedFT and the healthcare team or between the MedFT and her supervisor. Debriefing often helps providers to attend to strengths and challenges in handling an issue, but can also help to construct new policies when necessary.

Policy and Practice Implications

To date, there is very little guidance or explanation of healthcare policies related to confidentiality specifically for MedFTs in IPC settings. Although, more and more resources are emerging to clarify current laws and policies guiding practice (Collins, Hewson, Munger, & Wade, 2010), a more definitive interpretation is still needed. In addition, national- and state-level laws as well as professional ethical standards need to catch up with the evolving ethical issues presented by IPC models.

As it stands, confidentiality in IPC settings is governed by more than ethical codes. In all cases, the most restrictive guideline is the one in which the setting must adhere. When it comes to policy and practice implications, more than one source recommends consulting with an attorney or executing in-depth analysis of state and federal laws, in addition to professional ethics prior to developing any policy or protocol (Collins et al., 2010; OCCIC, 2010; Saviano, 2008). This step may help to avoid fines and other legal actions. Furthermore, due to the increased influence that IPC is wielding on state and federal law reform, sources across the board stress that it is critical for providers and stakeholders to stay abreast of changes related to confidentiality (Hudgins et al., 2013). Awareness of these changes in laws and other policies related to practice are central to providing competent care. In state-level legislation, there are few resources that draw direct comparisons between behavioral health and other healthcare laws. A clearer understanding of the relationship between these laws could help to provide a framework for additional policy changes, particularly when integrating behavioral health services into primary care settings.

It is clear that when IPC systems include substance abuse treatment in the array of services, 42CFR Part 2 compounds the challenges of exchange and release of information. The SAMSHA—HRSA Center for Integrated Healthcare Solutions and the LAC offer some of the most specific information and links to resources for providers treating patients who seek substance abuse treatment in integrated systems. These organizations offer recommendations and resources regarding many population-based patient care issues, including sample forms of agreement between providers and minors. However, formalized policies and guidelines grounded in best practices for confidentiality in IPC settings would be most beneficial for MedFTs when faced with complex patient situations, particularly situations with multiple family members and supports persons who are involved in the patient's care.

Informed Consent

Informed consent procedures also present quandaries when MedFTs and other BHPs partner with healthcare providers on IPC teams. Informed consent commonly refers to the process of providing information to a patient prior to treatment concerning patient rights and the provision of treatment information necessary to make informed decisions (Hudgins et al., 2013). Informed Consent is an ongoing procedure to ensure that the patient is aware of all of the potential risks and costs involved in a treatment or procedure. The elements of informed consent may include informing the client of the nature of the treatment, possible alternative treatments, and the potential risks and benefits of the treatment. It may also include the "notice" that is required by federal or state laws and/or professional ethical codes concerning the patient rights.

Federal and State Statutes

Guidance related to informed consent exists within federal laws, which prescribe specific kinds of notice necessary for patients receiving treatment (e.g., HIPAA & 42CFR Part 2 notices). HIPAA (1996), for example, has clear guidelines for provision of informed consent regarding notice to patients of their privacy rights. While traditionally considered apart from treatment decisions requiring consent, decisions concerning PHI sharing are arguably as important, and costs and benefits of releasing PHI should be part of the informed consent process.

Managing PHI and ensuring informed consent from all participating providers can become more challenging when primary care visits are integrated with sensitive issues such as behavioral health diagnoses or alcohol and drug use. In these instances, many providers may become involved in care but patients may not be clear that BHPs are part of the healthcare team, unless consent for treatment is especially clear. Therefore, consent documents must not only be written in accordance with HIPAA guidelines but should also be reviewed orally (when possible) so that patients can ask questions about consent processes, as well as questions about the providers who may be part of their care team. With widespread dissemination of information now possible through electronic health records, the potential harm and benefits are further magnified.

Given the ease of transferability in healthcare records, state laws are beginning to mandate more specific patient protection procedures (Koocher & Keith-Speigel, 2008). Such procedures are imperative given that front desk staff members are typically charged with providing patients with informed consent guidelines in healthcare settings (AMA, n.d., Curtis & Christian, 2012). Ultimately, it is up to MedFTs and other BHPs, as well as PCPs, to make clear the patient's rights to make an informed choice regarding care. As mentioned previously, in some instances it is not clear when, how, and from whom informed consent is attained in an integrated setting.

Seeking and receiving consent are ongoing processes that must be revisited with each new provider, procedure, or treatment option. Requesting consent rests on all providers and other IPC staff in a system; therefore, everyone in the healthcare context should know how to access legal counsel or at least be familiar with federal and state laws when developing informed consent policies, protocols, and forms, and keep abreast of these as states make changes to laws to accommodate IPC practices. A best case scenario is to defer to the most stringent requirements related to consent that pertain to the kind of services rendered and makeup of the healthcare context (Saviano, 2008).

Professional Code of Ethics

While many ethical guidelines across disciplines have some code related to informed consent, AAMFT Ethical Code 1.2 gives one of the clearest guidelines for relational providers . . .

> Informed Consent. Marriage and family therapists obtain appropriate informed consent to therapy or related procedures and use language that is reasonably understandable to clients. The content of informed consent may vary depending upon the client and treatment plan; however, informed consent generally necessitates that the client: (a) has the capacity to consent; (b) has been adequately informed of significant information concerning treatment processes and procedures; (c) has been adequately informed of potential risks and benefits of treatments for which generally recognized standards do not yet exist; (d) has freely and without undue influence expressed consent; and (e) has provided consent that is appropriately documented. When persons due to age or mental status, are legally incapable of giving informed consent, marriage and family therapists obtain informed permission from a legally authorized person if such substitute consent is legally permissible. (AAMFT, 2012)

An aspect of informed consent that is not as clear in this definition, but is also carried through other parts of professional codes of ethics, is appropriate representation of scope of practice and credentials. For example: "Marriage and family therapists do not represent themselves as providing specialized services unless they have appropriate education, training or supervised experience" (AAMFT Code of Ethics, Section 8.8). Individual state license regulations often guide behavioral health providers (i.e. psychologists and mental health counselors) to identify their scope of services, which includes specifying their background and training as well as the risks and benefits of the services they provide. Consents of this nature may be difficult for workflows to accommodate in the medical setting, especially at point of contact such as during warm handoffs or brief behavioral health encounters.

Consent quickly can become a bigger issue if the provider is not explicit and intentional about his role within an integrated care setting. Role identification may remove any question about the function of that provider within the integrated system (Curtis & Christian, 2012). Role expectations are influenced by a number of factors, including patient's prior experiences with healthcare providers, as well as how a provider introduces behavioral health service. An introduction by a PCP can influence a patient's expectations regarding the role of a MedFT, whether operating as a behavioral health consultant focusing on a lifestyle change or entering as a relational therapist to work on marital issues. A suggested introduction by a member of the IPC team might be: "we have a member of our team that specializes in helping people with [insert specific presenting problem here]." If the MedFT is introducing herself to the patient, she would want to identify her license and her role on the treatment team. This not only reduces false expectations but also additionally assists the MedFT to focus on a specific behavioral intervention and seek consent accordingly. This process is important via face-to-face interactions at the initial introduction and subsequent visits, but also in how provider services are advertised to the patient population in the waiting rooms, company brochures, and

Web sites. What follow is a case study and the corresponding decision-making model for informed consent.

Case Study: Informed Consent Decision-Making Model

A MedFT working in a small community health center is asked to go into the exam room to meet with a woman whom the PCP describes as "distraught." The woman is crying and visibly shaking. Initially, the patient is so upset that she is unable to verbalize her concerns. The MedFT acknowledges her emotions and waits until she is calm enough to explain. Upon discussion, the woman states that her PCP determined the need for a behavioral health consultation after she reacted to her diagnosis of Crohn's disease. The woman, who has a history of behavioral health problems, which have required that she be involuntarily committed several times, became anxious when the PCP stated that he was going to get the BHP to come in to assess her current behavioral status. In this case, the patient did not grant informed consent. Since the patient signed her consent when she entered into services with the PCP several months ago, the PCP believed that he did not need to ask for her permission to bring the MedFT to see her in the room.

Discussion: The first step in the decision-making model for a MedFT would be to clarify the facts regarding whether the patient consented to speak with the MedFT. In this case, the role of the MedFT, his credentials, scope of practice, and the intention and potential outcomes of the consult. This approach is consistent with both HIPAA and 42 CFR Part 2. Further guidance can be found in professional codes of ethics related to clarity on services provided and consent for services received. The policies and procedures of the practice ask that each patient be made aware of the presence and role provided by the MedFT and that the patient sign an acknowledgment that she understands and consents to this service, which this patient has done. An appropriate next step in creating an alliance with the patient would be to revisit the informed consent once the MedFT comes into the room and proceed only if the patient is interested in services. The MedFT may want to let the patient know that he is asked by providers to come in and meet with all consenting patients in the practice, when they receive a new diagnoses to ensure that patients have psychosocial support systems as they adjust to the new diagnosis. This is done to help the patient know that she is not singled out for behavioral health care. Documentation would then be completed based on outcomes from the appointment, including a note about the review of consent policies. This situation would then give the providers an opportunity to review policies about consent and encourage one another to bring up consent when other providers are involved in their patient's visit.

Policy and Practice Implications

In many of the IPC system manuals to date (Hudgins et al., 2013), the patient is given initial paperwork upon entering the system that describes the role and scope of behavioral health services. One blanket informed consent is commonly provided in initial paperwork during patient registration and justified by some practitioners through the notion that behavioral health is part of health, no different than provision of other services in the primary care setting. Hodgson et al. (2013) noted that a blanket consent process assumes that the patient has or can understand the consent and all that it encompasses, but that consent should not just occur prior to registration. A variety of sources agree with this perspective, asserting the belief that informed consent in any setting should occur through ongoing communication about treatment options (Barnett, 2007; Striefel, 2009). Once is not enough, especially if the provider does not take the time to make sure that the patient is making as much of an informed choice as possible regarding his or her care.

There are few prescriptions for language or method of delivery regarding consent in the literature. However, Curtis and Christian (2012) conducted a review of all of the professional codes of ethics for both BHPs and PCPs. Their review clarifies and provides important policy and practice recommendations pertaining to consent. They suggest that all patients receive an initial written informed consent, which would require not only a signature prior to service provision during registration but also a verbal consent during the initial interaction with the patient. These implications are perhaps especially important for patients who are illiterate or have lower level reading skills, speak or read in a language that is different than what is given to them via documentation, or experience physical challenges that impair their reading (e.g., poor eyesight, cognitive impairments). Curtis and Christian offered a sample script to highlight a way of introducing BHP services for verbal consent of treatment. What follows is an adaptation to their script, in order to better align with the role of a MedFT.

> Hello, Mr. Martin, I'm Jordan Smith, and as Dr. Fernandez explained, I am a medical family therapist and I have been working with this clinic to ensure that patients get comprehensive care. This care may include collaboration with your primary care provider on experiences in your life such as, sleep hygiene, pain management, or family stressors. I'd like to make sure you have this packet of information related to my education, areas of competency, confidentiality, and who to contact if you have grievances about the services I provide. All of this information is listed in this brochure, which is for you to take with you following this visit. Dr. Fernandez asked that I meet with you so that together we can find some strategies that might help alleviate some of the symptoms you mentioned. I know that I just gave you a lot of information, so please let me know what you understand and what questions you have. (See original script in Curtis & Christian, p. 129)

A final concern about consent, that is central to IPC systems, is the need to balance consent provision with efficiency of care. Most IPC settings are "busy and fast-paced and do not have the staff or infrastructure to maintain and coordinate multiple or detailed, time consuming consents" (Collins et al., 2010, p. 35). While MedFTs and other BHPs are charged with helping the system seek and maintain consent, MedFTs may also assist in creating policies or implementing changes that may ease flow or procedures pertaining to the consent process.

In addition to the information exchange and informed consent, there are additional ethical issues that arise in IPC settings. The most recent and comprehensive review of arising ethical concerns in IPC can be found in the special edition on ethics in the journal *Families, Systems & Health* (2013), including issues such as dual relationships and termination/provider abandonment as major concerns.

Exploitivė, Dual, and Multiple Relationships

Exploitive, dual, and multiple relationships relate to any situation whereby multiple roles exist between a therapeutic affiliation and an academic, supervisory, personal, or familial relationship. By nature, these relationships involve complications such as, a conflict of interest or a positive or negative bias that is able to influence treatment processes or outcomes. Dual relationships can occur when colleagues within a healthcare context request behavioral or medical treatments from other colleagues. This may be even more common in rural settings, where a child's coach may also be her healthcare provider (Smalley, Yancey, Warren, Naufel, & Pugh, 2010). In any case, MedFTs must be aware of boundaries that cannot be crossed when treating patients that they may know from other contexts.

Professional Code of Ethics

All of the major discipline-specific organizations (e.g., American Association for Marriage and Family Therapist, American Psychiatric Association, American Psychological Association, National Association of Social Workers, and National Board for Certified Counselors) provide ethical guidelines for therapeutic boundaries and dual relationships. For example, according to the AAMFT Code of Ethics 1.3. . .

> Marriage and family therapists are aware of their influential positions with respect to clients, and they avoid exploiting the trust and dependency of such persons. Therapists, therefore, make every effort to avoid conditions and multiple relationships with clients that could impair professional judgment or increase the risk of exploitation. Such relationships include, but are not limited to, business or close personal relationships with a client or the client's immediate family. When the risk of impairment or exploitation exists due to conditions or multiple roles, therapists document the appropriate precautions taken (AAMFT, 2012).

In contrast, guidelines provided for healthcare providers (American Medical Association, American Nurse Association, American Academy of Nurse Practitioners, and American Academy of Physician Assistants) view dual relationships differently. It is common practice for a healthcare provider to provide care to employees and colleagues. In addition, the nature of family practice is founded on seeing multiple members of the same family over time. AMA codes encourage PCPs to treat peers in healthcare settings (Kanzler, Goodie, Hunter, Glotfelter, & Bodart, 2013), while other ethical guidelines, such as those endorsed by the APA (2010), AMHCA (2010), and AAMFT (2012) recommend that the MedFT take considerate precautions when engaging in these types of dual relationships. This apparent difference in perspective may cause conflict within the IPC team, especially when a MedFT is asked to treat another staff member or his or her family members. Without clear communication about ethical guidelines, staff members and healthcare providers may not understand why a MedFT would refer a patient to another provider even though she is equipped to see the patient.

Case Study: Multiple Patients in a Rual Setting Decision-Making Model

Mr. Parker is a 53-year-old man presenting in his rural Federally Qualified Healthcare Clinic, for treatment of hypertension, diabetes, and panic attacks. His wife, an employed medical assistant at this healthcare facility, has encouraged her husband to become a patient in order to receive care for his medical conditions. She is working that day and becomes visibly anxious as she watches her husband walk into the exam room. After the initial exam, the physician and MedFT discuss a treatment plan in the exam room with the patient. The physician asks to be excused while the MedFT and patient work on specific goals. During a follow up visit with the MedFT, the patient arrives and states his wife wants to attend the session with him. She is not working that day and you see her sitting in the waiting room awaiting your decision.

Discussion: Reviewing the facts in relation to the ethical decision-making model shows there are several issues at play here. Clearly, there exists a potential of a dual relationship between the persons providing care for this patient (MedFT and PCP) and the patient's wife is also an employee at the same healthcare practice. There are no clear federal statutes relative to this dual relationship situation. Ethically, the MedFT must review his code of ethics relative to dual relationships and note that the MedFT will make every attempt to reduce the risk of exploitation of the client. Noting that the wife was not working at that time of the visit suggests that she would not be violating an agency policy or procedure by joining her husband in the session. The MedFT at this point must make very clear the patient's confidentiality rights with an explicit presentation of informed consent for treatment from the MedFT. Furthermore, a clear conversation regarding dual roles must be conducted with the patient's wife, clarifying that she is not the client but an agent providing supportive and relevant information for the accurate treatment of the patient. At that point, the MedFT could proceed with gleaning information from the couple as he may with any other couple and conduct the session in a similar fashion.

If the wife voices that she wishes to continue on as a client, a second phase of evaluation pertaining to dual roles must occur. After defining the problem,

Low Power	Mid-Range Power	High Power
Little or no personal relationship	Clear power differential present but relationship is circumscribed	Clear power differential with profound personal influence
Brief Duration	**Intermediate Duration**	**Long Duration**
Single or few contacts over short period of time	Regular contact over a limited period of time	Continuous or episodic contact over a long period of time
Specific Termination	**Uncertain Termination**	**Indefinite Termination**
Relationship is limited by time externally imposed or by prior agreement of parties who are unlikely to see each other again	Professional function is completed but further contact is not ruled out.	No agreement regarding when or if termination is to take place

Fig. 20.1 Dimensions for ethical decision-making (Gottlieb, 1993, p. 5)

resourcing state and ethical standards and consulting policy and procedure, the next step is to define options and consider clinical ramifications. Figure 20.1 on the following page provides a decision-making model to guide the MedFT in this situation. First the MedFT evaluates the level of power; in this case there seems to exist a mid-range power. The duration could be established by resourcing clinical policy. Many integrated facilities focus on short term (eight session or fewer) behavioral health models. If this was the case, the intermediate duration would be most appropriate with a specific termination agreement discussed. Using this model, the MedFT is able to deduce that this relationship has mid to low potential to negatively impact the patient and thus could reasonably proceed with integrated care.

Policy and Practice Implications

Dual relationships pose potential ethical complications in any setting; however, rural and IPC settings have been known to pose a higher risk for compromising the therapeutic relationship (Smalley et al., 2010). IPCs are similar to rural healthcare settings in that the providers all exist in a microcosm; a referral may be down the hall or across town. Either way, there is a high likelihood that both provider and patient relationships are complicated by overlapping roles (Davis & Roberts, 2009).

Unfortunately, sometimes the MedFT may be the only BHP for miles around. With high rates of depression, drug use, and suicide in rural areas (Smith, 2003; Zur, 2006), BHPs are greatly needed and, seemingly, equally avoided. Due to the high level of transparency (i.e., small talk and the likelihood that most people know one another) in small communities, many community members that would need services may avoid them due to the chance that they are known by most workers in a healthcare context (Eberhardt & Pamuk, 2004).

Linville, Hertlein, and Prouty-Lyness (2007) asserted that "the patient's interpersonal relationships are believed to play a key role and collaboration exists between the family therapist and the other health care practitioners" (p. 86). Taking this whole-person concept and placing it into a small, very cohesive, and transparent culture can make antiquated guidelines regarding therapeutic dual relationships literally impossible to follow. Contrary to current ethical guidelines, appropriate dual relationships may lead to more effective and rewarding healthcare outcomes (Davis & Roberts, 2009), and thus, current-day policies need to catch up with the potential for positive outcomes via these relationships in integrated care settings.

Although there are currently no ethical decision-making tools specifically developed for dual relationships in IPC, Gottlieb (1993) offered a decision-making matrix (see Fig. 20.1) that could prove useful when evaluating potential dual and multi-relationships. The basic premise of this model is to evaluate each dual relationship scenario by following the three dimensions shown below. The results provide insight into the potential dangers of the dual relationship according to three dimensions: power, duration, and termination. The further to the right each relationship falls (in each dimension), the more likely the dual relationship should be avoided.

Upon recognizing the potential for dual relationships, MedFTs must be careful in determining the next best options for the patient. While most medical providers are not restricted in who they can care for (e.g., someone that they know or work with), MedFTs may be perceived as abandoning their patients if they experience a dual relationship with an individual or family and are not able to serve as their provider. Terms pertaining to termination of services seem to be clearer in traditional behavioral health contexts, but could certainly still apply to IPC settings. Termination and provider abandonment refers to withdrawal from treatment of a patient without giving sufficient notice or providing a competent replacement within a reasonable amount of time to continue the therapeutic process. An abrupt disruption in treatment has the potential to harm the patient and taint their future therapeutic relationships or therapeutic outcomes. In contrast to the episodic nature of treatment in specialty behavioral care, the provider–patient relationship in IPC may be life-long. As such, patients may present episodically for treatment at critical junctures, such as with first diagnosis of healthcare conditions or when facing other stressful life events. In this sense, a patient may always be seen as a patient in primary care. Therefore, awareness that a dual relationship now exists can complicate care, particularly for those who have received healthcare services at this location for most of their life, but are just now receiving care from a MedFT.

Preparing in advance for potential dual relationship scenarios is important. Situations resulting in a termination may require risk management from both a clinical and legal perspective. Often, this is triggered by unilateral terminations from services, such as when providers discharge a patient for medication contract violations, overusing or diverting controlled medications, or exhibiting "abusive behavior" (e.g., yelling or threatening staff, stealing agency property, or repeated no shows). Bottom line is that policies should be created for each setting, such that patients know through their informed consent documents what circumstances are considered dual relationships and what scenarios may result in termination of services. When inevitable, termination should always include provisions for continuity of care. This is often achieved through a certified letter listing local alternative treatment options and an offer to manage emergencies for a defined length of time, and sufficient medications to cover a reasonable period to establish care with a new provider.

In response to common challenges associated with dual relationships, a new paradigm is emerging moving away from the complete avoidance of multiple and dual relationships to a more practical management of dual relationships, especially in rural communities (Barbopoulos & Clark, 2003; Schank & Skovholt, 2006). It is feasible to think that these types of policy and procedure shifts could be extended into IPC settings and other small communities, whereby providers may establish new policies related to managing the risks without impeding the therapeutic benefits. Solutions to these types of problems are not easily found; however, the current consensus in IPC literature is to consult with the team and communicate all of the potential risks to the patient prior to proceeding (Runyan et al., 2013). Until a unified IPC code of ethics is established, this type of collaborative decision-making allows all members of the team, including the patient, to determine the most ethical, informed choice for managing multiple and perhaps complex relationships.

Conclusion

Definitive ethical guidelines and policies for provider teams in IPC settings are developing as this model of care evolves. IPC literature and journals, such as the special edition on ethics in the journal of *Families, Systems, & Health* (2013), are being published as policy catches up to practice. In the meantime, MedFTs and other IPC providers should be aware of their profession's ethical codes and become more attuned to the codes that govern the work of their team members from other disciplines. Those practicing within an IPC system would benefit from open and ongoing collaborative interdisciplinary dialogues about federal regulations, state laws, and ethical standards along with healthcare protocols that may best address all considerations within their IPC system. Interdisciplinary cross-training and discussions will promote the highest level of ethical IPC (Hodgson et al., 2013). Ultimately, ethics are about protecting the rights of the patient and those most vulnerable in the system or relationship.

Discussion Questions

1. What happens if the wife, husband, and an adult child of the same family all are referred for behavioral health individually? As the only MedFT in this setting, how would you proceed?
2. If you treat this family as a unit, as well as the patient individually in IPC, into whose chart or charts would the notes be entered?
3. How would you document a patient's disclosure of drug use in an IPC setting, especially if he or she asks that you not tell the PCP or other members on the treatment team? What factors would you have to take into consideration?
4. What ethical guidelines governing your profession have the potential to impede the therapeutic processes in an IPC setting?
5. What steps would you need to take to develop a new policy in an IPC if an ethical challenge emerged?

References[1]

American Association for Marriage and Family Therapy. (2012). *User's guide to the AAMFT code of ethics*. Washington, DC: The American Association for Marriage and Family Therapy. Retrieved from http://aamft.org/imis15/Content/Legal_Ethics/Code_of_Ethics.aspx

American Medical Association. (n.d.). *Informed consent*. Retrieved from http://www.ama-assn.org/ama/pub/physician-resources/legal-topics/patient-physician-relationship-topics/informed-consent.page

American Mental Health Counselor Association. (2010). *AMHCA Code of Ethics*. Retrieved from http://www.amhca.org/assets/content/CodeofEthics1.pdf

American Psychological Association. (2010). *Ethical principles of psychologists and code of conduct*. Retrieved from http://www.apa.org/ethics/code/index.aspx

Barbopoulos, A., & Clark, J. M. (2003). Practicing psychology in rural settings: Issues and guidelines. *Canadian Psychology, 44*, 410–424. doi:10.1037/h0086962.

Barnett, J. (2007). Seeking an understanding of informed consent. *Professional Psychology: Research and Practice, 38*, 179–182. doi:10.1037/0735-7028.38.2.179.

Berg v. Berg. (2005). Retrieved from http://www.courts.state.nh.us/supreme/opinions/2005/berg112.htm

Collins, C., Hewson, D. L., Munger, R., & Wade, T. (2010). *Evolving models of behavioral health integration in primary care*. New York, NY: Milbank Memorial Fund.

Curtis, R., & Christian, E. (2012). *Integrated care: Applying theory to practice*. New York, NY: Routledge.

*Davis, R. & Roberts, R. (2009). *Handbook for rural healthcare ethics: A Practical guide for professionals*. Retrieved from http://geiselmed.dartmouth.edu/cfm/resources/ethics/chapter-05.pdf

Eberhardt, M. S., & Pamuk, E. R. (2004). The importance of place of residence: Examining health in rural and nonrural areas. *American Journal of Public Health, 94*, 1682–1686. doi:10.2105/AJPH.94.10.1682.

[1] An asterisk has been use to note references that the chapter authors recommend for further reading.

Gottlieb, M. C. (1993). Avoiding exploitive dual relationships: A decision-making model. *Psychotherapy, 30*, 41–48. doi:10.1037/0033-3204.30.1.41.
*Health Insurance Portability and Accountability Act of 1996, 46 C.F.R. 164.501–524 (2007).
Hodgson, J., Mendenhall, T., & Lamson, A. (2013). Patient and provider relationships: Consent, confidentiality, and managing mistakes in integrated primary care settings. *Families, Systems & Health, 31*, 28–40. doi:10.1037/a0031771.
*Hudgins, C., Rose, S., Fifield, P. Y., & Arnault, S. (2013). Navigating the legal and ethical foundations of informed consent and confidentiality in integrated primary care. *Families, Systems & Health, 31*, 9–19. doi:10.1037/a0031974.
Kanzler, K. E., Goodie, J. L., Hunter, C. L., Glotfelter, M. A., & Bodart, J. J. (2013). From colleague to patient: Ethical challenges in integrated primary care. *Families, Systems & Health, 31*, 41–48. doi:10.1037/a0031853.
Koocher, G., & Keith-Speigel, P. (2008). *Ethics in psychology and mental health professions: Standards and cases* (2nd ed.). New York, NY: Oxford University Press.
Legal Action Center. (n.d.). Alcohol and Drug Publications. Retrieved from http://lac.org/index.php/lac/130
Linville, D., Hertlein, K. M., & Prouty-Lyness, A. M. (2007). Medical family therapy; reflecting on the necessity of collaborative healthcare research. *Families, Systems & Health, 25*, 85–97. doi:10.1037/1091-7527.25.1.85.
Ohio Coordinating Center for Integrated Care and the Ohio Department of Mental Health. (2010). *Integrated care: Confidentiality and release of information fact sheet*. Retrieved from http://www.occic.org/documents/Integrated%20Care%20Confidentiality%20and%20Release%20of%20Information%20Fact%20Sheet%202-10.pdf
*Reiter, J., & Runyan, C. (2013). The ethics of complex relationships in primary care behavioral health. *Family Systems and Health, 31*, 20–27. doi:10.1037/a0031855.
Reitz, R., Common, K., Fifield, P., & Stiasny, E. (2012). Collaboration in the presence of an electronic health record. *Families, Systems, and Health, 30*, 72–80. doi:10.1037/a0027016.
*Reitz, R., Simmons, P. D., Runyan, C., Hodgson, J., & Carter-Henry, S. (2013). Multiple role relationships in healthcare education. *Families, Systems & Health, 31*, 96–107. doi:10.1037/a0031862
Runyan, C., Robinson, P., & Gould, D. A. (2013). Ethical issues facing providers in collaborative primary care settings: Do current guidelines suffice to guide the future of team based primary care? *Family Systems and Health, 31*, 1–8. doi:10.1037/a0031895.
Saviano, E. (2008). *Maintenance and disclosure of mental health records in the primary care clinic setting*. Retrieved from http://www.ibhp.org/uploads/file/MentalHealthRecordMaintenance_article.pdf
Schank, A. J., & Skovholt, T. M. (2006). *Ethical practices in small communities: Challenges and rewards for Psychologists*. Washington, DC: APA Books. doi:10.1037/11379-000.
Smalley, K., Yancey, C., Warren, J., Naufel, K., & Pugh, J. (2010). Rural mental health and psychological treatment: A review for practitioners. *Journal of Clinical Psychology, 66*, 479–489. doi:10.1002/jclp.20688.
Smith, A. J. (2003). Rural mental health counseling: One example of practicing what the research preaches. *Journal of Rural Community Psychology, 6*, 1–13. doi:10.1023/A:1025663311100.
*Striefel, S. (2009). Ethical behavior in medical settings. *Biofeedback, 37*, 119–122. doi:10.5298/1081-5937-37.4.119.
*Substance Abuse and Mental Health Services Administration U.S. Department of Health and Human Services. (2011). *Applying the substance abuse confidentiality regulations 42 CFR Part 2* (Revised). Retrieved from http://www.samhsa.gov/about/laws/SAMHSA_42CFRPART2FAQII_Revised.pdf
Zur, O. (2006). Therapeutic boundaries and dual relationships in rural practice: Ethical, clinical and standard of care considerations. *Journal of Rural Community Psychology, 9*, 1–49.

Chapter 21
How to Prepare a Medical Family Therapy Policy Brief

Peter Shin and Emily Jones

Background

Despite evidence indicating that Medical Family Therapy (MedFT) can improve patient health outcomes and help to mitigate adverse impacts of medical and behavioral health illnesses on families, they are not typically integrated into most clinical infrastructures (Phelps, Hodgson, Lamson, Swanson, & White, 2012; Phelps et al., 2009). This primarily stems from a lack in understanding the role and integration of MedFTs in healthcare settings (Fox, Hodgson, & Lamson, 2012). In fact, while low-income populations are most likely to benefit from the use of MedFT, due to their high risk for chronic medical conditions and co-morbid behavioral health issues, few understand the impact of providing MedFT to underserved populations (Petterson, Williams, Hauenstein, Rovnyak, & Merwin, 2009).

Given the novelty of MedFT in practice and research, much work is still needed regarding their impact on healthcare costs and revenues. By collecting, organizing, and simplifying disparate approaches to improving healthcare quality and health outcomes, policy briefs can provide an effective way to strengthen the relationship between research and health policy.

What Is a Policy Brief?

A policy brief is a short document that discusses a specific, focused issue for a non-academic audience. The purpose of a brief is to raise awareness about an issue and highlight the benefits of a specific course of action, as well as to inform and persuade the reader that the recommended action will reap benefits related to goals

---

P. Shin (✉)
George Washington University, Washington, DC, USA
e-mail: pshin@gwu.edu

J. Hodgson et al. (eds.), *Medical Family Therapy*, DOI 10.1007/978-3-319-03482-9_21,

that are relevant to the intended audience. For example, the policy brief may ask the question, "What is the level of unmet needs for MedFT?" Using survey data, the brief may highlight the overall need and then prioritize areas of the country, such as federally designated medically underserved areas, or subpopulations (e.g., low-income, racial and ethnic minorities, women) that may benefit from medical family therapy. Although informative, the intent is to translate knowledge into actionable recommendations for a policy and administrative audience. In addition to convincing the reader that the policy options recommended in the brief would be beneficial, effective policy analysis create a sense of urgency intended to engage and motivate the reader (Patton, Sawiki, & Clark, 2012).

Policy briefs should be written in plain or simple language with a minimum of jargon to make the topic accessible and understandable to audiences, such as policymakers, who are not proficient in the topic at hand. Given that few understand what MedFT is or how MedFTs are trained or financed, simple comparisons with well-known professional groups may be helpful. For example, a simple table that compares their roles with psychologists, social workers, and other peer groups who help with behavioral health issues, relationship problems, and other diagnoses may be more effective in conveying how MedFTs fill critical gaps between medical and psychosocial needs or better effectuate care delivery.

The problem should also be framed and policy options discussed in a way intended to strongly influence the stakeholders or administrators with power to change the status quo. Policy briefs that are succinct and coherent can be particularly important during the policy formulation phase, when a legislative or regulatory decision is being discussed. In general, the best time to prepare a policy brief is well before the anticipated policy debate takes place; in most cases, the policy formulation phase recurs at regular intervals, such as during discussion of budgets or legislation that periodically needs reauthorization due to sunset clauses.

Of course, the policy formulation phase is not the only time that a policy brief can be an effective way to communicate to decision makers. After a policy is adopted, the implementation phase typically contains even more decision points. This is a time when a policy brief will be useful to remind stakeholders of the value of MedFT. The target audience for follow-up policy briefs might shift from legislators to administrators after the policy is adopted, and the focus will shift to a new set of decisions facing implementers.

It is important to use a combination of in-person meetings and written materials such as policy briefs to cultivate champions for MedFT before any important decision is being debated and well before any relevant policies are implemented. In fact, policy changes are often the result of public attention on a problem, feasible solution(s), and politics. As a result, policy windows for a particular idea are infrequent and are not open for long. Policy entrepreneurs tirelessly work to create policy windows by educating the public on a particular issue while actively working to get their solution on the agenda (Kingdon, 2010).

The Art and Science of Policy Analysis

The tone, structure, and content of a policy brief might vary according to the purpose of the analysis. Views on the role of policy analysis have evolved over time. Traditionally, policy analysis was viewed as something best accomplished by a strictly impartial analyst using rigorous analytical methods (Wildavsky, 1979). According to this perspective, policy analysis is ideally free from the influence of politics, advocacy, interest groups, or the financial interests of the policy analyst. In the rational model, the policy analyst provides logical steps to get to the best possible solution. However, others argue that impartial policy analysis is a rarity in the real world due to the heavy influence of politics (Stone, 2001). Rather, policy analysis is argumentative in nature, in which policy analysis is not only based on rigorous methodology, but also depends on the art of argument to lace together strands of evidence to build toward a specific policy recommendation (Majone, 1992; Weimer & Vining, 2010; Teitelbaum & Wilensky, 2012).

As cliché as it may sound, policy analysis is both an art and a science. The policy brief should reflect some skill in building an argument based on the strongest evidence available. Peer reviewed studies are often equated as the gold standard when reporting and analyzing findings, given the rigorous review process involved, and the level of credibility generally tied to the name recognition in a particular journal. Refereed articles themselves do not make good policy briefs given that they are much longer and more technically detailed than the quick and easy consumption that a policy brief entails. As a result, policy briefs play a critical role in translating high quality research into policy by rendering timely and relevant peer reviewed findings more accessible to a general audience (White & Dudley-Brown, 2011).

Policy Briefs Rely on Strength and Source of Evidence

Use of recognized datasets and peer-reviewed articles generally confers greater credibility than non-peer reviewed research. The trend toward data-driven policymaking appears to be increasing, given greater adoption of health information technology, standardized reporting, and greater access to federal and state healthcare and census data. In fact, Weinick and Shin (2004) indicate that mining of relevant federal and state data for purposes of data-driven policymaking often helps to improve understanding of the problem, identifying a policy priority, and supporting policy, particularly as new data sources and measures become available. Federal agencies rely on varying national, state, and community data to continually identify medically underserved areas or where additional investments may be best served or needed.

Quantitative estimates, either directly from the data or estimated from literature, and projections of such factors as cost and return on investment can be particularly persuasive. During a legislative debate, it is not uncommon to find quantitative estimates from different perspectives being disseminated (Dor et al., 2009; Indiana State Department of Health, 2011; Rosenbaum & Shin, 2011). Differences largely stem from varying assumptions around pricing, per capita costs and savings, enrollment projections, and other factors related to consumption and use of services, such as the health status of new enrollees (CBO, 2012; The Child Health Business Case Working Group, 2004).

There are a number of federal datasets available that may help identify key opportunities in which MedFTs can engage. For example, the Health Resources and Services Administration (HRSA) houses the Geospatial Data Warehouse, which contains information across numerous agencies and programs. It includes identification of federally designated areas of underservice and, theoretically, the data may be overlaid with MedFT locations to assess their level of presence in these communities. Additional relevant data can be found from the Bureau of Health Professions (BHPR), which develops data on the National Health Service Corps (NHSC) placements and Heath Professional Shortage (HPSA) and Medically Underserved Area (MUA) designations. Beyond HRSA, data exists from other Department of Health and Human Services agencies, such as the Centers for Disease Control and Prevention's (CDC) Vital Statistics and National Health Insurance Survey, the Agency for Healthcare Research and Quality's (AHRQ) Medical Expenditure Panel Survey and Health Care Utilization Project, and the National Center for Health Statistics' (NCHS) Survey of Children with Special Health Care Needs. Such data can be used to assess costs, service utilization, and potential patient profiles. The US Census Bureau, the Centers for Medicaid and Medicare Services (CMS), and the Department of Labor also provide a vast array of potentially relevant statistics. These datasets can be used to assess the extent to which MedFTs can effectively help address disparities in health care and help reduce healthcare costs. Table 21.1 illustrates where some of these datasets may be used or need to be collected to improve understanding of MedFT and its impact. Examining the HRSA data alone, suggests MedFTs can help serve the growing number of underserved patients with behavioral health issues (Chow, Jafee, & Snowden, 2003; Shin, Sharac, & Mauery, 2013).

Policy briefs may rely on other sources of information, such as white papers or grey literature, to fill in gaps or provide more current or relevant information. White papers are informational documents which originate from government, businesses, or organizations and advocate for certain issues. Grey literature generally refers to unpublished or informally published studies and reports which include original research or unique findings, but are perceived as less methodologically rigorous (Conn, Valentine, Cooper, & Rantz, 2003; Cook et al., 1993). Although both white papers and grey literature are not peer reviewed, using non-refereed materials as part of policy analyses do not necessarily make policy briefs less credible, so long as they are consistent with the general literature and are from unbiased sources.

Given the nature of policy briefs, legislative research results are also often included to strengthen the analysis. These are generally legal and regulatory and focused on the precedents, cases, statutes, and regulations relevant to the issue being discussed. Like white papers and grey literature, policy briefs should be

Table 21.1 Key data needs

Profile of patients that MedFTs serve, by income, insurance status, age, marital status, and race and ethnicity
Description of the range of services provided, with particular focus on the chronic disease services provided
Assessment of the MedFT financing, including an assessment of barriers to increased use of third-party billing procedures
Summary and discussion of current payment methodology in each state and trends in State policies regarding reimbursement for MedFT services
Estimate of the "unmet need" for MedFT
Analysis of the impact of MedFT on the organizational performance, quality patient outcomes (and satisfaction), quality, and cost
Evaluation of technical assistance efforts centered on promoting MedFTs in safety net organizations

written in a timely fashion, and should take into account a publication process in which a polished product (in written and electronic form) can be distributed to appropriate policymakers.

Targeted Audiences

The policy brief should be targeted to the appropriate audience and tied to an existing agenda or to an audience who may share common priorities or ideas. Possible audiences for MedFT policy briefs are: (a) policymakers in federal, state, and local government: Legislative, Administrative, or Regulatory; (b) payers (e.g., Medicaid, private, Federal); (c) broader behavioral health community; (d) medical community (e.g., ambulatory care providers, hospitals, long-term and post-acute care facilities); or (e) foundations (e.g., Robert Wood Johnson Foundation, Kaiser Family Foundation, the Kresge Foundation, W. K. Kellogg Foundation).

A useful policy brief should take the opportunity to link the goals and programs to an issue that is already on the public agenda per the targeted audience. For example, if controlling rising expenditures in state budgets is important to decision makers, then it will be necessary to link MedFT to that goal.

Given that the federal government is heavily invested in the healthcare and public health infrastructure, there is no shortage of issues to which MedFT can be linked. In general, federal investments fund both population-based activities, such as health promotion and preventive services, and health services for low-income persons, persons with chronic illnesses and disabilities, and high-risk populations. Sources who currently invest in projects aligned with MedFT range from Medicaid and the Children's Health Insurance Program (CHIP), the Health Centers program, Centers for Disease Control and Prevention (CDC) project grants related to health promotion and disease prevention, the Substance Abuse and Mental Health

Services Administration's (SAMHSA) mental health and substance abuse programs, the Health Resources and Services Administration's (HRSA) programs for women and children and special populations (e.g., people with HIV/AIDS), and other Department of Health and Human Services (DHHS) programs and agencies that promote the development of community-based systems that are designed to support the coordination and integration of services for children, working-age adults, and elderly persons with disabilities. Even when funds become increasingly limited, the challenges the agencies face still relate to maximizing the value of these investments.

Policy and Programmatic Issues in Health Policy that May Be of Particular Interest

Despite numerous changes in health policy, policymakers will likely continue to face similar challenges in the short- and long-term. First, the healthcare infrastructure is likely to face significant strain with the surge of newly insured patients over the next few years. Additionally, care for the uninsured and underinsured is likely to continue as a major issue (CBO, 2012; Ku, Jones, Shin, Bryne, & Long, 2011). Therefore, MedFT policy briefs will likely span a broad range of population health issues, such as analyses of vulnerable and underserved populations, their healthcare needs, integrated care options, and the role of MedFTs in supporting public health goals and delivering healthcare services to these populations.

Second, improving the quality and efficiency of safety net providers serving low-income, publicly insured, and uninsured populations will remain paramount. In 2014, the Affordable Care Act (ACA) is expected to cover nearly 30 million more Americans through health insurance marketplaces, or Exchanges, and state Medicaid expansions. A key to the success of this expansion is the need to have a sufficient range and number of healthcare professionals to provide quality care. More notably is the expansion of the Health Centers Program, which is expected to double capacity in underserved communities over the next decade (Hawkins & Groves, 2011). Health centers serve a disproportionately low-income population with chronic healthcare needs that require greater scope and intensity of clinical services than for other populations. These patients often have multiple diagnoses, including chronic conditions such as HIV or diabetes as well as behavioral health problems.

Third, workforce and financing policies will need to be in place to ensure that as health reform is implemented, there is enough capacity to manage complex health conditions, to deliver quality care, and to create linkages to community providers for additional services. Billions of dollars are spent to develop, support, and operate systems of services that meet accepted standards of quality in the areas of both basic health care through the life cycle, as well as advanced, community-based long-term care services and support for children and adults with chronic physical and mental illness and disabilities. Implementation of complementary investment policies with MedFT will continue to be needed to aid in the success of such programs.

Fourth, adequately financing the healthcare safety net workforce will also be needed to better ensure success of the expansion initiative. Here, Medicaid and Medicare will be of special importance, not only because of the services it covers and the greater number of patients it will insure under health reform, but also because of its impact on provider reimbursement rates, staffing mix, and provider participation. Therefore, a brief should seek to identify and assess the types of state programs that effectively support and enhance MedFT performance, particularly in rural and inner-city safety net settings.

Finally, policies centered on quality improvement also present significant opportunities to add to the current conversation of medical home models or the triple aim goals of increasing the quality of health care, increasing the health of individuals and populations, and controlling per capita costs (Berwick, Nolan, & Whittington, 2008). Most notably, the Affordable Care Act includes a number of provisions to improve care coordination and integration of multi-disciplinary providers for vulnerable populations; and many states have already initiated Medicaid medical home projects (Ku, Shin, Regenstein, & Mead, 2011; Takach & Buxbaum, 2013). Therefore, better understanding of how effective integration of MedFT in primary care underserved settings can contribute to reducing disparities and generate cost-savings will be needed.

Steps for Developing Effective Policy Briefs

The hallmarks of effective policy briefs are brevity, clarity, and the persuasive use of evidence to make concrete recommendations. First, the title of the policy brief should be descriptive and clearly let the reader know what information is conveyed and why they should be interested in reading it. One way to make a title compelling is to use a question or a variation on a familiar phrase. The title should be brief and easily digestible, such as, "The Role of Medical Family Therapists in the Health Care Safety Net" or "Financing Options to Support MedFT Services in Underserved Communities." If a lengthy title is needed to convey the subject matter, consider using a subtitle to add clarifying detail to an abbreviated main title (see Table 21.2 as additional title examples).

Given that the audience often has competing priorities and might devote limited time to reading the brief, it must convey information in a visually appealing manner and be persuasive as quickly as possible. Instead of solid text, use tables and figures to convey information in a more reader-friendly way. In place of tables, consider displaying information using charts and graphs. Maps are another way to convey a lot of information without forcing the reader to sift through a sea of numbers. Diagrams or schematic illustrations might simplify the description of a complex process. Paragraphs should be short and headings and subheadings should be used liberally. Sidebars and text boxes can be used to highlight important points.

Table 21.2 Sample policy brief topics related to medical family therapy

Financial
Options for reimbursing on-site MedFT in primary care offices
Options for incentivizing on-site MedFT in inpatient, long-term care, and hospice settings
Options for enabling integrated care by funding provider-to-provider communication
Options for utilizing MedFTs to enhance access to behavioral health screening and prevention
Addressing same-day billing restrictions for behavioral and medical care
Workforce
Options for increasing the capacity of MedFT training programs
Options for enhancing the use of MedFTs to address the shortage and maldistribution of medical and behavioral health providers
Increasing equity and access for the underserved
Options to support access to translation, transportation, and other enabling services for patients in need of MedFT
Targeted brief on increasing MedFT capacity in community health centers
Policy options for incentivizing on-site MedFT for special populations: school-based clinics, homeless patients, migrant and seasonal farmworkers, patients in public housing
Miscellaneous
Policy options to incentivize electronic health record adoption among medical family therapists
Policy options to reduce barriers to health information exchanged

Information that is detailed might be included as an appendix, if necessary. Information on the methods used to generate evidence and information on the statistical significance of peer-reviewed findings should either be summarized in a footnote or added to the appendix. Although the methods and statistics are critical for purposes of transparency, they are not deemed necessary for main body of the brief.

Define the Problem and Provide Focused Background Information

The background of a policy brief should be as short as possible, with a targeted focus on the specific policy issue being discussed. It is important to set the context to ensure that the reader understands the importance of the message; if the background is not pithy and targeted, many readers might not make it to the message (Table 21.3).

The background should make it clear why the problem discussed in the brief is important and emphasize the urgency of addressing the problem. Linking the issue being discussed to the big picture and overarching goals will increase the effectiveness of the policy brief.

Table 21.3 Some questions to be addressed

What is the (potential) role of MedFTs in team-based care and in the patient-centered medical home?
Can employing or contracting with a MedFT help a primary care practice or hospital with accreditation and PCMH recognition?
How can MedFTs support accountable care structures?
Which financing options are available for sustaining MedFTs in inpatient and outpatient safety net settings?
What are the policy options for encouraging the use of MedFTs to prevent hospital readmissions?

Describe and Evaluate the Policy Options

Policy options should be based on the information provided in the background of the report. Policy options can be developed from diverse sources, from state and federal proposals to local programs. In general, policy options should have some measure of being tested or implemented elsewhere so that it can be considered actionable, technical, budget-friendly, and legally, financially, and administratively feasible. In addition to being politically feasible, the options should be effective on many levels, such as access, cost, quality, and health outcomes. At the least, options should indicate what changes are expected compared with the status quo. A useful format for providing information about several policy options at a glance is a side-by-side table with each dimension of the proposed policies described in a different row and column for each policy.

Use the Right Data and Evidence

Shine the spotlight on the information that makes the case. Since the policy brief has an abbreviated format, only include details that are directly relevant to the brief. Important details might include rationales for the need for MedFT, for example (a) evidence that family issues affect behavioral health (BH) and health status; (b) evidence that BH impacts overall health and management of chronic diseases; (c) evidence of effectiveness of MedFT in treating BH issues, as well as medical issues; (d) unmet need for behavioral health treatment, and the impact on society (e.g., absenteeism, presenteeism); or (e) impact on disparities (e.g., by race/ethnicity, income, payer-source).

Also, be sure to describe or allude to the benefits of expanding access to MedFT. It is especially useful to supply your audience with references and further readings that explain how MedFT can further their interests. Specific points might include (a) impact of meeting the need: cost and utilization offset effects; (b) return on investment of employing medical family therapists (c) different perspectives include insurers, state/federal payers, primary care practice, integrated delivery system, or accountable care organizations; (d) staff and provider satisfaction;

Table 21.4 Different audiences, different policy options

Audience	Policy "win" that you are seeking	Examples of effective messages
Policymakers in federal, state, and local government: Legislative, Administrative, Regulatory	Legislation that defines MedFT as a covered service under Medicaid	Triple Aim goals: Better care Better health Cost savings
	Regulations that eliminate same-day billing restrictions for medical and behavioral health services in Medicaid	Participate and be an innovator in health reform
	An administrative decision to include medical family therapists in the National Health Services Corps scholarship and loan repayment program	Better staff satisfaction in medical settings (ambulatory, inpatient, long-term care/palliative care)
	Funding for a pilot program that increases access to medical family therapists in ambulatory care, particularly in federally qualified health centers	Increased patient satisfaction
	Patient Centered Medical Homes	Reduce disparities
Payers (Medicaid, private, federal)	Coverage for MedFT services	
	Reduction in costs	
	Quality incentives	
The broader behavioral health and medical community	State licensure requirements	
	Collaboration with safety net providers	
Foundations	Funding for a pilot program	
	Family relationships and financial stability	
	Community health/social determinants	

(e) patient and/or family satisfaction; or (f) a possibility that medical family therapists can help alleviate behavioral health and medical workforce shortages and maldistributions.

The intended audience and purpose of the policy brief will dictate what to emphasize, the brief should be tailored to frame the evidence used for the audience and the relevant political context. If Medicaid reimbursement is the topic and the state Medicaid agency is the target, emphasizing benefits such as the cost offset effect and lower utilization would be effective. Other factors like staff satisfaction and patient satisfaction might be more effective if your target audience is a primary care clinic with whom you wish to partner (Table 21.4).

Recommendations and Conclusions

The conclusion should be brief. Although it is useful to revisit the policy problem and underline the urgent need for action in the concluding paragraph, in order to emphasize the connection with the proposed policy solutions and activate the reader, this section should remain concise.

Include a Short Executive Summary

The executive summary of a policy brief is usually a concise summary of the report. After the problem and need for change are briefly summarized, lay out the policy recommendations and rationale. Ideally, the summary can be digested at a glance, much like a fact sheet, so consider mixing bullet points with text, particularly for key points.

Develop Companion Documents, Dissemination Aids, and Promotional Materials

Companion documents might include fact sheets and other informational documents that contain a level of detail that might overwhelm the target audience of the policy brief. For example, details on implementation of several options may be included. In addition, the impact of the policy brief's release might be enhanced if you create dissemination aids such as slide decks, talking points, and Frequently Asked Questions (FAQs). Finally, promotional materials such as press releases and messages distributed via social media outlets should trumpet the release of your policy brief.

Short and focused documents such as fact sheets might serve as useful companion materials, particularly if the subject matter involves complexities and technical details that would not be familiar to someone who is not an expert in MedFT. When possible, informational material should be released in advance of the policy brief to build awareness of the policy issue. Fact sheets should not be longer than one sheet of paper, front and back, and should be written for a busy audience. Bullets, tables, and charts help convey information in an easy-to-digest format.

Other types of companion documents can also amplify the main messages conveyed in the policy brief. Tools should be developed to assist with the presentation of the policy brief for different audiences and in different venues. For an academic audience, a poster or podium presentation at conferences would be appropriate. For a policy audience, a one-page document with talking points can ensure that parties will help to disseminate the brief when interacting with policymakers. Another "leave-behind" version might be intended to be a handout in meetings with legislative staff or other decision makers.

Table 21.5 Checklist for effective policy briefs

Did you frame the policy problem with urgency? Does the reader know why they should pay attention to the topic?
Is the problem linked with the values and priorities of the target audience?
Is the writing clear and free of jargon? Double-check to make sure that acronyms are spelled out and terms of art are avoided.
Are the policy options clearly explained?
Is evidence of potential effectiveness presented?
Is the recommendation clear? Are the next steps concrete?
Is the brief summarized in an executive summary or text box?
Are tables, graphs, and text boxes used to break up solid text and enhance readability?
Are references and/or additional reading materials provided?

Sometimes it is possible to anticipate the types of questions that stakeholders will have about the policy issue. In this case, a FAQ document might be positioned on a Web site with the report, to highlight the information that should be emphasized in response to questions that are likely to arise. This might be particularly useful if the issue is controversial and thus prone to confusing messages.

Different types of promotional materials might also accompany the release of the policy brief to attract the attention of the media and the public. A press release can be used to capture the attention of the media. Leverage any partnerships and use personal or professional networks to promote the policy brief. For example, a short blurb and hyperlink to the policy brief should be distributed to organizations that might be persuaded to include the blurb in a listserv or newsletter. Using social media tools such as Twitter, Facebook, and LinkedIn can help to distribute the message, as well as writing a guest blog post or work with a blogger to distribute the message of the policy brief (Table 21.5).

Discussion

Most policy briefs are simple in structure, making them highly accessible and useful in the policy making process. Policy briefs are designed to be easy-to-read and action-oriented, with a clear set of options for policymakers and implementers to consider. Policy briefs should be coherent and concise at every step. While the art of argument is important in crafting an effective policy brief, credible policy briefs must be based on sound studies that employ rigorous methodology. However, the most effective way to package information depends on the purpose of the communication: what audience is it trying to reach, and why?

A number of federal health policy changes present significant opportunities for boosting the profile of MedFT. In general, the success of health reform expansion efforts depends heavily on attracting, coordinating, and integrating qualified personnel to provide a broad range of health care, behavioral health, and support services to enrollees. MedFT can play a critical role in serving high-risk populations that are of great concern to both public health and healthcare agencies. Although there is greater attention being paid to health professions programs, there remains little understanding of how MedFT can be used to address service and provider gaps.

As the health reform legislation continues to roll out, it will undoubtedly raise a series of implementation issues that may present additional opportunities for the MedFT community. Given that MedFTs seek to address population-wide health needs and concerns of entire communities, these policy briefs may also serve to promote collaborative arrangements with health centers and other safety net providers.

Discussion Questions

1. In what way can data be used to influence MedFT policy?
2. What kinds of policy options are available to improve integration of MedFT in primary care?
3. What are the major advantages and disadvantages of a MedFT policy brief vs. MedFT research article?

References[1]

*Berwick, D., Nolan, T., & Whittington, J. (2008). The triple aim: Care, health, and cost. *Health Affairs, 27*, 759–769. doi:10.1377/hlthaff.27.3.759.

Chow, J. C. C., Jafee, K., & Snowden, L. (2003). Racial/ethnic disparities in the use of mental health services in poverty areas. *American Journal of Public Health, 93*, 792–797. doi:10.2105/AJPH.93.5.792.

*Congressional Budget Office. (2012). *CBO and JCT's Estimates of the effects of the Affordable Care Act on the number of people obtaining employment-based health insurance*. Retrieved from http://cbo.gov/sites/default/files/cbofiles/attachments/03-15-ACA_and_Insurance_2.pdf

Conn, V. S., Valentine, J. C., Cooper, H. M., & Rantz, M. J. (2003). Grey literature in meta analyses. *Nursing Research, 52*, 256–261.

Cook, D. J., Guyatt, G. H., Ryan, G., Clifton, J., Buckingham, L., Willan, A., . . . Oxman, A. D. (1993). Should unpublished data be included in meta-analyses? Current convictions and controversies. *Journal of the American Medical Association, 269*, 2749–2753.

Dor, A., Richard, P., Tan, E., Rosenbaum, S., Shin, P., & Repasch, L. (2009). Community health centers in Indiana: State investments and returns. George Washington University Geiger Gibson/RCHN Community Health Foundation Research Collaborative. Retrieved from http://sphhs.gwu.edu/departments/healthpolicy/dhp_publications/pub_uploads/dhpPublication_A7BA8B9A-5056-9D20-3D3852F88AC4EF03.pdf

[1] An asterisk has been use to note references that the chapter authors recommend for further reading.

Fox, M. A., Hodgson, J. L., & Lamson, A. L. (2012). Integration: Opportunities and challenges for family therapists in primary care. *Contemporary Family Therapy, 34*, 228–243. doi:10.1007/s10591-012-9189-3.

Hawkins, D., & Groves, D. (2011). The future of community health centers in a changing health care landscape. *Journal of Ambulatory Care Management, 34*, 90–99. doi:10.1097/JAC.0b013e3182047e87.

Indiana State Department of Health. (2011). *2011–2016 Indiana state health improvement plan*. Retrieved from http://www.in.gov/isdh/files/Indiana_State_Health_Plan_FINAL_6_23_11.pdf

Kingdon, J. (2010). *Agendas, alternatives, and public policies, updated* (2nd ed.). New York, NY: Longman.

Ku, L., Jones, E., Shin, P., Bryne, F. R., & Long, S. K. (2011). Safety-net providers after health care reform: Lessons from Massachusetts. *Archives of Internal Medicine, 171*, 1379–1384. doi:10.1001/archinternmed.2011.317.

Ku, L., Shin, P. M., Regenstein, M., & Mead, H. (2011). *Promoting the integration and coordination of safety-net health care providers under health reform: Key issues*. New York, NY: The Commonwealth Fund.

*Majone, G. (1992). *Evidence, argument and persuasion in the policy process*. New Haven, CT: Yale University Press.

*Patton, C., Sawiki, D., & Clark, J. (2012). *Basic methods of policy analysis and planning* (3rd ed.). Upper Saddle River, NJ: Pearson.

Petterson, S., Williams, I. C., Hauenstein, E. J., Rovnyak, V., & Merwin, E. (2009). Race and ethnicity and rural mental health treatment. *Journal of Health Care for the Poor and Underserved, 20*, 662–677. doi:10.1353/hpu.0.0186.

Phelps, K., Hodgson, J., Lamson, A., Swanson, M., & White, M. (2012). Satisfaction with life and psychosocial factors among ethnic minorities with type 2 diabetes. *Social Indicators Research, 106*, 359–370. doi:10.1007/s11205-011-9811-z.

Phelps, K. W., Howell, C. D., Hill, S. G., Seemann, T. S., Lamson, A. L., Hodgson, J. L., & Smith, D.A. (2009). A collaborative care model for patients with type-2 diabetes. *Families, Systems, & Health, 27*, 131–140. doi:10.1037/a0015027

Rosenbaum, S. & Shin, P. (2011). *Community health Centers and the economy: Assessing centers' role in job creation efforts*. George Washington University Geiger Gibson/RCHN Community Health Foundation Research Collaborative. Retrieved from http://www.gwumc.edu/sphhs/departments/healthpolicy/dhp_publications/pub_uploads/dhpPublication_63C7B816-5056-9D20-3D6FC84132695FF2.pdf

Shin, P., Sharac, J., & Mauery, D. R. (2013). The role of community health centers in providing behavioral health care. *Journal of Behavioral Health Services and Research, 40*(4), 488–496.

*Stone, D. (2001). *Policy paradox: The art of political decision making* (3rd ed.). New York, NY: W.W. Norton & Company. revised.

Takach, M., & Buxbaum, J. (2013). *Care management for Medicaid enrollees through community health teams*. New York, NY: The Commonwealth Fund.

*Teitelbaum, J., & Wilensky, S. (2012). *Essentials of health law and policy* (2nd ed.). Burlington, MA: Jones & Bartlett Learning.

The Child Health Business Case Working Group. (2004). Exploring the business care for improving the quality of health care for children. *Health Affairs, 23*, 4159–4166. doi:10.1377/hlthaff.23.4.159.

*Weimer, D., & Vining, A. (2010). *Policy analysis: Concepts and practice* (5th ed.). London: Pearson.

*Weinick, R. M., & Shin, P. (2004). *Monitoring the health care safety bet: Developing data-driven capabilities to support policymaking. (AHRQ Publication No. 04-0037)*. Rockville, MD: Agency for Healthcare Research and Quality.

White, K. M., & Dudley-Brown, S. (2011). *Translation of evidence in nursing and health care practice: Application of nursing and health care*. New York, NY: Springer.

Wildavsky, A. (1979). *Speaking truth to power: The art and craft of policy analysis*. New York, NY: Little, Brown.

Part IV
Finance

Chapter 22
A Summary Report of Cost-Effectiveness: Recognizing the Value of Family Therapy in Health Care

D. Russell Crane and Jacob Christenson

Results from studies conducted over the past 30 years within established medical systems demonstrate that family therapy is an effective and relatively inexpensive modality of psychotherapy treatment (e.g., Crane & Payne, 2011). In addition, as a group of independently licensed treatment providers, Marriage and Family Therapists (MFTs) provide care that is as cost-effective as other behavioral health provider groups (Moore, Hamilton, Crane, & Fawcett, 2011). These providers are also associated with less therapy dropout, which suggests that patients are receiving at least average care (Hamilton, Moore, Crane, & Payne, 2011). The current chapter is an update and expansion of Crane (2008), which reviewed studies through 2007 that dealt with family therapy as a treatment modality, but did not summarize the findings regarding MFT as a behavioral health discipline. In particular, this chapter elaborates on findings that are relevant to health, health care, and health utilization (i.e., results that may be particularly informative for medical family therapists [MedFTs]). The authors focus most particularly on Marriage and Family Therapy because analyses for these studies were done according to type of license. Therefore, MFT is a more accurate descriptor than family therapy, relational therapy, or medical family therapy.

This chapter is organized into two sections. The first section presents a summary of the results for the 21 studies that make up this body of research. Within each subsection, studies are presented in chronological order according to where the data were collected. The level of significance is consistently valued at $p \leq 0.05$ throughout the chapter. The second section briefly touches on summary themes in the data and limitations and provides information for future directions in research and how this information can be used in advocacy efforts, especially as it relates to MFT and MedFT.

D. R. Crane (✉)
School of Family Life at Brigham Young University, Provo, UT, USA
e-mail: russ_crane@byu.edu

J. Hodgson et al. (eds.), *Medical Family Therapy*, DOI 10.1007/978-3-319-03482-9_22,

Findings from HMO Data

The first group of studies was derived from data gathered at a western United States Health Maintenance Organization (HMO) serving 180,000 subscribers and focused on "medical offset effect" (defined as the reduction in other healthcare services use after the provision of psychotherapy). Although this phenomenon had been well demonstrated for individual therapy, very little information previously existed specific to family therapy, family therapy in healthcare contexts, or MedFT.

Paper charts for behavioral health and physical health care were available for three discreet time periods: (a) 6 months before the start of therapy, (b) 6 months after the start of therapy, and (c) between 6 and 12 months after the start of therapy. A sample of 292 participants was selected from those who had used individual, couple, and family therapy services. Because of the archival nature of the data, little demographic information was available; however, it was determined that the average identified patient was 30 years old and the sample was largely made up of middle-income and White non-Hispanic individuals. Therapy type was the independent variable and outpatient care was the dependent variable in the studies. Participants were further separated into groups according to five different therapy types: (a) marital/couple therapy, (b) family therapy identified patient (FTIP), (c) family therapy other patient (FTOP), (d) individual therapy, and (e) a no therapy comparison group.

Study One (Law & Crane, 2000)

The first study was an attempt to apply medical offset research methods to family therapy specifically. When the three time periods were compared, it was found that there were significant reductions in healthcare use. In particular, those who participated in family therapy ($n = 172$) were found to have reduced healthcare use by 21.5 % 1 year after psychotherapy started, compared to a 10 % reduction for those who had individual therapy ($n = 60$). Additionally, the family therapy participant who was not the identified patient (FTOP) group ($n = 60$) also showed a reduction of 30 % in healthcare use after 1 year. This finding was notable because this group of participants was not the focus of therapy, suggesting that family therapy may produce a medical offset beyond just the identified patient. However, because this finding is unique to this study, further research should be conducted to verify this possibility. No study is known to have attempted replication of this finding at the present time.

Study Two (Law, Crane, & Berge, 2003)

This study focused on "high utilizers" of heath care ($N = 65$) within the larger Law and Crane (2000) sample. Little research has shown whether this population reduces healthcare use after psychotherapy, despite accounting for a disproportionate amount of costs. High utilization was defined as four or more healthcare visits during the first 6-month period. After therapy, those who received individual ($n = 22$), marital ($n = 15$), or family therapy ($n = 28$) all reduced healthcare use by about 50 %. The reductions in healthcare use were statistically significant at −57 % for the FTOP patients. The largest reductions of −50 to −57 % were seen among those who participated in some form of conjoint therapy. Individual therapy also produced a large and statistically significant reduction of −48 %.

Study Three (Crane, Wood, Law, & Schaalje, 2004)

This exploratory study examined the relationship between therapist characteristics (such as age, experience, gender, and profession) and use of health care with patients. The sample consisted of 197 patients who received services from 13 providers, who included: (a) marriage and family therapists ($n = 4$), (b) psychologists ($n = 2$), and (c) clinical social workers ($n = 7$). Logistic regression was used to analyze the data and the results supported the argument that psychotherapy, in general, contributed to reductions in healthcare use more than specific therapist characteristics or provider type. However, this study should be replicated with a larger sample for each of the provider types before drawing firm conclusions.

Study Four (Crane & Christenson, 2008)

Most offset studies combine various types of healthcare use into a single outcome variable such as "outpatient visits," which has the potential to mask patterns in reductions within specific subtypes of healthcare use. In this study, various types of outpatient care (e.g., health screening, illness visits, laboratory/X-ray, and urgent care) utilized by the 292 participants in the original Law and Crane (2000) study were separated out for analysis. Similar to the findings by Law et al. (2003), the most prominent reductions over the three time periods were found for high utilizers who participated in family therapy. For these participants, there was a 78 % reduction in urgent care visits, a 56 % reduction in laboratory/X-ray visits, and a 68 % reduction in health screening visits when T1 was compared to T2.

Findings from Kansas Medicaid Data

The second source of naturally occurring data was from the Kansas Medicaid system. Medicaid is a program funded by federal dollars intended to provide health care to lower-income children and families. Medicaid is administered at the state level and is one of the largest providers of health care to children in the United States.

Study One (Crane, Hillin, & Jakubowski, 2005)

The first use of these data was a longitudinal, retrospective study that looked at healthcare costs associated with treating conduct disorder for patients in Kansas. The youth in this study ($N = 3{,}753$) received comprehensive services (e.g., case management and pharmacological intervention), along with one of three types of therapy: (a) in-office family therapy ($n = 164$), (b) in-office individual therapy ($n = 3{,}086$), and (c) in-home family therapy ($n = 503$). The participants were mostly males (81 %), White non-Hispanic, (73 %), and had an average age of 14.4 years. The cost of healthcare use for a period of two and a half years after therapy was available for each participant. Over the two-and-a-half-year follow-up period, the cost of health care was $16,260 for the in-office individual therapy group, $11,116 for the in-office family therapy group, and $1,622 for the in-home family therapy group. These findings showed that, compared to healthcare costs for the individual therapy group, those who received in-office family therapy were 32 % lower and those who received in-home family therapy were 85 % lower. Accordingly, it appeared that when family therapy is included in treatment, there does not appear to be a resultant increase in costs.

Study Two (Christenson, Crane, Beer, Bell, & Hillin, in press)

Kansas Medicaid data were used to develop two structural equation models relating to the cost of treating patients ($N = 164$) diagnosed with schizophrenia. The participants were mostly males (55 %), White non-Hispanic (90 %), and had an average age of 30 years. The first model was based on extant literature (e.g., Lindström & Bingefors, 2000) and included only limited direct effects for family intervention (e.g., reductions in hospitalization costs). The second model reflected both direct and indirect effects (e.g., reducing hospitalizations by increasing medication compliance) and was shown to be a better fit to the data when the Akaike Information Criterion (AIC) for both models were compared. This second model showed a significant indirect relationship between family intervention and general medical costs that accounted for a savings of $586 for each session of family intervention provided. The total indirect effect of family intervention on costs was a savings of $796 for hospitalizations and $580 for general medical use for each session of family intervention provided.

Findings from Cigna Data

Data from the behavioral health division of Cigna, a large national health insurance company with over nine million members, were provided for the following 11 studies. Cigna initially provided cost data for all psychotherapy services in the United States and Puerto Rico during a 4-year period (2001–2004), producing a sample that included 490,000 unique patients. The majority of the sample was female (60 %), and the average age of participants was 32 years. Recently Cigna has provided additional data, including that from more recent years (2005–2006). Studies one through three, below, present results from the sample as a whole, whereas studies four through eleven focus on specific subsamples within the data (e.g., patients diagnosed with depression).

Study One (Crane & Payne, 2011)

Outpatient claims data for 489,649 unique patients were used to find the cost of therapy (individual and family) as provided by marital and family therapists (MFTs), master's level nurses, social workers, professional counselors (PCs), psychologists, and physicians (MDs). The results showed that family therapy alone was substantially more cost-effective than either individual therapy or "mixed" therapy (a combination of both individual and family therapy). Overall, 85 % of the patients required only a single episode of care, and services provided by PCs were the least expensive. The 86.6 % success rate and 13.4 % recidivism (i.e., returning for a second episode of care) rate shown by MFTs were the best in those categories among the various providers.

Study Two (Hamilton, Moore, Crane, & Payne, 2011)

The second study in this series examined dropout rates by provider type, modality (e.g., individual, family therapy), and diagnosis. Administrative claims data for 434,317 patients were examined. Results showed that individuals treated by MFTs had the lowest dropout rates. In terms of treatment modality, the lowest dropout rate was found with individual therapy, and when diagnosis was considered, the lowest dropout rate was found among those diagnosed with mood and anxiety disorders. It was also noteworthy that amid the DSM diagnoses, schizophrenia and substance use disorders were amongst those with the highest dropout rates.

Study Three (Moore et al., 2011)

This study sought to examine specifically whether having a MFT license affected outcomes in family therapy. The same provider types (e.g., MFTs, MDs, nurses, social workers) and outcome measures were used (i.e., dropout, recidivism, and cost-effectiveness). The final sample included a total of 31,488 men and 36,333 women. Results showed that LMFTs, again, had the lowest dropout rate. MFTs were also more cost-effective than nurses, MDs, and psychologists but, given the similar costs and lower dropout rates, were less cost-effective than social workers and professional counselors (PCs).

Study Four (Moore & Crane, in press)

The sample in this study consisted of 3,315 patients who had participated in psychotherapy for relational problems. These included those with a diagnosis of a partner relational problem or those with a parent–child relational problem. The outcomes of interest included total cost, cost-effectiveness, and recidivism. Psychotherapy dropouts (i.e., less than two sessions) were excluded from the analysis. Only services provided by psychologists, PCs, MFTs, and social workers were included due to the preliminary finding that MDs and nurses did not provide conjoint services for these types of problems. Results showed that those who received individual therapy for relational problems did not have a higher recidivism rate than those who participated in family therapy. Findings also showed that couples therapy was a relatively brief intervention that required an average of five sessions and cost approximately $280 for an episode of care (with recidivism of 8.43 %). These findings lend support to the contention that adding family services as a covered benefit to insurance plans would not be too costly.

Study Five (Chiang, 2011)

Cost-effectiveness of family and individual therapy was considered for those diagnosed with schizophrenia. Cigna provided 6 years of data (2001–2006) for this analysis, which included more than 2,000 unique patient claims for outpatient psychotherapy. The outcome measures of interest included recidivism and dropout rates, total treatment cost, and cost-effectiveness. Results demonstrated that family therapy was more cost-effective than individual therapy, largely due to lower recidivism rates and lower total treatment costs. However, family therapy also had higher dropout rates than individual therapy.

Study Six (Morgan, Crane, Moore, & Eggett, 2013)

This study looked at the cost of treating substance use disorders for more than 14,208 unique patients with individual and family therapy. Survival analysis revealed that family therapy on average used 2.41 sessions, individual therapy used 3.38 sessions, and mixed therapy (i.e., individual and family treatment) used 6.40 sessions. When the typical cost of each type of therapy was factored in, the analysis showed that each treatment episode cost $124.55 for family therapy, $170.22 for individual therapy, and $319.55 for mixed therapy. The recidivism rate was lowest for family therapy (8.9 %), mixed therapy (9.5 %) and highest for individual therapy (12 %). Not surprisingly, LMFTs used family therapy as a treatment modality three times more than other professionals.

Study Seven (Fawcett & Crane, 2013)

The sample for this study consisted of 230 men and 189 women who had received treatment for sexual dysfunction between 2001 and 2006. Differences in outcome (i.e., recidivism, dropout, cost of treatment, and number of sessions) were compared by provider type (i.e., psychologists, social workers, MFTs, and PCs) and modality (i.e., individual, family, or mixed therapy). Overall, the results showed that the average number of sessions was seven, and that MFTs use family and mixed modalities more often than other provider types. Additionally, it was found that mixed therapy had substantially lower dropout rates, suggesting that a combination of individual and family treatment may improve clinical outcomes.

Study Eight (Crane et al., 2012)

The same outcomes used by Fawcett and Crane (2013) were considered for 149 patients with somatoform disorder, both as a complete sample and based on provider type. Initial descriptive statistics for all patients revealed that those with somatoform disorder experienced higher than average recidivism and participated in more sessions (regardless of provider type), while dropout rates were consistent with previous studies (e.g., Hamilton et al., 2011). The analysis also showed that there was no significant difference in terms of total cost or dropouts between the various professions or between masters level vs. doctoral level providers.

Study Nine (Crane et al., 2013)

In this study, claims data for 164,667 patients diagnosed with depression were examined. Of interest was whether there would be differences in total cost and cost-effectiveness based on modality or provider type and whether various factors like age, gender, modality, provider type, etc., would account for differences in recidivism. Consistent with a number of the studies listed above (e.g., Crane & Payne, 2011), the results indicated that MFTs provided services that resulted in the lowest recidivism rate. However, contrary to the findings of Crane and Payne (2011), services provided by MFTs in this study were the least costly.

Study Ten (Fawcett, 2012)

This study explored the influence of practitioner license type, therapy modality, diagnosis, age, and gender on behavioral health therapy for children and adolescents. Participants included 106,374 boys (53.2 %) and 93,753 girls (46.8 %) ages 3–18 ($M = 12.1$, SD = 3.9), who were treated in outpatient facilities throughout the United States. Results indicate that there are differences in dropout, recidivism, cost, and treatment length by provider license, therapy modality, diagnosis, age, and gender. Specifically, results suggest that marriage and family therapists have the lowest percent recidivism and are among the lowest in terms of dropout and cost-effectiveness. The results also suggest that family therapy is more cost-effective than individual or mixed therapy and that mixed therapy has a much lower percent of dropout than individual or family therapy. Analysis by diagnosis suggests a potential severity scale based on dropout, recidivism, and number of sessions. There were also significant differences in dropout and recidivism by age suggesting that younger children are more likely to drop out of treatment. These results provide valuable information about behavioral health treatment of children and adolescents. Specifically, utilizing a family based approach may help reduce the total length of treatment while utilizing a mixed mode approach to therapy may help reduce the risk of dropout from treatment. Also, some diagnoses appear to be more difficult to treat, with higher percentages of dropout and requiring more time and money for successful treatment.

Study Eleven (Ballard, 2013)

This study examined the costs of pervasive developmental disorder (PDD) treatment in a large healthcare organization. Participants ($N = 2{,}095$) included individuals who had been diagnosed with a PDD, including autistic disorder (DSM IV 299.0) and pervasive developmental disorder—not otherwise specified (DSM IV

299.80)—and who received behavioral health care via Cigna during 2001–2006. Participants were seen in outpatient clinics. Participants' ages range from 1 to 61 ($M = 11.05$, $SD = 7.45$). Sixty-seven percent of participants were children (ages 1–12), 22 % were adolescents (ages 13–17), and 11 % were adults (18 or older). The majority of the participants were male (81.7 %, $n = 1{,}712$), 17.9 % ($n = 376$) of the participants were female, and gender was not reported for 7 participants. Almost 18 % ($n = 375$) of participants were diagnosed with autistic disorder and 79.1 % ($n = 1{,}657$) were diagnosed with pervasive developmental disorder—not otherwise specified. When compared to individual therapy and mixed therapy, family therapy had significantly fewer sessions, fewer episodes of care, and better cost-effectiveness. Individual therapy had significantly shorter treatment length than mixed therapy. There were no differences in treatment length or number of episodes by license, but dropout and cost-effectiveness were significantly different. MDs had the highest dropout and best cost-effectiveness, while MFTs had the lowest dropout and MSWs (e.g., LICSWs) had the poorest cost-effectiveness. Children had significantly higher dropout than other age groups. An autism diagnosis was associated with fewer sessions but additional episodes of care when compared to PDD. Having a comorbid diagnosis is associated with longer treatment length but slightly fewer episodes of care.

Findings from Training Clinic Data

This research took place in a university-based student training clinic that provides opportunities for masters and doctoral level students. Students from the Marriage and Family Therapy, Clinical Psychology, and Social Work programs served as providers to local individuals, couples, and families who requested psychotherapy services. Data were collected at therapy intake (prospective) and focused on the interrelationships between families and health, with the intent of investigating the potential for a medical offset effect after therapy. Retrospective data were also collected regarding healthcare use for 6 months before therapy, 6 months during therapy, and 6 months after therapy concluded.

Study One (Jakubowski et al., 2008)

One of the biggest issues with conducting research regarding healthcare services use and cost-effectiveness is the lack of access to medical records. In an effort to address this issue, this study sought to determine if self-reported medical use could be considered an accurate and valid measure in healthcare research. The sample in this study was 60 % female, 94 % White non-Hispanic, and had an average age of 31 years. Six months of medical records for 130 patients were gathered and compared to self-reported medical use for the same time period. Additionally, family members were asked to report on the healthcare use of their spouse and oldest children for the same period. In both cases, medical record and self-reported healthcare use were found to be highly correlated, suggesting that researchers can substitute self-report for medical records in research efforts. In addition, spouses were reasonably able to report their partners' and their children's healthcare use, suggesting that only one informant is necessary for healthcare research on families.

Study Two (Crane, Christenson, Shaw, Fawcett, & Marshall, 2010)

Although a significant number of researchers have investigated factors that predict healthcare service use for individuals, almost none have attempted to ascertain the impact of systemic influences. Two studies were conducted to investigate predictors of healthcare use among persons seeking help for relationship problems. In the first study, the dependent variable was children's healthcare use, and the independent variables were derived from a series of biopsychosocial measures administered to their parents ($N = 60$) at intake. Best subsets regression was used to determine the variable that accounted for the most variance in children's healthcare use. Results showed that parents' marital cohesion and life satisfaction were the strongest correlates and accounted for 46 % of the variance in healthcare use. In this model, a decrease in parent life satisfaction was associated with an increase in healthcare use by the child.

Study Three (Christenson, Crane, Hafen, Hamilton, & Schaalje, 2011)

The second study investigating correlates of healthcare use focused on a sample of adults seeking services for relationship problems and included 110 participants. The sample in this study was 66 % female, 96 % White non-Hispanic, and had an average age of 31 years. Given the dramatic reduction in healthcare use by high utilizers following therapy (Law et al., 2003), a subsample of these participants were selected out for analysis as well ($n = 40$). For the complete sample, the two variables that accounted for the most variance were "informational support" (i.e., the availability of advice and guidance) and "somatization." "Hostility" (e.g., having an urge to break things) was the strongest correlate for healthcare use in the high utilizer group. Interestingly, hostility accounted for as much as 36 % of the variance in healthcare use in the model for high utilizers. The findings of this study suggest that targeting certain psychosocial variables may promote greater reductions in healthcare use after therapy.

Study Four (Christenson, Crane, Law, Schaalje, & Marshall, under review)

This study considered healthcare use for 56 participants across three time periods (6 months before therapy, 6 months after the start of therapy, and 6–12 months after). Descriptive statistics showed that the sample was largely homogeneous in terms of race (96 % White non-Hispanic). Annual income was diverse, however, ranging from $2,500 to over $100,000. When healthcare use from the first time period (T1) was compared to the second 6 months (T2), persons who received family therapy showed a significant (44 %) decrease in healthcare use. There was also a slight increase in healthcare use during the third 6-month period (T3); however, from T1 to T3, there was still an overall decrease of 33 % in healthcare use. In addition, when biopsychosocial factors (e.g., behavior control, relationship satisfaction, and perceived criticism) were included in the analysis, participants who reported an improvement in general family functioning after treatment showed a significant 58 % decrease in healthcare use from T1 to T3, while those who did not improve in this regard showed no decrease in healthcare use.

Additional Findings Related to MFTs

In conjunction with the effort to argue for coverage of MFTs under Medicare, there was a need to demonstrate how much this additional coverage would add in terms of costs to the program (Christenson & Crane, 2004). Trends in healthcare use expenditures for Medicare were determined for a historical 3-year period. These trends were then used to make future projections for how the inclusion of MFTs as providers would affect the bottom line. Using established methods for estimating costs (including both induced costs and the substitution effect), it was determined that the true costs of including MFTs as providers would add less than $3 million per year to the Medicare budget. When compared against the entire Medicare budget, services provided by MFTs would account for less than 0.0015 % of total spending.

Morgan and Crane (2010) identified and reviewed eight cost-effectiveness family-based substance abuse treatment studies. The purpose of this review was to move past the limitations of considering clinical outcomes alone, instead focusing on the cost-effectiveness of family-based interventions and providing summary information across studies. The eight articles reviewed in this study were published between 1991 and 2006 and covered treatment for alcohol and substance abuse among both adolescents and adults. The outcomes for each study varied, though all studies included common indicators such as number of days sober and improvement in psychosocial functioning. The most relevant finding from this review was that despite encouragement from the research community to conduct cost-effectiveness analyses, to date few studies have done so in relation to substance abuse treatment. However, Morgan and Crane (2010) also showed that among studies with comparative data, three of the five studies showed that family-based treatment was more cost-effective than individual therapy.

Given the increasing amount of research showing that family therapy is an effective form of treatment, and sometimes the preferred intervention, Crane et al. (2010) deemed it prudent to investigate how much training each of the major behavioral health provider types receive in this modality. Content analysis was used to determine how much family therapy training is required in the standards for the six core behavioral health provider types (psychiatry, psychiatric nursing, clinical psychology, professional counseling, social work, and marriage and family therapy). Overall, the results for the 50 United States revealed that MFTs have three times more required systems-based coursework than any of the other professions and 16 times more face-to-face therapy hours required for licensure. Thus, MedFTs may wish to seek out programs or training opportunities that can maximize skills in relational assessment, diagnosing, intervening, and evaluation of utilization and effectiveness particularly as they relate to healthcare systems.

Themes and Implications

At the present time, there is a consensus that family therapy interventions are effective for a wide range of presenting problems (e.g., Sprenkle, 2012; Stratton, 2011) particularly those that are commonly seen in healthcare contexts. These types of interventions seem to be clinically effective and the studies within this review demonstrate that they are cost-effective. Thus, the results from these studies may be particularly relevant conversation points for MedFTs as they interface with healthcare administrators, financial reimbursers, and policy makers.

Despite showing good clinical results, there has been an overall inattention to costs when considering outcomes. This is especially troubling given that public and private discourse about the current healthcare market is dominated by cost considerations (Christenson & Crane, 2004; Cummings, O'Donohue, & Cummings, 2008). Much like what has been the case with medical offset research (Law et al., 2003), family therapy and medical family therapy have not yet fully realized the importance of demonstrating cost-effectiveness and how related findings may benefit market share. Cummings et al. (2008), approaching the issue from the perspective of Psychologists, argue that Psychologists' unwillingness to address costs has led to "a precipitous decline in their practices and in their incomes" (p. 32). Individual psychotherapy practitioners have awoken to this reality and have pushed to improve conditions for reimbursement (e.g., Kessler, 2008). Unless there is a commensurate and concerted effort to show that family therapy and MedFT are cost-effective, both are at risk (at best) of becoming marginalized in the healthcare market and (at worst) becoming irrelevant.

The research conducted by Crane and colleagues has sought to address this significant gap in the literature. Research outlined above shows that family therapy services are not very expensive to provide and may be less expensive than services provided by other professionals (e.g., MDs, psychologists) without any significant increases in recidivism or dropout. Additionally, family therapy appears to be associated with reductions in other types of healthcare use following therapy, especially for those who are considered high utilizers. Furthermore, MFTs and MedFTs are uniquely qualified to provide the couple and family services that have demonstrated effectiveness. The evidence presented here supports the argument that family therapy (as a distinct treatment modality) is a cost-effective means of delivering quality services to patients and that MFTs (as a distinct profession) are cost-effective providers of psychotherapy. Since systemically trained providers are cost-effective and systemically based psychotherapy is cost-effective, then it is likely that MedFTs are also cost-effective and provide medical cost-offsets to healthcare contexts.

However, despite the consistency of results across the studies, there are limitations that should be considered. Data presented here were archival, longitudinal, and retrospective (with the exception of the training clinic data). The strength of these data is that it is possible to investigate treatment as it occurs in the "real world" of healthcare delivery, as opposed to studies of tightly controlled laboratory studies of manualized treatment. The weakness of these data lies in the availability of various behavioral health providers being uneven. Some patients may have limited choices in what professional groups are available to them (e.g., perhaps there are not any, or only a few, MFTs or MedFTs on staff).

In addition, some patients may not be aware of differences in the professional training of the behavioral health disciplines or may select providers based upon unclear expectations about what they will receive. In these cases, one may be "comparing apples to oranges," but in the world of health services research, one must use the data that are available. In addition, there is no evidence that any of the results presented here are inherently biased for or against any treatment modality or for or against different professional groups.

Additionally, because the data from our HMO source, Medicaid, and Cigna are archival and based on claims reporting, it is impossible to link clinical outcomes as typically measured (e.g., standardized assessments) to cost data. Recidivism is one method for evaluating clinical outcomes, but not returning to therapy could also be related to dissatisfaction or with higher levels of treatment severity as with a remission of symptoms. In any case, although high dropout rates can be a driver of low-cost therapy, they almost certainly are not a good measure of clinical improvement or relief of human suffering.

Accordingly, cause and effect relationships cannot be determined from these data, and interpretations of the value of services by different provider types should be made with caution. Of course, the opposing view (as highlighted above) is that real-world demonstrations of cost-effectiveness are important because they represent what happens within naturally occurring behavioral health delivery systems. It is expected that this debate will continue for the foreseeable future.

Future Directions

Perhaps the most salient issue revealed by this review is what is still lacking in the cost-effectiveness research. Too often research in family therapy and MedFT demonstrate disconnects between clinical outcomes and costs. Numerous articles are produced to demonstrate that family therapy produces changes in psychosocial functioning without providing information on how much the intervention costs to deliver. In fact, a review of the recent 2012 special issue of the *Journal of Marital and Family Therapy* (Volume, 38, Number 1) revealed almost no information on costs in over 280 pages of information about MFT effectiveness and efficacy research.

In order to secure the place of MFT and MedFT in the healthcare market, researchers will need to simultaneously evaluate the costs and benefits of the interventions they develop. This is especially true in the case of MedFT, given the inclination of healthcare policy makers, hospitals, and insurance companies to see these specialized forms of treatment as simply an additional cost. Demonstrating effectiveness on this level would require that cost data be collected during the process of conducting outcome research and used to demonstrate cost-effectiveness.

One of the most basic methods of demonstrating cost-effectiveness is to take two interventions with similar outcomes (as demonstrated by effect sizes) and show comparative costs for delivering the intervention. If one is less expensive than the other, with equal outcomes, an argument can be made that the less expensive version is preferable. This method has been used effectively to demonstrate that cognitive behavioral psychotherapy is less expensive than psychopharmacological interventions for panic disorder (e.g., Gould, Otto, & Pollack, 1995). Cummings et al. (2008) make the persuasive argument that it is high time we learn the rules of a competitive market place, which dictate that if two products are equally good, the more costly one will soon disappear.

Although a simple comparative method would clearly support interventions that are less expensive to deliver initially, what about interventions that are inherently more expensive? Fortunately, there are ways to demonstrate that a substantially more expensive intervention produces far-reaching effects in terms of cost savings. This has been effectively demonstrated by proponents of Multisystemic Therapy (MST) such as Kleitz, Borduin and Schaeffer (2010), who used cost-benefit analysis to demonstrate that the net cumulative benefit of MST was a savings of $199,374 to victims and taxpayers (per participant), compared to a cost of $10,882 to provide the treatment (per participant).

This type of analysis requires that the researchers consider not only the costs associated with providing the treatment but also the factor in the benefits, usually by placing a monetary value on the identified benefits. MedFT research would be a particularly fruitful area to apply cost-benefit methodology. It is not difficult to imagine that cost savings from the medical offset effect, improved adherence to treatment recommendations, increased work productivity, and a decrease in malpractice suits (to name just a few) would far outweigh the perceived increased costs associated with an integrated care model. Some research within the field of Psychology has already shown that integrated care may be associated with a 20–30 % reduction in costs (beyond the cost of additional services) when a psychologist is included as part of the care team (Cummings et al., 2008). As MedFT grows, it will be imperative that researchers show similar benefits.

Advocacy

One final consideration is how policy can be shaped to encourage greater market share for family therapy and MedFT. Two approaches are most often considered in the literature. First, Crane (2008) discussed the importance of having satisfied consumers make the case to insurance companies that the services that family therapists provide are valuable. This type of grassroots effort has the potential to raise awareness among stakeholders about what services are in demand, which can ultimately affect decisions about which services to cover. Crane (2008) rightly pointed out, however, that clinicians must use caution and ensure that they are not unduly influencing patients to advocate for a profession. Nevertheless, it can be very helpful for patients to provide feedback about what services work and what they would like to see in their plans.

The second commonly described method is advocacy on the part of practitioners. When a particular service is not covered, practitioners can contact the insurance companies to argue for changes in their policies. Kessler (2008) described a number of examples of practitioners (armed with research) encouraging policy makers to modify their policies with positive results. These types of efforts are best carried out when the practitioner has at his or her disposal the evidence that (a) his or her services are as or more effective to what is already being provided and (b) that the services result in cost savings to the system. There are few policy makers who would not be interested in learning how to decrease costs, while also providing high quality services.

Research has made substantial progress on the first part of this argument (though less so for MedFT), and it is time to get started on demonstrating comprehensive cost savings. With this type of evidence available, practitioners will be well equipped to secure a place in the ever changing healthcare market.

Discussion Questions

All of the studies presented in this chapter use archival and retrospective data.

1. What are the strengths and weaknesses of this type of research?

2. In considering the chapter as a whole, what arguments can you make for including family therapy as a treatment option in healthcare management systems?
3. Similarly, what arguments can you make for including marriage and family therapists as a profession in healthcare management systems?
4. How can cost-effectiveness research inform clinical practice?
5. Please discuss the principles of the "medical offset." What theory would you use to understand the concept and present the evidence for and against the assumptions of the concept?

References[1]

Ballard, J. (2013). *Cost effectiveness of treating pervasive developmental disorders: A comparison by treatment modality*. (Unpublished master's thesis). Brigham Young University, Provo, UT.

Chiang, F. F. (2011). *The cost effectiveness of individual and family therapy for schizophrenia in managed care*. (Unpublished master's thesis). Brigham Young University, Provo, UT.

Christenson, J. D., & Crane, D. R. (2004). Estimating the cost of direct reimbursement of marriage and family therapy under Medicare. *Journal of Marital and Family Therapy, 30*, 515–525. doi:10.1111/j.1752-0606.2004.tb01259.x.

*Christenson, J. D., Crane, D. R., Beer, A. R., Bell, K. M., & Hillin, H. H. (in press). Family Intervention and Health Care Costs for Kansas Medicaid Patients with Schizophrenia. *Journal of Marital and Family Therapy*. doi:10.1111/jmft.12021

*Christenson, J. D., Crane, D. R., Hafen, M., Hamilton, S., & Schaalje, G. B. (2011). Predictors of health care use among individuals seeking therapy for marital and family problems: An exploratory study. *Contemporary Family Therapy: An International Journal., 33*, 441–460. doi:10.1007/s10591-011-9159-1.

Christenson, J. D., Crane, D. R., Law, D. D., Schaalje, B., & Marshall, E. (under review). *The effect of marital and family therapy on health care use*.

Crane, D. R. (2008). The cost effectiveness of family therapy: A summary and progress report. *Journal of Family Therapy, 30*, 399–410. doi:10.1111/j.1467-6427.2008.00443.x.

*Crane, D. R., & Christenson, J. D. (2008). The medical offset effect: Patterns in outpatient services reduction for high utilizers of health care. *Contemporary Family Therapy: An International Journal, 30*, 127–138. doi:10.1007/s10591-008-9058-2.

Crane, D. R., Christenson, J. D., Dobbs, S. M., Schaalje, G. B., Moore, A. M., Pedal, F. F. C., … Marshall, E. S. (2013). Costs of treating depression with individual versus family therapy. *Journal of Marital and Family Therapy 39(4)*, 457–469, doi:10.1111/j.1752-0606.2012.00326.x

Crane, D. R., Christenson, J. D., Shaw, A. L., Fawcett, D., & Marshall, E. S. (2010). Predictors of health care use for children of marriage and family therapy clients. *Journal of Couple and Relationship Therapy, 9*, 277–292. doi:10.1080/15332691.2010.515530.

Crane, D. R., Hillin, H., & Jakubowski, S. (2005). Costs of treating conduct disordered Medicaid youth with and without family therapy. *The American Journal of Family Therapy, 33*, 403–413. doi:10.1080/01926180500276810.

Crane, D. R., Morton, L. B., Fawcett, D., Moore, A. M., Larson, J., & Sandberg, J. (2012). Somatoform disorder: Treatment utilization and cost by mental health professions.

[1] An asterisk has been use to note references that the chapter authors recommend for further reading.

Contemporary Family Therapy: An International Journal., *34*, 322–333. doi:10.1007/s10591-012-9182-x.

*Crane, D. R., & Payne, S. H. (2011). Individual and family therapy in managed care: Comparing the costs of treatment by the mental health professions. *Journal of Marital and Family Therapy*, *37*, 273–289. doi:10.1111/j.1752-0606.2009.00170.x.

Crane, D. R., Shaw, A. L., Christenson, J. D., Larson, J. H., Harper, J. M., & Feinauer, L. L. (2010). Comparison of the family therapy educational and experience requirements for licensure or certification in six mental health disciplines. *The American Journal of Family Therapy*, *38*, 357–373. doi:10.1080/01926187.2010.513895.

Crane, D. R., Wood, N. D., Law, D. D., & Schaalje, B. (2004). The relationship between therapist characteristics and decreased medical utilization: An exploratory study. *Contemporary Family Therapy: An International Journal*, *26*, 61–69. doi:10.1023/B:COFT.0000016912.25239.52.

*Cummings, N. A., O'Donohue, W. T., & Cummings, J. L. (2008). The financial dimension of integrated behavioral/primary care. *Journal of Clinical Psychology in Medical Settings*, *16*, 31–39. doi:10.1007/s10880-008-9139-2.

Fawcett, D. (2012). *Mental health treatment for children and adolescents: Cost effectiveness, dropout, and recidivism by presenting diagnosis and therapy modality*. (Unpublished doctoral dissertation). Brigham Young University, Provo, UT.

Fawcett, D., & Crane, D. R. (2013). The influence of profession and therapy type for sexual dysfunction. *Journal of Sex & Marital Therapy*, *39*(5), 453–465. doi:10.1080/0092623X.2012.665814.

Gould, R. A., Otto, M. W., & Pollack, M. H. (1995). A meta-analysis of treatment outcomes for panic disorder. *Clinical Psychology Review*, *15*, 819–844.

Hamilton, S., Moore, A. M., Crane, D. R., & Payne, S. H. (2011). Psychotherapy dropouts: Differences by modality, license, and DSM-IV diagnosis. *Journal of Marital and Family Therapy*, *37*, 333–343. doi:10.1111/j.1752-0606.2010.00204.x.

Jakubowski, S. F., Crane, D. R., Christenson, J. D., Miller, R. B., Marshall, E. S., & Hafen, M. (2008). Marriage and family therapy research in health care: Investigating the accuracy of self and family reports of medical use. *The American Journal of Family Therapy*, *36*, 437–448. doi:10.1080/01926180701441320.

*Kessler, R. (2008). Integration of care is about money too: The health and behavior codes as an element of a new financial paradigm. *Families, Systems, and Health*, *26*, 207–216. doi:10.1037/a0011918.

Kleitz, S. J., Borduin, C. M., & Schaeffer, C. M. (2010). Cost-benefit analysis of multisystemic therapy with serious and violent juvenile offenders. *Journal of Family Psychology*, *24*, 657–666.

*Law, D. D., & Crane, D. R. (2000). The influence of marital and family therapy on health care utilization in a health maintenance organization. *Journal of Marital and Family Therapy*, *26*, 281–291. doi:10.1111/j.1752-0606.2000.tb00298.x.

Law, D. D., Crane, D. R., & Berge, J. (2003). The influence of marital and family therapy on high utilizers of health care. *Journal of Marital and Family Therapy*, *29*, 353–363. doi:10.1111/j.1752-0606.2000.tb00298.x.

Lindström, E., & Bingefors, K. (2000). Patient compliance with drug therapy in schizophrenia: Economic and clinical issues. *PharmacoEconomics*, *18*, 105–124.

Moore, A. M., & Crane, D. R. (in press). Relational Diagnosis and Psychotherapy Treatment Cost Effectiveness. *Contemporary Family Therapy: An International Journal*. doi:10.1007/s10591-013-9277-z.

Moore, A. M., Hamilton, S., Crane, D. R., & Fawcett, D. (2011). The influence of professional license type on the outcome of family therapy. *The American Journal of Family Therapy*, *39*, 149–161. doi:10.1080/01926187.2010.530186.

Morgan, T. B., & Crane, D. R. (2010). Cost-effectiveness of family-based substance abuse treatment. *Journal of Marital and Family Therapy*, *36*, 486–498. doi:10.1111/j.1752-0606.2010.00195.x.

Morgan, T. B., Crane, D. R., Moore, A. M., & Eggett, D. L. (2013). The cost of treating substance use disorders: Individual versus family therapy. *Journal of Family Therapy, 35*, 2–23. doi:10.1111/j.1467-6427.2012.00589.x.

Sprenkle, D. H. (2012). Intervention research in couple and family therapy: A methodological and substantive review and an introduction to the special issues. *Journal of Marital and Family Therapy, 38*, 3–29. doi:10.1111/j.1752-0606.2011.00271.x.

*Stratton, P. (2011). *The evidence base of systemic family and couples therapies*. London: Association for Family Therapy, United Kingdom.

Chapter 23
Getting Reimbursed for MedFT: Financial Models Toward Sustainability

Dan Marlowe, Jeff Capobianco, and Carl Greenberg

The 2010 Patient Protection and Affordable Care Act (ACA) has created the largest change to healthcare funding since the inception of Medicaid and Medicare over 40 years ago (Manchikanti, Caraway, Parr, Fellows, & Hirsch, 2011). In this chapter, financing integrated approaches to care will be discussed. Today's healthcare professional must understand that this new funding landscape is still evolving as providers, insurance companies, states, and the federal government test different approaches to bundling payments that tie care coordination, patient satisfaction, and healthcare processes and outcomes to funding. Until new bundled payment approaches are designed and implemented, the current fee-for-service approaches will remain in place.

In the United States, there are four primary funding mechanisms for health care: Medicaid, Medicare, commercial insurance, and out of pocket. The ACA has provisions for expanding Medicaid in all states (Patient Protection and Affordable Care Act, 2010). However, as a result of the US Supreme Court ruling in the case of *National Federation of Independent Business v. Sebelius* where the ACA was challenged, states were given a lot of latitude in how or whether Medicaid funding would be expanded. States were not allowed, however, to change provisions in the ACA impacting Medicare or commercial insurance.

For MedFTs working in primary care, it is imperative to understand how to bill for services in a logical, efficient way that best matches the needs of the patients and system. If a behavioral health service or the particular license of the MedFT is not billable, the MedFT needs to consider how to document and track services in order to be able to describe how his work creates other system-wide gains (e.g., how MedFT services assist a primary care provider (PCP) to be more productive, end her shift on time, generate lower recidivism or emergency room visits for the same diagnosis/complaint). Another possibility is to assess whether the inclusion of a MedFT leads to a cost-offset. For example, federally qualified health centers are

D. Marlowe (✉)
Campbell University's School of Osteopathic Medicine, Buies Creek, NC, USA
e-mail: marlowed@campbell.edu

J. Hodgson et al. (eds.), *Medical Family Therapy*, DOI 10.1007/978-3-319-03482-9_23,

paid a flat rate for a PCP service. So, if a PCP spends 15 min or an hour with a patient, they are paid the same amount. If a MedFT working in a primary care team cannot bill for some of her services due to state-specific billing restrictions, she can create cost-offsets by supporting the PCP with patients (e.g., those who are struggling with behavior change related to weight loss, pain, or who become emotional) and free up the PCP to see other billable patients. New approaches to reimbursement will emerge as health processes, outcomes, and patient satisfaction are aligned with integrated care and attributed to more productive ways of extending care. During this time of transition, it is important that MedFTs monitor the development of funding designs at the federal, state, and local levels.

As of this writing, a number of approaches to financing integrated care have been established that may be beneficial for MedFTs. Examples include the Health and Behavioral Health Assessment/Intervention 9,600 series (AMA, 2013) of Current Procedural Terminology (CPT) codes that allow for billing behavioral health services for nonmental health or non-substance-use-related conditions if indicated by the primary care provider. These codes are billable through Medicare, and states differ as to whether the codes can be billed through Medicaid. The Screening Brief Intervention and Referral for Treatment (SBIRT) codes allow for primary care providers to refer patients who screen positive for substance use disorders for treatment with a behavioral health clinician. The SBIRT codes are state-specific, meaning that the state Medicaid authority must "turn the codes on" in order for a provider in that state to bill for the services. Each state has a variety of Medicaid codes that are billable, if the state chooses to allow providers within that state to bill for services. Many states restrict what providers can bill for, or leave codes "turned off," to restrict the outflow of Medicaid dollars. For example, some states will not allow a primary care provider and a MedFT to bill for a service to the same patient on the same day, the so-called two services in one day rule. The federal government allows for this, but some states do not. All states that are marked in blue (see photo below) support same-day billing.

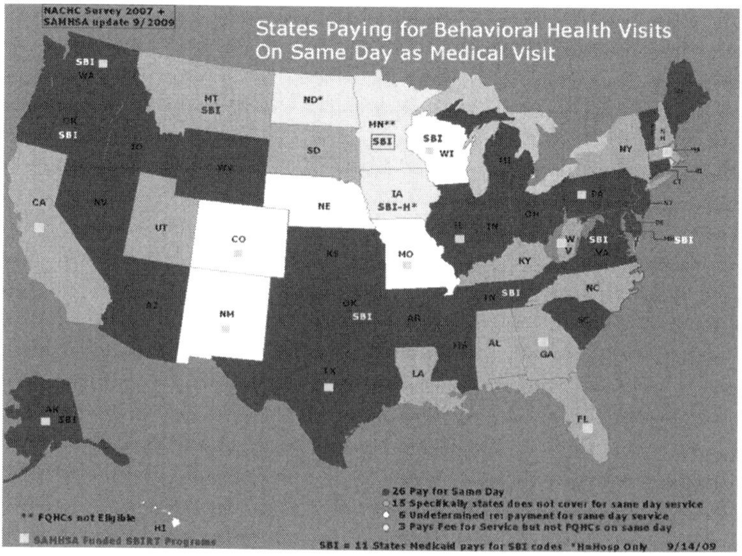

For instances, when two or more clinics are collaborating in order to integrate behavioral and primary care services, there are several options for how to best leverage funds. A community mental health (CMH) provider may collaborate with a federally qualified health center, hospital clinic, or primary care provider group by arranging for one or more primary care providers to rent space in the CMH clinic where primary care services can be provided in coordination with the CMH staff and providers. This allows for case management services, which are typically not billable through primary care, to be provided in direct consultation with the PCP(s). Or, conversely, a PCP might contract with a CMH clinic to have the MedFT work out of the primary care clinic. The specific funding design depends on the community (e.g., some communities have levies or local funding that can be used to offset the cost of the uninsured or underinsured) and the state (e.g., some states have waivers with the Federal Center for Medicaid and Medicare Services (CMS) or contracts with commercial insurance and/or managed care companies that allow for creative approaches to funding integrated services; see http://www.integration.samhsa.gov for additional resources pertaining to federally approved sate waivers and integration). Additional resources also exist on health reform by state (http://www.integratedcareresourcecenter.com), transformations that are underway for publicly funded health care (http://www.chcs.org), and frameworks to measure integrated care (http://integrationacademy.ahrq.gov/atlas).

Now more than ever, clinical and administrative staff must be able to explain how the cost of care is linked to care provision processes, patient outcomes, and satisfaction with their care. This will require that providers understand how preventative services, patient education, and activation (i.e., patient follow-through with treatment recommendations and health behavior change) can lead to reduced hospitalizations and emergency room visits which are the main targets for cost containment. Fortunately, the ACA mandates the moving away from the fee-for-service/fee-for-procedure-based approach and toward an approach which emphasizes prevention, patient education, and activation which can only be achieved if there is a strong provider-patient relationship. This leaves MedFTs uniquely positioned to increase the number and kind of services delivered, especially given their expertise in rapport building and ability to bridge medical and behavioral health services. These opportunities and services help to not only improve patient's health, but also improve the financial health of the healthcare system as a whole. The following are two examples of the ways in which MedFTs can succeed in a healthcare system in spite of the existing financial challenges and changing landscape. One example is from the western United States and the other from the eastern United States.

A Model from the West

My (CG) experience in Medical Family Therapy spans 30 years of practice that occurred in four different healthcare settings, all in the western United States. Each context has been different in terms of possible reimbursement options, including both strengths and challenges with public and private insurance companies for services provided. The settings have also been unique in determining the role of MedFT, based on patient needs and the model for sustainability.

A Private Practice Setting

My initial experience was in a private practice setting as a partner to a psychiatrist, who was trained as a family therapist by Carl Whitaker. As both of us saw patients that crossed the boundaries of medicine and family therapy, I began to get experience in what would later be called Medical Family Therapy. As a MedFT in this setting, I had to learn about psychiatric medications and began to understand the implications of how those meds impacted my patients. This was both a daily and weekly occurrence. The majority of my workload was clinical practice or paperwork pertaining to patients' needs through strong collaboration with the psychiatrist via traditional therapy sessions.

Getting paid for my services meant that I had to first be accepted on a particular insurance company's panel. At that time, getting on insurance panels was not often easy, as insurance companies could selectively choose who to accept. It was not until the Marriage and Family Therapy (MFT) Licensing Law was passed in Washington (which mandated insurance companies to accept MFTs on panels) that MFTs were able to be reimbursed for services similar to any other mental health discipline. In other words, if an insurance company decided they would accept Social Workers on their panels, they then also had to accept MFTs and Mental Health Counselors.

A Family Medicine Residency Setting

I left private practice to take the job of Behavioral Science Faculty in a family medicine residency program. My work there as a MedFT consisted of seeing patients in the clinic and teaching residents about (and how to assess for) depression, anxiety, and other mental health issues. This needed to be done in the context of a 10–15 min time slot (within patient appointments). This shift from traditional sessions to truncated appointment times demanded that I learn and become competent in healthcare culture. MedFTs must be bicultural, continuously crossing the bridge between mental and medical health care.

During a typical work week, I would be a part of the rounds for our patients within the hospital alongside the residents and faculty members who were in charge of the inpatient service. My responsibility in that setting was to ensure that any mental health issues were not only addressed, but that they became part of residents' normal thinking about hospitalized patients. This extended to incorporating family issues and concerns as well.

Given that I had already established myself on insurance panels, billing and getting reimbursement for patients was not an issue. However, many patients were either uninsured or were on Medicaid or Medicare, insurances that I could not bill directly. Fortunately, funding for my position did not rely on breaking even or making a profit, so there were many patients that were seen for either a low fee or no fee at all. As a result, residents would often provide integrated care with me when I saw patients, so that the resident could bill for the services that were provided as allowed by Medicaid. Through my 14 years with the program, finances became more and more of an issue and my caseload increased as the need to bill for all services became necessary. On average, behavioral science faculty spent at least 2 days a week seeing patients in order to fund a part of their salary line.

A Psychiatric Practice Setting

Following my tenure in a family medicine residency program, I went to work for a practice with five psychiatrists and three MedFTs. As part of a normal work week, I would often see patients who had medical issues and had been referred by their physician. It was important to keep the physician up-to-date on the progress of the therapy. Billing for the contact with the physician was not allowed, so that had to become something that was done during the session with the patient. I would sit with patients and discuss what we needed to tell their physicians and then compose that communication with them. The rest of the billing for my time was consistent with normal billing procedures in that I would document the sessions and fill out the necessary paperwork so that my biller could submit that to the patients' respective insurance companies.

Since this was a for-profit practice, there was an emphasis on billing for services. Most of the billing was fairly routine, but there was one significant difference that is worth mentioning. The largest HMO in the region recognized the importance of patients' needs for psychiatric care and agreed to pay therapists who saw their patients, even if they were not on the program's list of preferred providers.

A Cancer Treatment Center

After this, I transitioned to an oncology setting. The practice consists of 24 physicians, several mid-level providers and three full-time salaried therapists. The practice made it clear that they did not expect the therapists to break even, but rather were providing an on-site service to those in need of help in dealing with the emotional stress of cancer. Surprisingly, we did break even while also providing excellent patient care. This success was attributed to committed providers and diligent billing.

At this center, my typical day would involve seeing patients referred by one of the physicians within the system, often with their family members. It was typical to converse with several of the physicians either as curbside consults or to keep them informed as to what was transpiring with their patients. Practices that were helpful in my work included consistent communication with the physicians, learning about the medical side of the patients' struggles, language unique to oncology in order to better communicate between patients and their physicians, and being available on a moment's notice to help when the patient experienced a crisis that the physician did not feel comfortable handling.

There are two themes that emerged through the billing process that are worth discussing. First, it is important to get on as many insurance panels as possible, because that allows the therapist to bill independently when in an independent practice or to at least be more viable within diverse healthcare contexts. Without that ability, it may be difficult for a MedFT to be a financial asset to a team or to have sustainability in one's career. For example, I had to be able to bill for hospital visits which were often needed. To do so, I needed to become "privileged" at all four local hospitals. By becoming credentialed at these sites, I was reimbursed for my time at a greater rate than via regular clinic visits.

Second, there is the need for MedFTs to be fluent in the financial language and culture within healthcare systems. This facilitates the collegial relationship that must exist between providers, reimbursers, and financial officers. MedFTs must be able to understand and communicate about the costs for services, time, and space within their work contexts, while also recognizing the offset and benefits for lowered healthcare utilization, improved health outcomes, and better continuity in care. These elements toward financial sustainability are not unique to these settings in the west, but are equally relevant to models established in the eastern United States.

A Model from the East

As a MedFT, working in an integrated primary care (IPC) setting, billing for behavioral health services has always been a source of contention and consternation. Regardless of the venue, it seems that whenever and wherever I (DM) present on this topic, I am always faced with the same comment followed by the same question, "This all sounds great, it is just what we have been looking for, but how do we pay for it?" Many MedFTs who believe in IPC struggle with this question, because aside from providing the best standard of care (Robinson & Strosahl, 2009), an IPC model and the MedFT within it need to generate dollars and cents to thrive. If not, integrated care, regardless of its clinical worth, will be hard pressed to truly take hold in modern health care. The good news is that organizations willing to implement integrated care models are not necessarily looking to make a profit off of them. In fact, most organizations implement these models because they, too, believe IPC to be the best standard of care (Blount et al., 2007). However, while not necessarily looking to turn a profit, it has been my experience that these organizations do want to make sure that any model, at a minimum, is financially sustainable on its own merit.

While the billing process and structure discussed below occurred in a primary care setting, the general ideas and lessons learned are applicable regardless of the clinical setting itself. What follows is a discussion regarding how one organization's IPC model in the eastern United States was constructed to maximize financial sustainability while still improving the quality of patient care, along with a subsequent discussion of the specifics related to the billing process.

The Setting

This IPC model is based in a family medicine center that is part of a community-based family medicine residency program. At the time of this writing, there are 24 family medicine residents that clinically practice within the family medicine center, along with seven faculty physicians and three mid-level practitioners (e.g., physician assistants and nurse practitioners). Complementing the medical staff are both a PhD and master's level MedFTs who are also fully licensed as marriage and family therapists (i.e., LMFT), as well as an associate licensed predoctoral MedFT intern, all of whom function as behavioral health providers within the family medicine center. Of the 14,000 patients, there was a mix of payers, including Medicare, Tricare, Medicaid, commercial insurance, contract, and self-pay.

Model Development

The key to developing a sustainable model is making sure that the right people are involved from the very beginning and stay appropriately involved throughout the entire development process. Often, when designing a model, only the clinical and administrative staff are included, two of Peek's three worlds (2008). However, it is important to not confuse administrative policies and outcomes with financial needs, which often happens. To remedy this mistake, prior to the model's development, medical residents, clinical faculty, and the upper administration (e.g., CEO and VP) including the chief financial officer (CFO), business office manager, and coding specialist all met on a regular basis. Rather than developing and implementing the model first and only then trying to find ways to pay for the services, the team looked to the organization's financial experts to guide the initial development process. By including them from the very beginning, the team engendered a sense of ownership and buy-in from all participants, which is essential to implementing and sustaining any change to clinical practice.

The financial partners within the organization were generalists in terms of their expertise. They did not have the specific knowledge related to behavioral health or integrated care billing, which is much more complicated than traditional behavioral health billing alone. This lack of knowledge on their part meant that the MedFTs had to develop a fairly sophisticated working knowledge of both traditional behavioral health and integrated care billing from the very beginning. This was helpful for three reasons: (a) by working together, the team could clarify any incorrect information, (b) the MedFTs could give the billing office pertinent questions to ask when they began their own outside training (with external systems) related to behavioral health and IC billing, and (c) it took the guess workout of how to bill for an IC visit for the medical providers (described below).

It is also important to mention that the inclusion of the financial experts (i.e., CFO, business manager, and coding specialist) has continued throughout the implementation and evolution of the model. As the director, I (DM) meet monthly with the CFO to go over revenue. In addition, meetings take place with the business office manager to make sure that the charges in services were accepted for billing. The MedFTs also have a very good working relationship with the coding specialist, since she is the organizational expert on how notes needed to be written and services rendered for reimbursement.

The IPC Model

This IPC model follows the de facto recommendation of hybridizing traditional psychotherapy and consultation with a 40/60 split between the two-care delivery modalities (Robinson & Reiter, 2007). We maximize the MedFTs' traditional schedules by shortening their appointment times to 45 min, which in turn allows them to see one extra patient per half day. At any given time, there is at least one consultant available with two MedFTs seeing patients for traditional psychotherapy. Although ideally the MedFTs would be spending 60 % or more of their time engaged in consultation (Robinson & Reiter, 2007), the present reimbursement rates for integrated care services in North Carolina make sustaining a model like that impossible. Also, a large segment of the clinic's patient panel still requests traditional behavioral health services. So in effect, the team utilizes the highest reimbursable services (i.e., traditional psychotherapy) to subsidize the integrated half of the model.

Traditional Services. Medical providers within the family medicine center refer patients for mental health, behavioral health, and/or substance abuse issues. The MedFTs, like their family medicine counterparts, are generalists and treat patients regardless of age or presenting problem. From a documentation perspective, mental health issues are billed accordingly utilizing the Current Procedural Terminology (i.e., CPT) codes (AMA, 2013) related to both individual and family-oriented psychotherapy and are connected back to the appropriate mental health diagnosis (e.g., depression, anxiety, post-traumatic stress disorder). Providers are also encouraged to refer patients for behavioral health-related issues (e.g., treatment compliance, weight loss, smoking cessation) where MedFTs use either *Psychotherapy* or *Health*

Behavior Assessment and Intervention CPT codes depending on the nature of the presenting issue. It is important to remember that while psychotherapy codes must be tied to a mental health diagnosis, health assessment and behavior codes need to be tied to a medical diagnosis (e.g., diabetes, fatigue, back pain, congestive heart failure). The MedFTs also utilize the *Interactive Complexity* CPT add-on code, which is used when factors complicate the delivery of psychotherapeutic services (e.g., difficult communication patterns, family conflict in the room, developmental disabilities).

Integrated Services. Integrated services within the family medicine center typically involve consultation by the MedFTs during a patient's medical visit for behavioral and/or mental health-related issues. Only those consultations related to health behavior can be billed through the *Health Behavior and Assessment* CPT codes. However, even if a MedFT is consulted for a mental health issue (e.g., depression) yet the conversation deals with behaviorally addressing the physical symptom/s related to the diagnosis (e.g., fatigue), the MedFT can still bill for the consult through the *Health Behavior and Assessment* code, if the symptom is listed in the patient's chart. In some instances when the MedFT is consulted on mental health issues during a patient's visit, she is still able to bill under the *Psychotherapy* CPT codes. However, the patient will be charged a co-pay for these services whereas the *Health Behavior and Assessment* codes typically require no co-pay. Other codes that are utilized as a part of the IPC model are *Health Risk Assessment* (e.g., PHQ9), *Crisis Intervention*, and alcohol and substance use assessment (e.g., AUDIT and DAST) codes, although some of the assessments can mean a co-pay for the patient depending on the insurance carrier.

Caveats for Billing

One of the greatest barriers to implementing IC in this practice was the complexity of the billing structure for the IC services specifically, which is why it was imperative to involve the office manager and the coding specialist from the outset. Although the CPT code manual spells out the specifics of the service that is rendered, each insurance company has different rules regarding how and what can be billed in any individual visit as well as who can bill for the service. For example, while a private carrier might allow for a MedFT to bill for a health behavior assessment directly, another carrier (e.g., Medicaid) considers that a part of the medical provider's service (i.e., the medical visit). So, this means that the medical provider would need to *upcode* the level of their visit to include the MedFT's assessment/intervention, which essentially increases the overall cost of the medical visit due to the additional service. In this practice, when a medical provider needs to *upcode*, they use a *dummy code* within the EHR to capture the financial contribution of the MedFT. This is important, because a significant amount of the revenue generated though the behavioral health consultation was done this way, and without the coding system, it would be impossible to track.

Due to this level of complexity, the billing office created a spreadsheet of all the behavioral health codes used alongside the insurance company requirements for each code. The MedFTs memorized this form and when consulted by a medical provider, told him or her how they should code the visit based on the insurance and presenting problem. So, a MedFT tells the provider that he or she (a) upcodes their visit, (b) does nothing since the MedFT will bill directly, or that (c) this is a non-billable service. This way, the onus of knowledge is placed on the MedFT, which makes the model less cumbersome to the medical providers and more likely to be utilized regularly. The same protocol is used for the health risk and substance abuse assessments since they typically fall under the same reimbursement rules.

Incident to Billing. Another important aspect of billing in an IPC setting is the *incident to* provision for services, which are "services that are furnished incident to physician professional services in the physician's office. . .or in a patient's home" (Center for Medicare and Medicaid Services [CMS], 2013, p. 1). This allows for a MedFT to conduct psychotherapy with a patient that has an insurance carrier that the MedFT is not a part of, by billing under the primary care physician. This is especially important for IPC practices located in areas with closed mental health insurance panels or for providers who are not reimbursable for services via Medicare. However, in order to utilize this provision, the MedFT must be employed by the physician and/or group practice and the patient's primary physician must (a) provide the initial service (i.e., medical visit), (b) remain actively involved in the course of the treatment, and (c) provide direct supervision, meaning that they must be present in the building while the service is rendered (Center for Medicare & Medicaid Services, 2013).

Sustainability

In my experience, I have found that the key to sustaining integrated care is the same thing that allows for financial success when investing in the financial market—diversity. As previously mentioned, the MedFTs within our organization provide several different clinical services, all with varying degrees of profitability. By far, traditional psychotherapy is the most lucrative for our practice as well as the easiest in regard to the rules for billing and documentation. However, this is not to say that *integrated* services cannot be lucrative as well, albeit more complicated in terms of reimbursement. Below are some rough figures for each of the main services we provide utilizing Medicaid reimbursement rates in North Carolina (North Carolina Department of Health and Human Services, 2013; North Carolina Foundation for Advanced Health Programs, 2013); it is best to use Medicaid numbers because their rate is typically the lowest, thereby providing the most fiscally challenged circumstance for a MedFT.

The equation is as follows:

Number of encounters per week × $ for service × 50 weeks per year** = gross income.

A. Psychotherapy, 38–52 min: $50.89
 6 half days w/4 patients per half day = 24 patients per week
 24 × 50.89 × 50 = $ 61,068
B. Evidence-Based Screening (EBS; PHQ-9, GAD-7): $8.14
 20*** screenings per full day = 100 screenings per week
 100 × 8.14 × 50 = $40,700****
C. Health Behavior Assessment/Intervention, 15 min: $19.25
 5 per full day = 25 per week
 25 × 19.25 × 50 = $24,062.50

**This takes into account a small amount for vacation and/or sick leave.
***This is our average number based on our screening criteria.
****The MedFT typically only gets to half of the EBS in a given week.

Looking at the numbers above and taking into account a collection rate of 75 % (our department's rate is around 80 %) as well as halving the potential income from the Evidence-Based Screenings, a MedFT could potentially net almost $75,000 dollars per year. Taking this number and placing the cost of a MedFT at around $66,000 per year ($50,000 base income + 20 % for benefits), a practice could actually generate some income off of the clinician—a little under $10,000. It is also important to mention that the above figures are *best case scenarios* since they do not account for missed appointments and/or other variables (e.g., contractual adjustments). However, given the use of the lowest reimbursement rates, our practice has found that we outperform these numbers on a consistent basis. Another point to consider is that the Evidence-Based Screenings, and to a lesser extent the Health Behavior/Assessments, serve as pipelines that continually funnel patients into our traditional (more lucrative) services, which in turn allows for the subsidization of the integrated services.

In the end, the sheer enormity and complexity of designing, implementing, and most importantly sustaining an integrated care model cannot be overstated, especially when that model is purported to be constructed, overseen, and run by MedFTs. We are called a *burgeoning* field for a reason, and our academic and professional youth carries with it the need to *prove* our own worth both conceptually and practically. The epistemological view that MedFTs offer is essential to the functioning of any integrated care model because of its focus on relationships. For us, including the financial team was not only about conceptually wanting to cover all of Peek's three worlds (2008), thereby making the model financially sustainable, but the ultimate financial success of the model was the natural outcome of considering all the relationships within the organization. It was not enough to include the financial team at only one point in development or implementation, but their continued inclusion engendered a sense of ownership and buy-in on their part. It was this sense of buy-in that made them the financial champions of integrated care and even more importantly as champions for MedFT as a clinical practice and field.

The other piece of this model's financial success has to do with the MedFTs' willingness to learn about and consider the business and financial structures related to integrated care and traditional psychotherapy. Rather than sitting on the sidelines, only stepping in to discuss clinical flow, team, or care issues, we (the MedFTs) became savvy in our knowledge about reimbursement. It is this knowledge that allows us to find ways of billing for up to 90 % of our clinical encounters regardless of the type of service provided. If ever there was a setting where the stereotype of the business-inept behavioral health professional needed to change, integrated primary care would be that setting. MedFTs in these environments not only need to be able to demonstrate their clinical competency but also be able to demonstrate sound and reasonable financial and business competency or at least be open to developing that skill set.

Concluding Thoughts

There is no denying that the healthcare system in the United States is complicated in terms of care delivery and even more so when it comes to reimbursement for that care. However, despite its complexity, MedFTs must become versed in the various pathways of not only providing clinical services but also, and equally essential, is their need to become practical experts in how to pay for the services they provide. In order to achieve this degree of general expertise, MedFTs must be willing to find interest in both enacted and proposed state and federal laws (as it relates to healthcare reimbursement), the overarching methods of reimbursement (e.g., CPT codes and *incident to* billing), and the different possibilities of how care delivery systems can be organized. Make no mistake, this is no small feat and requires MedFTs to stretch themselves conceptually in ways that they might not be otherwise accustomed to. A feat made only more difficult by the mindset that many MedFTs and other behavioral health providers share one that sees good clinical care and profitable business practice as mutually exclusive. However, the best clinical practice is one that can continue to be available to its patients, which can only be achieved through a pragmatic outlook that views profitability as yet another avenue toward providing the highest quality of care possible (not one that detracts from it).

As it stands, there exists a paucity of practice management education in MedFT or any other mental health discipline's educational curriculum. Until behavioral health training programs move toward practice management as a core component of its students' education, as medical education has, it is incumbent upon each practitioner to seek out his or her own training in this area. Ultimately, the language of medicine is one of business as much as it is a language of treatment, and if MedFTs truly wish to coexist successfully in this context, they must become proficient in all aspects of that communication.

Discussion Questions

1. Given your state's laws on reimbursement, what distribution of traditional and integrated care visits would allow for a MedFT to be sustainable in a healthcare context?
2. What financial provisions should a MedFT consider in relation to changes made through the Affordable Care Act?
3. What cost-offsets can a MedFT bring to a healthcare context?

References[1]

American Medical Association. (2013). *Current professional terminology 2013: Professional addition*. Chicago, IL: American Medical Association.

*Blount, A., Kathol, R., Thomas, M., Schoenbaum, M., Rollman, B. L., & O'Donohue, W. (2007). The economics of behavioral health services in medical settings: A summary of the evidence. *Professional Psychology: Research and Practice, 38*, 290–297. doi:10.1037/0735-7028.38.3.290.

*Center for Medicare & Medicaid Services. (2013). *Incident to services*. Retrieved from http://www.cms.gov/Outreach-and-Education/Medicare-Learning-Network-MLN/MLNMattersArticles/downloads/se0441.pdf

*Manchikanti, L., Caraway, D., Parr, A. T., Fellows, B., & Hirsch, J. A. (2011). Patient Protection and Affordable Care Act of 2010: Reforming the health care reform for the new decade. *Pain Physician, 14*, e35–e67.

North Carolina Department of Health and Human Services. (2013, January 23). *Direct enrolled behavior health services: Licensed clinical social worker & licensed professional counselor & licensed marriage and family therapist*. Retrieved from http://www.ncdhhs.gov/dma/fee/mhfee/licensed_clinical_social_worker_012313.pdf

North Carolina Foundation for Advanced Health Programs. (2013, March 14). *Screening services with reimbursement handout*. Retrieved from http://www.ncfahp.org/Data/Sites/1/screening-svcs.-with-reimbursement-revised-03.14.13.pdf

Patient Protection and Affordable Care Act 111, 42 U.S.C. 18001, et seq. (2010).

Peek, C. J. (2008). Planning care in the clinical, operational, and financial worlds. In R. Kessler & D. Stafford (Eds.), *Collaborative medicine case studies: Evidence in practice*. New York, NY: Springer.

Robinson, P. J., & Reiter, J. T. (2007). *Behavioral consultation and primary care: A guide to integrating services*. New York, NY: Springer Science + Business Media.

Robinson, P. J., & Strosahl, K. D. (2009). Behavioral health consultation and primary care: Lessons learned. *Journal of Clinical Psychology in Medical Settings, 16*, 58–71. doi:10.1007/s10880-009-9145-z.

[1] An asterisk has been use to note references that the chapter authors recommend for further reading.

Chapter 24
Epilogue

Angela Lamson, Jennifer Hodgson, Tai Mendenhall, and D. Russell Crane

Epilogue

There have been numerous books, articles, and authors that have influenced us and our careers as MedFTs. We cited much of this work throughout our text and ensured that many of these scholars were direct contributors to its content. In thinking about the value of this epilogue, we reflected on the final chapters (specifically) from three books that have stood out most to us. These closing chapters are punctuated by and through the courage of their respective authors' writing. Our point is not for readers to necessarily agree with the content of these selections or even to agree with the recommendations that we put forth at the end of this epilogue. Instead, our hope is to challenge readers to be innovative, push envelopes, and serve as ambassadors of MedFT by advancing the field through best practices, research, and policy.

When we were first-year doctoral students in relationally based programs, many of us read Lynn Hoffman's (1981) book called *Foundations of Family Therapy*. Her epilogue challenged systemic thinkers to stretch beyond the role of conventional "clinician" and to position providers within the family as a seamless part of the system. Although this book was written over three decades ago, its message still stands true. As systemic providers become MedFTs, they are able to insert their work into lives beyond the traditional contexts of stand-alone mental health clinics and into healthcare settings, hospice rooms, and home health environments. Further, systemic work flourishes in integrated care practices, whereby relationships between providers and patients not only are relevant in the exam room but also have far-reaching implications for trainers, researchers, policy makers, and financial managers who all share in the responsibility of making our healthcare system the best it can be.

A. Lamson (✉)
College of Human Ecology, East Carolina University, Greenville, NC, USA
e-mail: lamsona@ecu.edu

J. Hodgson et al. (eds.), *Medical Family Therapy*, DOI 10.1007/978-3-319-03482-9_24,

A second memorable epilogue was that from Wright, Watson, and Bell's (1996) *Belief* text. Their concluding chapter communicated a passionate series of beliefs that the authors held to be true. Of course, the authors were also the first to pair spirituality with Engel's biopsychosocial model (1977, 1980). This epilogue was both courageous to share and humbling to read. At one level, the authors punctuated that families' and providers' beliefs matter, but on another level, they highlighted ways in which these beliefs influence the researchers', trainers', and providers' roles. As editors, we aligned with Wright, Watson, and Bell's writings so much that we included "spirituality" in most cited uses of BPS (i.e., BPSS) throughout this text. Whether working as researchers, trainers, supervisors, policy writers, or clinicians with underserved populations, those facing chronic conditions or devastated by natural or human-caused disasters and those who converse with us throughout our work week, we honor the meaning that these patients and families make out of any situation. We do this, whether it is grounded in religion, transcendence through nature, or any variety of other symbolic connections. Spirituality for us goes beyond the "social" in BPS; it stands in a higher order of meaning making within our lives as MedFTs.

Finally, Hardy's (2008) final chapter in *Re-Visioning Family Therapy* infused humility through our core. He discusses the *g*ood, *e*fficient, *m*ainstream, and *m*inority (GEMM) therapist. He described how minorities must be aware of invisible rules to appear to be "of the majority" when becoming a provider. While this chapter appears to be written for minority students and young professionals, it is the majority who most needed to read it. Dr. Hardy once described himself as being in the "hope manufacturing business." We imagine that he is a source of hope for many students and clients. His message must awaken MedFTs to strive for more awareness and sensitivity when working in a world that is diverse by culture, ethnicity, sex, sexual identity, sexual orientation, age, wellness, illness, disability, education, religion, employment, socioeconomic status, and citizenship. Accountability should come through in training, research, policy, and practice. MedFTs must engage in ethical practices that do not promote exploitation, but instead lead to policies that assure equal and safe treatment options for all persons.

MedFT Call to Arms

It is through each of the chapters in our text, the boldness in the closing chapters just described, and our passion as editors for MedFT that we draw energy to advance a call to arms. We must take action as MedFTs to be good consumers of, create, and disseminate biopsychosocial-spiritual care, training, research, and policies that govern health care for patients and their families. We must do this in collaborative partnership(s) with other behavioral health and healthcare professionals. We must maximize our roles and innovativeness across training, research, policy, and finance arenas and do so in a manner accountable to all healthcare populations, however, defined.

Duty to Innovation in Training, Research, Policy, and Finance

This is a call for MedFTs whose workload has been primarily comprised of clinical practice to get ignited and to begin tracking health or patient outcomes in their settings. MedFTs must not only stay informed about national trends that influence clinical practice, but they must also function on the front lines by providing the relational and BPSS outcomes that can systemically influence training, research, policy, and finance.

Innovations in training may include the need to further define and develop core competencies (see Chap. 3) in order to maximize the commonalities that employers and stakeholders can identify as associated with a MedFT. Because no universal license exists for MedFTs, they must be held to a standard in which stakeholders can be assured of their quality and competency in all work contexts. These competencies also hold trainers and supervisors accountable to the content and skills that a MedFT must have and incorporate into their work. Furthermore, training programs should be constructed and marketed in ways that best prepare MedFTs for a variety of healthcare contexts (e.g., primary and specialty care settings or clinical and teaching environments). These programs may then develop educators who are prepared to teach grand rounds or in clinics at medical schools or in MedFT master's, postgraduate, or doctoral programs. MedFTs may also receive some of their training in medical schools and residency programs in order to further their employment opportunities in these contexts. Fortunately, the training opportunities for MedFT are diverse (e.g., institutes, conference tracks, certificates, graduate degree programs) and growing each year; this affords MedFTs a variety of ways to pursue education that best meets their needs.

Secondly, MedFTs are made up of professionals from a variety of disciplines and must therefore attend and present at conferences or read and publish in journal articles from outside of their primary areas of expertise. To construct opportunities for innovation, MedFTs should be constant discoverers. MedFTs need to stretch outside of their disciplinary home bases by extending their work into and across multidisciplinary and integrated healthcare contexts.

The research innovation that is needed in MedFT must be grounded in ethics and diversity awareness and translational, so it can be quickly disseminated into the hands of researchers, trainers, and providers alike. In Crossing the Quality Chasm (2001), it was stated that it takes approximately 17 years to get research translated into practice. MedFTs must find ways to bolster communication with others in order to narrow this gap. For example, research outcomes should be disseminated through blogs and media outlets that are aligned with reputable guilds. It is also important that MedFTs critically review the professional healthcare literature on a regular basis to ensure that the leading evidence-based guidelines are being studied and integrated into practice. Likewise, it is the responsibility of MedFT clinicians and researchers to partner and develop studies that capture the outcomes of various therapeutic models and approaches. Program evaluation studies are one way that MedFTs can assist healthcare systems in advancing, redesigning, and disseminating their models.

Finally, MedFTs should not settle for professional development courses or conference sessions that capture clinical relevance alone; they must also demand attention to policy and financial implications through trusted and ethical professionals. MedFTs must learn how to construct policy briefs pertaining to relational and BPSS implications on health for diagnosis-specific organizations (e.g., American Diabetes Association, American Heart Association) and highly regarded health-related organizations (e.g., Agency for Healthcare Research and Quality). MedFTs must share financial models of sustainability as part of local, state, and national presentations and publications. The viability of MedFT and all behavioral health fields is dependent upon stakeholders who are aware of their effectiveness and sustainability.

Duty to Beliefs and Roles of a MedFT

We must acknowledge our past and enhance our future by announcing our beliefs and recognizing our roles as MedFTs. In order to recognize and then proclaim personal beliefs about what it means to be a MedFT, we should first understand the historical roots that ground our field. Chapter 2 helps to give some insight into this history. Certainly, McDaniel, Doherty, and Hepworth and McDaniel, Hepworth, and Doherty's texts (1992, 2014) provide even more depth. This is important for new MedFTs to recognize and honor, so that each new branch of research, teaching, practice, and policy innovation can be traced back to its roots.

While we encourage MedFTs to be bold in their work, or as our colleague Dr. Bill Doherty says, dare to have "Big, Hairy, Audacious Goals," each generation should also strive to maintain relationships with their predecessors. MedFTs should not lose sight of the importance of history, while at the same time be courageous enough to take their own steps as ambassadors of the field.

In honoring past legacies and constructing new innovations, MedFTs must be willing to share their beliefs and clarify their role(s). In reality, it is difficult to take a stand for MedFT, if one has not unveiled his or her personal biases and beliefs as a researcher, trainer, provider, and/or about policy pertaining to health care and behavioral health. These beliefs can help one to strive toward personal and professional missions. Furthermore, biases can be dissected such that MedFTs become more accountable to those who are served through their work.

The beauty about beliefs is that they have the capacity to change through each new encounter with others. While our beliefs (expressed mostly through the Chap. 1) represent what we as editors feel reflects MedFT (e.g., levels from those trained in relational or BPSS approaches to those who are proficient enough to train others), the ways in which these beliefs unfold may be unique to the role of any MedFT in his or her context. MedFTs are often a minority in the sea of healthcare providers, and therefore we must enfold our relational and BPSS lens and expertise into each of our unique roles and contexts. In the end, each of us must stand true to our beliefs and illuminate the roles we occupy.

Duty to be Humble

MedFTs are relational providers, whereby cultural humility in clinical practice is commonplace. However, we must stretch our awareness and humility to other realms of our work. As so beautifully described in Chap. 17, MedFTs must be accountable to who is recruited in research samples and how participants can become part of developing research designs, implementing programs, and disseminating results. MedFTs who are patient- or family-centered in their practice must become participant centered in their research, and outcomes must be relevant to more than the "majority." Policies must be constructed with key stakeholders at the table. Policy briefs should include authors from the community, not just those who hold a degree or title (e.g., community elders or those who have won or are losing their battle with a diagnosis). By including these voices, research and policies can be created by the community, not just for the community.

MedFTs must recognize cultural humility as a lifelong journey. It must be navigated alongside others, not a destination traveled to in isolation. Growing in cultural humility cannot just happen through reading a book or taking a class. MedFTs must engage with their communities through participating in local functions, listening for strengths and challenges instead of talking about personal agendas, and coming in as learners instead of as experts. MedFTs are relational thinkers and doers; we must work in conjunction with communities to eradicate health disparities, particularly those due to injustices from power differences in culture, sexual identity and orientation, age, sex, wellness, illness, disability, education, religion, race, employment, and citizenship. Ultimately patients, families, participants, and stakeholders deserve to know that MedFTs, in all work roles, serve as agents for change in culturally humble ways.

Conclusion

This text reflects many things for us as editors: a hope, a vision, and a passion to strengthen the advanced applications of MedFT. It also reflects the synergy of many generations and disciplines that came together in shared interests to further MedFT. We want to applaud and thank all of the authors who contributed to this text for recognizing the importance of MedFT across training, leadership, policy, and finance arenas. We now call current and future MedFTs to go forth and innovate. Boldly state your beliefs. Create new knowledge. Advance best practices. Inform change. And do so with humility.

References

Engel, G. L. (1977). The need for a new medical model: A challenge for biomedicine. *Science, 196*, 129–136.

Engel, G. L. (1980). The clinical application of the biopsychosocial model. *American Journal of Psychiatry, 137*, 535–544.

Hoffman, L. (1981). *Foundations of family therapy: A conceptual framework for system change*. New York, NY: Basic Books.

Institute of Family Medicine. (2001). *Crossing the quality chasm: A new health system for the 21st century*. Washington, DC: National Academy Press.

McDaniel, S. H., Doherty, W. J., & Hepworth, J. (Eds.). (2014). *Medical family therapy and integrated care*. Washington, DC: American Psychological Association. doi:10.1037/14256-000.

McDaniel, S. H., Hepworth, J., & Doherty, W. J. (Eds.). (1992). *Medical family therapy: A biopsychosocial approach to families with health problems*. New York, NY: Basic Books. doi:10.1080/01926189208250882.

McGoldrick, M., & Hardy, K. V. (2008). *Re-visioning family therapy: Race, culture, and gender in clinical practice* (2nd ed.). New York, NY: Guilford Press.

Wright, L. M., Watson, W. L., & Bell, J. M. (1996). *Beliefs: The heart of healing in families and illness*. New York, NY: Basic Books.

Author Bios

Steve Arnault, M.A., is CEO and Lead Consultant of Healthcare Systems Align and Vice President of Quality, Compliance and Integrated care at the Center for Life Management in Derry, New Hampshire. He has taught at the graduate and undergraduate level at New England College for the past 20 years.

Macaran (Mac) Baird, M.D., M.S., is Professor and Head of the Department of Family Medicine and Community Health at the University of Minnesota (UMN). This large department with over 150 residents and multiple practice locations sponsors eight family medicine residencies in both rural and urban locations across Minnesota. Baird was trained as both a family physician and family therapist as he began his career in 1978 as a rural physician and therapist. He and Bill Doherty coauthored *Family Therapy and Family Medicine* in 1983 which launched his academic and leadership career. Since his rural days he has held a number of leadership positions including family medicine residency director at the University of Oklahoma; Professor and Chair of Family Medicine at Upstate Medical University at Syracuse, New York; Associate Medical Director, for HealthPartners where he helped integrate behavioral health services into 24 primary care clinics; and Medical Director of Mayo Medical Services (now MMSI) for Mayo Clinic, Rochester, Minnesota. Since 2002 he has been in his current position at the UMN Medical School. He was a coauthor for the Institute of Medicine's 2001 *Health and Behavior Report* and has been a member of advisory panels for the Robert Wood Johnson Foundation and the MacArthur Foundation as well as for other organizations. His current research and clinical focus is in the integration between behavioral medicine and primary care and identifying the social and care system factors that inhibit positive outcomes for patients and families.

Jerica Berge, Ph.D., M.P.H., L.M.F.T., C.F.L.E., is an assistant professor, researcher, and behavioral medicine provider in the Department of Family Medicine and Community Health at the UMN Medical School. Dr. Berge's research interest is in examining risk and protective factors for childhood and adolescent obesity in the home environment. She also conducts research on integrated care in primary care settings, with a focus on interprofessional collaborations

J. Hodgson et al. (eds.), *Medical Family Therapy*, DOI 10.1007/978-3-319-03482-9, between mental health, medicine, and pharmacy. She has been awarded several National Institutes of Health (NIH) grants (grant mechanisms include K12; R21; R03; R56), has published widely (journals include JAMA Pediatrics; Pediatrics; Obesity; Journal of Behavioral Medicine; Families, Systems and Health), and has presented nationally and internationally on these topics. She is also the associate director of the Citizen Professional Center at the UMN which conducts community-based participatory research with community members/citizens to increase dissemination and sustainability of research projects and results. Dr. Berge is also a licensed marriage and family therapist and an approved marriage and family therapy (MFT) supervisor who specializes in collaborative care and family health issues. She supervises both doctoral level medical family therapists and medical residents in primary care settings regarding collaborative care.

Dr. Tommie Boyd, Ph.D., is the chair of the Family Therapy department at Nova Southeastern University. Her career interests combine clinical/professional education and medical family therapy (MedFT). She has published and presented widely on MedFT topics, including work with Parkinson's, diabetes, chronic pain, death and dying process (including the withdrawing of mechanical ventilation), and autism. She has conducted funded research in the areas of autism, Parkinson's, sexuality, and mental health needs of returning veterans. In addition, she has also published and presented widely on clinical/professional training, including the collaboration of family therapists and physicians, and family-related training for both family therapists and physicians. She is an ad hoc reviewer for Journal of Marital and Family Therapy and Journal of Systemic Therapies. Recent publications include an edited book, "Family Therapy Review: Contrasting Contemporary Models" (Rambo, West, Schooley, & Boyd, 2012); a book chapter on supervision in nontraditional settings (Rambo & Boyd, 2013); a book chapter on the scholarship of engagement (Boyd, Hibel, & Yang, 2012); a book chapter on diabetes education; and a book chapter on the need for auditory/verbal practitioners working with cochlear implant recipients to work with families (Rambo, Rhoades, Boyd, & Bello, 2009). Dr. Boyd is the recipient of the American Association for Marriage and Family Therapy (AAMFT) Leadership Award (2007) as well as the recipient of leadership awards from both the Florida Association for Marital and Family Therapy (FAMFT) and the Broward County Association for Marriage and Family Therapy (BAMFT). She has served as a division leader for AAMFT and has been president, board member, licensure chair, and consultant to the FAMFT board. She presents nationally and internationally on her research and training interests. She is currently involved with the creation of a joint biannual family therapy conference with the family therapy department of Beijing Normal University.

Dr. Jeff Capobianco, Ph.D., has over 20 years of clinical, administrative, and healthcare research experience, with extensive background in primary and behavioral healthcare integration, evidence-based practice implementation, Lean Six Sigma methodologies, and learning community approaches to organizational change and practice improvement. Prior to joining the National Council for Behavioral Healthcare where he is a Senior Consultant and Director of Practice

Improvement for the Center for Integrated Health Solutions, he held positions as a Research Investigator at the University of Michigan School of Social Work and as the Director of Research and New Program Development for the Washtenaw Community Health Organization (WHCO). Dr. Capobianco has published in national journals including Social Work in Healthcare, Journal of Evidence-Based Social Work, Administration and Policy in Mental Health, and Family, Systems, & Health. He is the author of two books and is currently an institutional review board member for the National Research Institute, Inc., a journal review member of the Journal of Behavioral Health Services & Research, and a member of the advisory council for Centerstone Research Institute Knowledge Network.

Jacob Christenson, Ph.D., is an Assistant Professor and Clinical Director for the MFT program at Mount Mercy University in Cedar Rapids, Iowa. He received his Doctorate in MFT from Brigham Young University. He is an editorial board member for Contemporary Family Therapy: An International Journal and has published numerous articles in professional journals. Among the journals he has published in are the Journal of Marital and Family Therapy, the American Journal of Family Therapy, and Contemporary Family Therapy. Dr. Christenson is a Licensed Marriage and Family Therapist as well as a Clinical Fellow and Approved Supervisor in the AAMFT. He is an active board member for the Iowa Association for Marriage and Family Therapy. His professional areas of interest include interventions for treatment-resistant children and adolescents, families and health, and family therapy training.

Russell Crane, Ph.D., is a Professor of MFT in the School of Family Life at Brigham Young University. He is the editor of *Contemporary Family Therapy: An International Journal* and an editorial board member for a number of other professional journals. He has published over 80 journal articles and book chapters. His primary research concerns the cost-effectiveness of the profession and practice of MFT and the influence of family interaction on health outcomes. His work has been translated and published in Portuguese, German, and Czech. He is the author of four books including *Fundamentals of Marital Therapy*, the *Handbook of Families and Health*, *Handbook of Families and Poverty*, and the *Handbook of Families and Work*. He received the AAMFT, Cumulative Contributions to Marriage and Family Therapy Research Award in 2007. He was elected Scholar of the AAMFT Research and Education Foundation in 2012. He is also a Fellow, Approved Supervisor, and Clinical Fellow in that organization and a licensed Marriage and Family Therapist. He is also a former Chair of AAMFT's Commission on Accreditation for Marriage and Family Therapy Education.

Maureen Davey, Ph.D., is an Associate Professor in the Department of Couple and Family Therapy at Drexel University. She is a licensed clinical member and approved supervisor in the AAMFT. She is a frequent presenter at AAMFT, the Collaborative Family Healthcare Association (CFHA), NIMH Annual International Research Conference, National Council on Family Relations (NCFR), and the International Congress of Behavioral Medicine. Dr. Davey is a productive scholar whose program of research focuses on mixed-method clinical research to develop culturally relevant interventions for minority cancer patients and their families and training providers to use more family-centered approaches to care. She is an author on over 40 peer-reviewed articles (e.g., Psycho-oncology, Family Process, Journal of Marital and Family Therapy, Families, Systems, and Health), book chapters, and an edited volume (Bean, R.A., Davis, S., & Davey, MP (Eds.) (in press, 2013). Exercises and Activities for Clinical Supervision: Cultivating Self-Awareness and Competence. Wiley Press, Inc.) focusing on training culturally sensitive providers in order to overcome health disparities.

Emilee Delbridge, Ph.D., received her doctorate from the University of Nebraska-Lincoln and is a Licensed Marriage and Family Therapist (LMFT) in Indiana. She is a Behavioral Science faculty member at Indiana University Purdue University-Indianapolis Family Medicine Residency in Indianapolis, IN. She teaches Behavioral Science curriculum to Family Medicine residents and medical students, provides therapy to patients in the residency clinic, and supervises family therapy students. Her research interests include the practices and benefits of interdisciplinary training, spirituality education and curriculum development in family therapy, and Behavioral Science curriculum development and assessment, including addressing professionalism development of healthcare providers.

Wayne Denton, M.D., Ph.D., is Professor of MFT and Director of the MFT Program at Florida State University. He is a board-certified psychiatrist, has a Ph.D. in MFT, and is a licensed MFT. He is a clinical fellow of, and approved supervisor with, the AAMFT. He has conducted NIMH-supported research on the use of emotionally focused therapy (EFT) for couples in the treatment of depression and is interested in the application of EFT to psychiatric and medical conditions as well as basic couple research.

William Doherty, Ph.D., is Director of the Citizen Professional Center at the UMN where he is Professor of Family Social Science and Adjunct Professor of Family Medicine and Community Health. In addition to his work in MedFT, he has been a pioneer in Citizen Health Care which uses community organizing strategies to build democratic engagement of individuals and families in health care. He has 35 years of experience working in health care as a teacher, family therapist, consultant to primary care physicians, and community organizer. His most recent book, with Susan McDaniel and Jeri Hepworth, is *Medical Family Therapy and Integrated Care* (second edition).

Todd Edwards, Ph.D., is a Professor and Director of the Marital and Family Therapy program at the University of San Diego and a Voluntary Assistant Clinical Professor in the Department of Family and Preventive Medicine at the University of California, San Diego. Dr. Edwards is a Clinical Member and Approved Supervisor in the AAMFT and an Associate Editor of the journal *Families, Systems, & Health.*

Peter Fifield is the Behavioral Health Services Manager at Families First Health and Support Center, a fully integrated FQHC in Portsmouth, NH. He has a master's degree in counseling psychology and is a licensed clinical mental health counselor and masters licensed alcohol and drug counselor in the state of New Hampshire. He is currently pursuing a doctoral degree from University of New England investigating how team-based care is impacted by the use of an integrated electronic medical record (iEMR).

Melissa Fox, M.A., M.S., L.M.F.T., is a MedFT doctoral candidate in the Department of Child Development and Family Relations at East Carolina University. She received master's degrees in MFT from East Carolina University and in psychology from Wake Forest University. She is a licensed marriage and family therapist and an AAMFT-Approved Supervisor Candidate. She has coauthored in areas related to coping with chronic illness and the junction of MedFT and integrated primary care. She is currently working in private practice in Charlotte, North Carolina.

Bobbi-Ann Gordon, M.S., M.F.T.I., holds a master's degree in MFT from Loma Linda University (LLU). She is currently in her second year of pursuing a Doctorate of Marital and Family Therapy at LLU. She is specializing in Program Development and Evaluation with a concentration in MedFT. Bobbi-Ann is a research staff member of the Department of Counseling and Family Sciences Evaluation Team that conducts evaluations and helps develop programs for the Riverside County of Education. She is also involved in research to develop an evidence-based multifamily group curriculum for a pilot study currently being tested in the public housing communities in CA. Bobbi-Ann is passionate about developing a career in program evaluation and looks forward to completing her doctoral project that is an evaluation of a family-centered treatment program for maternal substance abuse.

Carl Greenberg, Ph.D., has recently retired from practicing MedFT in a variety of settings for 31 years. These have included private practice with a psychiatrist as a partner, teaching in a family practice residency, solo private practice, working in a psychiatric clinic, and most recently as an oncology family therapist. His primary interest in his career has been practicing MedFT as well as teaching and training other therapists and healers. Toward that end he has taught many workshops, locally, regionally, and nationally including the ones at the Collaborative Family Health Conference, the Family in Family Medicine Conference, and the AAMFT. He is a long-time member of AAMFT having joined in 1986 and is currently a Clinical Fellow and an AAMFT-Approved Supervisor. He was elected to the Board of Directors of AAMFT in 2011 for a 3-year term which will end in December 2014. He has served in the Washington Division of AAMFT in a variety of positions including Legislative Chair, Board Member, and President. He is currently licensed in both Washington as an MFC and in California as an MFCC. His favorite hobby is working on his golf game.

Carrie Hanson, M.S., L.A.M.F.T., is a fourth-year Ph.D. student in the Couple and Family Therapy at the UMN. She works as a family therapist for Joining Hands Child and Family Counseling Services in Roseville, Minnesota, where she specializes in providing clinical care to children, individuals, and families. Her primary research interest is understanding systemic influences on childhood and adolescent obesity as well as community-based participatory research around child and family health issues. Carrie is an active member of AAMFT, MAMFT, and NCFR.

Jennifer Hodgson, Ph.D., LMFT, is a Professor in the Departments of Child Development and Family Relations. She has reappointed time in the Department of Family Medicine at East Carolina University where she holds a clinical, supervision, and teaching role. She received her doctoral degree from Iowa State University, specializing in MFT, and completed a postdoctoral fellowship in MedFT at the University of Rochester, New York. She coauthored the nation's first doctoral program in MedFT. She is a Clinical Member of AAMFT, an AAMFT-Approved Supervisor, and served two terms as a Commissioner and 1 year as Chair for the Commission on Accreditation of Marriage and Family Therapy Education. She is Chair of the North Carolina Marriage and Family Therapy Licensure Board and is a recent past President for the CFHA. She serves as a reviewer for several journals is on the advisory board for the Journal of Marriage and Family Therapy. She has published numerous articles, book chapters, and research studies involving MedFT, interprofessional collaboration initiatives. biopsychosocial-spiritual health, and integrated care. Her funding record is extensive in these areas as well.

Cathy Hudgins, Ph.D., is the Director of the Center of Excellence for Integrated Care under the North Carolina Foundation for Advanced Health Programs. Dr. Hudgins has experience in integrated care management and development, crisis assessment and intervention, community-based and college-based outpatient counseling, in-patient assessment and intervention, and community mental health consulting. She received her doctorate in MFT from Virginia Tech and has practiced in community mental health agencies, hospital and healthcare settings, as well as private practice. She has also held a variety of posts in higher education administration and student affairs. Dr. Hudgins is a cofounder and prior Director of the Radford University Center for Integrated Care Training and Research. Through this post, she trained and developed integrated systems and participated in research and grant writing initiatives. Her research interests and publications are related to integrated care include policy, ethics, workforce development, and evidence-based practice models. She is an active member of the Collaborative Family Health Association and AAMFT and presents locally and nationally on integrated care topics.

Tom Irons, Ph.D., is Professor of Pediatrics, Brody School of Medicine, and Associate Vice Chancellor for Health Sciences, East Carolina University. He is a graduate of Davidson College and the University Of North Carolina School Of

Medicine, where he graduated in 1972 with the highest academic honors. He completed his pediatric internship at the University of California, San Francisco, and residency at the North Carolina Memorial Hospital. From 1975 to 1978, he served in the US Army in West Germany and practiced pediatrics in Raleigh, NC, from 1978 to 1981. He joined the faculty of the ECU (now Brody) School of Medicine in 1981 and has continued an active teaching practice since that time. In 1999, he founded HealthAssist, a health improvement and healthcare program for low-income and uninsured residents of Eastern North Carolina. Beginning in 2005, he spearheaded the construction of the James D. Bernstein Community Health Center and now serves as its medical director. The center provides comprehensive medical, dental, and behavioral health services, pharmacy, and a broad range of educational programs for community members and health professionals. In 2008, he was honored by the UNC Medical Alumni Association with its Distinguished Service Award. He was most recently recognized in October 2011 by the University of North Carolina System Board of Governors with its Award for Excellence in Public Service. Dr. Irons serves on a number of state and national boards and presents frequently throughout the country and abroad on the subjects of leadership, institutional service commitment, service learning, community health, and a wide variety of topics related to child and adolescent health. Since 2007, he has been actively involved with the Medical Marriage and Family program at ECU.

Barry Jacobs, Psy.D., is a clinical psychologist, family therapist, and the author of the book, *The Emotional Survival Guide for Caregivers—Looking After Yourself and Your Family While Helping an Aging Parent* (Guilford, 2006). As a clinician, he specializes in helping families cope with serious and chronic medical illnesses. As an educator, he works as the Director of Behavioral Sciences for the Crozer-Keystone Family Medicine Residency Program in Springfield, PA, and has had adjunct faculty positions with the Temple University School of Medicine, University of Pennsylvania School of Nursing, and the Institute for Clinical Psychology of Widener University. He is the national spokesperson on family caregiving for the American Heart Association and a member of the AARP Caregivers Advisory Panel. He was a member of the American Psychological Association Presidential Task Force on Caregiving that produced the Caregiver Briefcase website. A former journalist, he writes an advice column for Take Care!, the newsletter of the National Family Caregivers Association, and was the long-time editor of the "In Sickness & Health" column for the APA journal Families, Systems, & Health. He is a past board member of the CFHA, a national organization dedicated to the integration of physical and mental healthcare, and contributes frequently to its "Families and Health" blog. He is also an honorary board member of the Well Spouse Association and is on the expert panel for the Caregiving Crisis Great Challenge for TEDMED.com. Dr. Jacobs received his bachelor's degree from Brown University and his doctorate in clinical psychology from Hahnemann/Widener Universities. He lives with his wife and two children in Swarthmore, PA. He maintains a website—www.emotionalsurvivalguide.com.

Emily Jones, Ph.D., is the Team Lead for *Health Information Technology for Economic and Clinical Health* Act (HITECH) Evaluation at the Office of Economic Analysis, Evaluation, and Modeling at the Office of the National Coordinator for Health Information Technology in the Department of Health and Human Services. Previously, she served as the Associate Director of the Geiger Gibson/RCHN Foundation Research Collaborative at GW University and gained research experience at the Urban Institute and the Georgetown Health Policy Institute. She worked for 2 years at the Health Resources and Services Administration as part of the team administering the federally qualified health center program and for 4 years at the Federal Trade Commission, performing investigative duties on healthcare antitrust cases and serving as the Assistant Director of the Outstanding Scholar Program in the Bureau of Competition. She holds a Doctorate in Health Policy from George Washington University, a master's in Public Policy from Georgetown, and a bachelor's in Organizational Behavior and Management from Brown University. The views expressed in this publication are solely the opinions of the authors and do not necessarily reflect the official policies of the Department of Health and Human Services or the Office of the National Coordinator for Health Information Technology nor does mention of the department or the agency names imply endorsement by the US government.

Sharon Knight, Ph.D., R.N., is a professor of health education and promotion at East Carolina University and former Associate Dean of the College of Health and Human Performance. Her research interests are in the area of professional development and the application of qualitative research methods in health-related areas. She holds a certificate in qualitative research from the University of North Carolina, Chapel Hill, teaches graduate-level courses on qualitative research, and has had over two decades' experience as a qualitative researcher. She has published over 40 refereed journal articles and two books.

Aubry Koehler, M.A., L.M.F.T.A., is a MedFT doctoral student at East Carolina University. She received her Master's of Arts in MFT from Antioch University, New England. Aubry has interned as a behavioral health specialist in integrated care settings serving underserved and minority populations in both New England and eastern North Carolina. She is especially interested in the impact of chronic illness on the family system, culturally sensitive care, and closing health disparities.

Katherine Kueny, Ph.D., is an assistant professor and the Director of Behavioral Medicine of the General Internal Medicine Division at University of Nebraska Medical Center (UNMC). She has her LIMHP and LMFT in the state of Nebraska and is an AAMFT-Approved Supervisor. Dr. Kueny obtained her master's degree from East Carolina University in 2004 and her Ph.D. from Kansas State University in 2008, both in MFT. She has been working at UNMC, since her doctoral internship in the Family Medicine Department in 2006. Dr. Kueny began in 2007, as the first mental health practitioner and behavioral medicine provider in the Internal Medicine Department. She has built a behavioral medicine program for the General Internal Medicine residents at UNMC. Dr. Kueny conducts therapy and research as part of a patient-centered medical home model and is the director of the MedFT Certificate Program at UNMC. She and her husband are happy to live in Omaha, NE, with their vibrant 20-month-old daughter and their second child on the way.

Angela Lamson, Ph.D., L.M.F.T., C.F.L.E., is a Professor in the Department of Child Development and Family Relations within the College of Human Ecology at East Carolina University. She is the Program Director for the MedFT doctoral program and Director of the Redditt House: Medical Family Therapy Research Academy. She has served as a Division President for the North Carolina Association for Marriage and Family Therapy and member of the Elections Council for the AAMFT. In addition, she is on the Executive Committee for the Alliance of Military and Veteran Family Behavioral Health Providers at the national level. Dr. Lamson's teaching, funding, and publications have been devoted to MedFT and integrated care, particularly in areas of trauma, chronic illness (Alzheimer's, obesity, and diabetes), loss, and compassion fatigue in the lives of individuals, couples, families, and providers. Her training and research initiatives have been housed in community health, primary care, and specialty care contexts as well as on military bases.

Melissa Lewis, Ph.D., is a licensed marriage and family therapist and an AAMFT-Approved Supervisor. Dr. Lewis earned her doctorate from East Carolina University in MedFT and is an assistant professor at the UMN Medical School, Duluth campus. Her research focuses on the social/relational (e.g., couple, family, community) determinants of health. Specifically, she studies the stress transmission model between military couples and integrated care interventions aimed to increase biopsychosocial-spiritual health in both military and indigenous communities.

Zephon Lister, Ph.D., L.M.F.T., is an Assistant Clinical Professor and Director of the Collaborative Care Program at the University of California, San Diego. He earned his doctorate in MedFT from LLU with an emphasis in MedFT and completed his postdoctoral training at the Chicago Center for Family Health, an affiliate of the University of Chicago. His clinical and research interests have focused on the recursive influences of family relationships and lifestyle-related chronic health conditions and the integration of behavioral health into healthcare settings. As the director of the UCSD family medicine collaborative care program he facilitates behavioral science training for family medicine residents, directs MFT clinical training, facilitates learning groups and lectures for the UCSD medical school, and serves as affiliate faculty in the University of San Diego MFT program. Dr. Lister serves on the research committee for the CFHA. He also is a contributor and journal reviewer for the Journal of Marital and Family Therapy, Family, Systems, and Health, and Contemporary Family Therapy. His research has been presented at the several national and international conferences including AAMFT, CFHA, International Family Therapy Association, NCFR, and Society of Teachers of Family Medicine.

Laura Lynch, M.S., is a doctoral candidate in her third year at Drexel University's Couple and Family Therapy Department. She received her master's degree in MFT at the University of Rochester and completed internships at a community mental health center, an OB-GYN practice, and a community hospital. Laura's clinical research focuses on developing interventions to help couples and families facing chronic illness. She is currently conducting her dissertation study which was designed to pilot an emotionally focused therapy group intervention with a diverse sample of couples who are coping with cancer in a partner or in a spouse. She is also completing her doctoral clinical internship at Drexel Medicine's primary care practice. Her research interests include addressing health disparities by developing culturally sensitive relational interventions, examining how chronic illness affects couple relationships, and children's experience of parental illness, in particular cancer and diabetes. She has published in *Contemporary Family Therapy,* the *Journal of Behavioral Health, Psycho-Oncology,* and the *Journal of Cancer Education* and has presented at AAMFT and AFTA.

Dan Marlowe, Ph.D., L.M.F.T., is a North Carolina-licensed Marriage and Family Therapist. He received his master's degree in MFT and doctorate in MedFT at East Carolina University in Greenville, NC. Over the course of his career, Dr. Marlowe has helped develop and implement integrated/collaborative care programs at a federally qualified health center, patient-centered medical home, family medicine residency program, and major university cancer center. Currently, he is the director of Behavioral Health at Campbell University's School of Osteopathic Medicine in Lillington, NC, where he oversees the psychosocial health of medical student body and faculty. In his prior position as director of Applied Psychosocial Medicine for Southern Regional AHEC in Fayetteville, NC, Dr. Marlowe oversaw integrated care education for family medicine, pharmD, and MedFT residents. Dr. Marlowe has published both nationally and internationally on integrated/collaborative care and MedFT as well as presented at regional, state, and national levels on integrated care program development, teaching integration in graduate medical education, and the use of family therapy as a practice change model in healthcare settings.

Patrick Meadors, Ph.D., L.M.F.T., is the Manager of Psychosocial Oncology at the Levine Cancer Institute within Carolinas Healthcare System. He is an AAMFT-Approved Supervisor and has served as an Assistant Professor within a COAMFTE program. Dr. Meadors earned a doctorate in MedFT from East Carolina University and has studied and published articles on compassion fatigue and burnout with healthcare providers (i.e., pediatric intensive care, neonatal intensive care, behavioral health, and oncology). Dr. Meadors has worked in various medical settings in the area of oncology, internal medicine, behavioral health, and the emergency department and has experience teaching on the theories of MFT, sexuality, human development, and MedFT.

Tai Mendenhall, Ph.D., L.M.F.T., is a Medical Family Therapist and Assistant Professor at the UMN in the Department of Family Social Science, Director of the UMN's Medical Reserve Corps' Mental Health Disaster-Response Teams, and

Associate Director of the UMN's Citizen Professional Center. He works actively in the conduct of collaborative family healthcare and community-based participatory research (CBPR) focused on a variety of public health issues. His principal clinical efforts center on working with families who are coping with chronic illness (e.g., dementia, diabetes, chronic pain), and his principal research efforts center on health disparities (e.g., the Family Education Diabetes Series—the "FEDS"—with an urban-dwelling American Indian community) and behaviors (e.g., Students Against Nicotine, Tobacco, and Alcohol Abuse—the "SANTAA" project—with the St. Paul Job Corps). Dr. Mendenhall's and his colleagues' work through the UMN's Citizen Professional Center encompasses more than a dozen community-based projects that involve active partnerships between professionals and community members.

Laurelle Myhra is a licensed marriage and family therapist. She practices at the Native American Community Clinic in Minneapolis, MN, where she is also the head of the counseling department. She is an adjunct assistant professor in the MFT master's degree program at St. Mary's University of Minnesota. Dr. Myhra completed her doctoral degree at the UMN's Couple and Family Therapy Program. Her clinical and research interests include family strengths, integrated health care, and intergenerational patterns of substance abuse and traumatic stress among American Indian families.

Beth Nolan, Ph.D., is an Assistant Professor of Public Health and the Senior Associate Director for the Evaluation Institute at the Graduate School of Public Health, University of Pittsburgh. She is a program evaluator trained in applied behavior analysis, and implementation, which she combines to evaluate and provide implementation assistance to a number of health services including behavioral health crisis response, quality improvement initiatives, senior living communities, and integrated care practices.

Jo Ellen Patterson, Ph.D., is a Professor in the Marital and Family Therapy program at the University of San Diego and a Clinical Associate Professor in the Departments of Family Medicine and Psychiatry at the University of California School of Medicine. Dr. Patterson has published numerous articles and books, including *Essential Skills in Family Therapy*. She is on the editorial boards of the *Journal of Marital and Family Therapy* and *Families, Systems, & Health.*

Kenneth Phelps, Ph.D., is an Assistant Clinical Professor and Outpatient Clinic Director in the Department of Neuropsychiatry and Behavioral Science at the University of South Carolina School of Medicine. Dr. Phelps earned his undergraduate in psychology as well as graduate degrees in MFT and MedFT from East Carolina University. He completed a doctoral internship in Behavioral Medicine at Concord Hospital, Dartmouth, Family Practice Residency Program. His specialty involves the treatment of couples with co-occurring physical, relational, and sexual difficulties. He has a particular interest in neurological disorders, including multiple sclerosis and tic disorders. In his administrative role, Dr. Phelps works closely with the Faculty Development Office to deliver conflict management presentations to various clinical departments and residency programs. He is a member and past committee chair of the CFHA as well as member of the AAMFT and the American Association of Sexuality Educators, Counselors, and Therapists (AASECT). Past grants and publications involve the impacts of diabetes, cancer, and sleep apnea on personal and relational health.

Jodi Polaha, Ph.D., is Associate Professor of Psychology at East Tennessee State University. Her career has been devoted to innovation in delivering behavioral health services to children and families in rural areas, including through integrated care. She is best described as a "pracademic," with one foot firmly planted in real-world pediatric primary care clinics, working with patients and healthcare teams and training doctoral students in clinical psychology from ETSU as well as medical residents, nursing students, and other interprofessional trainees. Her other foot is well established in research engaging end-point use, particularly work that strives to provide evidence-based treatments better "reach." She is funded by the National Institute of Mental Health and has completed extensive training in dissemination and implementation science. Dr. Polaha is an active member of the CFHA.

Keeley Pratt, Ph.D., I.M.F.T., is an assistant professor in the couples and family therapy program in the Department of Human Sciences at The Ohio State University, an independently licensed marriage and family therapist, and an AAMFT-Approved Supervisor. Her research focuses on family-based factors (i.e., parenting and feeding styles, family functioning) that contribute to or are modifiable in the treatment of child/adolescent obesity. She has presented at local, national, and international conferences and has published on topics related to child and adolescent family-based or integrated obesity treatment, MedFT, and supervision in healthcare settings. Currently, Dr. Pratt is working to expand family therapy education to include clinician training on systemic weight-related behaviors in families and training to work with clients and families who are struggling with overweight and obesity.

Randall Reitz, Ph.D., L.M.F.T., is the Director of Behavioral Sciences at the St. Mary's Family Medicine Residency in Grand Junction, CO. He trains family physicians and MedFT fellows in an integrated care model. His scholarly interests include collaborative care, professional identity development, healthcare ethics, and stewing about the next big idea. He considers Jennifer Hodgson his academic older sister.

John Rolland, M.D., M.P.H., is Professor of Psychiatry and Behavioral Neuroscience at the University of Chicago Pritzker School of Medicine and Executive Co-Director of its affiliate postgraduate training institute the Chicago Center for Family Health (http://www.ccfhchicago.org). He received his training in medicine and psychiatry at the University of Michigan and Yale University and earned a master's degree from the Harvard School of Public Health. He was the founding Director of the Center for Illness in Families affiliated with Yale University. Widely recognized for his conceptual model and clinical work with families facing serious physical disorders, his publications include his landmark book, Families, Illness, and Disability: An Integrative Treatment Model (1994); coauthored Individuals,

Families, and the New Era of Genetics: Biopsychosocial Perspectives (2006); and Treating Illness and Disability in Families: An Integrative Model (in press). He is a Distinguished Fellow of the American Psychiatric Association and a former Fellow of the Institute for Social and Policy Studies at Yale. Past President of the American Family Therapy Academy (AFTA), his professional honors include AFTA's Innovative Contributions to Family Therapy Award. He serves on the Editorial Boards of a number of journals including Families, Systems, & Health and has been active on the Boards of the CFHA, Physicians for Social Responsibility (PSR), and Physicians for a National Health Program (PNHP). From 2000 to 2003 he co-led a multi-year international project in Kosovo, the Kosovar Family Professional Education Collaborative, addressing family-centered training and service delivery needs in the aftermath of trauma, genocide, and loss.

Sandra Rose, Ph.D., is a psychologist and the Director of Behavioral Health at Goodwin Community Health, a federally qualified health center in Somersworth, New Hampshire. She helped to establish the integrated behavioral health program at GCH and is currently leading the clinical implementation of the Screening, Brief Intervention and Referral to Treatment (SBIRT) program at the Center. She is a past President of the New Hampshire Psychological Association, a two-term past member of the Council of Representatives (the governing body of the American Psychological Association), and a former long-term member of the Psychology Advisory Committee for NH's Board of Mental Health Practice. She has presented at the CFHA's annual meeting and published in its journal, Family, Systems, and Health on ethical issues in integration and has also presented at the Intermountain Healthcare annual integration retreat on integration issues and ethics.

Joseph Scherger, M.D., M.P.H., is Vice President for Primary Care & Academic Affairs at Eisenhower Medicine Center in Rancho Mirage, California. Dr. Scherger is Clinical Professor of Family Medicine at the University of California, San Diego School of Medicine (UCSD), and the Keck School of Medicine at the University of Southern California (USC).

Peter Shin, Ph.D., M.P.H., is an Associate Professor of Health Policy at George Washington University and Gibson Program in Community Health Policy and RCHN Community Health Foundation Research Director. Dr. Shin focuses on the study of community health systems and integration of care for vulnerable populations and is author of over 100 health policy reports on the access to care, the health care safety net, medically underserved populations, and health information technology. He teaches courses in public health management and policy analysis and is an expert in the management and analysis of data, healthcare financing, and regulatory and policy analysis and regularly provides technical assistance to federal state agencies and organizations.

Laura Sudano, M.A., is a MedFT Fellow at St. Mary's Family Medicine Residency in Grand Junction, CO. Laura received her Master's of Arts from the University of San Diego and is a Doctoral Candidate at Virginia Tech. Laura's research interests include collaborative care and sports medicine. She enjoys transdisciplinary training and teaching family-oriented care to physicians.

Janie Taylor, Ph.D., L.M.F.T., is regional director of CareNet Counseling East (CNCE), Greenville, NC. CNCE is an affiliate of Wake Forest Baptist Health, Winston-Salem, NC, and is a faith-integrated center. Taylor earned her Ph.D. from the MedFT Program at East Carolina University. Her areas of interest include spirituality, integrated behavioral health, family and relationship issues, as well as healthy living.

Stephanie Trudeau-Hern, M.S., is a doctoral student at the UMN in the Department of Family Social Science's Couple and Family Therapy Program. Her clinical and research interests include family coping with chronic illness and end of life, provider self-care within collaborative healthcare teams, and collaborative healthcare delivery model design and development.

Lisa Tyndall, Ph.D., L.M.F.T., is a Clinical Faculty member in the Department of Child Development and Family Relations. She serves as the Clinic Director of the East Carolina University Family Therapy Clinic. She received her doctoral degree in MedFT and her master's in MFT. She is a Clinical Member of AAMFT and an AAMFT-Approved Supervisor candidate.

Susanna Vakili is a graduate student in the Marital and Family Therapy program at the University of San Diego and a family therapy trainee at St. Vincent De Paul Village in San Diego, CA.

Monique Walker is a doctoral candidate at Drexel University in the Couple and Family Therapy Department. She is in the process of completing her dissertation focusing on the intersections of attachment and minority stress in understanding Black families' experiences and acceptance of lesbian, gay, bisexual, transgender, and queer (LGBTQ) youth. Ms. Walker earned her master's degree in MFT from East Carolina University. Her clinical and research interests target Black individuals, couples, and families, particularly within communities. She is the counseling services coordinator at the Attic Youth Center, which is Philadelphia's only independent LGBTQ youth center. She is also clinically active at the Women's Therapy Center, a nonprofit feminist-based psychotherapy center in Philadelphia.

Mark White, Ph.D., LMFT, is a Core Faculty Member in the School of Marriage and Family Sciences at Northcentral University. He received his doctoral degree in Human Ecology (specialization: Family Therapy) from Kansas State University. Dr. White is a Clinical Member of the AAMFT and an AAMFT-Approved Supervisor. He has served as an Associate Editor for the Journal of Marital and Family Therapy and is currently on the editorial board for Contemporary Family Therapy. He has held faculty positions at Auburn University, Kansas State University, and East Carolina University. His research interests include clinical process and outcome research, coping with an acquired brain injury, and technology and relationships.

Jackie Williams-Reade, Ph.D., L.M.F.T., holds a doctorate in MedFT from East Carolina University and is currently an Assistant Professor and Director of MedFT at LLU in Southern California. Jackie has over 15 years' experience in developing, implementing, and evaluating social support services for families who have a child with a chronic or a critical illness. As part of her dissertation, she carried out a program evaluation of a pediatric palliative care program using ethnographic research methods in order to further explore the institutional resources and challenges related to providing appropriate end-of-life care for infants. During her postdoctoral fellowship at Johns Hopkins University, Jackie continued working in the implementation and evaluation of an interdisciplinary training program aimed at increasing the understanding and application of pediatric palliative care concepts. Currently, she is working on developing a family therapy-based intervention for children with complex medical needs into an evidence-based practice.

Alison Wong, M.A., is a doctoral candidate in MFT at the University of Connecticut, with a specialty in MedFT. With her supervisor, she created a 3-year longitudinal doctoral internship in the Family Medicine residency program at the University of Connecticut School of Medicine. This has enabled her to have continuity with patients and develop collaborative relationships with residents, faculty, clinical teams, and other healthcare institutions within the community. She helps teach family medicine residents through a longitudinal behavioral health curriculum, which focuses on psychosocial issues in medicine and integrated care. Alison's research is in the area of psycho-oncology, with specific interests in improving relational and behavioral health and wellness during cancer treatment and survivorship.

Wendella Wray, M.S., M.Ed., M.F.T.I., holds master's degrees in Education Curriculum Instruction from National Louis University and in MFT from LLU. She is currently a second-year Ph.D. student in MFT at LLU with a concentration in MedFT. She presently works as a MedFT at the local community health center providing behavioral health services. Wendella has over 10 years of experience in curriculum development and evidence-based teaching practices in addition to assisting community and church organizations in completing needs assessments and program development. She is also working with a research team at LLU to develop an evidence-based multi-family group curriculum for a pilot study currently being tested in public housing communities in CA. Our goal is to help marriage and family therapists develop partnerships with the community to help families achieve self-sufficiency.

Felisha Younkin is a doctoral candidate in the Couple and Family Therapy Program at the Ohio State University. She has experience in the medical setting and an interest in pursuing MedFT. She currently works with Dr. Keeley Pratt discussing collaborative and integrative care and also as an intern at Nationwide Children's Hospital in their Eating Disorder Program. She believes that working from a biopsychosocial model within a multidisciplinary team provides the best care for patients.

Lisa Zak-Hunter, Ph.D., L.M.F.T., is behavioral science faculty with the Via Christi Family Medicine Residency Program and a Clinical Instructor with the University of Kansas, Wichita School of Medicine. She received her Ph.D. in MFT from the University of Georgia and completed a MedFT doctoral internship with St. John's Family Medicine Residency at the UMN. She is currently (2013–2014) completing a Behavioral Science/Family Systems Educators fellowship through the Society of Teachers of Family Medicine. Dr. Zak-Hunter's main clinical, teaching, and research interests lie in collaborative health care and increasing biopsychosocial-spiritual understanding of mental and medical health conditions. She has a particular interest in the systemic impact of adult eating disorders.

Max Zubatsky, Ph.D., L.M.F.T., is a licensed marriage and family therapist and a speaker on medical topics in couples and families. He received his master's degree from the University of San Diego in MFT and his doctoral degree from the UMN in Family Social Science, specializing in MedFT. He is currently pursuing a postdoctoral fellowship at the University of Chicago-affiliated Center for Family Health, with clinical responsibilities at the Illinois Masonic Family Practice. His clinical interests include chronic illness in families, dementia, end-of-life issues, and couples therapy. Dr. Zubatsky has authored several peer-reviewed journal and media articles in publications such *as Families, Systems & Health, Journal of Aging and Mental Health, Journal of Couple and Relationship Therapy*, and *Minnesota Physician*. Dr. Zubatsky received the MAMFT student of the year award while attending the University of Minnesota, honoring clinical, research, and community achievements as a doctoral student. He contributes to the "Families and Health" blog for the CFHA and maintains a personal website—maxzubatsky.com.

Index

J. Hodgson et al. (eds.), *Medical Family Therapy*, DOI 10.1007/978-3-319-03482-9,

C

T